Chest Wall Surgery

Volume 1

Verses Kindler Publication

Verses Kindler Publication
Website: www.verseskindlerpublication.com

Chest Wall Surgery: Volume 1
By: Mr. Wenlin Wang
ISBN: 978-93-49532-68-7
1st Edition
Price: INR 6000/$78

Disclaimer

This book is intended solely for educational and scholarly purposes. It is written for qualified healthcare professionals and assumes a foundational knowledge of medical and surgical practice. The content is not intended to provide medical advice, establish a standard of care, or replace independent clinical judgment, professional training, or institutional protocols.

The editors and contributors have made every reasonable effort to ensure that the information presented is accurate and consistent with accepted practice at the time of publication. However, medical knowledge, surgical techniques, device availability, and regulatory requirements evolve continuously. The editors, contributors, and publisher make no representations or warranties regarding the completeness, accuracy, or applicability of the content and disclaim responsibility for any adverse outcomes resulting from the use or interpretation of information contained in this book.

All surgical procedures described should be performed only by appropriately trained and credentialed clinicians in properly equipped clinical settings, with appropriate patient selection, informed consent, and adherence to applicable local regulations and institutional guidelines. Readers are strongly encouraged to consult current literature, manufacturer instructions, and regulatory guidance before applying any technique or using any device described herein.

References to specific products, devices, instruments, or commercial entities are provided for informational purposes only and do not constitute endorsement or recommendation by the editors, contributors, or publisher. All trademarks and registered trademarks are the property of their respective owners.

Clinical images, case descriptions, and patient-related information included in this book have been anonymized or reproduced with appropriate permission in accordance with ethical standards. Any resemblance to identifiable individuals is unintentional.

Editor's Introduction

Chest wall surgery has gradually emerged as a focused area of surgical practice, encompassing a wide range of congenital and acquired conditions that affect both form and function. While advances in surgical techniques and perioperative care have expanded what can be achieved, knowledge in this field remains scattered across multiple specialties and sources. As a result, surgeons often rely on fragmented information rather than a unified reference dedicated specifically to the chest wall.

This book was developed in response to that need. *Chest Wall Surgery* brings together current understanding and surgical practice related to chest wall disorders in a single, structured volume. The goal is not only to describe operative techniques, but also to place them within a clear clinical context that supports sound decision-making.

The chapters address a broad spectrum of chest wall conditions, including congenital deformities, acquired deformities, trauma, tumors, infections, and reconstructive challenges. Both traditional and minimally invasive approaches are discussed, with attention to indications, technical execution, perioperative considerations, and outcomes. Where newer methods are presented, they are discussed alongside established practices to allow readers to evaluate their role critically.

Rather than advocating a single approach, this volume reflects the collective experience of contributors working in different healthcare settings and surgical traditions. This diversity is intentional and mirrors the realities of clinical practice, where patient factors, resources, and expertise vary widely.

This book is intended for surgeons involved in the management of chest wall conditions, including thoracic surgeons, pediatric surgeons, trauma surgeons, orthopedic surgeons, and plastic surgeons, as well as trainees seeking a focused reference. Each chapter is designed to stand alone, allowing the reader to use the book as both a comprehensive resource and a practical reference when needed.

We hope that this volume will help clarify existing knowledge, encourage thoughtful and well-informed surgical care, and support the continued development of chest wall surgery as a clearly defined area of surgical practice.

Wenlin Wang
Rajkamal Vishnu
Editors

Preface – 1

Director Wang Wenlin was an undergraduate student of the 1985 class at the Third Military Medical University. In 1989, he interned in the Department of Thoracic Surgery at Daping Hospital, where I was his supervising instructor. At that time, he showed a strong interest in thoracic surgery, and after graduation, he indeed became a thoracic surgeon. for a clinical doctor, the level of passion for their specialty often determines their professional performance. It was precisely his love for this field that laid a solid foundation for his future career.

After graduating from the Third Military Medical University, Dr. Wang Wenlin pursued postgraduate studies at Nanfang Hospital, affiliated with the First Military Medical University. He later completed a postdoctoral fellowship at Sun Yat-sen University. Following this, he was assigned to the General Hospital of the Guangzhou Military Region, where he specialized in cardiothoracic surgery, with a particular focus on heart procedures. In 2009, he transitioned to his current institution, continuing his work in the same specialty. Up until 2012, Dr. Wang had achieved significant success in cardiac surgery. However, in an unexpected move, the hospital decided to separate the cardiothoracic department into distinct cardiac and thoracic units, assigning him to thoracic surgery. Though initially surprised by the change, Dr. Wang quickly adjusted and embraced the new direction with determination and resilience.

for Dr. Wang Wenlin, whose background was in cardiac surgery, the shift to a new specialty posed significant challenges. Yet, it was precisely these challenges that paved the way for an even more remarkable chapter in his career. In the face of adversity, he carved out a new path for himself, one that led to the creation of an entirely new medical specialty: chest wall surgery.

The emergence of chest wall surgery stems from both objective and subjective reasons. Thoracic surgery itself is a traditional clinical specialty that encompasses the treatment of diseases within the thoracic cavity as well as those affecting the chest wall. In earlier times, thoracic surgery was a combined field addressing both internal thoracic and chest wall conditions. However, in recent years, with the continuous advancement of thoracoscopic techniques, treatments for intrathoracic diseases have made significant progress, while the treatment of chest wall diseases has relatively lagged behind. This trend has become increasingly apparent with the introduction of various advanced technologies. Despite this, chest wall diseases are not uncommon, and patients with these conditions equally require up-to-date, advanced treatments. The demand from patients has provided a strong driving force for the development of chest wall surgery and ultimately led to the establishment of this specialty. Director Wang Wenlin keenly recognized this opportunity and has become a leading figure and pioneer in this field.

After the separation of thoracic and cardiac surgery departments, considering the intense competition in treating common thoracic diseases, Director Wang Wenlin focused his work on a very special condition—pectus excavatum. At that time, the treatment for pectus excavatum was not ideal. Although the Nuss procedure had become the mainstream minimally invasive treatment for this disease, it was only effective for patients with relatively standard and simple chest wall deformities. for those with complex or irregular chest wall deformities, the Nuss procedure had poor outcomes and often failed to achieve therapeutic goals. Moreover, it carried significant risks, such as serious cardiac injury. Director Wang, with his solid foundation and rich experience in cardiac surgery, was able to skillfully perform the Nuss procedure. He quickly mastered the technique and made numerous improvements, significantly enhancing the treatment outcomes for pectus excavatum. After mastering these mature techniques, he also solved many complex and difficult problems that the Nuss procedure alone could not address. His achievements soon gained recognition within the professional community. However, he did not stop there. In his subsequent work, he undertook extensive efforts to address other chest wall deformities and ultimately became a nationally renowned expert in the diagnosis and treatment of chest wall deformities.

Director Wang Wenlin has not only achieved remarkable success in the field of chest wall deformities but has also turned his attention to the surgical treatment of other chest wall diseases, including common tumors, trauma, infections, and defects. Through relentless effort, he has made significant progress in these areas as well. By 2018, the patients admitted to his department had developed a distinct focus almost exclusively on chest wall diseases. This situation led him to make a historic decision: on May (5) 9th of that year, he established the first independent Chest Wall Surgery Department, thus beginning the formal development of chest wall surgery as a specialized field.

Looking back at the history of the emergence of chest wall surgery, it is first and foremost an inevitable trend in the development of the traditional field of thoracic surgery. Any established specialty, upon reaching a certain stage of maturity, inevitably evolves toward greater depth and specialization. Traditional fields such as orthopedics and general surgery have already branched into more focused subspecialties. Similarly, thoracic surgery has the need to develop subspecialties as well. It is foreseeable that in the near future, further divisions may occur, leading to subspecialties such as pulmonary surgery, esophageal surgery, and mediastinal surgery. The emergence of chest wall surgery marks a decisive and pioneering first step forward from the traditional thoracic surgery field.

In the emergence of chest wall surgery, Director Wang Wenlin undoubtedly played a crucial role. This role was both accidental and inevitable. The hospital's unintended decision changed Wang Wenlin's destiny but ultimately led to his even more remarkable career. This might be an unexpected coincidence for anyone. However, it was precisely the solid foundation he had built earlier in cardiac surgery that greatly facilitated his later work. This, in turn, became an essential and inevitable factor in the development of chest wall surgery.

Through his dedicated efforts in the past, Director Wang Wenlin has not only significantly advanced the clinical practice of chest wall surgery but also personally established its theoretical framework. Chest Wall Surgery, as the first monograph in this field, comprehensively presents the concepts, theories, and techniques of chest wall surgery. These valuable contributions will provide strong theoretical support for the development of the discipline. As Director Wang's teacher, I sincerely congratulate him on his achievements and feel deeply gratified.

When our former department head, Professor Jiang Yaoguang, was alive, he often spoke of Wang Wenlin's story, saying that his passion for his career and fighting spirit serve as a role model for young doctors. The remarkable achievements Wang has made today are the greatest comfort to Professor Jiang's spirit in heaven.

Congratulations on the successful publication of *Chest Wall Surgery*, and best wishes for the future of chest wall surgery in China!

Wang Ruwen
Daping Hospital, Army Medical University
1 2023

Preface II

Thoracic surgery is an ancient discipline that treats all diseases occurring in the chest. Chest diseases include both those within the thoracic cavity and those affecting the chest wall. In the early development of thoracic surgery, due to the limited advancement of anesthesia techniques, much of the work focused on the chest wall, especially during wartime, when chest wall trauma was a major area of treatment. With continuous technological progress, surgeries within the thoracic cavity gradually developed and eventually became the mainstream of thoracic surgery.

However, for a considerable period, the treatment ofchest wall diseases was carried out simultaneously. At that time, thoracic surgery was more like a comprehensive discipline, meaning that both diseases inside and outside the thoracic cavity received equal attention. This period is known as the era of open surgery, primarily characterized by all kinds of operations being performed through conventional incisions in the chest wall. Due to the ideal exposure provided by these techniques, various classic surgical procedures emerged rapidly and soon became standardized. At this time, thoracic surgeries mainly focused on treating diseases. Although some aesthetic considerations were taken into account when choosing incisions, the length of the incisions was often long, so aesthetics was not the primary concern. By the 20th century 90 the concept of minimally invasive surgery gradually began to appear in clinical practice.

As trauma and aesthetic factors gained more attention, thoracic surgery quickly entered the era of minimally invasive surgery. Early minimally invasive procedures mainly involved small-incision surgeries, with the primary focus on reducing the length of the incision. However, due to the lack of effective tools, small-incision surgery was short-lived and was soon replaced by an even less invasive technique: thoracoscopic surgery (video-assisted thoracic surgery). Thoracoscopy is a revolutionary tool in the field of thoracic surgery. After its introduction into clinical practice, it became possible to perform operations through extremely small incisions. Especially with the continuous development of various supporting instruments, thoracoscopic surgery gradually became the mainstream technique in the field of thoracic surgery. This technology has continued to develop up to the present day, bringing about revolutionary changes in the treatment of thoracic diseases. Compared to traditional open surgery, thoracoscopic surgery offers unparalleled advantages. It is precisely because of these advantages that nearly all thoracic surgeons actively participate in performing this type of surgery.

However, the widespread use of thoracoscopic surgery has brought about another serious issue: the neglect of chest wall diseases. Thoracoscopy is a tool designed for surgeries inside the thoracic cavity. When too many doctors focus on using this tool for surgeries, those procedures that do not use thoracoscopy, namely surgeries for chest wall diseases, inevitably become overlooked. This phenomenon is very prominent in today's field of thoracic surgery. The most common sight nowadays is that the larger the hospital and the more famous the specialists, the less attention is paid to the treatment of chest wall diseases. This trend is intensifying and directly affects the overall development of thoracic surgery. From a macro perspective, although thoracic surgery appears bustling on the surface, it is actually in a state of distorted development, mainly manifested as an imbalance in the treatment of diseases inside and outside the thoracic cavity. This situation not only impacts the development of thoracic surgery but also affects the treatment of a large number of patients. In fact, the incidence of chest wall diseases is not low; some data even show that their overall incidence is higher than that of intrathoracic diseases. A large number of patients with chest wall diseases do not receive effective treatment, which has clearly become a significant social issue. The root cause of this problem is quite obvious: it lies in the distorted development of thoracic surgery.

Since the problem objectively exists, it must be acknowledged and addressed. fortunately, while many thoracic surgeons were enthusiastic about the hot topic of thoracoscopic surgery, one clear-headed thoracic surgeon chose the opposite path. He keenly identified chest wall diseases, a major condition collectively forgotten, dedicated himself to research and hard work in silence, and ultimately brought these diseases back into focus, enabling patients to receive better treatment. He integrated the clinical work on chest wall diseases, proposed new concepts, improved related theories, and invented numerous new surgical techniques. Ultimately, he established a new clinical specialty chest wall surgery and rightfully became the founder of this specialty. He is Director Wang Wenlin.

My relationship with Director Wang Wenlin can be described as both teacher and friend. He completed his undergraduate studies at the Third Military Medical University and after graduation, he was admitted to the Southern Hospital of the First Military Medical University for his master's and doctoral degrees, which he completed over six years. I was his mentor during this time. Director Wang is an exceptionally diligent doctor during his clinical work, he practically lived in the ward, working tirelessly and never once complaining regardless of how many surgeries he performed or how exhausted he was. He is also a very intelligent physician; even as a student, he demonstrated outstanding thinking and was often praised by his teachers. After graduating from the First Military Medical University, he first did a postdoctoral fellowship at the First Affiliated Hospital of Sun Yat-sen University, then was assigned to the Guangzhou Military Region General Hospital. In his practical work, he gradually became an outstanding surgeon.

Director Wang Wenlin's original specialty was not thoracic surgery but cardiac surgery; strictly speaking, he is a cardiac surgeon. After transferring to his current institution in 2009, because the department was cardiothoracic surgery, he began to truly engage in thoracic surgery work. During this period, he achieved remarkable results starting almost from scratch in cardiac surgery, and by 2012, he had completed a total of 306 cardiac surgeries in that year alone, which is an impressive accomplishment. If he had continued on this trajectory, his cardiac surgery skills would undoubtedly have reached a new level. However, fate played a cruel joke on him—the hospital decided to separate the cardiothoracic department, assigning him to focus solely on thoracic surgery. for a specialist trained in cardiac surgery, this decision posed significant challenges for his future work. Nevertheless, Director Wang Wenlin promptly adjusted his mindset, faced the difficulties head-on, and embraced the challenge. He keenly identified thoracic wall diseases as a weak spot and devoted himself fully to tackling them. The first condition he conquered was pectus excavatum, followed by pectus carinatum, and later various complex chest wall deformities. Thanks to his solid theoretical foundation and strong research capabilities, he not only mastered surgeries for common deformities but also developed numerous innovative surgical techniques. Among these surgical techniques, the most famous is the Wang procedure. Once introduced, it immediately attracted widespread attention, and many hospitals quickly adopted the technique. Because the Wang procedure fundamentally transformed the treatment of pectus excavatum, it received official recognition and was ultimately included in the National Clinical Version 3.0 of the Surgical Operation Classification Codes. His surgery became the only procedure named after a Chinese doctor to be included in the classification. In addition to surgeries for chest wall deformities, he has performed a large number of other chest wall disease operations, such as those for chest wall tumors, defects, and infections. The development of these surgeries gave his department a distinctive character and gradually shaped the prototype of chest wall surgery as a specialized field.

Director Wang Wenlin's unique focus was precisely on a disease area overlooked by others, which quickly attracted widespread attention from his peers. Within just a few years, he visited over 300 hospitals across the country to assist in performing surgeries. During this process, he not only spread advanced surgical techniques but also introduced new concepts. Thus, a brand-new specialty was born, Chest Wall Surgery.

On 9-5-2018, Director Wang Wenlin established the first specialized Department of Chest Wall Surgery in China. He subsequently founded the Professional Committee on Chest Wall Surgery, and later initiated the China (Chest Wall Surgery) Alliance. His work gained widespread recognition among his peers and earned him great respect.

Under his leadership, chest wall surgery in China developed from scratch growing from a small spark into a widespread movement. He has made outstanding contributions to the establishment and advancement of this medical field. The book Chest Wall Surgery, which he has now compiled, is the culmination and comprehensive summary of his many years of dedicated work.

This book has six chapters. The first chapter presents the fundamental theories of chest wall surgery. The following five chapters each focus on one of the five major categories of chest wall conditions: deformities, tumors, defects, trauma, and infections.

The most notable highlight of the book lies in its introduction of numerous new concepts, theories, and techniques. What makes it especially valuable is the inclusion of extensive experience with complex and high-difficulty surgical procedures, which will serve as a vital resource for the treatment of such conditions.

As the first academic monograph dedicated to the specialty of chest wall surgery, the publication of this book will provide valuable technical guidance for clinical practice in the field.

Congratulations on the publication of (Chest Wall Surgery)!

Best wishes for the continued development and success of chest wall surgery in our country!

Kai Can Cai
Southern Hospital, Southern Medical University
1 2023

Preface - III

Thoracic surgery is an ancient and broad discipline. Clinically, its work can generally be divided into two parts: surgeries inside the thoracic cavity and those outside it. In the early days, the distinction between these two was not clear; they developed simultaneously and were closely interconnected, forming an organic whole. for a long time, thoracic surgery did not have a clear separation between intrathoracic and extra-thoracic procedures. In the 20th century 90 the concept of minimally invasive surgery began to emerge in clinical practice. We were among the first in China to perform thoracoscopic surgery. Since then, we have made great efforts to advance thoracoscopic techniques, gradually bringing them to maturity. Over the past twenty-plus years, we have trained a large number of thoracoscopic surgeons nationwide, ushering traditional thoracic surgery in China into a completely new era, the era of minimally invasive surgery. The hallmark of this era is the widespread application of thoracoscopic technology. Its use has brought about a revolutionary transformation in thoracic surgery, with two major advantages: minimal invasiveness and improved cosmetic outcomes. These benefits have maximally met patients' treatment needs, making thoracoscopic surgery widely welcomed by both patients and doctors. Consequently, more and more thoracic surgeons have joined the ranks of thoracoscopic surgery specialists, to the extent that thoracic surgery in recent years is increasingly resembling thoracoscopic surgery itself.

The thoracoscopic technology we have vigorously promoted has brought about a sweeping technological revolution in thoracic surgery. With the continuous development of various instruments and devices, this technology has become increasingly mature. However, a significant drawback has gradually emerged: the neglect of chest wall diseases. Thoracoscopy is a tool designed for intrathoracic surgeries. As its use has expanded widely in clinical practice, surgeries that do not require thoracoscopy, namely, chest wall procedures have been increasingly overlooked. Before the advent of thoracoscopy, chest wall surgeries were commonly performed at many medical centers. But in recent years, such procedures have become rare even in large hospitals. This phenomenon is highly abnormal and can be considered a sign of distorted development. In fact, chest wall diseases are not uncommon; the incidence of chest wall deformities alone reaches as high as 1%. As living standards improve and more people become concerned about the appearance of their chest wall, an increasing number of patients desire corrective chest wall surgery. This growing patient demand stands in stark contrast to the current state of thoracic

surgery, creating a significant and urgent contradiction that must be resolved.
Dr. Wang Wenlin was originally a cardiac surgeon, with most of his previous surgeries focused on cardiac procedures. However, in 2012, his hospital decided to split the original cardiothoracic surgery department into two separate divisions, assigning him to lead the thoracic surgery department. Fate played a cruel joke on him but, in doing so, entrusted him with an even greater mission—launching the field of chest wall surgery in China.
After the department was split, considering the fierce competition in thoracic surgery in Guangzhou, Dr. Wang Wenlin did not choose the most popular field intrathoracic surgery. Instead, he focused on a neglected condition: pectus excavatum (funnel chest). In the early days, pectus excavatum surgeries were mainly performed by pediatric surgeons, and thoracic surgeons rarely undertook these operations. Although the Nuss procedure was popular at the time, it carried risks of heart injury, which made the treatment outcomes for pectus excavatum less than ideal.
Since Dr. Wang's background was in cardiac surgery, he had a natural technical advantage. He quickly overcame the surgical challenges associated with pectus excavatum, significantly reducing surgical risks and improving outcomes. Through his relentless efforts, pectus excavatum surgery soon became his signature procedure, earning him widespread recognition. He then turned his attention to other chest wall deformities such as pectus carinatum (pigeon chest), flat chest, and barrel chest, achieving remarkable success in these areas. The most challenging surgeries he performed were for asphyxiating thoracic dystrophy (Jeune syndrome). Not only did he invent new surgical techniques for this condition, but he also completed the highest number of cases worldwide. By the end of 2021, he had performed 28 such surgeries, including on the oldest surviving patient globally, who was 36 years old at the time. Dr. Wang repeatedly broke world records with his outstanding surgical skills. In addition to completing numerous complex surgeries, he invented many new surgical methods. His most famous procedure, known as the Wang procedure, has been officially included in the National Clinical Version 3.0 of the Surgical Operation Classification Codes, further cementing his reputation.

From the very beginning, Dr. Wang Wenlin focused on diseases that others had overlooked, which became the key to his success. In his subsequent work, he expanded his efforts to other chest wall conditions, including chest wall tumors, infections, and defects. In 2018, he established China's first dedicated chest wall surgery department, marking the official birth of a new clinical specialty.

Over the following years, Dr. Wang led his team in intensive research and development of chest wall surgery techniques. They not only performed numerous complex surgeries but also introduced many new concepts and designed several innovative surgical procedures. Ultimately, they developed a comprehensive theoretical system for chest wall surgery. These achievements have laid a solid foundation for the development of chest wall surgery in China.

Over the past several years, Dr. Wang Wenlin has assisted numerous hospitals across China in performing various chest wall surgeries. This not only facilitated the exchange of surgical techniques but also helped spread the concepts of chest wall surgery. Thanks to his persistent efforts, the field of chest wall surgery in China has developed rapidly and achieved remarkable success. Dr. Wang himself has rightfully become the founding figure of this specialty. (Chest Wall Surgery) is the first monograph in the field of chest wall surgery, authored by Dr. Wang Wenlin. This book represents the culmination of his years of dedicated work. It systematically explains the fundamental theories of chest wall surgery and details many surgical techniques. The publication of this monograph will provide theoretical guidance for clinical practice in chest wall surgery. With the joint efforts of colleagues nationwide, it is believed that the chest wall surgery field in China will continue to overcome challenges, forge ahead courageously, and achieve even greater accomplishments.

He Jianxing
The First Affiliated Hospital of Guangzhou Medical University
1 2023

Preface - IV

Thoracic surgery has achieved remarkable progress to date and has fully entered the era of minimally invasive surgery. A wide range of advanced technologies, represented by thoracoscopic techniques, have become the mainstream in thoracic surgical practice. Compared with traditional thoracic surgery, these modern techniques are less invasive, result in smaller and more concealed postoperative scars, and significantly improve the patient experience. With continuous breakthroughs in scientific research, we have good reason to believe that thoracic surgery will make even greater leaps forward. However, some challenges remain in the field's development. One major issue is the uneven progress within the specialty. Since thoracoscopic techniques are primarily used to treat diseases inside the thoracic cavity, as more hospitals and surgeons focus their attention on intrathoracic procedures, diseases of the chest wall tend to be neglected. This has become a significant problem facing thoracic surgery today.

Thoracic surgery is originally a comprehensive and integrated specialty, encompassing not only the treatment of intrathoracic diseases but also diseases of the chest wall. In the early days of thoracic surgery, these two areas developed simultaneously and were closely interconnected, playing a positive role in advancing the entire discipline. However, in recent years, the treatment of chest wall diseases has clearly lagged behind, leading to a distorted development within the field of thoracic surgery.

However, the incidence of chest wall diseases is not low. According to the classification of surgical diseases, chest wall diseases include deformities, tumors, defects, trauma, and infections. Apart from the common trauma cases, the other diseases have relatively high incidence rates. Take pectus excavatum, a type of chest wall deformity, For example the incidence rate ranges from 0.2% - 0.8%, which is quite significant on its own. Some rough estimates suggest that when other deformities are included, the total incidence may even exceed 1%. and that's just the incidence of deformities. When chest wall tumors, infections, defects, and other conditions are added, the overall incidence becomes even higher surpassing that of many intrathoracic diseases. As living standards improve and more people become concerned about the appearance of their chest wall, the number of individuals seeking treatment is increasing. Despite such a large patient population, thoracic surgeons have not given sufficient attention to these conditions. This clearly represents a major social issue that urgently requires effective solutions.

Director Wang Wenlin graduated early from the Third Military Medical

University, earned his master's and doctoral degrees at the First Military Medical University, and completed his postdoctoral work at Sun Yat-sen University. His major was cardiac surgery, so strictly speaking, he is a specialized cardiac surgeon. Given his background, he was expected to make significant achievements in cardiac surgery. However, fate played a surprising trick on him. Just as he was becoming proficient in cardiac surgery, his hospital suddenly decided to split the original Department of Cardiothoracic Surgery into two separate departments, assigning him to lead the thoracic surgery division. This change of specialty brought him considerable challenges. But instead of following the conventional path of thoracic surgery development, he chose an unexpected new direction, one that led him to break new ground and achieve even greater success.

At the beginning of his journey, Director Wang Wenlin did not set ambitious goals for himself. Instead, he chose relatively unremarkable condition pectus excavatum (funnel chest). Although this disease has a relatively high incidence, it was mostly treated by pediatric surgeons, and thoracic surgeons were rarely involved in such procedures. At that time, the Nuss procedure had already been introduced in China, but its clinical application was clearly limited due to the risk of cardiac injury. Director Wang Wenlin, with his background in cardiac surgery, had a technical advantage that made him better suited to perform this operation. After intensive technical research and development, he not only mastered the procedure proficiently but also quickly gained recognition for his work on pectus excavatum. In the following years, he successfully tackled surgeries for various other deformities, gradually becoming a renowned expert in chest wall deformity surgery. However, he did not stop at these achievements; he set his sights on the treatment of the entire spectrum of chest wall diseases. Through relentless efforts, his department gradually became a recognized center for the treatment of chest wall diseases. Chest wall disease treatment became the hallmark of his department. Once everything was progressing smoothly, Director Wang Wenlin made a major decision in 2018, he established China's first independent Chest Wall Surgery Department, marking the official beginning of the development of chest wall surgery in the country.

Over the past decade, Director Wang Wenlin and his team have made tremendous contributions to the field of chest wall surgery. They have not only performed a large number of complex chest wall surgeries but have also gradually developed a comprehensive theoretical framework for the specialty. This body of work has provided crucial guidance for clinical practice and helped establish chest wall surgery as an emerging, distinct discipline.

Clinical medicine is a rapidly evolving field, and no traditional surgical specialty can afford to remain stagnant. One of the main directions of development is moving toward greater specialization and refinement. for specific clinical disciplines, this means the emergence and growth of subspecialties. Among various clinical fields, general surgery and orthopedics have taken the lead in developing subspecialties, while thoracic surgery's progress in this regard seems comparatively slower. However, from the perspective of overall discipline development, the rise of subspecialties is an unstoppable trend. It is foreseeable that thoracic surgery will eventually divide into subspecialties such as pulmonary surgery, esophageal surgery, and mediastinal surgery. The establishment of chest wall surgery undoubtedly marks a pioneering step in this direction. If this momentum continues, it will not only improve treatment for subspecialty diseases but also revitalize the traditional field of thoracic surgery, promoting a more comprehensive and vibrant development.

(Chest Wall Surgery) is the culmination of years of dedicated research by Director Wang Wenlin. This book provides a comprehensive introduction to the theories and techniques of chest wall surgery, supported by numerous detailed surgical case studies. Its content is thorough and rich, making it a seminal work in the field of chest wall surgery. The successful publication of this book also carries the hopes of thoracic surgery colleagues nationwide. With the dedicated efforts of Director Wang Wenlin and many like-minded professionals, it is believed that the cause of chest wall surgery in China will achieve leapfrog development and make significant contributions to the health of society as a whole.

Jiang Gening
Shanghai Pulmonary Hospital
1 2023

Preface - V

The year 2008 was a special one for me. I was transferring from Guangzhou Military General Hospital to a local hospital, and I had to make plans for my future work. At that time, a special technique in thoracic surgery was quietly emerging, the increasingly popular thoracoscopic surgery. I was not very interested in this technique initially because I was a cardiac surgeon. However, the new department I joined was not purely cardiac surgery but cardiothoracic surgery, which involved general thoracic surgery as well. Therefore, I had to pay attention to thoracoscopic technology and seriously consider its potential impact on the future work of the department.

My thought was that since this technique was very popular, it would undoubtedly become highly sought after. Thoracoscopic surgery is primarily used for procedures within the thoracic cavity, and its widespread adoption would greatly improve the treatment outcomes of lung, esophageal, and mediastinal diseases. However, I was also certain that another category of diseases—those affecting the chest wall would be neglected because their treatment does not require thoracoscopy. I clearly realized that the use of thoracoscopic surgery would cause a division within traditional thoracic surgery, splitting it into two camps: thoracic cavity surgery and chest wall surgery. The neglect of chest wall diseases, paradoxically, presented a rare opportunity. If this opportunity could be seized and developed as a subspecialty, there would certainly be a lot of work to do. This was my initial vision for chest wall surgery.

This idea occupied my mind for a long time, and I shared it with many experts. Unfortunately, at that time, the allure of thoracic cavity surgery was so strong that no one was willing to give up the popular surgeries to focus on the less common chest wall surgeries. Nonetheless, I did not stop paying attention. Even though I was a cardiac surgeon, I knew I had to prepare for the future of cardiothoracic surgery.

In 2009, I officially started working at the new institution. The department mainly focused on cardiac surgery but also performed general thoracic surgeries. Although these were not the main focus, we attached great importance to chest wall surgeries. By 2013, the hospital made an adjustment to the department's work, and I no longer handled cardiac surgeries, instead focusing entirely on general thoracic surgery. This change became a major turning point in my career. Because of this shift, I devoted myself wholeheartedly to chest wall surgery, helping this specialty take root, grow, and eventually become independent.

Thoracic surgery is a traditional and highly competitive specialty. for someone like me, entering thoracic surgery midway through my career, finding a clear departmental role was almost as difficult as climbing a mountain. But I had no other choice. I had to press forward with no retreat. After a long period of observation and reflection, I finally discovered a breakthrough—a disease that few paid attentions to at the time: pectus excavatum (funnel chest). Although this is a relatively common chest wall deformity, it had traditionally been treated mostly by pediatric surgeons, with thoracic surgeons rarely performing these operations. Because thoracic surgeons paid little attention to this disease, I saw a potential opportunity. Through persistent effort, my department quickly achieved remarkable results in treating this condition. We not only completed a large number of Nuss procedures for pectus excavatum, but building on this foundation, I made significant improvements and ultimately designed a safer and more reliable procedure, which became known as the Wung operation.

This laid a solid foundation for the smooth progress of subsequent clinical work.

During the treatment of patients with pectus excavatum, many patients with non-pectus excavatum deformities also came seeking treatment. Although these patients had some form of chest depression, their deformities were not typical pectus excavatum. Some of these patients came after failed surgeries at other hospitals; nearly all had undergone the Nuss procedure, but their deformities were not pectus excavatum. These failed cases prompted me to reflect deeply. I eventually realized that not all chest wall depressions are pectus excavatum; they are entirely different deformities, which deserve their own names and require distinct surgical approaches.

This reflection directly led to the naming of several new deformities. Early on, I named several new deformities, such as sulcus chest, saddle chest, and lateral chest wall depression deformity. Naming deformities is not only about understanding them but, more importantly, about guiding their treatment. I also designed multiple new surgical techniques specifically for treating these deformities, achieving very satisfactory results.

Because effective treatments were developed for various deformities, my patient base gradually expanded. These patients were no longer limited to pectus excavatum but included nearly all types of deformities. This allowed me to accumulate extensive experience in treating a wide range of deformities. To better address deformity correction, I designed multiple specialized surgeries, including the Wenlin procedure, Willine procedure, Wang procedure, Tesla procedure, and others. I also proposed several novel surgical concepts, such as clean surgery, bleeding less surgery, and band-aid surgery.

During this period, I focused on treating some special deformities, including barrel chest surgery, rib arch surgery, thoracic dysplasia syndrome surgery, asphyxiating thoracic dysplasia surgery, Poland syndrome surgery, and secondary chest wall deformity surgery. These operations were nearly all pioneering procedures that filled gaps in the field.

These efforts earned me a strong reputation, and my department became known as a professional center for chest wall deformity correction. I personally transformed from a cardiac surgeon into a specialist in chest wall deformity surgery.

for a long time, I dedicated myself wholeheartedly to deformity correction without considering other fields. Due to the success of my work, I received many invitations from other institutions to assist in developing their surgical capabilities. As my reputation grew, some institutions invited me to join them permanently. These invitations forced me to confront a practical issue: the structure of the department. Focusing solely on deformity surgeries made it difficult for a department to survive, at least in the early years when I lacked sufficient confidence.

At this time, I recalled the concept I had considered years earlier chest wall surgery. I believed that the only way forward was to combine all chest wall diseases into one independent department. Thus, the idea of establishing a dedicated chest wall surgery department emerged. Originally, this idea was planned for my future new institution, but when that plan fell through, it instead became a reality at my own institution on 9-5-2018, when the first independent chest wall surgery department was established.

With the establishment of the department as an independent clinical unit, many tasks had to be undertaken. The first very concrete task was patient admission. After repeated consideration, I limited the scope of admissions to five basic types of diseases, including deformities. My department already had a solid foundation in deformity treatment, and now with new disease types included, although experience was limited, the areas were interconnected. Therefore, the work proceeded quite smoothly and quickly achieved good results. After establishing the first independent chest wall surgery department, I went on to found the first specialized chest wall surgery committee the Chest Wall Surgery Committee of the Guangdong Thoracic Disease Society as well as China's first nationwide academic organization dedicated to chest wall surgery the China Chest Wall Surgery Alliance. These efforts gradually brought attention to the concept of chest wall surgery. To familiarize more people with this new specialty, I undertook extensive theoretical work, writing a large number of articles to explain and promote the concepts and theories of chest wall surgery.

These efforts played a strong role in advancing the field. Many doctors across the country began to join the work in chest wall surgery, and numerous hospitals established their own chest wall surgery departments. From nothing, chest wall surgery gradually took shape as an independent specialty.

for a long time, my articles primarily discussed the basic concepts of chest wall surgery, patient admission criteria, surgical principles, and surgical techniques. Many colleagues relied on these writings to carry out clinical work. However, the content was scattered across various places, making it difficult to access systematically. Some enthusiastic individuals repeatedly reminded me that it was necessary to compile these articles into a book to guide clinical practice. To meet this need, I began the work in early 2019, and after more than four years, finally completed it in early 2023. This was an extremely arduous task, with all content personally written by me. Because of my busy clinical work, I had to use every possible spare moment to work on it. Some suggested inviting several experts to co-author the book, which was a valuable suggestion, but I ultimately declined. My reasoning was that chest wall surgery is a completely new specialty, and its concepts and principles are not yet fully unified. Having multiple authors could lead to differing viewpoints within the same book, which would not only affect the book's seriousness but might also misguide the development of the specialty. Therefore, I decided to complete it on my own.

The book first defines the research scope of chest wall surgery, which includes the five basic disease categories mentioned earlier: deformities, tumors, defects, trauma, and infections. This classification draws reference from general surgery disease divisions; although not entirely scientific, it meets practical needs in department operations and is therefore very useful.

Regarding concepts, the book provides detailed discussions of the fundamental ideas of chest wall surgery, as well as introducing numerous theories and surgical methods. To make the explanations as comprehensive as possible, I included many images, mostly from patients in my department and a few from patients I assisted at other institutions. Additionally, I drew numerous schematic diagrams to provide detailed explanations of related content.

Most of the concepts and theories in the book have been gradually published in recent years on various online platforms, rather than traditional print media. To provide verifiable references, I cited articles previously published online. However, due to inherent limitations of online platforms, readers may not always be able to access the original texts, which is somewhat regrettable.

The publication of this book is itself an attempt, much like the many attempts experienced during the development of this specialty. I do not wish for regrets, but they are unavoidable. Therefore, if readers find any issues while reading, these represent challenges that we all need to address together moving forward. Finally, I want to express my gratitude to many individuals involved in this work. First are my team members: Chen Chunmei, Long Weiguang, Liu Yang, Cai Bin, Wang Wenjie, Gong Wen, Luo Juan, Chen Kai, and others. During the process of collecting and organizing materials, they have made tremendous contributions. I also want to thank numerous experts from peer institutions across the country, who have provided valuable encouragement and support for the writing of this book and offered many precious suggestions. Additionally, I am grateful to the leaders of my hospital, who have always cared about the development of chest wall surgery and offered us selfless assistance.

The cause of chest wall surgery is just beginning and has a long way to go. As a new specialty, it possesses strong vitality. I believe that through the joint efforts of all those who are passionate about the chest wall surgery field, this specialty will surely ride the wind and waves, continuously mature and grow, and ultimately become a fully independent clinical specialty.

Wang Wenlin
Guangdong Second Provincial People's Hospital
1 2023

Index

Chapter 1: Summary

Chapter 2: Chest Wall Deformities (Part 1)

CHAPTER 1
SUMMARY

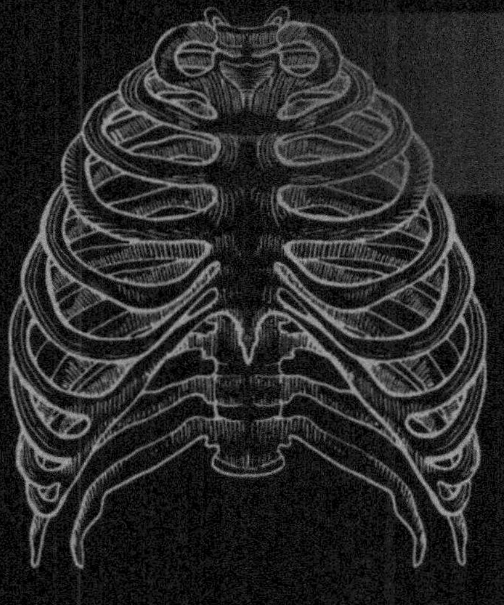

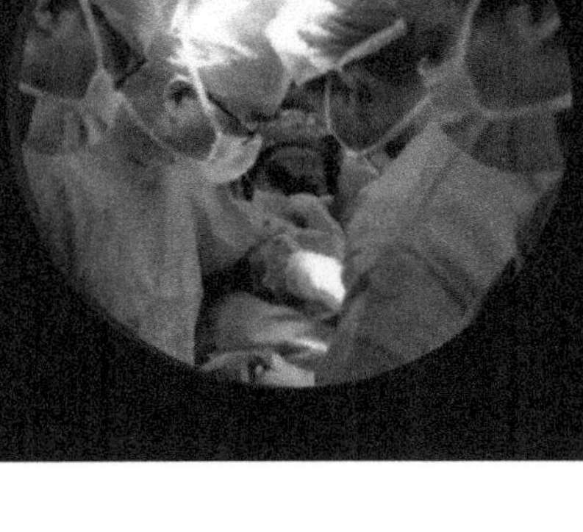

Section 1

ORIGIN OF CHEST WALL SURGERY

Traditional thoracic surgery is an ancient discipline, with its research subjects including all diseases of the chest, encompassing both intrathoracic and extra-thoracic diseases [1]. Extra-thoracic diseases mainly occur in the chest wall. In the early practice of thoracic surgery, due to limitations in anesthesia and respiratory support techniques, much of the work was performed on the chest wall. At that time, surgeries for chest wall trauma and infections were frequently carried out. Therefore, thoracic surgery back then was more like chest wall surgery, although no one had yet proposed the concept of chest wall surgery as a separate field.

With the overall advancement of anesthesia and surgical techniques, intrathoracic surgeries gradually developed. Lung surgery, esophageal surgery, and mediastinal surgery became the main focus of thoracic surgery. At this time, thoracic surgery became a true surgery of the chest, with diseases both inside and outside the thoracic cavity receiving widespread attention. Nearly all diseases traditionally considered thoracic surgical diseases could be seen in thoracic surgery wards [1,2].

By the 20th century 90 the concept of minimally invasive surgery began to emerge in the surgical field, and minimally invasive thoracic surgery also started to take shape. The earliest form was small-incision surgery. As thoracoscopic techniques became more widely used in clinical practice, small-incision surgeries gradually faded away, replaced by thoracoscopic surgery. Thoracoscopic surgery soon became synonymous with minimally invasive surgery. With its small and discreet incisions, minimal trauma, quick recovery, and reduced patient discomfort, it offered many advantages and was quickly welcomed by patients. Thanks to the efforts of many forward-thinking individuals, thoracoscopic techniques rapidly spread and gradually became the mainstream approach in thoracic surgery [2].

Thoracoscopic surgery is a technically demanding procedure that is not easy to master. However, with increased surgical opportunities and the establishment of extensive training programs, more and more surgeons have acquired this skill. The growing participation of physicians created a positive feedback loop, ultimately leading to the rapid development and increasing refinement of thoracoscopic techniques. Due to its high technical content, it also became a focal point for basic research and scientific studies in thoracic surgery. With significant human and material resources invested in this field, thoracoscopic surgery eventually became a trend. The larger the hospital, the more renowned its thoracic surgery department tends to be, and the more successful its thoracoscopic surgeries become. This undoubtedly created a "star effect." Driven by this effect, senior specialists at major hospitals took pride in mastering thoracoscopic surgery, while junior specialists at smaller hospitals felt ashamed if they could not perform it. This clear distinction between honor and disgrace became a powerful driving force, pushing thoracoscopic techniques to new heights. Eventually, robotic-assisted thoracoscopic surgery began to replace conventional Thoracoscopy, bringing the technology to an unprecedented level [3-5].

The development of thoracoscopic surgery has led to significantly improved treatment for many thoracic diseases; this is its great achievement. However, the blind worship of Thoracoscopy has also brought about another issue: the distorted development of thoracic surgery. Thoracoscopy is a tool designed for performing intrathoracic procedures. Thoracoscopic surgery is limited to operations on the lungs, esophagus, or other structures within the thoracic cavity. If surgeons focus solely on performing thoracoscopic surgeries, it means that only intrathoracic procedures are being emphasized, while others are neglected. The neglected surgeries are extra-thoracic, located in the chest wall and can be performed without the use of Thoracoscopy. Precisely because Thoracoscopy is not required for these procedures, many surgeons have simply stopped performing them.

In recent years, with the unchecked development of thoracoscopic technology, an extremely bizarre phenomenon has emerged: the majority of thoracic surgeons have become obsessed with thoracoscopic procedures, while other types of surgery are rarely addressed. In many large hospitals today, thoracic surgery departments present a strikingly uniform scene ward filled almost exclusively with patients undergoing lung or esophageal surgeries, with perhaps a few mediastinal cases scattered among them. These have come to represent the entirety of thoracic surgery patients. Common conditions mentioned in textbooks such as rib fractures, chest wall tumors, and pectus excavatum have long disappeared from these wards. Some departments may not see a single case of such conditions throughout the entire year. This phenomenon is highly abnormal.

The contributors to the thoracic surgery chapters in surgical textbooks are often theoretical experts who tirelessly compile volumes of material on extra-thoracic diseases to educate generation after generation of medical students, teaching them that thoracic surgery includes not only diseases of the lungs, esophagus, and mediastinum, but also many chest wall conditions. Yet, ironically, these same experts rarely perform such surgeries themselves or don't know how to perform them at all. This has become a real-life version of "armchair strategizing." Perhaps they do perform some simple chest wall procedures, but their technical skill leaves much to be desired. Once top specialists at major hospitals began to disdain chest wall surgeries that don't involve Thoracoscopy, the responsibility for such procedures fell to doctors at lower-tier hospitals. These surgeons may be highly skilled and efficient in the operating room, but they lack influence. They are unable to advocate for or publicize the importance of extra-thoracic procedures. Thus, a reality of arrogance and prejudice has taken shape: well-known doctors look down on non-thoracoscopic surgeries, while lesser-known doctors feel embarrassed to admit they perform them. One group refuses to do the work, while the other does it in silence and as a result, extra-thoracic surgeries have been increasingly overlooked. For many years, while thoracoscopic surgery was flourishing, its counterpart, non-thoracoscopic surgery, namely extra-thoracic procedures, was pushed into a dead end.

A thoracic surgeon should be called a thoracic surgeon because they are expected to be capable of performing all types of thoracic surgeries. If a doctor can only perform lung surgeries, then they should be called a lung surgeon, not a thoracic surgeon. Similarly, if a doctor only performs esophageal surgeries, they should be called an esophageal surgeon not a thoracic surgeon. Objectively speaking, once thoracoscopic surgery came to dominate the entire field of thoracic surgery, the specialty ceased to be thoracic surgery in the true sense of the term. It effectively became thoracoscopic surgery or intra-thoracic surgery. These names may sound awkward, but they accurately reflect the current state of modern thoracic surgery.

When the vast majority of thoracic surgeons are racking their brains trying to develop thoracoscopic procedures, does that mean non-thoracoscopic patients are extremely rare? Quite the opposite, these patients are actually more numerous, in greater need of treatment, and more deserving of public attention. Data shows that pectus excavatum alone has an incidence rate of 2% to 8%. When all thoracic deformities are considered together, the incidence is astonishingly high. and that doesn't even include other extra-thoracic conditions. If all of these diseases are taken into account, their combined incidence may even exceed that of intrathoracic diseases. These high-prevalence conditions urgently require the attention of thoracic surgeons, yet most surgeons devote their limited energy solely to an endless stream of intrathoracic operations. This is clearly no longer just a medical issue; it has become a significant social issue. The problem needs to be addressed. The patients need treatment. Yet this objective need has been forgotten by most thoracic surgeons and ignored by many well-known thoracic experts. However, in every era, there are always clear-eyed observers who keenly identify problems and propose solutions. And so, the era of chest wall surgery has arrived [6].

The emergence of chest wall surgery has a profound historical background. The aforementioned state of thoracic surgery laid a solid foundation for the birth of chest wall surgery, yet its emergence still required a certain opportunity. Although this opportunity was accidental, it was also a historical inevitability. What surprised me was that I myself became the protagonist of this opportunity [7-10].

I was originally a cardiac surgeon, with my master's, doctoral, and postdoctoral research all focused in the field of cardiac surgery. After graduation, I worked exclusively in cardiac surgery. In 2008, my workplace changed, and the new department was cardiothoracic surgery. Besides cardiac surgeries, I had to prepare to perform general thoracic surgeries. At that time, thoracoscopic surgery was the hottest technique, but I personally did not want to pursue that technology. Regarding the future work of the department, my thought was that if the majority of thoracic surgeons in most hospitals were performing thoracoscopic surgeries and my department did not, we would definitely fall behind. However, we could focus on what others were not doing, that is, surgeries on the chest wall. These types of surgeries do not require Thoracoscopy and naturally attract little attention, but if we focused on them, we would surely attract many patients. If the patient volume became sufficient, it could even form an independent department dedicated to treating such cases. At that time, I also considered the name for this department and eventually came up with "Chest Wall Surgery." I pondered this for a long time and later discussed the idea with many experts. Unfortunately, none were willing to give up the popular thoracoscopic surgeries to focus on the less common chest wall procedures. However, I had to pay attention. Although I am a cardiac surgeon, I must plan for the future of cardiothoracic surgery. On 1.1.2009, I officially became the director of the Cardiothoracic Surgery Department at Guangdong Second Provincial People's Hospital. The work in the department mainly involved cardiac surgery. I loved the cardiac surgery specialty and had devoted a long time to working hard in this field, never once considering giving it up. However, since the department was cardiothoracic surgery, I had to perform some general thoracic surgeries as well, with a focus on surgeries for chest wall diseases.

Before officially joining the department, the clinical work situation was not ideal, with the number of cardiac surgeries performed each year only in single digits. To change this backward situation, I made great efforts. After a short period of hard work, the cardiac surgery level in the department improved dramatically, and the number of cardiac surgeries rapidly increased from single digits per year to 306 cases in 2012. The cardiac surgery team was established, and the foundation was solidified. I should have been able to relax and enjoy the fruits of my labor, but at that time the hospital made a major decision to separate the cardiothoracic surgery department. After careful consideration, the hospital ultimately decided that I would be responsible for the thoracic surgery work. I was originally a cardiac surgeon, and the hospital's decision was equivalent to asking me to give up the beloved specialty I had worked hard for many years. This was undoubtedly a difficult choice. However, for the hospital to develop and the specialty to progress, the separation was inevitable. I had to consider the bigger picture, face reality, and accept the challenge. When I first entered the field of thoracic surgery, thoracoscopic technology was extremely popular, and I couldn't help but be influenced by this prevailing trend. At that time, Guangzhou was filled with experts. Many major hospitals had very famous doctors who did nothing else but specialize in thoracoscopic surgery. They performed lung surgeries, esophageal surgeries, and mediastinal surgeries, all as top experts in the field of thoracoscopic surgery. As a newcomer, if I wanted to squeeze in and get a share of the pie, I was destined to hit a wall facing such fierce competition. I was very clear that if I followed the conventional path, I would never be a match for these institutions and experts. To carve out my own space, I had to take a shortcut and find a path uniquely my own. So naturally, I thought of chest wall surgery, which I had been focusing on for many years. The breakthrough I chose was a special chest wall condition, namely pectus excavatum. Pectus excavatum is an ancient disease, well known to many thoracic surgeons. However, for a long time, the treatment of this disease was not ideal because many hospitals had pediatric surgeons performing pectus excavatum surgeries, and the vast majority of thoracic surgeons did not perform these operations. Pediatric surgery has its own professional limitations, which inherently affect the treatment of pectus excavatum. After analyzing the situation, I realized that if I took on this work, I would definitely be more competitive.

In 2010, Dr. Nuss personally came to Guangzhou and held a large-scale surgical promotion event. I participated in that event and gained a very deep understanding of the Nuss procedure. By 2013, when it was time to reconsider my professional direction, the first thing I thought of was the Nuss procedure for pectus excavatum. I clearly realized that, as a former cardiac surgeon, I was better suited to perform this surgery and would have more advantages than the average thoracic surgeon. My reason is: First, I can skillfully manage the risks of the Nuss procedure. The Nuss procedure was introduced in 1998, and although many have performed it since then, it has often not been done with full confidence. The main reason is that surgery carries significant risks. During the placement of the steel bar, any injury to the heart could be life-threatening for the patient. Because of this risk, many thoracic surgeons are not brave enough to perform this surgery. As a cardiac surgeon, I am able to skillfully avoid the risk of injuring the heart. From this perspective, compared to the average thoracic surgeon, I have a clear advantage. Second, I can skillfully perform various complex pectus excavatum surgeries. Besides having greater risks, complex pectus excavatum surgeries also involve increased technical difficulty. These surgeries share certain similarities with complex congenital heart defect surgeries, which gives me, as a cardiac surgeon, better capability to handle complicated deformities. This is an advantage that ordinary thoracic surgeons do not possess. Third, the hospital I work at has advantages in patient intake. The hospital where I work is a comprehensive top-tier hospital, capable of treating pectus excavatum patients of all ages, which gives it a greater capacity for patient intake compared to general children's hospitals. This advantage is more conducive to advancing my career. After rationally recognizing these advantages, I began my new work. I made the treatment of pectus excavatum my sole focus.

After I devoted nearly all my energy to treating this disease, I quickly achieved results. A clear sign of this success was that everyone had forgotten I was once a cardiac surgeon; they only knew me as a doctor who specialized in pectus excavatum surgery. Achieving this outcome was exactly the result I longed for.

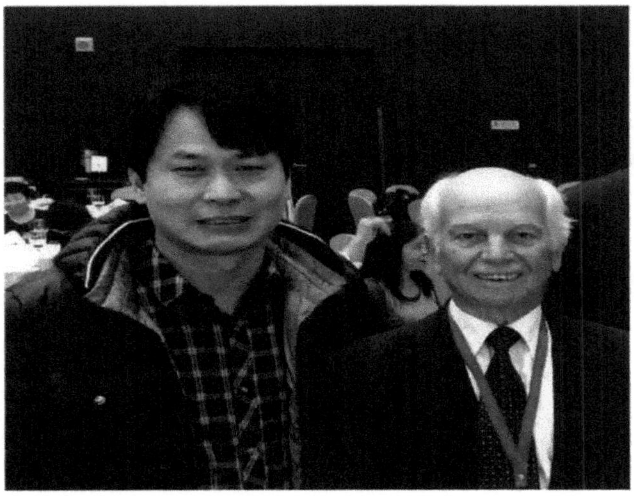

Figure 1-1-1: The author with Dr. Nuss in 2015.

My goal was to make everyone know that, aside from pectus excavatum surgery, I couldn't do any other surgeries. As I got closer and closer to this goal, I became an expert in this field. My goal was realized, and pectus excavatum patients from all directions both domestic and international came seeking my help. This provided me with more practical opportunities. My skills continuously improved and advanced, and my reputation grew even stronger. Not only did pectus excavatum patients come for consultation, but patients with other deformities also arrived, those with pectus carinatum, barrel chest, flat chest, and various other complex deformities that are difficult to name. I did not disappoint my patients. I devoted a lot of effort to studying these deformities, the surgeries, and the various issues related to these conditions. As a result, not only did I perform pectus excavatum surgeries very successfully, but I also did quite well with surgeries for other deformities.

While striving to complete clinical work, I devoted a great deal of effort to related theoretical research. During this time, I named several new deformities, including groove chest [11], saddle chest [12], lateral chest wall depression deformity [13], Wenlin chest [14], and flat pectus carinatum [15]; designed a large number of new surgical techniques such as the Wang procedure [16-18], Wang procedure [19], Wenlin procedure [14,20], Willine procedure, and Tesla procedure [21]; proposed new concepts including the adhesive bandage surgery [22], clean surgery[23,24], and bleeding less surgery [25]; and carried out a comprehensive classification of all thoracic deformities [26]. In addition, I conducted research on some fundamental theories, such as the basic principles of Nuss procedure operation [27], the mechanism of scoliosis occurrence in thoracic deformities [28], the mechanism of pectus excavatum development [29], and the mechanism of pectus carinatum development [30]. These studies ultimately converged into a complete theoretical system for surgical treatment of thoracic deformities.

Alongside theoretical research, I also completed a large number of pioneering surgeries. I was the first in the world to perform minimally invasive surgeries for barrel chest [31], Wenlin chest [14], and rib arch deformity [32]; completed the largest series of surgeries for asphyxiating thoracic dystrophy (Jeune syndrome) [33], the largest series of minimally invasive surgeries for Poland syndrome [34], and the largest series of reoperations for thoracic deformities; and was the first to use chest wall surgery techniques to successfully treat multiple cases of thoracic dysplasia syndrome [35]. The development of these achievements quickly made my department a nationally renowned center for thoracic deformity correction.

Once a surgeon gains a reputation, other hospitals will invite them to perform surgeries. I was no exception; many hospitals began to send me invitations. I didn't want to disappoint anyone, so I tried my best to accept whenever asked. Performing surgeries at other hospitals was a great opportunity for promotion. As I operated more frequently outside my home hospital, my reputation grew, and I gained increasing attention. Finally, one day, I received a call from the assistant of Professor He Jianxing at the First Affiliated Hospital of Guangzhou Medical University. He told me, "Professor, he would like to invite you to assist in a surgery. At the moment I received the call, I knew my fate was about to change.

Professor He Jianxing's name is known by every contemporary thoracic surgeon; he was the one who introduced the concept of thoracoscopic surgery to China. He is regarded as the pioneer of modern thoracoscopic surgery and a true master surgeon. for my surgery to be recognized by Professor He was equivalent to receiving approval from the most authoritative expert in the field. I realized then that I had truly gained widespread attention.

In the days that followed, I performed several surgeries at Professor He's hospital. Among them, the most important was jointly performing a bilateral lung transplant combined with severe thoracic deformity correction alongside Professor He. The surgery was a tremendous success, and after being reported, it attracted widespread social attention [36]. This was the world's first surgery of its kind.

During my multiple interactions with Professor He, he offered valuable advice on my work [37]. He mentioned several times that deformity surgeries are not limited to congenital deformities; there are many secondary deformities in clinical practice that no one has operated on yet. He encouraged me to pay more attention to these cases. Later, he also told me that, in fact, many diseases involving the chest wall are not well managed. If these diseases could be grouped together, there would be a lot of work to be done.

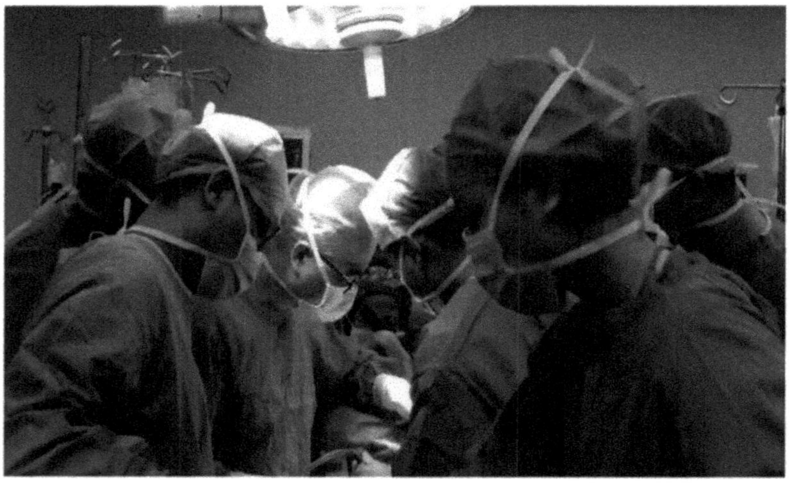

Figure 1-1-2 On 14.4.2018, the author and Professor He Jianxing at the First Affiliated Hospital of Guangzhou Medical University jointly completed the world's first double lung transplantation combined with severe thoracic deformity surgery.

Although Professor He did not directly suggest that I establish a Chest Wall Surgery department, his words reminded me of my own ideas about chest wall surgery from many years ago. After returning to my hospital, I deeply reflected on the development of the specialty. However, considering the realities of the hospital, I was unable to make more in-depth attempts. Soon after, another event occurred. Professor Cai Kaican from Nanfang Hospital of Southern Medical University invited me to join their hospital. Shortly after, Professor He Jianxing also extended an invitation, hoping I would join his team. Both hospitals are top-tier and well-known in China, and both experts are prominent thoracic surgeons. Naturally, receiving invitations from these two distinguished professors should have made me very happy, but I soon found myself caught in a happy dilemma. I was unable to decide and didn't know how to choose. Soon, official transfer request letters from both hospitals arrived at my current hospital. Upon learning this, the leadership at my hospital naturally did not want me to leave. To ensure that I would continue working at the hospital, Secretary Tian Junzhang personally had a heartfelt conversation with me, expressing his hope that I would stay. He also promised to provide all favorable conditions to help me expand and strengthen my specialty. After careful consideration, I decided to remain at the hospital and continue contributing to the institution that nurtured me. At this point, I had a clear goal for the development of my specialty. I was no longer satisfied with just treating pectus excavatum and various deformities; I wanted to grow this field into a major undertaking. I shared my idea with Secretary Tian, who immediately decided to act. The very next day, 9.5.2018, my new department was officially established, and it was named the Chest Wall Surgery Department [38].

On the day of the unveiling, reporters from all directions swarmed in as Guangdong Second Provincial People's Hospital held a press conference to announce the establishment of the world's first independent Chest Wall Surgery Department. From the very moment this plaque was hung, a new member was added to the big family of clinical surgery. Although this member was small and young, it possessed a powerful vitality.

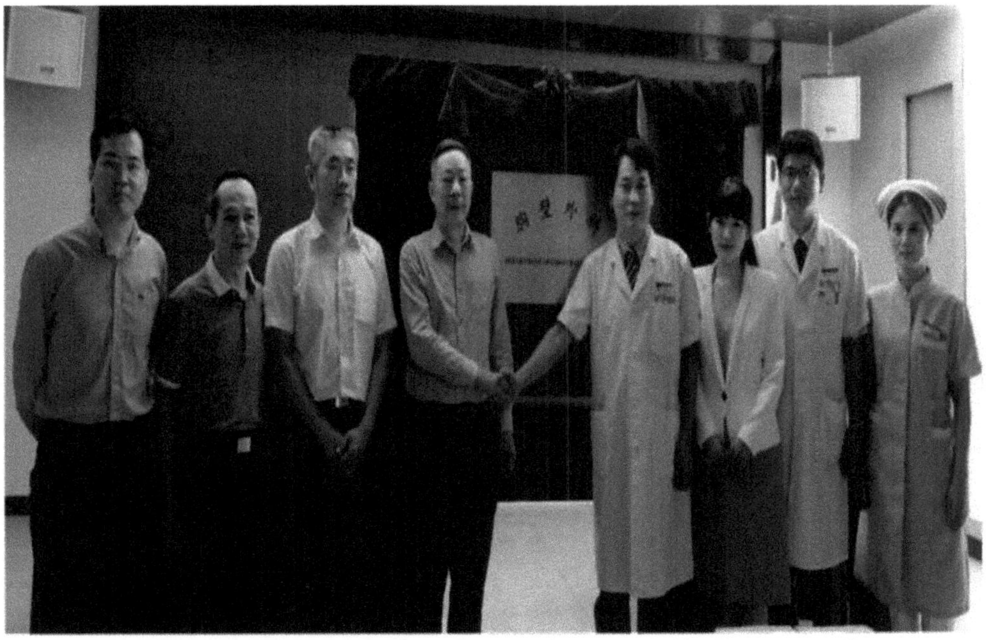

Figure 1-1-3 09.05.2018, the first Chest Wall Surgery Department was officially established at Guangdong Second Provincial People's Hospital.

Starting from the conception of chest wall surgery in 2008, after 10 years of hard struggle, I transformed from a cardiac surgeon into a thoracic surgeon, and personally established the first Chest Wall Surgery Department. The journey was full of hardships and obstacles, and I put in tremendous effort. What brings me comfort is that these efforts have finally paid off. I brought chest wall surgery into existence and proudly branched out from traditional thoracic surgery. I have carved out a significant share from the old, conventional thoracic surgery field, bringing joy to many, envy to some, and, most importantly, benefits to countless patients.

As a brand-new specialty emerging in clinical practice, chest wall surgery must

first have its fundamental framework. My initial concept
was to focus on treating five categories of diseases: deformities, trauma, infections, tumors, and defects. This concept was based on the general classification of surgical diseases. Although this idea was formulated rather hastily, subsequent clinical practice has shown that it is quite appropriate. After the establishment of the first chest wall surgery department, it received widespread attention from domestic peers. Soon, other hospitals also took action and successively established their own chest wall surgery units. Although these units were not necessarily independent departments, they reflected a strong consensus and desire. Many doctors recognized the existing drawbacks in contemporary thoracic surgery and hoped to change the status quo through their own efforts.

Since 2018, I have been invited to over 300 hospitals across China to assist in performing surgeries. Beyond simply spreading surgical techniques, much of my work has involved promoting the concept of chest wall surgery. Influenced by this concept, many colleagues have actively started chest wall surgery programs in their own institutions and have expressed the hope for a professional platform dedicated to chest wall surgery where everyone can learn and exchange ideas. In response to these demands, on 27.10.2018, China's first professional organization dedicated to chest wall surgery the Chest Wall Surgery Committee of the Guangdong Provincial Thoracic Disease Society was established in Guangzhou [39]. The founding of this committee has made an indelible contribution to the development of chest wall surgery in China.

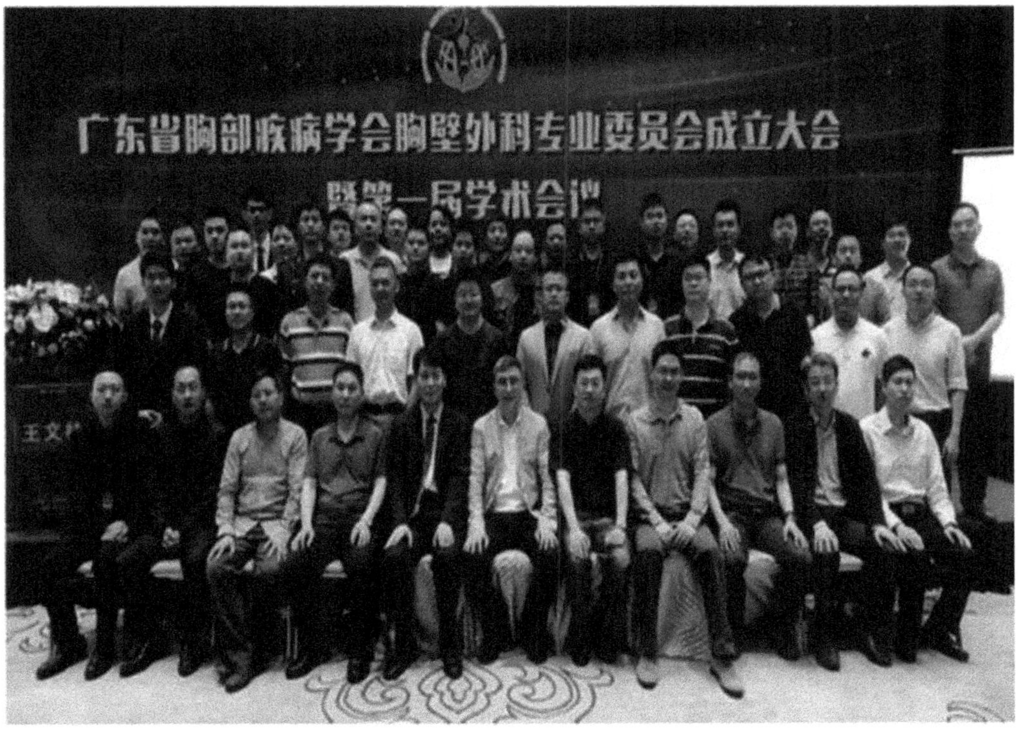

Figure 1-1-4 27.10.2018, China's first professional organization for chest wall surgery the Chest Wall Surgery Committee of the Guangdong Provincial Thoracic Disease Society was established in Guangzhou.

After the establishment of the Chest Wall Surgery Committee, the concept of chest wall surgery was spread more widely. More hospitals across China began to establish their own chest wall surgery departments, and an increasing number of thoracic surgeons started to pay attention to this field. With growing recognition of chest wall surgery nationwide, there was an urgent need for a larger platform to facilitate communication and learning among peers. To meet this demand, on 2.11.2019, the first national professional organization for chest wall surgery, the China Chest Wall Surgery Alliance, was founded in Guangzhou [40]. The establishment of the Alliance marked a significant step forward in the development of chest wall surgery in China.

After the establishment of the China Chest Wall Surgery Alliance, regional alliances were subsequently formed in various parts of the country. In addition, many regions also established their own professional chest wall surgery organizations. These organizations regularly hold academic events, which have greatly promoted the further dissemination of the concepts and techniques of chest wall surgery.

On 5.12.2020, at the 2020 annual meeting of the China Chest Wall Surgery Alliance, after extensive discussions between the alliance and social

organizations, May 9th, the anniversary of the establishment of the first chest wall surgery department was officially designated as "Chest Wall Care Day" to raise public awareness of chest wall diseases [41]. On 9.5.2021, the first "Chest Wall Care Day" saw numerous hospitals nationwide actively participate in the promotion and public education of
chest wall diseases, generating a significant response throughout society [42]. This played a crucial role in further advancing the development of the chest wall surgery field.

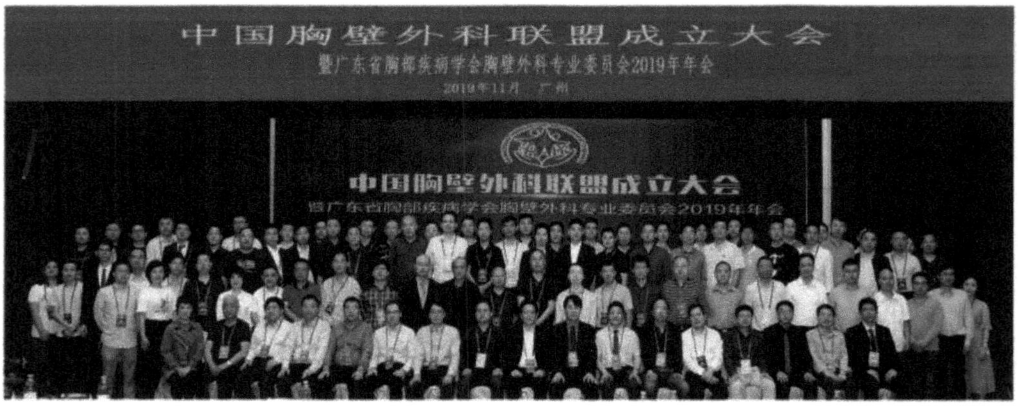

Figure 1-1-5 02.11.2019 Establishment of the China Chest Wall Surgery Alliance

Alongside the clinical development of chest wall surgery, the related theoretical framework has also been continuously refined. Through the joint efforts of numerous colleagues nationwide, the concept of chest wall surgery has gradually become clearer, its scope of treatment more defined, and various surgical techniques have been basically standardized. The specialty's unique characteristics have become increasingly distinct [43]. After years of hard work, what was once a minor concept has grown into a relatively complete clinical specialty. More and more hospitals now have their own chest wall surgery departments, and an increasing number of doctors are joining this field. Chest wall surgery is demonstrating increasingly strong vitality.
On 9.2.2023, in order to further develop and strengthen chest wall surgery, the hospital leadership decided to establish a specialized chest wall surgery hospital within one of the hospital campuses. This became the Chest Wall Surgery Research Institute of Guangdong Second Provincial General Hospital. The founding of this institute marks the birth of the world's first specialized chest wall surgery hospital [44,45].

The development of chest wall surgery from nothing to something, from a small subspecialty to an increasingly complete and independent clinical specialty cannot be separated from the selfless dedication of many domestic experts. They include Professor He Jianxing from Guangzhou Medical University, Professor Cai Kaican from Southern Medical University's Nanfang Hospital, Professor Li Jun from Shandong Provincial Hospital, Professors Zhou Huafu and Liang Guanbiao from the First Affiliated Hospital of Guangxi Medical University, Professor Wei Gaoxiang from the Second Affiliated Hospital, Professor Wang Wenzhang from Hebei Yanda Hospital, Professor Shang Hongwei from Tianjin 983 Hospital, Professor Xu Quan from Jiangxi Provincial People's Hospital, Professor Gao Bingyu from the First Affiliated Hospital of Hainan Medical University, Professor Zhou Zhiming from the Central Hospital Affiliated to Shenyang Medical College, Professor Li Dingbiao from Kunming Yan'an Hospital, Professor Qu Yi from Qinghai Cardiovascular and Cerebrovascular Specialty Hospital, Professor Jiang Jianqing from the Western Theater Command General Hospital, Professor Jing Lihua from Xi'an Red Cross Hospital, Professors Zhang Shuanglin and Zhang Guoyu from the First Affiliated Hospital of Henan University, Professors Qian Rulin and Zhang Binbin from Henan Chest Hospital, Professor Dong Xinwei from Nanyang Central Hospital of Henan Province, Professor Xiao Gongzheng from Ningxia Third People's Hospital, Professor Chen Hang from Guiyang First People's Hospital, Professor Shen Yuguang from Zunyi People's Hospital, Professor Zhang Dongsheng from Shijiazhuang Third People's Hospital, Professor Hong Qiongchuan from Shenzhen Ninth People's Hospital, and many others. Besides these experts, numerous passionate individuals have silently contributed enormous efforts to the development of chest wall surgery. Without the tireless work of these insightful and dedicated people, chest wall surgery would not have achieved what it has today.

Looking back at the development of chest wall surgery, there was a significant element of chance—but more importantly, it was a historical inevitability. With the advancement of science, every traditional clinical specialty is bound to evolve. The subdivision of specialties is an inevitable trend in the development of disciplines. Take traditional general surgery, for example: it has long since branched into subspecialties such as hepatobiliary surgery, gastrointestinal surgery, colorectal surgery, and breast and thyroid surgery. These subspecialties have gradually matured and are now established specialties in their own right. The same holds true for traditional orthopedics. Today, well-known specialties such as spinal surgery, trauma surgery, plastic surgery, joint surgery, and hand surgery all originated from traditional orthopedics. These fields, too, have developed into independent disciplines. Thoracic surgery, as old as general and orthopedics surgery, has clearly lagged behind in subspecialty development.

Although major medical centers today show a trend toward specialization, none of the sub-specialties have truly emerged as fully independent disciplines. On the surface, this situation appears relatively calm, but beneath it lies an undercurrent of development. The emergence of chest wall surgery is precisely a manifestation of this undercurrent breaking through. We have every reason to believe that as chest wall surgery continues to mature, more sub-specialties will gradually separate from traditional thoracic surgery and embark on paths of rapid development.

REFERENCES

[1] Ren, H., and L. Xu. 2010. "History of Thoracic Surgery." In *Peking Union Medical College Thoracic Surgery*, 2nd ed., edited by Z. Y. Zhang, 1–12. Beijing: Science Press.

[2] Gao, S. Z., Y. G. Liu, Q. Geng, et al. 2015. "A Brief History of Thoracic Surgery in China." *Chinese Journal of Surgery* 53 (1): 27–32.

[3] Wang, W. L. 2019. "The Inevitable Path of the Development of Thoracic Wall Surgery in China." Medical Science and Technology Channel, February 17.

[4] Wang, W. L. 2018a. "A New Path for Thoracic Surgery: The Future of Chest Wall Surgery." 365 Medical Network, May 8.

[5] Wang, W. L. 2018b. "The Road to Independence: The Break Between Chest Wall Surgery and Thoracic Surgery." 365 Medical Network, August 17.

[6] Wang, W. L. 2019b. "The Current Situation and Future of Chest Wall Surgery in China." 39 Health Network, November 25.

[7] Jiang, R., and L. Liao. 2019. "Wenlin Wang: A 'Weird Doctor' in Defiance of the Matthew Effect." *Journal of Thoracic Disease* 11 (7): E90–E95.

[8] Wang, D. B. 2021a. "Founder of Chest Wall Surgery, Wenlin Wang: Carving Out a Unique Specialty in a Narrow Field." *Southern Metropolis Daily*, January 19.

[9] Gao, L., and B. N. Xue. 2019. "Founder of Chinese Chest Wall Surgery Wenlin Wang: Doing One Small Thing Well." 39 Health Network, May 17.

[10] Wang, D. B. 2021b. "National Leader in Chest Wall Surgery, Now a Key Influencer in a Specialized Online Field." *Southern Metropolis Daily*, August 17.

[11] Wang, W. L. 2016. "Naming and Morphological Characteristics of Groove Chest." *Journal of Practical Medicine* 32 (2): 335–336.

[12] Wang, W. L. 2017. "Naming and Morphological Features of Saddle Chest." *Journal of Practical Medicine* 33 (Suppl): 380–381.

[13] Wang, W. L. 2015a. "Naming of Localized Depression in the Lateral Chest Wall." *Journal of Practical Medicine* 31 (Suppl): 196.

[14] Wang, W. L. 2019c. "Wenlin Chest and Wenlin Procedure." Medical Science and Technology Channel, June 22.

[15] Wang, W. L. 2019d. "Naming of Flat Pigeon Chest: A Special Type of Chest Wall Deformity." Medical Science and Technology Channel, May 23.

[16] Wang, W. L., C. M. Chen, W. G. Long, et al. 2018. "Wang Procedure: A Novel Minimally

Invasive Procedure for Pectus Excavatum Children with Low Age." *Case Reports and Images in Surgery* 1 (1): 1–2.
[17] Wang, W. L., W. G. Long, and C. M. Chen. 2019. "Wang Procedure: A Novel Minimally Invasive Procedure for Pectus Excavatum Children with Low Age." *Journal of Southern Medical University* 39 (2): 249–252.
[18] Wang, W. L. 2020a. "The Working Principle of the Wang Procedure." 365 Medical Network, September 25.
[19] Wang, W. L. 2020b. "The Wang Procedure." 365 Medical Network, July 31.
[20] Wang, W. L., W. G. Long, C. M. Chen, et al. 2015b. "Ultra-Minimally Invasive Surgery for Pectus Carinatum." *Journal of Practical Medicine* 31 (5): 863–864.
[21] "Tesla Procedure: The Ultimate Surgery for Pectus Excavatum." 2018. Zhihu, July 8.
[22] "Sticker Surgery vs Traditional Surgery." 2018. Health World, October 7.
[23] "Three Dimensions of Clean Surgery." 2019. China.com Medical Channel, January 24.
[24] "The Four Realms of Clean Surgery." 2019. Health World, January 26.
[25] "The Basic Concept of Bleedingless Surgery." 2019. Health World, January 14.
[26] Chen, C. M., X. J. Li, et al. 2018. "A Systematic Classification Method for Chest Wall Deformities." *Chinese Journal of Clinical Thoracic and Cardiovascular Surgery* 25 (11): 981–985.
[27] Wang, W. L. 2018c. "Reverse Thinking: From the Nuss Procedure to the Wang Procedure." 365 Medical Network, August 21.
[28] Wang, W. L. 2018d. "Chest Wall Deformity and Scoliosis: Mechanical Principles." 39 Health Network, February 28.
[29] Wang, W. L., W. G. Long, C. M. Chen, et al. 2015c. "Preliminary Exploration of the 'Thoracic Defect Hypothesis' in the Pathogenesis of Pectus Excavatum." *Journal of Practical Medicine* 31 (Suppl): 200–201.
[30] Wang, W. L., W. G. Long, C. M. Chen, et al. 2015d. "Analysis of the Pathogenesis of Pectus Carinatum." *Journal of Practical Medicine* 31 (Suppl): 313–314.
[31] Wang, W. L. 2018e. "Minimally Invasive Surgical Technique for Barrel Chest." *Surgical Case Reports* 1 (2): 1–2.
[32] Wang, W. L. 2018f. "Minimally Invasive Operation for Costal Arch Deformity." *Surgical Case Reports* 1 (2): 1–3.
[33] Wang, W. L., W. G. Long, C. M. Chen, et al. 2021. "Surgical Treatment of Asphyxiating Thoracic Dystrophy." *Chinese Journal of Clinical Thoracic and Cardiovascular Surgery* 28 (8): 984–989.
[34] Wang, W. L. 2019e. "Minimally Invasive Wenlin Procedure for Poland Syndrome with Protrusion Deformity." 365 Medical Network, April 25.
[35] Wang, W. L. 2019f. "Making History Again: Curative Surgery for Thoracic Dystrophy Syndrome." iWen Doctor, January 23.
[36] Wang, W. L. 2018g. "Reflections on the World's First Successful Double Lung Transplant Combined with Chest Wall Deformity Correction." Southern Media Platform, November 10.
[37] Wang, W. L. 2020c. "Professor He Jianxing's Outstanding Contributions to the Development of Chest Wall Surgery in China." Thoracic Surgery, December 26.
[38] Xue, B. N. 2018. "China's First 'Chest Wall Surgery' Department Established at Guangdong Second Provincial General Hospital." 39 Health Network, May 14.
[39] Gong, W. 2018. "The First Chest Wall Surgery Professional Committee in China's Medical Sector Established." Medical Science and Technology Channel, October 30.
[40] Zhou, Y. 2019. "China Chest Wall Surgery Alliance Established in Guangzhou." CNR News, November 2.
[41] Gong, W. 2020. "China Chest Wall Surgery Alliance Proposes Establishing 'Chest Wall

Awareness Day.'" Medical Science and Technology Channel, December 5.
[42] Li, N. 2021. "Chest Wall Awareness Day: Focusing on Chest Wall and Eliminating Deformities." North News Network, May 8.
[43] Wang, W. L. 2018h. "Contents of Chest Wall Surgery Research." 365 Medical Network, August 12.
[44] Gong, W. 2023. "15 Years of Chest Wall Surgery: Expert in Thoracic Deformity Surgery." Thoracic Deformity Surgery Specialist, June 17.
[45] Jiang, X., and Y. Huang. 2023. "Guangdong Second Provincial General Hospital Establishes Chest Wall Surgery Research Institute." People's Daily Client (Guangdong Edition), February 10.

In an era when all thoracic diseases were equally valued, thoracic surgery functioned as a unified specialty, and it was unlikely that any specific part of the chest would receive disproportionate attention. However, in recent years, intrathoracic diseases have garnered unprecedented focus, while diseases outside the thoracic cavity have been largely neglected. At first glance, this neglect appears detrimental to the development of chest wall–related conditions. Yet paradoxically, it is precisely this lack of attention that created an opportunity for others to focus on these overlooked areas. As a result, chest wall surgery, a brand-new medical specialty, was born.

The recognition of chest wall diseases as independent conditions initially arose through comparison with intrathoracic diseases. Chest wall diseases occur in a specific anatomical region, the chest wall itself. While much attention has been given to intrathoracic diseases, chest wall diseases have not decreased due to this neglect. In fact, the incidence of chest wall diseases is even higher than that of intrathoracic diseases [1]. Such a high incidence means a large number of patients require care and treatment. This demand is the most practical driving force that has motivated some insightful individuals to focus on these patients and their diseases. Therefore, the emergence of chest wall surgery is not only a historical choice but also a logical inevitability.

The emergence of chest wall surgery in clinical practice represents not only a concept but also a tangible entity. To accurately define chest wall surgery, one can refer to the traditional methods of defining surgical specialties. For example, neurosurgery, abdominal surgery, orthopedics, and even thoracic surgery are all defined primarily by a specific anatomical region. Once the region is identified, all surgical-related conditions within that area become the focus of that specialty. Therefore, the precise definition of chest wall surgery should be a clinical specialty that provides surgical interventions for various diseases occurring in the chest wall.

To accurately understand the connotation of chest wall surgery, it is essential to clarify three fundamental concepts: first, the concept of the chest wall; second, the concept of chest wall diseases; and third, the concept of chest wall surgical procedures. Only when all three concepts are clearly defined can the meaning of chest wall surgery become clear.

1. The Concept of the Chest Wall

The chest wall is an anatomical region. Although traditional anatomy has not provided an exact delineation, understanding it conceptually is not difficult. The concept of the chest wall can be referred to in the same way as other anatomical regions: as the name suggests, it should be understood as the totality of the external structures surrounding the thoracic cavity. According to this understanding, the chest wall should first include the skin and soft tissues, and secondly, the bony structures. These tissues and structures all contribute to the composition of the chest wall. However, understanding the chest wall also requires considering some historically inherited issues, such as the classification of the mammary gland [2]. If we do not take into account the already established field of breast surgery, the mammary gland could fully be classified under chest wall surgery. However, as breast surgery has already developed into a mature specialty, it is unlikely to be subsumed under chest wall surgery. Another structure is the spine [3]. From the perspective of structural composition alone, the spine should also be included in the chest wall. However, because it involves more aspects of orthopedics and neurosurgery fields, and since spinal surgery is also a highly developed specialty, it likewise cannot be forcibly classified under chest wall surgery. As chest wall surgery originated from traditional thoracic surgery, its scope can only encompass the relevant parts of the original thoracic surgery. In other words, the mammary gland and spine cannot be included. Such a delineation is not only conducive to the structuring of specialties but also beneficial for the conduct of clinical work. According to the traditional thoracic surgery definition of the chest wall, besides the breast and spine, there is another relatively special area that needs to be specifically mentioned: the posterior chest wall, which is anatomically referred to as the back. Although this area also contributes to the structure of the chest wall, it is not called the chest wall. This distinction is largely due to customary usage in daily life. In previous literature, it has been customary to refer to the anterior chest wall as the "chest," while the posterior chest wall is called the "back" [4]. Although there is no clinical specialty known as back surgery, the back is clearly considered separate from thoracic surgery. This separation is largely due to a unique structure: the scapula. Although the scapula is located on the chest wall, it is a structure belonging to orthopedics. This anatomical fact often complicates thoracic surgery work and makes the back a somewhat awkward region to categorize. Although nominally classified as the back rather than the chest, many procedures in this area still require thoracic surgeons to perform them. Even when this region is considered part of the chest wall surgery scope, the challenges remain. Since the scapula is also not within the domain of chest wall surgery, its complicating influence persists and continues to affect the work of chest wall surgeons [5].

From the analysis above, it can be seen that while the concept of the chest wall can be understood as the entirety of structures surrounding the thoracic cavity, in practice, it primarily refers to the anterior and lateral chest wall. When the back is involved, it is mainly limited to the ribs and surrounding structures; the areas containing the spine and scapula are not considered part of the chest wall surgery domain.

Regarding the concept of the chest wall, in addition to discussing the major regions as mentioned above, attention must also be given to the boundaries of the chest wall. There are two aspects to these boundaries: one is the boundary with the intrathoracic structures, and the other is the boundary with structures belonging to other surgical specialties. The first boundary is relatively easy to define and can be understood as the structures outside the parietal pleura. The second boundary is more ambiguous. The lower boundary of the chest wall can be understood as the xiphoid process, costal arch, and the 12th rib, while the upper boundary can be understood as the thoracic inlet. However, the upper boundary at the front is more difficult to define due to the presence of the clavicle. When boundaries are unclear, it can create challenges in treating certain diseases. This is why diseases in this area require special attention. In addition to the upper and lower boundaries, another important consideration is the boundary between the chest wall and adjacent structures such as the breast, spine, and scapula mentioned earlier. Under normal physiological conditions, the boundaries between these structures and the chest wall are relatively clear. However, once pathological changes occur, the situation becomes more complicated. Diseases may simultaneously involve these related structures, making them cross-disciplinary in nature. This undoubtedly increases the complexity and difficulty of managing such diseases.

2. The Concept of Chest Wall Surgery Diseases

After clarifying the concept of the chest wall, the next concept to define is chest wall surgical diseases. Literally, any disease occurring in the chest wall should be considered a chest wall disease. However, diseases are divided into medical (non-surgical) and surgical categories. There are chest wall diseases that are not suitable for surgical treatment, so it is necessary to specify what constitutes a surgical disease. According to common classification, any disease requiring surgical treatment should be classified as a surgical disease. Similarly, chest wall surgical diseases refer specifically to those chest wall diseases that require surgical intervention. All other diseases fall outside this scope.

There are many specific types of surgical diseases. However, referring to the classification of diseases based on the nature of surgical specialties, chest wall surgical diseases can roughly be divided into five categories: trauma, tumors, defects, deformities, and infections [6–10] (Figure 1-2-1). This classification may not be entirely comprehensive or perfectly accurate, and it may not include all disease types, but judging from classifications in other surgical specialties, this division is generally reasonable and can therefore be adopted as a working standard.

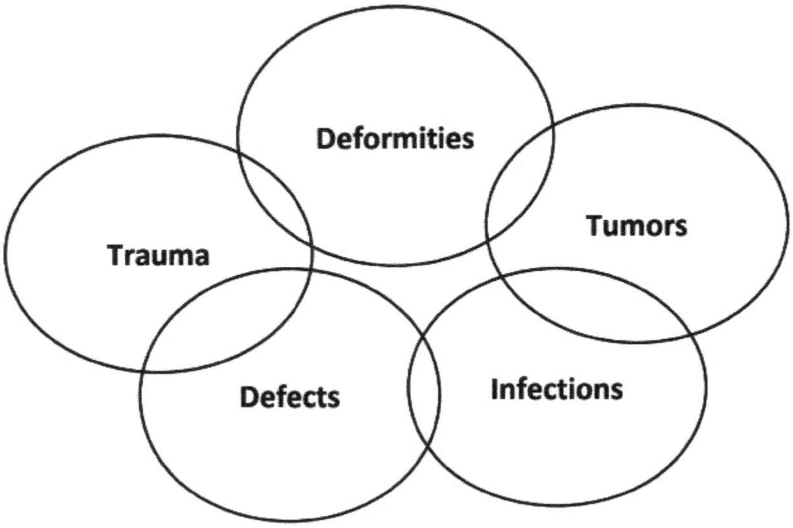

Figure 1-2-1 The Five Basic Diseases of Chest Wall Surgery.

Since the concept of chest wall surgery was proposed, especially after clinical practice began, clinical work has consistently followed this orderly classification. Existing practical experience has shown that this classification is both scientific and quite practical.

(1) Chest Wall Trauma

Trauma is one of the most common conditions treated in chest wall surgery [11]. It can be divided into soft tissue injuries and injuries to bony structures. Soft tissue injuries are relatively straightforward to manage. However, injuries to bony structures may lead to serious complications and therefore require special

attention. The main bony structures involved in trauma include the ribs, costal cartilage, and sternum. In most cases, treatment of these injuries is not complicated, but severe trauma can make management more challenging.
When managing chest wall trauma, one important issue to clarify is its relationship with intrathoracic trauma. In traditional thoracic surgery, both types of injuries are treated simultaneously. After the concept of chest wall surgery was introduced, the focus appeared to be only on trauma involving the chest wall itself. However, because intrathoracic injuries often coexist with chest wall trauma, treatment must still address both aspects concurrently. It is not sufficient to consider only the chest wall injury without taking intrathoracic damage into account.

(2) Chest Wall Tumors

Chest wall tumors are common in chest wall surgery [12]. They can be benign or malignant and are classified as either soft tissue or bony tumors based on location. Bony tumors may originate in the thoracic cage and invade nearby tissues or grow into the chest cavity. These tumors pose three main risks: direct harm from the tumor, impact on thoracic organ function, and changes in chest wall appearance. The primary treatment is surgical removal, including both the tumor and surrounding healthy tissue. After tumor resection, defects of varying sizes may remain on the chest wall. Small defects may not require intervention, but large ones often need chest wall reconstruction. Reconstruction involves two key components: restoration of the bony structures and reconstruction of the skin and soft tissue. Bony reconstruction requires special materials, with the primary goal of restoring the structural integrity of the thoracic cage. for skin and soft tissue reconstruction, specialized flaps are used not only to ensure proper wound healing but also to preserve the function and contour of the affected area.

(3) Chest Wall Defects

Chest wall defects mainly refer to defects caused by the absence of certain chest wall structures [13]. These defects may exist independently or occur during other surgeries, such as those left after chest wall tumor resection. Since such defects are typically addressed during surgery, they are not considered true defects and are not included in the discussion of chest wall defects. The defects discussed here are those that exist independently and can be divided into two types: primary defects and secondary defects. Primary defects have no clear cause and are mostly characterized by the absence of bony structures in the chest wall. These defects can occur in any location and may involve the sternum, ribs, or costal cartilage. Sternal defects may present as sternal clefts, where the sternum is severely malformed or damaged, leading to an incomplete chest wall structure [14]. Defects of the ribs and costal cartilage are directly manifested as the absence of these structures, resulting in defects in the corresponding areas. Primary defects can be independent diseases or manifestations of other conditions. Diseases commonly associated with such defects include Poland syndrome [15] and thoracic dysplasia syndrome [16]. In Poland syndrome, when there is a loss of ribs or costal cartilage, it can manifest as localized defects and depressions in the chest wall. This condition also occurs in thoracic dysplasia syndrome, where rib loss similarly leads to chest wall depressions. Primary chest wall defects have no fixed shape or location, and their specific presentations can vary greatly. Due to the lack of bony structures in the defect area, paradoxical respiration may occur, which is the most typical sign of this type of disease.

Secondary defects have clear causes, which can be trauma or other factors. Chest wall defects caused by trauma are often more severe and require urgent treatment. Defects caused by other factors have more complex origins and may include infections or certain treatments such a s radiotherapy. Radiotherapy is a highly invasive treatment method that, while eliminating lesions, may also damage surrounding healthy tissue. This is especially true for ribs and costal cartilage, where radiotherapy can lead to aseptic necrosis of these structures. At this time, once skin ulceration occurs, a defect will appear. The affected area lacks blood supply, making healing extremely difficult. Due to prolonged non-healing, repeated necrosis and infection of the local structures occur, making the defect very stubborn. Defects after radiotherapy are commonly seen in patients who have undergone radiotherapy following breast cancer surgery. These defects remain a clinical challenge and require special techniques to achieve surgical success [17].

Other secondary defects may occur in special situations, such as patients who have undergone thoracic surgery through a rib bed incision. This surgical approach was more common in earlier thoracic surgeries but is now rarely encountered. Another situation involves patients who previously had chest wall lesion resection without chest wall reconstruction, resulting in large residual chest wall defects. There is also a situation related to an earlier procedure, the thoracoplasty, which was more commonly performed in the past [18]. To eliminate lesions within the thoracic cavity, destructive procedures were deliberately performed on the chest wall to cause its collapse. This process could not only result in deformities of the chest wall but also lead to defects. Due to the significant surgical trauma involved, this procedure is now rarely

performed.
Chest wall defects are a relatively complex type of chest wall surgical disease. However, the treatment principle is very clear: reconstruction. of course, reconstruction not only involves the restoration of bony structures but also includes the reconstruction of skin and soft tissue defects if they are present.

(4) Chest wall deformity

Chest wall deformities are an important category of chest wall surgical diseases, mainly referring to abnormalities in the appearance of the chest wall. When discussing this disease, it is important to distinguish between chest wall deformities and thoracic deformities. Chest wall deformities refer to abnormalities in the appearance caused by pathological changes in all structures of the chest wall. These abnormalities can involve bone structures or soft tissues. In a broad sense, chest wall deformities even include abnormalities in appearance caused by all chest wall surgical diseases, such as deformities resulting from chest wall tumors, which strictly speaking also fall under the category of chest wall deformities. Thoracic deformities specifically refer to chest wall appearance abnormalities caused by bone structure abnormalities; these deformities are limited to bone structures and are unrelated to soft tissues [19]. Chest wall deformities cover a wide range and are difficult to clearly define. Due to the potential for conceptual ambiguity, they are not discussed as an independent disease category. In contrast, the concept of thoracic deformities is clear, and the treatment methods are well-established and mature. Thoracic deformities constitute a major part of chest wall surgical diseases.
Thoracic deformities can be caused by abnormalities in local thoracic structures or by multiple structural abnormalities, leading to visible deformities. These deformities may present as localized lesions or multiple lesions, occurring individually or in combination. Due to differences in lesion location, nature, and severity, various specific types of deformities can manifest.
The main characteristic of thoracic deformities is the abnormal appearance of the chest wall. This deformity may cause two types of harm: one is psychological damage caused by the abnormal appearance, and the other is physiological functional impairment due to the impact on intrathoracic organs [20]. Although these two types of harm are different in nature, both are unavoidable injuries that require attention.
Thoracic deformities are caused by abnormalities in the shape of the bony structures, and therefore their treatment involves corrective surgery that alters the shape of the bones. These surgeries can be open procedures or minimally

invasive ones; correction can be achieved directly through reshaping or indirectly using implants or materials.

(5) Chest Wall Infection

Infectious diseases are among the most common surgical conditions and can be caused by various pathogens. Clinically, infections can be classified in different ways based on different criteria. Superficial infections are relatively localized and usually involve infection of the local soft tissues. Deep infections can involve the full thickness of the chest wall, including the bony structures. Infections lead to various pathological changes, such as localized redness and swelling, or abscess formation. Abscesses may rupture, causing skin ulcers or even defects. Deep infections can cause inflammation of the ribs or costal cartilages and may result in full-thickness chest wall necrosis, which can also lead to defects.

Primary chest wall infections are relatively rare. More commonly encountered are secondary infections, which mainly occur as surgical site infections following various chest surgeries, with infections after cardiac surgery incisions being the most frequent [21]. This situation is influenced by multiple factors, among which poor blood circulation and the limited soft tissue coverage in front of the sternum are important contributors. Once a surgical site infection occurs, clinical management is often very challenging. Improper treatment may lead to serious consequences.

Chest wall infections can exist independently or coexist as complications alongside other diseases. For example, patients with defects often have infections when skin defects are involved. Tumor patients may also develop infections if skin necrosis and ulceration occur. When trauma involves the skin, infection is the most common complication. This shows that infection can appear in nearly every type of chest wall surgical disease. The effectiveness of infection control is closely related to the final treatment outcome of the disease.

3.The Concept of Chest Wall Surgery

Chest wall surgery refers to the surgical treatment methods applied to chest wall diseases. Since each disease has different characteristics, the specific surgical approaches also vary. Overall, chest wall surgery has two common attributes: one is disease treatment, and the other is reconstruction. The treatment attribute directly addresses the physiological damage caused by the disease, while the reconstruction attribute focuses on correcting external deformities. These attributes distinguish chest wall surgery clearly from intrathoracic surgery. The goals of treatment and reconstruction are basically aligned, but sometimes they conflict. Treatment requires removing or reshaping the diseased area as much as possible, while reconstruction aims to restore the normal shape as much as possible. These two goals often clash. To achieve the best outcome, a balance between them must be carefully considered.

The basic requirement of reconstruction is to achieve as normal a shape as possible. Its highest level is cosmetic, meaning to attain an appearance that meets the patient's expectations. Reconstruction imposes specific requirements on the surgical procedure. To accomplish reconstruction successfully, two key aspects must be focused on: first, the remodeling of the overall shape; second, the execution of the surgical incision. Remodeling the overall shape primarily involves the correction of bony structures and the reconstruction of soft tissues. The execution of the incision entails detailed considerations during the incision process, including the incision's location, length, direction, and suturing method. By thoroughly addressing both shape and incision requirements, a more ideal reconstructive outcome can be achieved.

4. The Relationship Between Thoracic Wall Surgery and Traditional Thoracic Surgery

Thoracic wall surgery originates from traditional thoracic surgery. This special "blood relationship" means that the emergence of thoracic wall surgery is first based on inheritance, and only then on development and innovation. All thoracic wall diseases were originally part of traditional thoracic surgery. Although managing these diseases with the conventional concepts of thoracic surgery has certain limitations, it has laid a solid foundation for their treatment. Theories and experiences from the past are extremely valuable and cannot be disregarded; they form the foundation for the existence of thoracic wall surgery. From the current clinical practice of thoracic wall surgery, many clinical procedures are still carried out following the concepts and techniques of traditional thoracic surgery. Since thoracic wall surgery originated from thoracic surgery, it is impossible to completely reject these established concepts and techniques.

However, as a brand-new clinical specialty, its independence relies on having its own unique characteristics. These characteristics are clearly different from traditional thoracic surgery. Specifically, they are reflected in the following aspects: ① Intersection with other specialties. One important aspect of chest wall surgery is reconstruction. To better accomplish this work, it is necessary to extensively draw on the experience and techniques of plastic surgery; therefore, the two fields may overlap. Additionally, to better manage diseases of the bony structures of the chest wall, experience and techniques from orthopedics are also needed, which causes chest wall surgery to potentially overlap with traditional orthopedics work. Moreover, since many chest wall diseases involve the spine, there is also overlap with spinal surgery. Such cross-disciplinary interactions clearly do not exist in traditional thoracic surgery. This interdisciplinary crossover and integration may give rise to entirely new concepts and techniques. ② Development and innovation within the specialty itself. In traditional thoracic surgery, chest wall diseases received little attention and lacked in-depth research. Without research, development is impossible, and innovation even less so. However, once chest wall surgery became an independent specialty, chest wall diseases became the sole focus of its work. This provided specialists with dedicated research subjects and opportunities, thereby creating chances for development and innovation. By adopting a fresh perspective to examine and address chest wall diseases, groundbreaking achievements are bound to emerge—something that was not possible within traditional thoracic surgery.

The development and innovation of chest wall surgery are reflected in multiple aspects. First, there is innovation in theory. As an independent clinical specialty, chest wall surgery must establish its own distinct theoretical system. Such a system can only emerge with the existence of chest wall surgery; it is impossible to develop this theory within the broader framework of thoracic surgery. This theoretical foundation is crucial as it guides the discipline's development and lays the groundwork for its progress. Secondly, there is innovation in concepts. When a new specialty arises, it inevitably brings new concepts. These concepts form the cornerstone of the discipline, enriching it and enhancing its practical significance. Third, innovation in techniques. One of the most evident signs of chest wall surgery becoming an independent specialty is the rapid advancement of surgical techniques. These techniques are developed under the guidance of new theories and concepts, making such innovations highly practical and meaningful. This represents the true significance of chest wall surgery's independence. Fourth, innovation in materials. Chest wall surgery is not only about removing lesions but, more importantly, about reconstruction and reshaping. These procedures require specialized materials to be successful. The emergence of new techniques creates new demands for materials, which in turn drives the design and development of new materials, leading to the introduction of many new materials into clinical practice.

Chest wall surgery has inherited and developed the chest wall disease content from traditional thoracic surgery, emerging as a fully independent specialty. This evolution is an inevitable trend in the development of thoracic surgery and a practical necessity for the treatment of chest wall diseases. However, it must be emphasized that although chest wall surgery is no longer the same as traditional thoracic surgery, the inherent connection between the two cannot be severed. This connection is evident in almost every aspect of clinical practice. Each type of chest wall surgical disease may involve intrathoracic organs, and every chest wall surgery may affect the structures within the thoracic cavity. Chest wall surgery and thoracic surgery form a closely connected organic whole, and this connection will persist throughout the discipline's development. Valuing this organic relationship not only enables better completion of related work but also creates more opportunities for development, leading to greater achievements in building the specialty.

REFERENCES

[1] Wang, Wenlin. 2016. "The Alarming Incidence of Thoracic Deformities." *Expert in Thoracic Deformity Surgery*, December 21.
[2] Wang, Xiangyi, Chun Zhong, Yunfei Nie, et al. 2005. "Anatomy of Breast Fixation Structures." *Journal of Zhengzhou University (Medical Edition)* 40 (4): 637–639.
[3] Liu, Hucheng, Shizhang Zong, Yi Xu, et al. 2009. "Anatomical Study of Intravertebral Rib-Joint Fixation through the Mid-Upper Thoracic Vertebra." *Journal of Jiangxi Medical College* 49 (6): 7–10.
[4] Zhu, Zhiping, Junyan Yue, Juan Wang, et al. 2017. "CT and MRI Diagnosis of Back Elasticity of Fibroma." *Journal of Practical Radiology* 33 (2): 258–261.
[5] Greiffenstein, P., M. Q. Tran, and L. Campeau. 2019. "Three Common Exposures of the Chest Wall for Rib Fixation: Anatomical Considerations." *Journal of Thoracic Disease* 11 (Suppl 8): S1034–S1043.
[6] Wang, Wenlin. 2018a. "Content of Chest Wall Surgery Research (Part 1)." 365 Medical Network, August 12.
[7] Wang, Wenlin. 2018b. "Content of Chest Wall Surgery Research (Part 2)." 365 Medical Network, August 12.
[8] Wang, Wenlin. 2018c. "Content of Chest Wall Surgery Research (Part 3)." 365 Medical Network, August 16.
[9] Wang, Wenlin. 2018d. "Content of Chest Wall Surgery Research (Part 4)." 365 Medical Network, August 16.
[10] Wang, Wenlin. 2018e. "Content of Chest Wall Surgery Research (Part 5)." 365 Medical Network, August 16.
[11] Caragounis, E. C., Y. Xiao, and H. Granhed. 2021. "Mechanism of Injury, Injury Patterns and Associated Injuries in Patients Operated for Chest Wall Trauma." *European Journal of Trauma and Emergency Surgery* 47 (4): 929–938.
[12] Sanna, S., J. Brandolini, A. Pardolesi, et al. 2017. "Materials and Techniques in Chest Wall Reconstruction: A Review." *Journal of Visualized Surgery* 3: 95.
[13] Bille, A., L. Okiror, W. Karenovics, et al. 2012. "Experience with Titanium Devices for Rib Fixation and Coverage of Chest Wall Defects." *Interactive Cardiovascular and Thoracic Surgery* 15 (4): 588–595.
[14] Eigellar, A., and J. H. Beitel. 1970. "Congenital Cleft Sternum." *Thorax* 25 (4): 490–498.

[15] Revanna, K. G. Chandan, D. Ari, et al. 2013. "Lung Herniation: An Uncommon Presentation of Poland's Syndrome in a Neonate at Birth." *BMJ Case Reports* 2013: bcr2013200106.
[16] Gronefeld, B., and A. K. Hella. 2013. "Ossifications after Vertical Expandable Prosthetic Titanium Rib Treatment in Children with Thoracic Insufficiency Syndrome and Scoliosis." *Spine (Phila Pa 1976)* 38 (13): E819–E823.
[17] Raz, D. J., S. L. Clancy, and L. J. Erhunmwunsee. 2017. "Surgical Management of the Radiated Chest Wall and Its Complications." *Thoracic Surgery Clinics* 27 (2): 171–179.
[18] Perikiliou, P., S. Rathinam, and D. A. Waller. 2017. "VATS and Open Chest Surgery in Diagnosis and Treatment of Benign Pleural Diseases." *Journal of Visualized Surgery* 3: 84.
[19] Mak, S. M., B. N. Bhaludin, S. Naaseri, et al. 2016. "Imaging of Congenital Chest Wall Deformities." *British Journal of Radiology* 89 (1061): 20150595.
[20] Wang, Wenlin. 2014. "Harms of Thoracic Deformities." *Thoracic Deformity Surgery Expert*, December 8.
[21] Dubert, M., A. Pourbaix, S. Alkholder, et al. 2015. "Sternal Wound Infection after Cardiac Surgery: Management and Outcome." *PLOS ONE* 10 (9): e0139122.

Section 3

STRUCTURE AND FUNCTION OF THE CHEST WALL

Chest wall diseases occur in the structures of the chest wall, and chest wall surgery refers to surgical procedures performed on these structures. To successfully carry out clinical work in chest wall surgery, it is essential to first understand the structure and function of the chest wall. This knowledge forms the foundation for all clinical activities in chest wall surgery. The structure of the chest wall pertains to anatomy and mainly involves the study of the structural characteristics of its various components and their internal relationships [1]. The function of the chest wall relates to physiology and involves the study of the physiological functions of the chest wall as a whole and of its individual components [2]. The structure and function are closely interconnected, and a thorough understanding of their intrinsic relationship will greatly facilitate the clinical work in chest wall surgery [1].

1.Structure of the Chest Wall

The chest wall is a unique region of the human body. While some anatomical texts provide basic descriptions, there is no precise definition [1]. This lack of a clear definition poses challenges for in-depth study of the chest wall's structure. However, for thoracic surgeons, this is not particularly difficult, as such terms frequently appear in their daily work, and they generally have a clear understanding of the general meaning. Therefore, descriptions of the chest wall may seem familiar. Nevertheless, the concept of the chest wall in chest wall surgery inevitably differs from that in traditional thoracic surgery; otherwise, there would be no need to divide them into two separate specialties. From the perspective of chest wall surgery, understanding the chest wall requires approaching it from three aspects: first, the scope of the chest wall; second, the composition of the chest wall; and third, the relationships between its various structures. These are the fundamental requirements for a comprehensive understanding of the chest wall's structure.

(1) The Scope of the Chest Wall

The chest wall comprises the external structures of the thorax, including all the components that enclose the thoracic cavity. Its inner boundary is formed by the parietal pleura, and everything from this layer outward to the body surface is considered part of the chest wall [3]. Generally, the chest wall is divided into three regions: the anterior chest wall, the lateral chest wall, and the posterior chest wall. The anterior chest wall refers to the front of the chest, the lateral chest wall to the sides, and the posterior chest wall commonly called the back is located opposite the anterior part. These three regions do not have clearly defined borders but are separated by approximate boundaries. The upper boundary of the anterior chest wall is formed by the lower edges of both clavicles and the upper edge of the manubrium, while the lower boundary is defined by the xiphoid process and the lower edges of the two costal arches. The upper boundary of the lateral chest wall lies at the top of the axilla, and its lower boundary corresponds to the lower edge of the costal arch. The posterior chest wall is bounded superiorly by the shoulder and inferiorly at the level of the 12th rib. Overall, the chest wall occupies a unique anatomical position: it connects superiorly with the superficial structures of the neck, inferiorly with the abdominal wall, laterally with the upper limbs, and lies deeply adjacent to the thoracic organs. This distinctive location underlines the vital significance of the chest wall.

(2) Composition of the Chest Wall

The main components of the chest wall consist of three types: skin, soft tissue, and bony structures [1]. The soft tissues primarily include the superficial mammary glands, muscle tissue, fat tissue, and intercostal structures. The bony structures mainly comprise three elements: the sternum, costal cartilage, and ribs [1,4]. In addition to these three bony structures, there is a special structure called the xiphoid process, which can be considered a downward extension of the sternum. The soft tissues and bony structures are integrated, forming an organic whole.

The main structures of the anterior chest wall include the superficial mammary glands, pectoralis major, and pectoralis minor muscles. The deeper bony structures mainly consist of the sternum, costal cartilages, and portions of the ribs. The lateral chest wall's important superficial structure is the serratus anterior muscle, while its deeper structure is primarily composed of ribs. The posterior chest wall is covered superficially by muscles such as the latissimus dorsi and trapezius. The scapula lies freely over the posterior chest wall, with the posterior halves of the ribs beneath it, and the spine positioned medially.

The bony structures of the chest wall form a three-dimensional thoracic cage, which serves as the skeletal framework of the chest wall. The thoracic cage provides attachment points and leverage for the chest muscles and serves as the internal structural foundation that maintains the shape and appearance of the chest wall. To study chest wall diseases and perform related surgeries, it is

essential to be familiar with the basic anatomy of the thoracic cage.
The thoracic cage is a funnel-shaped, cage-like structure that is narrower at the top and wider at the bottom, with two openings: an upper and a lower aperture. The upper aperture is smaller and is bordered by the upper edge of the sternum, the 1st ribs, and the anterior edge of the spine. The lower aperture is larger and mainly formed by the xiphoid process, the costal arch, the floating ribs, and the anterior edge of the spine. The anteroposterior diameter of the thoracic cage is shorter, while the transverse diameter is wider, creating the characteristic physiological shape of the chest wall (Figure 1-3-1).

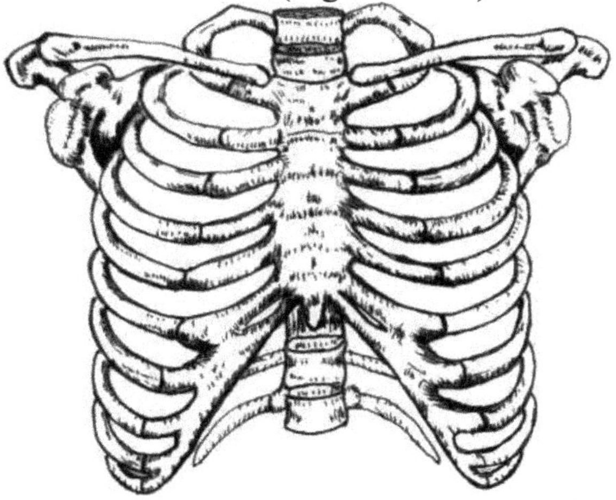

Figure 1-3-1 Shape of the Normal Thoracic Cage

When studying the basic structure of the chest wall, it is necessary to consider the impact of several special structures on thoracic surgery. The three main structures are: first, the spine; second, the scapula; and third, the clavicle. Traditionally, these three structures have been the focus of orthopedics, with the spine being particularly unique. In fact, some institutions have even established spine-related diseases as a separate specialty, known as spine surgery.
The spine is a structure studied primarily by orthopedics or spine surgery and is not traditionally associated with thoracic surgery. However, from a functional perspective, the spine contributes to the composition of the thoracic cage and should be considered an important part of the chest wall. In many thoracic wall diseases, spinal factors are involved, making it an indispensable subject of study[5,6]. For example, complications of pectus excavatum often include scoliosis. Scoliosis in this context is generally a secondary condition, with its root cause being the depression of the anterior chest wall. Conversely, certain spinal disorders involving abnormal spinal shape can also lead to changes in

the shape of the thoracic cage, resulting in various types of thoracic deformities. There is also another type of disease in which pathological changes involve both the spine and the thoracic cage. This disease is known as thoracic dysplasia syndrome [7]. This disease was initially recognized and managed primarily by spinal surgeons, and for a long time, its treatment remained within the scope of spine surgery. However, spine surgery mainly focused on correcting spinal deformities without addressing the pathological changes of the thoracic cage. Since abnormalities of the thoracic cage are the fundamental cause of the disease, it is more reasonable for chest wall surgery to take the lead in its treatment.

The scapula is located on the posterior chest wall and is traditionally considered part of orthopedics anatomy. Due to its significant impact on surgeries involving the posterior chest wall, it is also a key focus in chest wall surgery. The scapula mainly affects surgical exposure and access to the posterior chest wall, and many procedures in this area require special adjustments or techniques because of its presence.

The clavicle also falls under the domain of orthopedics and seems to have little direct connection with chest wall surgery. However, when performing procedures targeting lesions of the upper chest wall, the clavicle often becomes involved. For example, tumors in the upper part of the sternum often invade the sternoclavicular joint and may even extend into the clavicle. In such cases, surgery involves not only removing the tumor but also addressing the sternoclavicular joint and the clavicle. All of this falls within the scope of chest wall surgery.

In addition to the three bony structures mentioned above, another structure warrants attention—the breast on the anterior chest wall. Although the breast is an important component of the chest wall, clinical work related to breast diseases has already developed into a separate and well-established specialty. Therefore, it is not appropriate to include it within the scope of chest wall surgery. However, much like the bony structures, the presence of the breast can significantly affect various clinical procedures in chest wall surgery, and thus it must also receive adequate consideration.

(3) The Relationships Among the Structures of the Chest Wall

The soft tissue of the chest wall is located in the superficial layer. Aside from the breast, the main component is muscle tissue. The pectoralis major and pectoralis minor muscles cover the upper part of the anterior chest wall, with fibers attaching to specific areas of the clavicle, sternum, costal cartilages, and parts of the ribs. The serratus anterior attaches to the ribs on the lateral chest wall. There are distinct gaps between the bony structures of the chest wall, which are filled by the intercostal muscles. Blood vessels and nerves pass through these intercostal muscles. The bony structures of the chest wall are tightly connected to each other, with the gaps filled by soft tissue. These bones are also closely integrated with the surface muscles and other soft tissues, thus forming an organic whole. The structural integrity of the chest wall is of great clinical importance, as it provides the foundation for the chest wall to perform its normal physiological functions [1].

(4) Clinical Significance of Chest Wall Structures

Every structure in the human body exists for a reason that is, it serves a specific function. The functions of the chest wall will be analyzed separately in a later section. Here, the focus is on the relationship between the chest wall's structure and clinical practice. While the link between structure and function is inherent and natural, the relationship between structure and clinical work is man-made rather than innate. Therefore, understanding this relationship holds greater significance.

(1) The Influence of Chest Wall Structure on Disease Onset: Every disease has an objective cause. A careful analysis of the causes of disease often reveals structural explanations behind their development [8]. For example, pectus excavatum most commonly occurs near the xiphoid process. From a pathogenic perspective, the primary cause of pectus excavatum is an external downward pulling force, with the chest wall serving as the structural basis for this force. If the chest wall is sufficiently rigid, no depression can occur. Conversely, if the chest wall is relatively weak, a depression may develop. Among all areas of the chest wall, the region near the xiphoid process is the weakest. Because there is no bony structure between the two coastal arches, this area represents a natural defect. When subjected to internal forces from the thoracic cavity, it can lead to a depression, ultimately resulting in pectus excavatum. Other parts of the chest wall are very rigid and rarely experience such depressions. The occurrence of pectus carinatum (pigeon chest) is also closely related to structural factors. Its pathological basis is the softening of the chest wall, with the direct cause being the continuous positive pressure from the heart. Combining these two factors shows that pectus carinatum most commonly develops in the midline of the anterior chest wall, slightly left of center directly in front of the heart. This is the most distinctive feature of pectus carinatum [9]. The development of secondary pectus carinatum follows a similar mechanism. For example, young children who undergo median sternotomy for heart surgery are prone to developing pectus carinatum [10]. The underlying cause is the

disruption of thoracic stability, which illustrates the influence of chest wall structure on disease occurrence. Additionally, among postoperative chest wall infections, infections of the median sternotomy incision have the highest incidence. This situation is closely related to the local structural characteristics of the chest wall. The area in front of the sternum lacks muscular coverage and has very little subcutaneous tissue. Additionally, the placement of steel wires during surgery may further damage blood supply, all of which affect incision healing. In contrast, the risk of infection in lateral chest wall incisions is much lower. At the most fundamental level, the influence of structure on disease is essentially a cause-and-effect relationship. Normal structures do not develop diseases, but once structural abnormalities occur, various problems inevitably arise that manifest as clinical diseases. In clinical practice, tracing a disease back to its origin is essentially looking for causes based on observed outcomes. If the focus is placed on structure, the cause is much easier to identify.

(2) The Impact of Chest Wall Structure on Examinations: Each diagnostic method is based on different principles that directly target chest wall structures, and the properties of these structures influence the examination results. X-ray imaging is the most basic diagnostic tool in chest wall surgery and can directly visualize structures with higher density. For this reason, bony structures are best examined using X-rays. However, its limitation is well known; it is not effective for soft tissue evaluation, and costal cartilages are not visible. These limitations arise from the inherent characteristics of the chest wall structures themselves CT scanning is a more advanced diagnostic method. As a cross-sectional imaging technique, it provides good visualization of some solid lesions. However, it lacks a holistic view. For example, when examining bony structures, it is difficult to display the entire structure on a single plane. From this perspective, its effectiveness can be less than that of X-rays. To obtain a comprehensive view, 3D reconstruction imaging is performed based on CT scans. Because there is a significant difference in density parameters between cartilage and bone, cartilage often remains invisible, which undoubtedly affects the diagnostic outcome. For example, in some patients with pectus excavatum, the most severely affected areas often involve the costal cartilages, which are precisely the regions that are difficult to visualize. This undoubtedly impacts the overall effectiveness of the examination. Clinically, to achieve better results, specialized software is often used for advanced image processing. While this can produce more satisfactory images, it significantly increases the cost and time required for imaging. Thus, it is evident that the differing characteristics of various chest wall structures have distinct effects on diagnostic examinations.

(3) The Impact of Chest Wall Structure on Treatment Methods: Generally speaking, all treatment strategies are designed based on the characteristics of the structure. Without considering the chest wall's structure, surgical planning loses its meaning. For example, the Nuss procedure is fundamentally based on the lever principle [11]. To elevate the depressed area, a suitable fulcrum must be found for the steel bar.

The fulcrum must have some fundamental characteristics: first, it must have a certain height; second, it must possess sufficient hardness; and finally, it must provide adequate stability. Height is relatively easy to meet and can be located at the highest point around the depression. Hardness is more difficult to satisfy. Here, hardness refers not only to the rib's own rigidity but also to the firmness of the local chest wall serving as the fulcrum. If the local mobility of the rib is high, it is difficult to meet the hardness requirement. Using such a site as a fulcrum can easily affect the surgical outcome. The stability of the fulcrum depends on many factors, one important factor being the relationship between the steel bar and the rib. Ideally, this relationship should be perpendicular, but such a condition is almost never achieved. In many cases, the angle between the rib and the steel bar near the fulcrum is very small, sometimes nearly parallel. This relationship is extremely unfavorable for the surgery. Many surgical failures are related to this factor. The design of the Wenlin procedure for pectus carinatum is also closely related to the chest wall structure [12]. After the protruding chest wall is flattened by the steel bar, the key step is to firmly fix the steel bar. Because the compression force is strong, the fixation must be very secure. If stress factors are ignored and the steel bar is fixed arbitrarily to certain ribs, sudden increases in stress after surgery may cause wire or rib fractures, leading to surgical failure. Therefore, during the procedure, it is crucial to consider stress distribution. After fully considering the spatial arrangement of the lateral chest wall ribs, the success of the surgery depends on the reasonable design of both the number of steel bars and their fixation points. The design of the Wang procedure also reflects a thorough consideration of chest wall structure [13]. This surgery is performed on the surface of the depression. Since the depressed area needs to be lifted, a fulcrum is also required to support the steel bar. In this case, the fulcrum is not a single rib but multiple ribs, turning the fulcrum from a point into a surface. This support becomes much more solid, making the surgery more feasible and providing a structural foundation for operations on young children. There is a very special clinical deformity characterized by both a deep depression and a sharp angular protrusion on one side. Many people mistakenly treat this deformity as pectus excavatum and perform the Nuss procedure, but the results are disappointing:

not only does the depression remain, but the protrusion becomes more severe. This deformity is actually an angular deformity, and its biggest challenge is the extremely high local stress, making indirect remodeling almost impossible. To correct it, special methods must be used, which clearly fall outside the scope of the Nuss procedure. Beyond deformity surgeries, operations for other diseases are also influenced by chest wall structural features. For example, when designing flaps for incisional infections, the blood supply to the flap must be carefully considered; this is the same principle. In other words, any surgery must be based on a solid structural foundation, which is the prerequisite for surgical success. Without this foundation, successful surgery is very difficult.
Studying the chest wall structure from the perspective of clinical application belongs to the field of clinical anatomy and can also be considered part of applied anatomy. This type of research is purpose-driven, focusing on identifying and solving problems, and holds significant value. By closely integrating structural studies with clinical issues, it can guide basic research directions and provide practical guidance for clinical practice.

2. Functions of the Chest Wall

The major organs in the chest are the heart and lungs. When discussing the physiological functions of the chest, cardiopulmonary function must be addressed. The chest wall, as the outer structure of the chest, is not an integrated part of the heart and lungs. Without an in-depth study, it is difficult to link its function directly to that of the thoracic organs. However, no organ exists or functions in isolation. The chest wall exists as an independent, integrated structure within the body and therefore must have its own significant purpose. Its significance is ultimately reflected through various specialized functions not only its own functions but also its interactions with surrounding organs, especially the heart and lungs.

(1) Respiratory Function

The chest wall is anatomically part of the thorax, and an important function of the thorax is respiration; therefore, the chest wall inevitably participates in this function [4]. The respiratory function of the chest wall is indirect and manifests in two aspects: maintaining negative pressure and increasing negative pressure. The maintenance of negative pressure comes from the rigid structure of the thorax. Under normal physiological conditions, negative pressure is generated by the difference between the volume of the thoracic cavity enclosed by the thorax and the volume of the lung tissue. The greater the difference, the greater the negative pressure produced. To maintain this difference, the thorax must have sufficient strength. If the strength is inadequate and local or overall collapse occurs, the negative pressure cannot be maintained, severely impairing respiratory function. Clinically, chest wall softening is common; conditions such as chest wall defects or multiple rib fractures can damage the chest wall's rigid structure. This damage alters the negative pressure inside the thoracic cavity and affects breathing. The increase in negative pressure is mainly achieved through respiratory muscle movement, which increases thoracic volume and thus enhances negative pressure. This increase in negative pressure improves respiratory work and is an active way to enhance respiratory function.

(2) Protective Function

The protective function of the chest wall comes from two aspects: its isolating effect and its rigid supportive role. The chest wall's isolation separates the internal structures of the thoracic cavity from the external environment, allowing them to perform their physiological functions independently. The supportive role mainly refers to the rigid thorax providing an ideal space for the thoracic organs, preventing important organs like the heart and lungs from being compressed, thereby enabling them to function normally. The organs within the thoracic cavity differ in structure and function from those in other body regions, and their proper functioning depends on having a specialized working space. The heart itself is a pump-like structure that requires contraction and relaxation to function properly, and the lungs work similarly, relying on expansion and contraction to complete gas exchange. These functional characteristics objectively require a relatively enclosed space. The chest wall provides exactly such a space, not only allowing the heart and lungs to have an independent existence but also creating the necessary conditions for their proper function. This role of the chest wall not only protects the thoracic organs but also directly participates in their functional performance.

(3) Function of Maintaining Normal Chest Wall Appearance

The chest wall has a normal shape, which is maintained by the various structures of the chest wall. Strictly speaking, this is not a function. However, broadly speaking, if abnormal appearance is considered a disease, then maintaining normal shape naturally becomes part of its physiological function. The appearance of the chest wall depends on the shape of its structures, and any local or overall structural problem will inevitably affect the chest wall's shape. The chest wall's role in maintaining shape is not only reflected in preserving the shape of the chest itself but also in influencing the shape of other structures. One of the most important influences is on the shape of the spine. The spine and chest wall form an integrated whole. Changes in the shape of the chest wall inevitably led to changes in the shape of the spine, which in turn affect the shape of the chest wall. Thus, the appearance of the chest wall is the result of the combined effects of multiple factors. To maintain a normal shape, the chest wall itself must have a normal structure.

3. Relationship Between Chest Wall Structure and Function

The relationship between structure and function is dialectical. Structure is the basis of function, and function is the purpose of structure's existence. Studying the relationship between structure and function is of great significance for the diagnosis and treatment of chest wall diseases.

From the relationship between structure and function, it is evident that the integrity of the chest wall structure is the foundation for its proper function. When the chest wall structure is intact and free of defects, its functions can be normally performed, and various diseases will not occur. However, once the chest wall structure is damaged, its function will be impaired, leading to various functional abnormalities. The five basic diseases in chest wall surgery can all lead to abnormalities in chest wall structure. The symptoms that appear are ultimately manifestations of the impact on chest wall function. For example, in pectus excavatum, the most direct structural abnormality is the compression of the heart and lungs, which destroys the protective function of the chest wall, resulting in various symptoms. In contrast, anterior protrusion deformities do not compress the heart and lungs, so the chest wall's protective function remains unaffected. However, the function of maintaining normal chest appearance is impacted. This can harm the patient's aesthetics and lead to psychological issues, which in severe cases may develop into mental illness. Chest wall trauma causes the most direct damage to chest wall structure, affecting all functions and ultimately presenting through various symptoms.

Understanding the relationship between structure and function not only helps better explain the mechanisms of disease occurrence but also aids in treating various chest wall diseases. Diseases manifest certain symptoms, which are the direct result of functional abnormalities in the body. By tracing these functional abnormalities back to structural causes, the true nature of the pathology can be revealed. From a treatment perspective, every reasonable surgical method in clinical practice is a perfect understanding and interpretation of the relationship between structure and function. For example, various surgeries for pectus excavatum are based on recognizing that the depression of the anterior chest wall damages its function, and they approach the correction from different angles to ultimately eliminate the depression. Treatments for other types of diseases also reflect this relationship well. Therefore, fully understanding the relationship between structure and function not only improves comprehension of basic surgical principles but also helps design new surgical techniques.

The Nuss procedure is a common surgical method for treating pectus excavatum, and its design fully reflects the relationship between structure and function. However, its underlying mechanism was not clearly explained for a long time. After extensive analysis, we found that the principle of this surgery can actually be simplified to the lever principle. This conclusion was reached through a thorough analysis of the relationship between chest wall structure and function. The discovery of this mechanism is of great significance. Without awareness of this principle, the surgery is prone to failure. Conversely, if the principle is truly understood, the surgery is almost impossible to fail. This is a concrete example of the significance of the relationship between structure and function.

In fact, for any surgery, a general understanding is usually sufficient to guide its implementation. However, to perform the surgery with precision and achieve better outcomes, a deeper understanding of the relationship between structure and function is essential. Take the Wang procedure as an example many doctors initially see it as a simple, minor surgery, but when they start performing it, they encounter many detailed challenges. Failing to manage these details makes it difficult to obtain good results. This principle applies to all other surgeries as well. What truly tests a surgeon's skill is always the handling of details, and the root of these challenges lies precisely in the understanding of the relationship between structure and function. This is the important significance of this relationship.

In summary, understanding the anatomical structure of the chest wall is the cornerstone for conducting chest wall surgery, while understanding its function gives meaning to this cornerstone. For the specialized clinical field of chest wall surgery, both the structure and function of the chest wall form the foundation for basic research and clinical practice. Only by fully comprehending the structure and function of the chest wall can the demands of clinical work be adequately met.

REFERENCES

[1] Clemens, M. W., K. K. Evans, S. Mardini, et al. 2011. "Introduction to Chest Wall Reconstruction: Anatomy and Physiology of the Chest and Indications for Chest Wall Reconstruction." *Seminars in Plastic Surgery* 25 (1): 5–15.

[2] Mendes, L. P. D. S., D. S. R. Vieira, L. S. Gabriel, et al. 2020. "Influence of Posture, Sex, and Age on Breathing Pattern and Chest Wall Motion in Healthy Subjects." *Brazilian Journal of*

Physical Therapy 24 (3): 240–248.
[3] Charalampidis, C., A. Youroukou, G. Lazaridis, et al. 2015. "Pleural Space Anatomy." *Journal of Thoracic Disease* 7 (Suppl 1): S27–S32.
[4] Wang, Wenlin. 2014. "Defects of the Bony Structure of the Thorax." *Expert in Chest Wall Deformity Surgery*, June 19.
[5] Wang, Wenlin. 2018a. "First Law of the Relationship between Spine and Thorax." 365 Medical Network, December 14.
[6] Wang, Wenlin. 2018b. "Second Law of the Relationship between Spine and Thorax." 365 Medical Network, December 14.
[7] Wang, Wenlin. 2018c. "Conceptual Issues of Thoracic Dysplasia Syndrome." Haodaifu Online, February 5.
[8] Wang, Wenlin, Chunmei Chen, Weiguang Long, et al. 2015a. "Preliminary Study on the 'Thoracic Defect Hypothesis' of Pectus Excavatum Pathogenesis." *Journal of Practical Medicine* 31 (Suppl): 200–201.
[9] Wang, Wenlin, Weiguang Long, Chunmei Chen, et al. 2015b. "Analysis of the Pathogenesis of Pectus Carinatum." *Journal of Practical Medicine* 31 (Suppl): 313–314.
[10] Wang, Wenlin. 2016. "Pectus Carinatum after Cardiac Surgery." *Expert in Chest Wall Deformity Surgery*, July 17.
[11] Wang, Wenlin. 2019. "Wang Procedure and NUSS Procedure." Medical Science and Technology Channel, June 21.
[12] Jiang, R., and L. Liao. 2019. "Wenlin Wang: A 'Weird Doctor' in Defiance of the Matthew Effect." *Journal of Thoracic Disease* 11 (7): E90–E95.
[13] Wang, W. L., C. M. Chen, W. G. Long, et al. 2018. "Wang Procedure: Novel Minimally Invasive Procedure for Pectus Excavatum Children with Low Age." *Case Reports and Images in Surgery* 1 (1): 1–2.

A condition is considered a disease because various pathological changes have occurred. These changes are abnormal and differ entirely from normal physiological structures and functions. Such changes arise due to pathogenic causes. Through certain mechanisms, these causes lead to pathological alterations that manifest as disease. Chest wall surgical diseases are categorized into five main types, encompassing numerous specific disorders. Each disease may have distinct causes and corresponding pathogenic mechanisms, making it nearly impossible to fully elucidate the pathogenesis of every individual disease. However, by examining these diseases from a macroscopic perspective and studying their causative factors, it is possible to identify some common patterns and broadly clarify their mechanisms of onset.

1. The Role of Mechanical External forces

Diseases caused by mechanical external forces are mainly related to changes in anatomical structures, which are more commonly seen in chest wall deformities. Under normal circumstances, the development of the chest wall follows a fixed timeline and shape. For example, during childhood, the thorax appears barrel-shaped; as age increases, the anteroposterior diameter gradually shortens while the transverse diameter widens, forming what is considered the normal shape [1]. The shape of the thorax at different ages reflects physiological changes, the reasons for which will not be discussed here. However, under the influence of external forces, the shape of the chest wall can undergo various related changes, leading to different types of thoracic deformities, which are typical pathological alterations.

Among various deformities, pectus excavatum is the most common. There has been extensive research on its pathogenesis, with multiple hypotheses proposed, but none has been definitively confirmed. However, one mechanism that is relatively clear is the role of external forces. Pectus excavatum typically occurs near the xiphoid process, where the sternum is absent in the midline and the costal arches on both sides are not directly connected, creating a large triangular defect area in the center (Figure 1-4-1). Some believe that if there are fibrous structures exerting traction in this deep area, it can cause the chest wall to depress, leading to the formation of pectus excavatum [2]. Fibrous traction is clearly a manifestation of mechanical external force. This mechanism can

relatively clearly explain the occurrence of pectus excavatum. However, some patients do not have abnormal fibrous tissue, suggesting that other mechanisms may also be involved in the formation of pectus excavatum. Clinically, there are two situations that can be regarded as direct evidence of pectus excavatum caused by external forces. The first is pectus excavatum following congenital diaphragmatic hernia surgery[3]. After diaphragmatic hernia repair, two possible outcomes may occur: one is local shortening at the site of diaphragm suturing, which directly pulls on the anterior chest wall structures; the other is that after the intrathoracic organs are returned to the abdominal cavity, the negative pressure within the thoracic cavity increases, and this negative pressure directly acts on the weak areas of the anterior chest wall, leading to the development of a depression deformity. Both outcomes are secondary pathological changes related to mechanical external forces, with these forces being the sole cause of the depression formation (Figure 1-4-2). Besides diaphragmatic hernia surgery, there is another clinical procedure neonatal pulmonary cystadenoma surgery that can also lead to pectus excavatum [4]. In this surgery, a large amount of lung tissue is resected, which increases the negative pressure inside the thoracic cavity and can result in the formation of funnel chest
(Figure 1-4-3). Additionally, funnel chest occurring after median sternotomy is related to mechanical traction caused by postoperative deep fibrous tissue proliferation [5]. In many failed pectus excavatum surgeries, the depression may deepen further due to the effect of deep fibrous traction, leading to more severe deformities, which is also a result of mechanical external forces (Figure 1-4-4) [6].

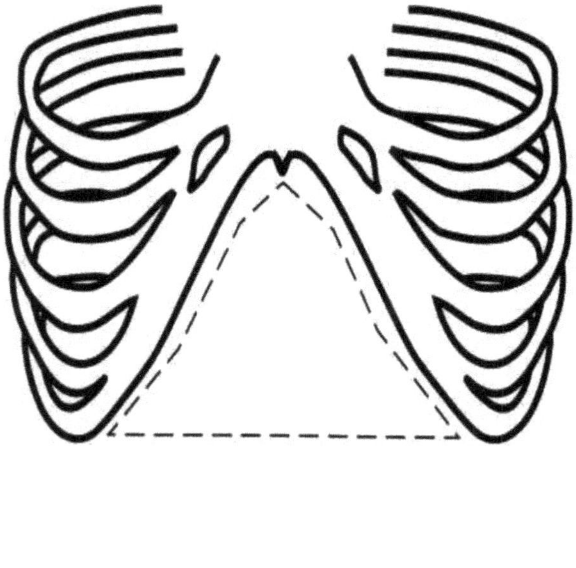

Figure 1-4-1 Structure near the xiphoid process (The area between the bilateral costal arches and the xiphoid process lacks bony structures. If this region is considered part of the chest wall, it should be the weakest area. When subjected to external forces, this site is the most prone to positional changes, which can lead to deformities.)

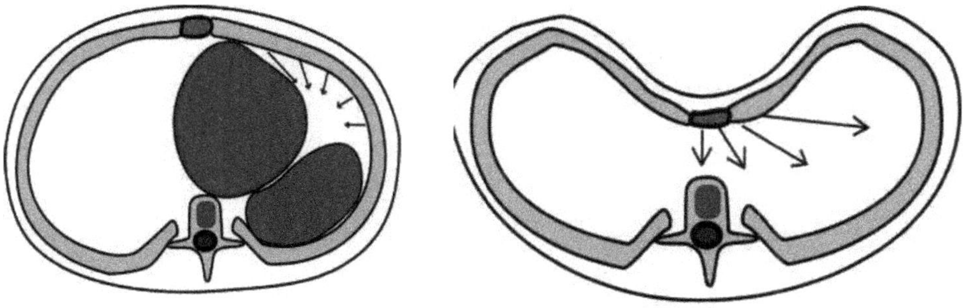

A B

Figure 1-4-2 Mechanism of pectus excavatum formation after congenital diaphragmatic hernia surgery (A. After abdominal structures are removed from the thoracic cavity, the intrathoracic negative pressure increases. Under this pressure, because the lateral chest wall is entirely bony, depressions generally do not occur. However, near the xiphoid process, due to the absence of bony structures, it is prone to depression caused by the negative pressure. B. During diaphragmatic hernia repair, direct suturing of the diaphragm is often necessary. Even when repair materials are used, postoperative diaphragmatic contraction frequently occurs. The diaphragm attaches directly to the lower chest wall, with the area near the xiphoid process being the weakest. When contraction is severe, traction from the diaphragm causes depression near the xiphoid process, resulting in pectus excavatum.)

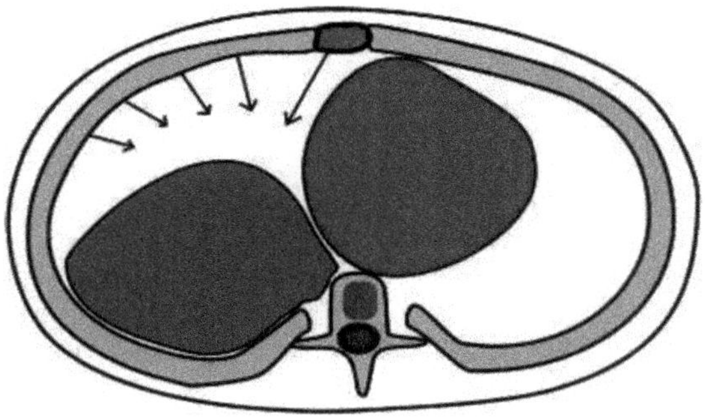

Figure 1-4-3 Mechanism of pectus excavatum formation after pulmonary cystadenoma resection (The cystadenoma itself has a relatively large volume, and during resection, a certain volume of normal lung tissue may also be removed. The removal of these structures results in an increased postoperative intrathoracic space. Although the remaining lung tissue may expand to some extent, it cannot fill the newly created space. This leads to an increase in the negative pressure within the thoracic cavity. The increased negative pressure acts on the chest wall. The lateral chest wall, supported by intact bony structures, does not collapse. However, near the xiphoid process, where bony structures are absent, depression is likely to occur, leading to pectus excavatum. Additionally, pulmonary cystadenoma resection is an intrathoracic surgery, and postoperative connective tissue proliferation may occur. If the proliferated tissue pulls on the

lower anterior chest wall, it may also cause pectus excavatum.)

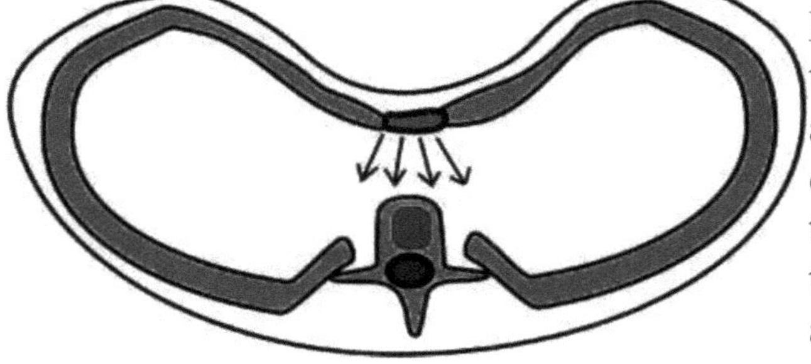

Figure 1-4-4 Fibrous tissue in the midline pulling on the anterior chest wall, causing a depressed deformity. After thoracotomy or other surgeries through a midline incision, adhesions can form inside the mediastinum. The main feature of these adhesions is the proliferation of fibrous tissue. Since there is an absence of bony structures near the xiphoid process, fibrous traction in this area can lead to the formation of pectus excavatum.

The influence of mechanical external force on pectus excavatum is also observed in a very specific scenario namely, in cases of monozygotic twins with pectus excavatum [7]. Logically, monozygotic twins should develop identically, yet it is possible for one child to develop pectus excavatum while the other remains completely normal. The most reasonable explanation for this discrepancy is mechanical compression, which is almost certainly the only plausible cause.

The causes of pectus excavatum mentioned above are relatively clear and can effectively explain its general pathogenesis. However, in other cases, the connection appears less obvious, For example, the relationship between pediatric asthma and the development of pectus excavatum. At first glance, it seems difficult to link asthma with this deformity [8]. In reality, this too results from the action of mechanical external forces. During asthma attacks, children experience intense and exaggerated respiratory movements. These vigorous movements themselves are a direct manifestation of mechanical external force. The force can originate from the chest wall muscles or from changes in intrathoracic pressure. When such forces continuously act on the anterior chest wall, positional changes in the chest wall may occur. The overall direction of displacement depends on the magnitude and vector of the resultant force. In cases of asthma, the dominant force is directed toward the center of the thoracic cavity, leading to the development of a depression deformity. This provides a reasonable explanation for the occurrence of pectus excavatum in children with asthma. In this process, the role of mechanical external force is a direct pathogenic factor (Fig. 1-4-5).

Figure 1-4-5 Mechanism of Asthma-Induced Pectus Excavatum: (During an asthma attack, the airways narrow due to various causes. When inhaling forcefully, the intrathoracic negative pressure increases significantly. The lateral chest wall may expand outward under the action of chest wall muscles, but due to local weakness near the xiphoid process, a depression may occur. A brief asthma episode is unlikely to cause a permanent depression, but if asthma attacks occur frequently, a permanent depression, pectus excavatum may form)

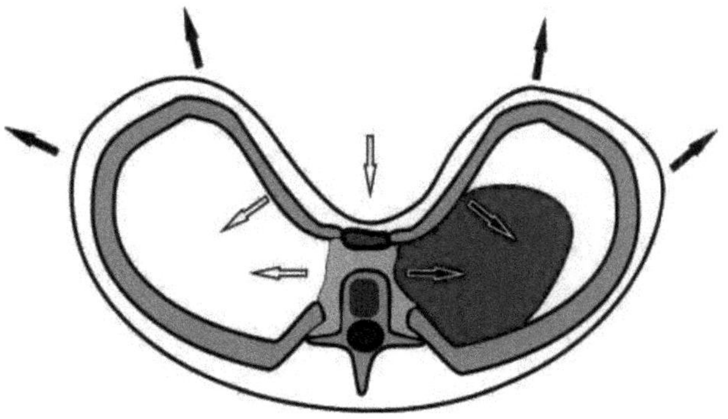

In clinical practice, there are other conditions For example, cases of chronic empyema characterized by fibrous plaque proliferation within the thoracic cavity. After such fibrous proliferation occurs, it can exert traction on chest wall structures, resulting in collapse of one side of the chest wall[9]. This is also a type of depression deformity. Clearly, such deformities are likewise the result of mechanical forces. While there are many hypotheses regarding the formation of pectus excavatum or chest wall depressions, only the mechanical force hypothesis can be supported by direct evidence. The same mechanism may also play a role in the development of other deformities.

The mechanism of pectus carinatum (pigeon chest) formation is different from that of pectus excavatum, but it is also related to the action of mechanical forces [10]. There are two fundamental elements in the development of pectus carinatum: first, a weakened chest wall; and second, the presence of external forces. Chest wall weakness may have some objective causes; some believe it is related to calcium deficiency. This explanation is plausible, as the incidence of pectus carinatum is significantly higher in children with rickets, whose overall bone strength is compromised, including that of the chest wall. This condition directly affects the rigidity of the chest wall. The mechanical force involved is primarily the sustained impact of the heart. These two factors can perfectly explain the pathogenesis of pectus carinatum. However, there may also be other contributing causes, as some patients present with extremely severe anterior chest protrusion despite the heart not being in contact with the anterior chest wall. Such cases may involve a different underlying mechanism. In addition, clinical observations have shown that some monozygotic twins both develop pectus carinatum, which clearly suggests a genetic component.

Barrel chest is a specific type of deformity that can be regarded as a generalized anterior protrusion of the anterior chest wall. Clinically, the most common cases of barrel chest are secondary deformities, typically seen in elderly patients with chronic pulmonary diseases [11]. Due to prolonged hypoxia, these patients must exert extra respiratory effort to meet physiological demands, and over time, this increased work leads to compensatory changes in the shape of the thoracic cage. From this mechanism, it can be seen that the occurrence of barrel chest is also directly related to mechanical forces, which originate from the forces exerted by the respiratory muscles. Besides elderly patients with lung diseases, barrel chest is frequently seen among residents living in high-altitude areas. Due to long-term exposure to a hypoxic environment, their chest walls may undergo changes similar to those caused by chronic lung disease, ultimately resulting in barrel chest. The onset of the barrel chest can be secondary or primary. Primary barrel chest is more common in younger patients, with unknown causes and an unclear relationship to mechanical forces.

The above analysis discusses the relationship between mechanical forces and the occurrence of chest wall deformities. In fact, the role of mechanical forces is not limited to inducing deformities; it can also manifest as causing complications of chest wall deformities. For example, scoliosis occurring in patients with pectus excavatum is a result of mechanical forces [12,13].

The spine is the main load-bearing structure of the human trunk, and it remains straight because the forces on both sides are balanced. In patients with pectus excavatum, the depression of the anterior chest wall directly compresses the heart, causing the heart to shift toward the left thoracic cavity. As the heart moves leftward, the related mediastinal structures also shift to the left side of the chest. Since all these structures are suspended from the spine, their leftward movement causes an imbalance in the forces acting on both sides of the spine, which can result in scoliosis. Thus, scoliosis in patients with pectus excavatum is entirely the result of mechanical forces [14]. In patients with thoracic dysplasia syndrome, in addition to chest wall issues, scoliosis often occurs. This scoliosis is also related to mechanical forces. When ribs on one side are missing or fused, the forces on both sides of the spine become uneven, similarly leading to scoliosis [15].

In addition to the effects mentioned above, mechanical forces also directly cause certain specific clinical manifestations in patients with various deformities. Patients with pectus excavatum have two particular habits: one is disliking lying flat [16], and the other is frequent hunching of the back [17]. Both habits are also results of mechanical forces. When pectus excavatum patients lie flat, the depression in the anterior chest wall directly compresses the heart, causing significant discomfort. To relieve this, patients tend to lie on their sides. The hunchback posture arises from a similar mechanism. When patients straighten their chest and raise their heads, the depression presses more heavily on the heart, worsening their symptoms. As a result, they must adopt a protective posture to relieve discomfort. This posture bending forward with a hunched back is characteristic of patients with pectus excavatum. When the anterior chest wall is depressed, the pressure exerted on the heart and lungs is the most direct manifestation of mechanical forces. Once this pressure acts directly, various related clinical problems naturally arise.

In addition to the many effects mentioned above, mechanical forces also impact chest wall deformities through complications that arise after various chest wall deformity surgeries. The Nuss procedure is the most commonly used surgery to treat pectus excavatum, but it is also the one most prone to failure. The fundamental reason for these surgical failures is also related to the action of mechanical forces. The most common failure in the Nuss procedure is displacement of the metal bar [18]. The bar should be correctly positioned at the lowest point of the chest wall depression. Once displacement occurs, the bar moves away from this lowest point, allowing the depression to revert to its original state, resulting in surgical failure. The fundamental cause of the bar displacement is an issue with fixation, and the root of this fixation problem remains mechanical forces. Besides bar displacement, another possible complication of the Nuss procedure is abnormal support or pressure on the chest wall, which is mainly related to improper placement of the bar. If the metal bar presses on one side of the depression instead of directly underneath it, the depression may be pushed toward the opposite side, causing the edge of that side's depression to bulge forward, resulting in a sharp-angled deformity [19]. This is an extremely serious complication. From the process of its occurrence, it is clear that mechanical forces play a fundamental role.

The Nuss procedure has been in use for many years and is performed by doctors worldwide. Unfortunately, until recently, no one had studied the fundamental principle behind its mechanism. In 2017, after extensive observation and research, we discovered that its basic principle is the lever principle (Figure 1-4-6) [20]. This discovery provides theoretical guidance for the proper execution of the surgery. From this principle, it is clear that the Nuss procedure itself is a process involving the application of force. A successful surgery can be seen as a success of mechanical force application, while a failure can be understood as a failure of mechanical force application. Every successful or failed case can be explained by the lever principle itself.

Besides the Nuss procedure, many other surgeries for thoracic deformities are also related to mechanical forces. Although these forces differ in nature from those that cause the deformities, improper use of these forces can lead to a series of complications. Such complications can be regarded as secondary thoracic deformities. This means that mechanical forces also play a decisive role in the formation of secondary thoracic deformities.

After the occurrence of chest wall surgical diseases, various symptoms may manifest, some of which are related to the effects on the heart and lungs, primarily caused by mechanical compression. This mechanism is completely different from the impact of intrathoracic diseases on cardiopulmonary function; mechanical force plays a direct role. Mechanical force can also affect other organs, such as the trachea and esophagus, causing related symptoms due to external pressure. This situation can be seen with large tumors on the anterior chest wall, as well as in certain special conditions, such as pectus excavatum combined with straight back syndrome. The mechanical pressure not only causes obvious symptoms in patients but also worsens the original condition [21].

In summary, mechanical forces are an important factor in the occurrence of chest wall surgical diseases, and they continue to play a crucial role throughout the development and treatment of these diseases.

2. Abnormal Blood Supply

The occurrence of chest wall diseases, besides the action of external forces, is often related to blood supply. This situation can happen in certain special diseases. The first case is infectious diseases, especially infections occurring at surgical incision sites, such as infections in the median chest incision [22]. This area has little subcutaneous tissue and poor blood circulation. If blood flow is further damaged before closing the incision, healing is easily affected, eventually leading to infection. Once infection occurs, because blood supply cannot improve, it will impair incision healing, and in severe cases, can even be fatal. This situation also frequently happens in patients undergoing radiotherapy after breast cancer surgery [23]. Radiotherapy causes significant damage to normal tissues, and the chest wall may develop aseptic necrosis. The necrotic tissue almost completely lacks blood supply. Once skin ulceration occurs, it often fails to heal due to insufficient blood supply. When the wound cannot heal, it gradually becomes an infectious focus, exposing deep necrotic tissue and ultimately leading to more severe consequences

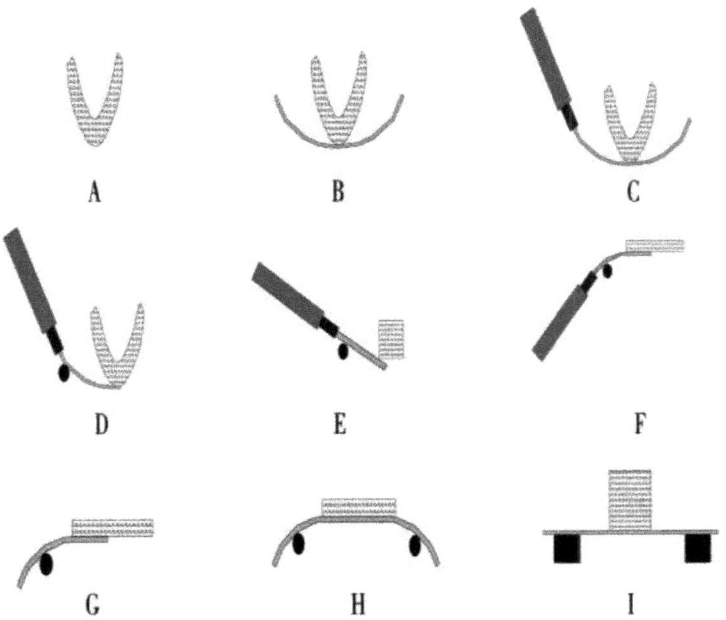

Figure 1-4-6 Basic Principle of the Nuss Procedure: (A) In the Nuss procedure, the movement of the steel bar and the surgical device is three-dimensional. To study this movement, it needs to be decomposed into components of motion and force. This decomposition is a simplification process. To better reveal the movement pattern, the trajectory on the horizontal plane is selected for observation. The figure shows the shape of the local depression on the horizontal plane of the pectus excavatum.(B) When the steel bar is placed at the bottom of the depression, the curved side of the steel bar faces the bottom of the depression.(C) One end of the steel bar is connected to a flipping wrench; at this point, the movement pattern is still not obvious.(D) The steel bar has a symmetrical bilateral structure. To clearly show the movement pattern, the steel bar is divided into two symmetrical parts, and one side is observed. At this point, the wrench and the steel bar are combined as one object. The relationship between this object and the depressed chest wall becomes clearer, revealing traces of a lever. (E) To analyze the principle more clearly, it is standardized into an ideal lever model for analysis. From this model, it can be seen that the combined unit of the steel bar and the wrench is actually a lever. The process of flipping the steel bar in the Nuss procedure is a lever motion process. The chest wall is the object that needs to be lifted, and the fulcrum is exactly the ribs of the lateral chest wall.(F) After the anterior chest wall is lifted, it is equivalent to the lever raising the target object to the required height.(G) After fixation is completed, the wrench is removed, ending the lever movement.(H) Restoring the appearance of the two halves of the steel bar, it can be seen as two levers operating simultaneously on both sides. Observing both halves simultaneously does not affect the explanation by the

lever principle. (I) The final position of the steel bar is similar to another idealized model, where a heavy object is loaded on two fulcrums by a plate-like structure. This model does not contradict the lever principle and can be regarded as a result of lever action.

Abnormal blood supply can directly lead to the occurrence of chest wall surgical diseases. During the treatment process, blood supply is equally important. If it is inadequate, various complications may arise, resulting in more severe chest wall conditions. This situation is often seen in flap transplantation surgeries [24]. At this time, blood supply is the key to surgical success. Without adequate blood supply, the flap cannot survive, and the chest wall disease may worsen, potentially leading to other types of chest wall conditions. For example, during chest wall tumor surgery, if there is a problem with the flap's blood supply during chest wall reconstruction, the flap will necrotise, resulting in a large local defect. On top of this defect, an infection may develop. This is a severe consequence caused by poor blood supply.

In addition to the examples mentioned above, there is another disease in clinical practice closely related to abnormal blood supply, which is Poland syndrome [25]. The occurrence of this syndrome is believed to be caused by blood supply disruption to one side of the chest wall and the ipsilateral upper limb during the fetal period. Due to insufficient blood supply, various structures of the affected chest wall and the distal part of the ipsilateral upper limb develop slowly or even abnormally, eventually resulting in permanent deformities and dysfunction. The specific manifestations of these lesions include hypoplasia or absence of the unilateral breast and pectoralis major muscle, absence or fusion of the upper rib cartilages and ribs, and deformities of the ipsilateral fingers, while the contralateral chest wall and fingers remain completely normal. The patient's chest wall appearance shows severe asymmetrical deformity, with the affected side sometimes exhibiting a noticeable localized depression. The patient's chest wall shows severe asymmetrical deformity, with the affected side sometimes exhibiting a noticeable localized depression. This depression is directly related to abnormalities in the development of the bony structures.
In summary, blood supply is directly related to the development and growth of tissue structures. Without an adequate blood supply, normal tissues cannot develop properly, and pathological changes become more severe. Throughout the occurrence and progression of various chest wall surgical diseases, blood supply remains a crucial and decisive factor.

3. Genetic Factors

Genetic factors are another important cause of disease occurrence, and many diseases are related to these factors. In chest wall surgical diseases, congenital diseases are often associated with genetic factors. For example, in pectus excavatum, many patients have a family history, with multiple family members exhibiting the same deformity, showing clear signs of heredity [26]. Asphyxiating thoracic dystrophy (Jeune syndrome) is also influenced by genetic factors; it is often seen affecting multiple family members, and genetic testing has confirmed that this disease is related to definite genetic factors [27]. Other various deformities also show familial hereditary tendencies. The occurrence of deformities within the same family is mostly related to genetics; this is common knowledge. However, this phenomenon is not absolute. If a certain deformity is related to acquired factors, such as nutritional or environmental factors, family members living in the same environment may also develop the deformity simultaneously. In such cases, the deformity is clearly unrelated to genetics. However, there is one situation that serves as direct evidence of genetic causation, which is mainly manifested by the simultaneous occurrence of the disease in monozygotic twins. The deformity they suffer from may be pectus excavatum, pectus carinatum, or other deformities [28]. In such cases, it is almost certain that genetic factors are the sole cause of the disease.

In addition to chest wall deformities, chest wall defects can also be congenital, and these diseases may likewise be related to genetic factors. The occurrence of chest wall tumors is complex and is unlikely to be influenced by genetic factors. Other chest wall diseases also appear to have no relation to genetic factors.

The relationship between genetic factors and the occurrence of chest wall surgical diseases can be directly confirmed through genetic material testing. However, studying the true pathogenesis is not easy. From genetic-level variations to the onset of clinical diseases, there are many steps and processes in between, making it an extremely complex undertaking to thoroughly investigate.

4. Other Congenital Causes

Genetic factors can be regarded as congenital pathogenic factors. However, many children are born with thoracic deformities but lack clear genetic evidence. Therefore, it is reasonable to believe that their deformities are caused by some non-genetic congenital factors. The specific causes of these factors remain unclear. Referring to common fetal teratogenic causes, the following are some possible factors [29,30]: ①Microbial infection: Certain maternal microbial infections, especially viral infections, may cause fetal deformities. This is a relatively common teratogenic factor. ② Drugs or chemical agents: Many drugs have severe side effects that can cause congenital deformities. The risk of teratogenicity is higher if these drugs are taken during early pregnancy. Some chemical agents also have obvious teratogenic effects, such as alcohol, formaldehyde, and other toxic chemicals, which may lead to fetal malformations. ③ Heavy metals: Certain heavy metals, like mercury and lead, can also cause deformities. ④ Severe maternal diseases: When the mother suffers from certain serious illnesses, fetal development can be affected, leading to malformations. ⑤ Maternal nutritional factors: Deficiency of certain dietary elements can cause deformities. For example, folic acid deficiency may result in specific malformations. Conversely, excess intake of certain elements, such as vitamin A overdose, can also lead to deformities. ⑥ Direct injury to the fetus [31]: The maternal womb is generally a safe environment for fetal growth; however, in extreme cases, direct harm to the fetus can occur, causing chest wall surgical diseases. We have treated 4 cases where injuries occurred before birth, with lesions located on the chest wall. After birth, these children gradually developed chest wall inflammation and infection, ultimately resulting in permanent chest wall deformities. These deformities affected not only the thorax but also the soft tissues, causing extremely severe consequences.

Non-genetic congenital factors affect fetal development through various pathways. When these influences impact the chest wall, they can cause various related thoracic deformities. Besides deformities, other congenital diseases may also develop, such as chest wall defects or congenital chest wall tumors. It must be noted that congenital factors often affect multiple systems or organs; thus, when chest wall deformities are present, there may be concurrent malformations of other organs or structures, making the fetal condition more complex and severe.

5. Infectious Factors

In chest wall surgical diseases, chest wall infection is a special type of disease. Infections are almost entirely acquired (not congenital) and are often secondary, while primary infections are relatively rare. Primary infections can be hematogenous or arise from direct local infection. Secondary infections may result from trauma or surgery. Infections caused by trauma can occur due to untimely or incomplete debridement. Surgical infections are related to many factors and often occur at the incision site; in severe cases, they may involve the surgical field or even a larger area. Infections after surgeries through lateral

chest wall incisions are relatively less common, mainly due to good local blood supply and abundant soft tissue. However, infections are more common with median incisions and can be complicated by mediastinal infections [32]. If chest wall infections are not treated promptly, they can spread into the thoracic cavity, leading to more severe consequences.
The direct cause of chest wall infections is various pathogens, with bacterial infections being the primary causative factor. Localized features of chest wall infections are obvious and may present as abscesses, local tissue necrosis, or ulceration. Infection is the definite cause of chest wall infections; however, whether other chest wall diseases are related to infection factors remains unclear. The occurrence of some chest wall tumors may be associated with viral infections, but no direct causal relationship has been reported.
The pathogenic mechanism of infection factors is relatively clear: on one hand, it comes from the direct damage caused by pathogens, and on the other hand, it is related to toxins secreted by the pathogens. After pathogen invasion, the body exhibits various protective responses, leading to inflammation and the appearance of various clinical symptoms. This is the general mechanism of infection development.

6. Traumatic Factors

Chest wall trauma is also a type of thoracic surgical disease. Its occurrence is related to many factors, but fundamentally, it is caused by violent forces. The essential characteristic of traumatic factors is the destruction of the normal structure of the chest wall. Once the chest wall structure is damaged, its function is directly affected, leading to various symptoms [33]. This is the basic mechanism of injury caused by trauma.
In real life, there are many types of traumatic factors. When various external injurious forces reach a certain intensity, they can all become traumatic factors, leading to serious consequences. After chest wall trauma occurs, the respiratory function and protective function of the chest wall will be affected, and the function of maintaining appearance will also be impaired. Patients may exhibit a variety of related clinical manifestations.
Traumatic factors, besides directly causing chest wall injuries, can also lead to other conditions such as chest wall defects, which are often manifestations of severe chest wall trauma. If trauma is not treated promptly and properly, it may result in chest wall infections and other chest wall surgical diseases. Additionally, chest wall deformities can develop after trauma; these deformities can be both a sign of the injury and an independent disease caused by the trauma. Thus, traumatic factors represent a complex pathogenic factor whose

consequences are not only complicated but also relatively severe.

7. Nutritional Factors

Nutritional factors are frequently mentioned as pathogenic factors, especially in some congenital chest wall deformities, and are even considered definite causes. For example, many pediatricians believe that chest wall deformities are related to calcium deficiency or vitamin D deficiency. Their evidence often comes from low levels in various nutritional element tests [34]. The simultaneous presence of abnormal indicators and deformities may suggest a causal relationship, but it could also be completely unrelated. If abnormal test results are directly taken as the cause of the deformity, it may lead to serious misjudgments. This situation is most common in young children with pectus excavatum. Many patients are diagnosed with calcium deficiency by doctors and then given large amounts of calcium supplements, cod liver oil, or vitamin D, but ultimately these treatments have no effect and cannot change the chest depression. This phenomenon indirectly demonstrates that the occurrence of pectus excavatum is not necessarily related to nutritional factors. Of course, this conclusion may not be entirely accurate. After all, nutritional issues can affect the development of the thorax. If the hardness and strength of the thorax are indeed related to nutritional factors, malnutrition will lead to localized weakness. If this occurs in the anterior chest wall, especially near the xiphoid process, then continuous external force acting on that area may cause the chest wall near the xiphoid to collapse, eventually resulting in a concave deformity. Obviously, such deformities are also related to malnutrition, but this is only an indirect effect.

Regarding the role of nutrition, it seems to be even more important in the formation of certain protrusive deformities. The specific mechanism is that nutritional factors can cause poor development of the chest wall, leading to localized areas lacking sufficient strength and becoming softened. When such a weakened chest wall is subjected to outward pressure from within the thoracic cavity, it may result in a localized protrusion, forming a convex deformity. This situation can occur in the precordial region of the chest wall, where the heart lies directly beneath, and since the heart is a positive-pressure organ, it can push outward against the softened chest wall. The continuous and repetitive beating and impact of the heart directly act on the softened chest wall, which can cause the chest wall to protrude forward and form a deformity. This is the mechanism behind the formation of certain types of pectus carinatum.

In addition to playing a decisive role in the formation of deformities, nutritional factors may also influence the development of other chest wall diseases. For example, in chest wall infections, if a patient is malnourished and has weakened immunity, the risk of infection increases and the spread of infection may be accelerated. For example, in cases of chest wall trauma, if the patient is malnourished, their ability to withstand the injury will be reduced, which may lead to very severe consequences. The situation is similar to chest wall tumors. Tumors themselves are wasting diseases, so if the patient already has nutritional problems, it only worsens the condition. In these cases, although nutritional factors are not direct causes of disease, they can accelerate the pathogenic process caused by other factors and exacerbate the disease outcomes.

8. Other Factors

Besides the aforementioned factors, there may be many other pathogenic factors that lead to the occurrence of chest wall surgical diseases. People come into contact with various factors in daily life, and these factors may influence the development of disease. These factors may originate from nature or from the human environment; they can be physical, chemical, or biological; they can be natural or man-made. Although in-depth research on these factors may not always clarify the exact mechanisms, it is beneficial for avoiding these factors and preventing the occurrence of chest wall surgical diseases.

REFERENCES

[1] Bastir, M., D. G. Martinez, W. Recheis, et al. 2013. "Differential Growth and Development of the Upper and Lower Human Thorax." *PLOS ONE* 8 (9): e75128.

[2] Brochhausen, C., F. K. P. Turial, et al. 2012. "Pectus Excavatum: History, Hypotheses and Treatment Options." *Interactive Cardiovascular and Thoracic Surgery* 14 (6): 801–806.

[3] Wang, Wenlin. 2019. "Pectus Excavatum after Congenital Diaphragmatic Hernia Surgery." Medical Science Channel, November 29.

[4] Wang, Wenlin. 2020a. "Why Does Pectus Excavatum Occur after Pulmonary Cystadenoma Surgery?" China Medical Channel, April 13.

[5] Wang, Wenlin. 2018. "Wang Surgery for Pectus Excavatum after Cardiac Surgery." Zhihu, July 1.

[6] Wang, Wenlin. 2020b. "Analysis of Causes for Pectus Excavatum Surgery Failure." 365 Medical Network, April 20.

[7] Wang, Wenlin. 2020c. "Wang Surgery for Monozygotic Twins with Pectus Excavatum." 365 Medical Network, November 9.

[8] Wang, Wenlin. 2020d. "The Relationship between Pectus Excavatum and Paradoxical Respiration." 365 Medical Network, February 18.

[9] Wang, Wenlin. 2019b. "Correction Surgery for Secondary Thoracic Deformity (Empyema Combined with Chest Wall Collapse)." 365 Medical Network, November 29.

[10] Wang, Wenlin. 2017. "Why Do Patients with Rickets Tend to Develop Pectus Carinatum Rather than Pectus Excavatum?" iAsk Doctor, March 8.

[11] Fry, J. 1954. "Chronic Bronchitis in General Practice." *British Medical Journal* 1 (4855): 190–194.
[12] Wang, Wenlin. 2018a. "Thoracic Deformities and Scoliosis: Mechanical Principles." 39HealthNet, February 28.
[13] Wang, Wenlin. 2021a. "Another Serious Hazard of Pectus Excavatum: Scoliosis." 365 Medical Network, May 16.
[14] Wang, Wenlin. 2021b. "Unlucky Girl: Surgery for Scoliosis Combined with Pectus Excavatum." 365 Medical Network, May 18.
[15] Campbell, R. M. 2013. "VEPTR: Past Experience and the Future of VEPTR Principles." *European Spine Journal* 22 (Suppl 2): 106–117.
[16] Wang, Wenlin. 2021c. "Sleeping Posture Issues in Children with Pectus Excavatum." *Thoracic Deformity Surgery Expert*, July 21.
[17] Wang, Wenlin. 2021d. "Pectus Excavatum and Kyphosis." *Thoracic Deformity Surgery Expert*, June 7.
[18] Simon, N., S. Kolvekar, and A. Khosravi. 2020. "Extra-Thoracic Migration of the Nuss Bar in Corrective Surgery for Pectus Excavatum: A Very Rare Late Complication." *Journal of Surgical Case Reports* 2020 (10): rjaa388.
[19] Wang, Wenlin. 2021e. "Sharp Angle Deformity." *Thoracic Deformity Surgery Expert*, August 18.
[20] Wang, Wenlin. 2017b. "Basic Principles of Nuss Surgery (2)." *Thoracic Deformity Surgery Expert*, December 2.
[21] Wang, Wenlin. 2020e. "The World's First Case: Straight Back Syndrome Combined with Severe Tracheal Stenosis Digital Material Repair Surgery." *Thoracic Deformity Surgery Expert*, December 29.
[22] Dohmen, P. M., T. Markou, R. Ingemansson, et al. 2014. "Use of Incisional Negative Pressure Wound Therapy on Closed Median Sternal Incisions after Cardiothoracic Surgery: Clinical Evidence and Consensus Recommendations." *Medical Science Monitor* 20: 1814–1825.
[23] Raz, D. J., S. L. Clancy, and L. J. Erhunmwunsee. 2017. "Surgical Management of the Radiated Chest Wall and Its Complications." *Thoracic Surgery Clinics* 27 (2): 171–179.
[24] Harati, K., J. Kolbenschlag, B. Behr, et al. 2015. "Thoracic Wall Reconstruction after Tumor Resection." *Frontiers in Oncology* 5: 247.
[25] Hashim, E. A. A., B. H. Quek, and S. Chandran. 2021. "A Narrative Review of Poland's Syndrome: Theories of Its Genesis, Evolution, and Its Diagnosis and Treatment." *Translational Pediatrics* 10 (4): 1008–1019.
[26] Wu, S., X. Sun, W. Zhu, et al. 2012. "Evidence for GAL3ST4 Mutation as the Potential Cause of Pectus Excavatum." *Cell Research* 22 (12): 1712–1715.
[27] Bosakova, M., S. P. Abraham, A. Nita, E. Hruba, M. Buchtova, S. P. Taylor, I. Duran, J. Martin, K. Svozilova, T. Barta, and M. Varecha. 2020. "Mutations in GRK2 Cause Jeune Syndrome by Impairing Hedgehog and Canonical Wnt Signaling." *EMBO Molecular Medicine* 12 (11): e11739.
[28] Wang, Wenlin. 2017c. "Evidence for Heredity of Pectus Carinatum: Ji Sheng Brothers and Their Family's Pectus Carinatum." *Thoracic Deformity Surgery Expert*, February 20.
[29] Kaleelullah, R. A., and N. Garugula. 2021. "Teratogenic Genesis in Fetal Malformations." *Cureus* 13 (2): e13149.
[30] Sebastiani, G., C. Borras-Novell, M. A. Casanova, et al. 2018. "The Effects of Alcohol and Drugs of Abuse on Maternal Nutritional Profile during Pregnancy." *Nutrients* 10 (8): 1008.
[31] Wang, Wenlin. 2020f. "Wang Surgery for Severe Secondary Complex Thoracic Deformities." *Thoracic Deformity Surgery Expert*, October 26.

[32] Suelo-Calanao, R. L., R. Thomson, M. Read, et al. 2020. "The Impact of Closed Incision Negative Pressure Therapy on Prevention of Median Sternotomy Infection for High-Risk Cases: A Single Centre Retrospective Study." *Journal of Cardiothoracic Surgery* 15: 222.
[33] Dogrul, B. N., I. Kiliccalan, E. S. Asci, et al. 2020. "Blunt Trauma Related Chest Wall and Pulmonary Injuries: An Overview." *Chinese Journal of Traumatology* 23 (3): 125–138.
[34] Wang, Wenlin. 2016b. "Misconceptions about Pectus Excavatum (1): Is Calcium Supplementation Effective?" *Thoracic Deformity Surgery Expert*, July 20.
[35] Wang, Wenlin. 2017d. "Pathogenesis of Pectus Carinatum and Metabolic Diseases." *Thoracic Deformity Surgery Expert*, August 30.
[36] Wang, Wenlin. 2014. "Pathogenesis of Pectus Carinatum." *Thoracic Deformity Surgery Expert*, December.

Section 5

CLINICAL MANIFESTATIONS OF CHEST WALL SURGICAL DISEASES

Although chest wall surgery is a relatively new specialty, most chest wall surgical diseases originate from traditional thoracic surgery [1]. Since the chest wall and the intrathoracic organs form a functional whole, the clinical manifestations of related diseases may influence one another. Intrathoracic diseases can manifest through certain signs on the chest wall, and chest wall diseases can affect intrathoracic organs, presenting with corresponding symptoms or physical signs. Therefore, when studying the clinical manifestations of chest wall surgical diseases, a broad perspective is necessary, one that consistently considers the impact on intrathoracic organs. Only with this approach can clinical signs be used more accurately to guide diagnosis and treatment.

1. Symptoms

Symptoms are the patient's subjective feelings and experiences of a disease essentially, the patient's own description of their condition [1]. Because symptoms are subjective, different patients may describe the same disease differently. However, some primary symptoms are directly related to specific pathological changes or damage, and therefore show common patterns, forming characteristic symptoms of certain diseases. Thoracic wall surgical diseases are confined to the chest wall, and because the chest wall has unique structural and functional features, the symptoms of these diseases also exhibit distinct characteristics.

(1) Pain

Pain is the most common symptom of thoracic wall surgical diseases, and almost every such condition may involve pain. The location of the pain varies depending on the site of the lesion; it can be localized or involve a large area of the chest wall. Compared to intrathoracic diseases, thoracic wall surgical conditions have more precise localization; the location of the pain generally corresponds closely to the site of the lesion [2]. Different types of diseases may present with different qualities of pain, such as sharp pain, dull pain, or aching pain. Chest wall trauma often causes severe pain [2,3]. If a fracture is present, the pain tends to worsen with breathing or movement [2]. In the early stages of chest wall infection, pain may be present; however, once the infection becomes chronic, the pain may lessen or even disappear. Patients with chest wall defects may not necessarily experience pain especially those with congenital bony structural defects, who may be entirely pain-free. However, if the defect is secondary to other causes, such as trauma, pain is usually present. Additionally, if the defect results from radiotherapy following breast cancer surgery, pain is also commonly reported. Chest wall tumors may present without pain or with varying degrees of pain. The intensity and nature of the pain can differ significantly between individuals. Chest wall deformities themselves generally do not cause pain. Some patients may experience chest pain after physical activity, but this pain is likely due to cardiac compression rather than being a direct symptom caused by the deformity.

Pain is a subjective symptom influenced by many factors, including [1]: ① Nature of the disease. Different diseases cause varying pain experiences. For example, pain caused by trauma is often more severe, mainly related to the injury stimulus and the patient's fear of the trauma. Deformities generally do not cause direct pain, which is also related to the patient's focus of concern. ② Subjective willpower. Some patients have strong willpower and higher pain tolerance, so they often do not feel excessive pain. Conversely, patients who are more fragile and have lower pain tolerance will feel the pain more intensely. ③ External environmental cues. Before seeking medical help, some patients may learn about the disease and can be easily influenced by this information, affecting their experience of pain. If the information received is positive, they may not fear pain much; otherwise, they might become overly sensitive to pain and have reduced tolerance. ④ Treatment methods. Different treatments cause different pain sensations. Open surgery causes greater injury and thus more pain; minimally invasive surgery significantly reduces trauma and pain accordingly. Surgeries involving bone structures tend to be more painful and have longer-lasting pain. Pain from other surgeries is usually shorter and disappears quickly after the operation. ⑤ Pain relief measures. Many patients actively or passively receive pain management, and the effectiveness varies depending on the method used. The choice of pain relief directly affects the pain experience.

For chest wall surgical diseases, pain is an important warning sign, and its presence greatly aids in diagnosis. Since pain is a symptom reflecting the patient's experience of suffering, timely management is necessary. When treating this symptom, relying solely on painkillers is insufficient. If the underlying cause is not addressed, or if the subjective factors influencing pain are ignored, not only will effective pain relief fail to be achieved, but there is also a risk of drug dependency, which can cause greater harm to the patient.

(2) Cough, sputum production, and hemoptysis

Chest diseases often cause coughing, which can have many causes, the most common being irritation of the respiratory tract. Chest wall surgical diseases are limited to the chest wall and generally do not directly involve the respiratory tract, so coughing usually should not occur. However, since chest wall diseases are not isolated conditions and the chest wall forms the outer structure of the thoracic cavity, it naturally relates to the internal structures of the chest. Therefore, the appearance of symptoms like coughing is not surprising. Among various chest wall surgical diseases, patients with primary deformities lack the pathological basis that causes coughing, so they almost never exhibit this symptom. Patients with secondary deformities usually have primary diseases inside the thoracic cavity, such as chest wall collapse deformity caused by chronic empyema. Due to irritation from lesions inside the chest cavity, coughing may occur. Similarly, chest wall trauma that affects intrathoracic structures or irritates the pleura can also cause coughing. Chest wall defects are similar to deformities in that isolated defects generally do not cause coughing; however, coughing may occur if the defect is secondary to other diseases. If a chest wall infection involves a surgical incision, it usually indicates the presence of intrathoracic pathology, and coughing may be present. Chest wall tumors confined to the chest wall without pleural involvement or invasion into the thoracic cavity typically do not cause coughing. If coughing does occur, the possibility of involvement of intrathoracic structures should be considered.

Coughing is often accompanied by sputum production. Sputum mainly results from increased secretions or inflammation in the lungs, with the root cause located in the pulmonary system. If sputum appears in chest wall surgical diseases, it indicates that the chest wall lesion has involved the lungs, reflecting a worsening of the condition.

Hemoptysis is a sign of injury to the airways or pulmonary blood vessels. It is a rare but serious symptom, often accompanied by coughing. Common chest wall surgical diseases generally do not cause hemoptysis. However, if the disease involves the lungs or airways, hemoptysis may occur. This situation can be seen in severe chest wall trauma or tumors. Once hemoptysis occurs, it requires prompt treatment; otherwise, it may lead to more serious consequences.

(3) Dyspnea

Dyspnea is a general term for symptoms caused by impaired respiratory function and can manifest as chest tightness, shortness of breath, or rapid breathing. Many factors can affect respiratory function, including those related to the airways, tissues distal to the airways, and various structures of the thorax. The chest wall consists of many structures involved in respiration, such as ribs, costal cartilages, sternum, and various respiratory muscles. If any of these structures are damaged, respiratory function will be affected. Therefore, for chest wall surgical diseases, dyspnea is a relatively common symptom.

Simple chest wall surgical diseases generally affect respiratory function through three mechanisms: ① Compression of intrathoracic organs. Chest wall diseases can compress the heart and lungs in various ways. Depressed deformities mainly compress the heart and lungs through the indentation of bony structures. When the compression is mild and does not exceed the cardiopulmonary functional reserve, no symptoms appear. However, when the compression becomes severe, cardiopulmonary insufficiency occurs, and symptoms manifest. Another form of compression comes from lesions, with the most common example being chest wall tumors. Large chest wall tumors directly compress the heart and lungs, impairing respiratory function. Besides directly affecting the diastolic function of the heart and lungs, compression can also reduce thoracic volume, a mechanism often overlooked. Both depressed deformities and chest wall masses may reduce thoracic volume, thereby restricting the lungs and affecting pulmonary function. ② Pain limiting respiratory movement. Breathing is a complex movement that involves not only lung expansion and contraction but also chest wall motion. Chest wall movement is an important part of respiration. When chest wall surgical diseases cause severe pain, this pain can inhibit chest wall movement, ultimately impairing respiratory function. ③ Abnormal chest wall movement. Normal chest wall motion during breathing follows a fixed pattern, which depends on the intact structure of the chest wall. If the structure is damaged, such as in large-area injuries, abnormal chest wall movement can occur. This abnormal motion can impair respiratory function and cause breathing difficulties.

Abnormal chest wall movement can occur in various conditions. The first and most common condition is flailing chest caused by trauma, which usually involves extensive damage to the bony structures of the chest wall, commonly referred to as multiple rib fractures in multiple locations. The second condition is chest wall defects, mainly involving defects in the bony structures. At this time, the chest wall may be softened, showing obvious paradoxical breathing. The third situation involves thoracic deformities, such as in young children with pectus excavatum, where paradoxical movement occurs in the sunken area. Abnormal chest wall movement directly counteracts the work of breathing and severely affects respiratory function.

Overall, when chest wall surgical diseases are not severe, there may be no difficulty breathing. However, regardless of the type of disease, if left untreated and it progresses to a certain severity, it will affect respiratory function through various mechanisms, ultimately leading to breathing difficulty. The onset of respiratory distress is a direct indication of worsening chest wall surgical disease.

(4) Asphyxia

Asphyxia is not actually an independent symptom but a severe form of respiratory distress. Its main characteristic is extreme difficulty in breathing, to the point where breathing is nearly impossible. This symptom occurs in some extreme situations, such as major airway obstruction or tension pneumothorax. In most cases, chest wall surgical diseases do not cause such changes. But there are exceptions. The exceptional cases mainly include two types of conditions: ① Severe chest wall trauma combined with tension pneumothorax. This can be either closed chest wall trauma or open chest wall trauma; it can be isolated chest wall trauma or chest wall trauma combined with lung injury. These traumas may all lead to tension pneumothorax [4]. ② Some extremely severe thoracic constrictive diseases, such as asphyxiating thoracic dystrophy (Jeune syndrome) [5]. In this condition, the thorax is severely collapsed, compressing lung tissue and causing lung atelectasis. If accompanied by lung inflammation, lung function cannot meet the body's needs, resulting in severe respiratory distress, i.e., asphyxia. If not corrected in time, this situation may be life-threatening.

(5) Palpitations

Palpitations are a specific symptom related to various factors, primarily the heart rate and rhythm. Since the heart is an organ within the thoracic cavity, if a chest wall disease does not affect the heart, this symptom generally should not occur. However, many chest wall diseases can impact the heart, which makes the occurrence of this symptom possible.

The most common way chest wall diseases affect the heart is through direct compression. This is often seen in concave deformities. For example, in patients with pectus excavatum, when the depression is deep enough, the heart can be noticeably compressed, causing abnormalities in heart rate and rhythm, which leads to the sensation of palpitations. Additionally, direct compression from a lesion can also cause palpitations; For instance, if a tumor on the anterior chest wall is large enough to significantly compress the heart, palpitations may occur. When discussing the issue of cardiac compression, it is necessary to introduce

a special disease called straight back syndrome [6]. Strictly speaking, this disease belongs to spinal surgery and is not part of chest wall surgery. However, because the normal physiological curvature of the spine disappears, the heart is compressed jointly by the sternum and the spine, causing many patients to seek medical attention primarily for cardiac symptoms. Because of this characteristic, the disease is also called “pseudo-cardiac disease.” The root cause of this condition lies in the compression of the heart. So far, spinal surgery has no better method to treat it. However, if treatment is approached from the anterior chest wall, this disease can achieve very good therapeutic outcomes.
The symptom of palpitations primarily reflects the direct clinical impact on the heart. However, besides compression, another situation can cause palpitations systemic injury resulting from chest wall disease. For example, massive bleeding caused by chest wall trauma can reduce overall blood volume, leading to an increased heart rate and causing the person to feel palpitations.

(6) Asthma

Asthma is also a symptom closely related to respiratory function. Its typical manifestations include increased respiratory rate, intensified breathing effort, and rapid, deep breathing. The occurrence of asthma is associated with many factors, mainly originating from within the thoracic cavity. If chest wall diseases involve internal thoracic organs, asthma can also occur. Clinically, the most common occurrence of asthma happens in chest wall trauma. If the chest wall trauma also involves lung tissue, it can lead to acute respiratory distress and result in severe asthma.

2. Signs

Signs are objective manifestations present at the site of the lesion. Compared to subjective symptoms, signs more accurately reflect the characteristics of chest wall surgical diseases and therefore play an important role in disease diagnosis.

(1) Changes in Skin Color

Under normal circumstances, the skin color of the chest wall does not show obvious changes. After a local lesion occurs, if the lesion infiltrates toward the skin surface, it may affect the skin and cause changes in skin color. In the early stage of infectious lesions, local redness and swelling of the skin can appear, while chronic lesions may cause darkening of the skin color. Lesions after radiation exposure may show characteristic pigmentation of the skin. Chest wall deformities generally do not cause local skin color changes, but some patients may have associated pigmented spots on other parts of the body, which is a relatively common characteristic skin lesion.

(2) Skin Ulceration

When chest wall infection progresses to a certain extent, local skin ulceration may occur, with the ulcer possibly discharging necrotic tissue and pus. Tumors with local necrosis can also cause skin ulceration. Once ulceration occurs, it indicates a very severe condition requiring further treatment; otherwise, healing is difficult. In cases of severe chest wall trauma complicated by infection, skin ulceration may also develop. This situation is similar to chest wall infection and is considered a secondary chest wall infection.

Chest wall deformities themselves generally do not cause skin ulceration. However, such signs may appear after surgery for deformities. This situation is related to three factors: The presence of metal plates within the incision. Because metal plates are foreign bodies, they can interfere with wound healing. Insufficient local soft tissue at the incision site. After suturing, soft tissue is needed to cover the metal plates. If the soft tissue is inadequate, the metal plates may lie directly beneath the skin, affecting healing. Even if the wound initially heals, the plates can gradually erode through the skin over time, causing local ulceration. Poor blood circulation. Proper wound healing requires adequate blood supply. When blood flow is insufficient, healing is impaired, leading to local ulceration. A typical example is recurrent skin ulceration after reoperation on chronically infected wounds. At this time, due to poor blood circulation around the incision, even if it is sutured again, healing is difficult, ultimately leading to recurrent local skin ulceration.

(3) Skin Defects

Skin defects refer to the loss of a large area of skin and can occur in various situations. In chest wall trauma, severe injuries may cause large areas of skin loss, directly resulting in defects. After breast cancer surgery and radiotherapy, local skin may undergo necrosis, eventually leading to extensive skin defects [7]. Skin defects represent a serious form of damage and generally require prompt treatment; otherwise, the lesion may extend deeper, causing more severe consequences.

When skin ulceration occurs, there will be local breaks in the skin. If these breaks gradually enlarge and fail to heal, they can lead to permanent skin defects. Therefore, skin defects are more severe than skin ulceration and represent a more serious clinical sign.

(4) Mass

Chest wall masses are one of the most common signs and represent localized growth of lesions. Masses are most frequently seen in chest wall tumors and are mainly solid masses [8]. Infections can also present with masses, which may be cystic if pus is present. Local deformities in the bony structures of the chest wall can also result in the formation of masses.

Masses are generally exophytic structures that protrude from the body surface. However, it must be clearly understood that as a mass grows outward on the surface, it inevitably also grows into the surrounding tissues and even into the thoracic cavity. Therefore, once a mass is found, the possibility of infiltration into the surrounding and deeper areas must be considered. When examining a mass, it is important to carefully observe multiple aspects, including the color of the overlying skin, size, texture, hardness, mobility, boundaries with surrounding structures, presence or absence of tenderness, and whether fluctuation is present. This information will help in determining the nature of the mass.

(5) Flail Chest

Flail chest is a very important physical sign in chest wall surgery [9]. As mentioned above, it can be seen in three basic conditions involving three fundamental diseases: trauma, defects, and deformities. Besides these three basic diseases, flail chest may also occur after some special surgical procedures. For example, in the resection of chest wall tumors, if the removed tissue includes bony structures and no reconstruction is performed afterward, a flail chest may occur. Additionally, it must be pointed out that even if reconstruction is done, a flail chest can still develop if the reconstruction is not effective.

The main harm of a flail chest is paradoxical respiration, which damages breathing by canceling out the work of breathing. Therefore, the most important treatment for this sign is local fixation. Effective fixation can eliminate the flail segment and control its harmful effects.

(6) Chest Wall Edema

The skin of the chest wall can become swollen, presenting as localized or extensive edema. The occurrence of edema may be related to impaired venous return from the chest wall and can be caused by tumors of the chest wall or inside the thoracic cavity, as well as chest wall infections. Additionally, localized edema may also occur in cases of closed chest wall trauma.

(7) Subcutaneous Emphysema

Subcutaneous emphysema is a special sign in chest wall surgery [10]. It manifests as widespread swelling under the skin, but unlike edema, pressing the area does not cause indentation. It may produce a crackling sensation to the touch, and a crackling sound can be heard on auscultation. Subcutaneous emphysema can start from the chest wall but may spread to the neck, face, abdominal wall, and other subcutaneous areas, causing extensive swelling. The cause is the continuous entry of high-pressure gas into the subcutaneous tissue. It can occur in closed chest wall trauma or secondary to certain chest wall surgeries. Subcutaneous emphysema is usually transient and will gradually resolve if no more gas enters.

(8) Depression

Under normal physiological conditions, the chest wall is full and does not have any form of depression. Once a depression appears, it becomes a pathological sign, that is, a clinical sign. Depression is one of the most common characteristic manifestations of chest deformities (Figure 1-5-1) [11]. These deformities can be primary or secondary. The most common type of depressed deformity is pectus excavatum. Different locations of the depression present different characteristics and can manifest as various types of deformities.

Most deformities present as localized depressions. Patients with flat chest often show no visible depression on the anterior chest wall. However, if the entire anterior chest wall is compared to various depressed deformities, it can be regarded as an overall depression of the anterior chest wall. Although this concept may be difficult to understand, it helps in surgical planning. Many people choose the Nuss procedure to treat flat chest, which in itself actually acknowledges the presence of depression.

However, when understanding the characteristics of depression, it is important to recognize the difference between the depression in flat chest and typical localized depressions. Only by recognizing this difference can variously mistakes during the Nuss procedure for flat chest be avoided.

Besides the depression unique to pectus excavatum, there are other types of depressions, such as groove-like depressions. These deformities should not be classified as pectus excavatum but rather as sternal groove deformity [12]. The depression can be located in one area or multiple areas, existing alone or combined with other deformities, thus forming various types of complex deformities.

In addition to thoracic deformities, other thoracic wall diseases can also cause chest wall depression. For example, severe chest wall trauma may damage the chest wall structure, leading not only to chest wall softening but also localized depression. Chest wall depression can also result from intrathoracic diseases, such as thickened fibrous membranes in chronic empyema, which may cause localized chest wall depression. Furthermore, certain surgical procedures, like traditional thoracoplasty may intentionally disrupt the chest wall structure, causing it to collapse to eliminate pulmonary cavities and achieve therapeutic goals. In such cases, the chest wall exhibits more severe depression.

Depression is a pathological sign and a typical clinical manifestation. Its presence indicates the existence of thoracic wall disease, which may originate primarily in the chest wall or be secondary to diseases in other regions. Regardless of the underlying cause, surgical intervention is typically required for such conditions

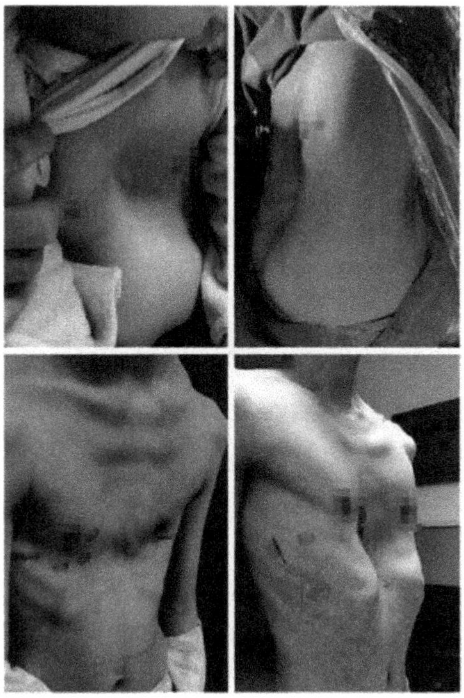

Figure 1-5-1 Various Types of Depressions (Depressions can appear in every part of the chest wall, present in different

(9) Protrusion

Protrusion is also a common clinical sign in thoracic wall surgery, characterized by a localized area of the chest wall that is significantly raised compared to the surrounding area. It differs from a mass. A mass refers to a solid or cystic structure that is not part of the normal chest wall anatomy, whereas a protrusion indicates an outward bulging of the chest wall structure itself, where the bony components and contours of the chest wall can be seen or palpated. A mass consists of pathological tissue, while a protrusion is formed by the bony framework of the chest wall. Protrusions can be localized or involve a large area, even extending to the entire anterior chest wall. The extent of protrusion varies, leading to different manifestations of deformity (Figure 1-5-2). Localized protrusion is characteristic of pectus carinatum [13], but the protrusion can also be extensive and severe in degree. A protrusion involving the entire anterior chest wall is generally not perceived as a localized protrusion but rather as a hallmark feature of barrel chest. This understanding is instrumental in guiding surgical planning for such specific deformities.

(10) Angular Deformity

When discussing various clinical signs, one specific manifestation warrants dedicated attention, a distinct feature we have termed "angular deformity" (Figure 1-5-3) [14]. This clinical sign is relatively uncommon and is typically observed only in severe thoracic deformities. It may manifest as either a protrusion toward the body surface or a depression into the thoracic cavity. The hallmark feature of this sign is an extreme localized distortion of the chest wall's bony structure, presenting as a sharp-angled protrusion or depression within a confined area of the anterior chest wall. Angular deformity can be either primary or secondary. Primary angular deformity is seen in severe thoracic deformities, which may present as either pectus excavatum or pectus carinatum. Secondary angular deformity may occur in some failed Nuss procedure cases if the pectus bar is misplaced and deviates from the deepest part of the depression, it can create an angular deformity along one edge of the indentation. Angular deformity represents the most severe form of malformation. Once this sign appears, it often indicates that unconventional surgical techniques will be required for successful correction.

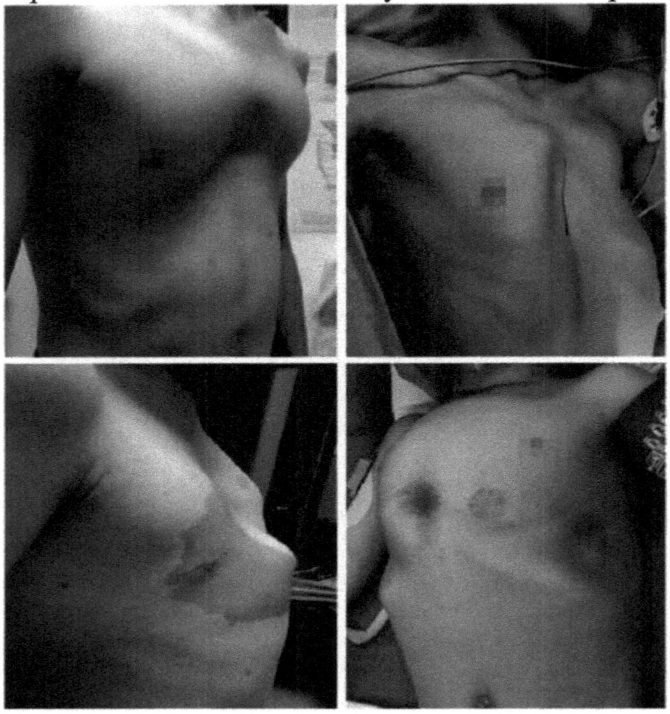

Figure 1-5-2 Various Types of Protrusions (Protrusions may exhibit diverse shapes, varying degrees of severity, and occur at different locations; they can present in isolation or coexist with other deformities.)

The preceding sections have provided a concise overview of the symptoms and signs associated with thoracic wall disorders. In clinical practice, however, each disease entity manifests with distinctive clinical features that may demonstrate considerable variability. Certain presentations may extend beyond the spectrum described, while others might lack even fundamental symptomatology or physical signs. Clinicians must therefore adopt a case-specific analytical approach, leveraging all available clinical data to guide diagnostic and therapeutic decision-making. While proficiency in recognizing disease symptoms and signs constitutes an essential foundation for clinical work, it remains merely the preliminary phase of patient evaluation. To establish precise diagnoses, comprehensive ancillary investigations are invariably a subject that will form the focus of discussion in the subsequent section.

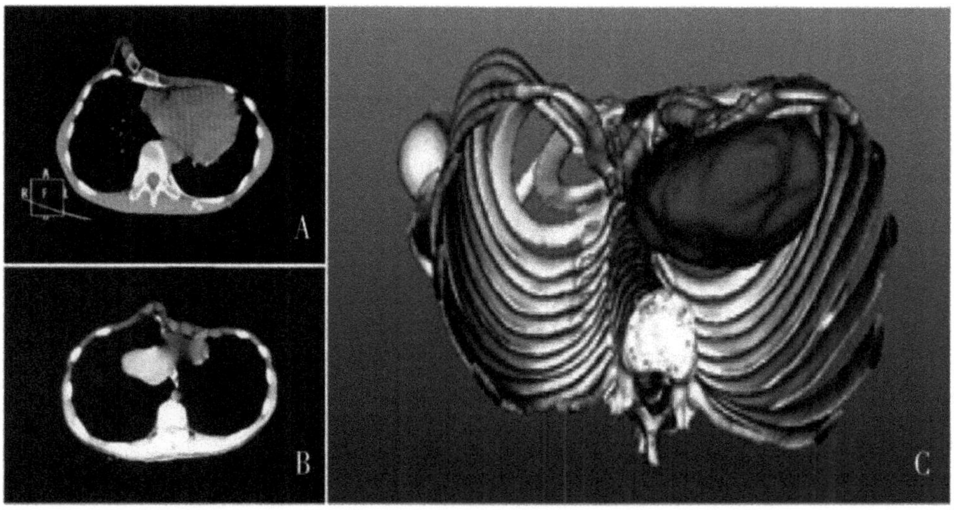

Figure 1-5-3 Angular Deformity (A) Lateral chest wall protrusion with distinct sharp-angled projection; (B) Midline protrusion exhibiting localized acute-angled prominence;(C) Focal anterior chest wall depression forming a sharp inward angulation toward the thoracic cavity.

REFERENCES

[1] Wang, W. L. 2021. "Clinical Manifestations of Thoracic Wall Diseases: Symptoms and Signs." *Pectus Deformity Surgery Expert*, August 20.
[2] Tulay, C. M., S. Lardiz, and A. Bilge. 2018. "Do We Really Know the Duration of Pain after Rib Fracture?" *Kardiochirurgia i Torakochirurgia Polska* 15 (3): 147–150.
[3] Zhang, J. P., L. Sun, W. Q. Li, et al. 2019. "Surgical Treatment of Patients with Severe Non-Flail Chest Rib Fractures." *World Journal of Clinical Cases* 7 (22): 3718–3727.
[4] Robert, D. J., S. Leigh Smith, P. D. Faris, et al. 2014. "Clinical Manifestations of Tension Pneumothorax: Protocol for a Systematic Review and Meta-Analysis." *Systematic Reviews* 3: 3.
[5] de Vries, J., J. L. Yntema, van Die, et al. 2010. "Jeune Syndrome: Description of 13 Cases and a Proposal for Follow-Up Protocol." *European Journal of Pediatrics* 169 (1): 77–88.
[6] Hasegawa, K., T. Takaya, S. Mori, et al. 2016. "Compression of the Right Ventricular Outflow Tract due to Straight Back Syndrome Clarified by Low-Dose Dual-Source Computed

Tomography." *Internal Medicine* 55 (22): 3279–3283.
[7] Billington, A., D. Dayicioglu, P. Smith, et al. 2019. "Review of Procedures for Reconstruction of Soft Tissue Chest Wall Defects Following Advanced Breast Malignancies." *Cancer Control* 26 (1): 1073274819827284.
[8] Bacheri, R., S. Z. Haghi, M. R. Kalantari, et al. 2014. "Primary Malignant Chest Wall Tumors: Analysis of 40 Patients." *Journal of Cardiothoracic Surgery* 9: 106.
[9] Beks, R. B., M. B. de Jong, R. M. Houwert, et al. 2019. "Long-Term Follow-Up after Rib Fixation for Flail Chest and Multiple Rib Fractures." *European Journal of Trauma and Emergency Surgery* 45 (4): 645–654.
[10] Hardy, B., N. Sunderland, M. Perera, et al. 2016. "Traumatic Hemopneumothorax and 'Whole-Body' Subcutaneous Emphysema: Successful Use of a Small-Bore Chest Drain." *BMJ Case Reports* 2016: bcr2016216329.
[11] Wang, W. L., C. M. Chen, W. G. Long, et al. 2018. "Wang Procedure: Novel Minimally Invasive Procedure for Pectus Excavatum in Children with Low Age." *Case Reports and Images in Surgery* 1 (1): 1–2.
[12] Wang, W. L. 2016. "Nomenclature and Morphological Characteristics of Sulcus Chest." *Journal of Practical Medicine* 32 (2): 335–336.
[13] Wang, W. L., W. G. Long, C. M. Chen, et al. 2015. "Analysis of the Pathogenesis of Pectus Carinatum." *Journal of Practical Medicine* 31 (Suppl): 313–314.
[14] Wang, W. L. 2021. "Angular Deformity." *Pectus Deformity Surgery Expert*, August 17.

Thoracic Wall Surgery originates from traditional thoracic surgery, and most of the examination methods used in thoracic surgery can also be applied to the diagnosis of thoracic wall surgical diseases. These examinations include both basic physical examinations and various advanced instrumental investigations. However, the examination of thoracic wall diseases has its own particularities, mainly due to the anatomical location of the thoracic wall. First, thoracic wall surgical diseases are located very superficially. All such diseases are found on the surface of the chest. Even lesions that occur deeper within certain special structures such as the breast or scapula (shoulder blade) are still considered superficial (body surface) lesions. Since they are located on the surface, the examination methods differ from those used for internal diseases. Second, thoracic wall surgical diseases often involve the bony structures of the chest wall [1]. In the composition of the chest wall, the ribs, costal cartilage, and sternum form the skeletal framework and are the main components of the chest wall. Any type of chest wall surgical disease may involve these structures, which in turn gives rise to specific clinical features associated with such diseases. These characteristics necessitate that examinations also include assessment of the bony structures. Lastly, chest wall surgical diseases may be related to intrathoracic conditions. The chest wall and the thoracic cavity are inherently a unified whole, with natural anatomical connections. While mild chest wall surgical diseases may exist solely within the chest wall, once the disease progresses to a certain extent, it may extend into the thoracic cavity, eventually developing into more complex pathological conditions. This characteristic requires that examinations also take into account the internal organs within the thoracic cavity. The three features of chest wall surgical diseases mentioned above place specific demands on diagnostic approaches, making it necessary to conduct examinations on three levels [1]: First, since chest wall surgical diseases primarily occur on the surface of the chest, physical examination should be given the greatest attention, as it is the most fundamental diagnostic method. Second, as most of these diseases involve the bony structures of the chest wall, and because these structures have particular diagnostic requirements, the second level of examination should consist of X-ray or CT scans, which are essential for assessing chest wall conditions. Third, because chest wall surgical diseases may be associated with intrathoracic structures, it is necessary to also perform examinations of the thoracic cavity to obtain more detailed and comprehensive information. The specific methods can include standard CT scans or more advanced three-dimensional reconstruction imaging. From the characteristics of these three levels of examination, it is clear that to obtain the most comprehensive information about the disease, all three levels of examinations need to be conducted simultaneously. However, performing all these tests at once can not only impose a significant financial burden on the patient but also make the preoperative preparation extremely complicated. Therefore, to make the examination process more reasonable, a stepwise approach must be adopted by conducting examinations according to the patient's specific needs. Only in this way can the examinations become more practical and better meet clinical requirements.

1.Physical Examination

Physical examination is the most basic and fundamental method of examination, and it is also one of the important examination techniques. Especially for certain chest wall surgical diseases, this type of examination is almost the most crucial diagnostic tool. General chest wall surgical diseases often present with obvious signs on the body surface, so important firsthand information can be obtained through physical examination. The main physical sign of chest wall deformities is an abnormal appearance.

For the vast majority of these deformities, a final diagnosis can be made solely based on physical examination unless medical protocols require otherwise; even proceeding directly to surgery is often acceptable. However, in clinical practice, not everyone recognizes the importance of physical examination. Many doctors prefer to rely on instrumental tests rather than trust their own eyes, ears, or hands. On the surface, this approach may seem very professional, but in reality, it is exactly the opposite; it reflects a lack of professionalism.

Physical examination is equally important for chest wall tumors, infections, defects, trauma, and other diseases. Through simple examination, one can obtain key information about the disease that often cannot be replaced by instrumental tests. For example, understanding the relationship between the lesion and important surface structures, as well as designing the incision and the extent of lesion removal, all require the aid of a physical examination.

Among the various physical examination methods, visual inspection is very important for the diagnosis of all chest wall surgical diseases. Especially for patients with deformities, visual inspection alone can almost confirm the majority of diseases. For other types of chest wall diseases, if the lesion is clearly visible on the surface, visual inspection also aids in the diagnosis. Palpation and percussion are also important physical examination methods, playing a significant role in diagnosing conditions such as trauma, tumors, and deformities. Among all physical examination techniques, auscultation is often overlooked because its primary focus is the heart and lungs, which seem unrelated to chest wall diseases. However, this is not the case. Many chest wall diseases can involve the heart and lungs, and auscultation can indirectly assess the severity of the chest wall condition. This is very helpful for both diagnosis and treatment. Among the five types of chest wall diseases, auscultation is especially important for the diagnosis and management of chest wall deformities, particularly concave deformities, and should be considered a routine part of their examination.

For patients with chest wall deformities, one of the purposes of auscultation is to examine the condition of the heart. If there is a general abnormality in the heart rhythm, it should be considered as a result of the deformed chest wall pressing on the heart. If a murmur is present, two possibilities need to be considered: one is a functional murmur, and the other is a structural murmur. The former is generally the result of excessive compression, while the latter indicates the presence of a structural heart defect. Patients without heart murmurs may not require further examination. However, if a murmur is heard, a cardiac ultrasound should be performed to clarify the nature of the heart lesion [2]. If a structural heart defect is present, the cardiac surgery should be performed simultaneously with the deformity correction surgery. Therefore, the presence and nature of heart murmurs directly determine the choice of surgical method, making the detection of murmurs especially important. Auscultation can also provide information about the lungs; if crackles are detected, further evaluation with additional tests is necessary to make a proper diagnosis.

2. Instrumental Examinations

Physical examination is a relatively basic and subjective method of assessment. To obtain more objective and detailed information, advanced examinations using instruments are necessary. There are various types of instrumental examinations, each operating based on specific scientific principles. As a result, each has its own characteristics and can provide different types of diagnostic information.

(1) X-ray Examination

X-ray examination is the oldest and most basic form of instrumental inspection.

While this method has poor imaging capability for soft tissues, it provides excellent imaging results for bony structures. For chest wall surgical diseases, the primary imaging targets are the ribs and sternum. Additionally, the spine, scapula, and clavicle which are related to chest wall diseases can also be well visualized through X-ray examination. These characteristics make X-ray examination extremely important in the clinical management of chest wall surgical diseases [3]. Since X-ray examination is widely available and can be conducted in most general hospitals, it is considered the most basic diagnostic tool for chest wall surgical diseases. The diagnosis of many chest wall conditions can essentially be made based on this examination alone. For example, in cases of rib fractures, X-ray examination is almost the gold standard. This type of imaging not only clearly reveals the condition of the fracture but also allows for the assessment of air and fluid within the chest cavity. Therefore, X-ray examination is the most important diagnostic tool for patients with chest wall trauma.

For patients with chest wall deformities, in many cases, a physical examination alone can complete the diagnosis. However, considering certain specific regulations, an X-ray examination may be performed as well. This examination is generally sufficient. If there are no signs of intrathoracic disease, no further tests are necessary. The role of X-ray examination in chest wall deformities mainly has two aspects:

First, to understand the shape of the anterior chest wall, primarily observed through lateral views to see if there is any protrusion, depression, or other complex shapes; Second, to determine the position of the heart and the spatial relationship between the anterior chest wall and the heart. The latter is assessed through the frontal view. A normal heart is located slightly left of the midline. In patients with depression-type deformities, the heart is compressed and shifts to the left. If the heart remains centered despite a severe depression, this results in a serious type of depression deformity called malignant pectus excavatum. The relationship between the anterior chest wall and the heart can be understood through lateral X-ray views. In depression-type deformities, due to the heart being compressed, the deepest shadow of the anterior chest wall overlaps with the cardiac silhouette on the imaging. Protrusion-type deformities do not show signs of heart compression. Overall, X-ray examination is of high value for depression-type deformities; however, for protrusion-type deformities, since X-rays are mainly used to observe the shape of the anterior chest wall, their practical effectiveness is less intuitive than visual inspection.

Besides the various characteristics and conveniences mentioned above, X-ray examination has two other obvious advantages: First, it can reveal the overall structure of the thoracic skeleton. This is the simplest, cheapest, and most convenient method. While many advanced examinations can show details of lesions from different perspectives, which is important for understanding the lesion's nature, X-ray remains the absolute first choice for comprehensively displaying the thoracic contour and general details. Second, it can show the shape of the spine. Although the spine is not directly part of thoracic wall surgery clinical work, it is a component of the thorax. Many thoracic wall diseases involve spinal issues, so understanding the spine's shape is necessary, especially for thoracic wall deformities, where this information is even more critical. Other methods can also provide spinal information, but compared to them, X-rays are more practical and valuable.

(2) CT Examination

Besides X-ray examination, CT scanning is the most important diagnostic tool in traditional thoracic surgery, with the vast majority of diseases being clearly diagnosable through CT scans [3,4]. The advantage of CT examination lies in its detailed depiction of lesions, making it especially suitable for examining structures such as the lungs, esophagus, and mediastinum. For chest wall diseases, this advantage remains significant, and CT is indispensable particularly for conditions like chest wall tumors, infections, and defects. Compared to X-ray examination, CT scans are clearer and more detailed, and their superiority is obvious. However, for chest wall trauma patients, especially those suspected of bone structure damage, since the main targets of the examination are the costal cartilage, ribs, or sternum, CT is not as effective as X-ray. For chest wall deformities, CT not only clearly shows the cross-sectional shape of the chest wall and the spatial relationship between the chest wall, heart, and lungs, but can also detect potential lung lesions, giving it special value. However, it must be emphasized that for many chest wall deformity patients, this examination is unnecessary. For example, in protruding deformities like barrel chest or pectus carinatum, the chest wall cannot compress the heart or lungs. If there is no suspicion of lung disease, CT examination is completely redundant.

Although CT examination in chest wall surgery focuses only on chest wall diseases, it is impossible to perform a CT scan exclusively on the chest wall in isolation. General CT scans are usually chest examinations that include not only the chest wall but also the thoracic cavity. Therefore, for certain chest wall surgical diseases, CT scans can also help provide information about the thoracic cavity, which is equally meaningful for improving the diagnosis of chest wall diseases. For example, in cases of chest wall tumors, infections, trauma, and defects, since these conditions may involve thoracic structures, a CT scan can simultaneously obtain information about both the inside and outside of the thoracic cavity, making such information very valuable. For these types of diseases, CT scans are almost indispensable. However, for chest wall deformities, since in many cases it is not necessary to understand the condition inside the thoracic cavity, CT scans are not always required. Of course, if there is a need to rule out the possibility of concurrent diseases within the thoracic cavity, CT scans can be routinely performed.

When considering whether to perform a CT scan, there is one disease that is regarded as requiring this examination: pectus excavatum. Performing a CT scan on such patients can provide a lot of information about depression. However, the reason some doctors consider this examination indispensable is that the CT scan is used to measure a special value called the Haller index (see Figure 1-6-1) [5]. This value is recognized by many people, especially certain experts, as the key indicator for assessing the severity of pectus excavatum, and it is considered the most important metric [6,7]. Currently, various so-called consensus statements and guidelines on pectus excavatum surgery have made specific provisions regarding this value. The Haller index is so important and indispensable that general doctors dare not skip this examination, and such an assessment can only be completed through a CT scan. As a result, CT has become a mandatory examination for all patients with pectus excavatum. On the surface, this practice seems undisputed. However, if there are problems with the Haller index itself, then this approach is worth re-examining.

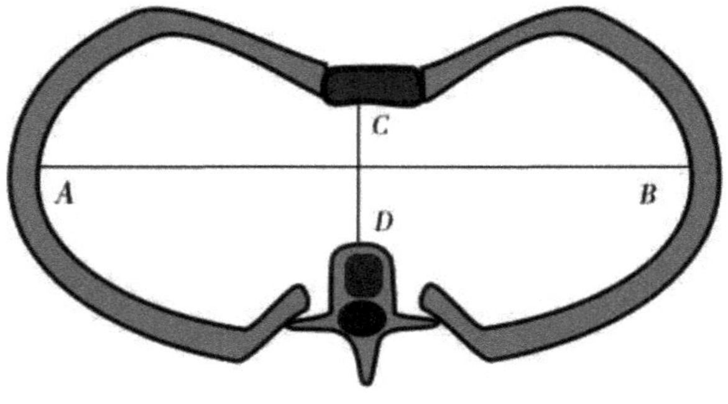

Figure 1-6-1 Measurement of the Haller Index (AB is the transverse diameter of the chest cavity, CD is the distance from the bottom of the depression to the anterior edge of the spine. The practical significance of this index is to standardize the degree of chest depression, allowing for comparability of depression parameters between different individuals. However, due to many influencing factors, this index has

several limitations.)

The Haller Index is the ratio of the transverse diameter of the chest cavity to the distance from the anterior edge of the spine to the bottom of the anterior chest wall on a CT cross-section. This ratio is a relative value and is considered to reflect the severity of the chest depression. Many people believe that the average Haller Index for a normal person is about 2.52, mild chest depression deformity is less than 3.2, moderate depression ranges from 3.2 ~ 3.5, and values greater than 3.5 indicate severe chest depression deformity [8]. While this classification of severity appears objective on the surface, it actually has significant problems. The issues mainly arise from the following aspects:

The Haller Index itself does not necessarily reflect the true severity of chest depression. For typical or standard pectus excavatum patients, the Haller Index can roughly indicate the severity of the deformity. However, in many special cases, it fails to serve this purpose. Such situations can be seen in the following special cases [8,9]: ① Some patients with predominantly flat chest walls may have a Haller Index identical to that of some pectus excavatum patients. In such cases, the Haller Index cannot objectively reflect the true severity of the depression. In other words, the actual deformities of the two are completely different (Figure 1-6-2) and cannot be directly compared. ② During the measurement of the Haller Index, as the denominator decreases, the value increases indefinitely. However, even if the value approaches infinity, it does not necessarily indicate the most severe deformity. This is because there is a situation where the bottom of the depression continues to sink and actually goes beyond the anterior edge of the spine, reaching below one side of it. In such cases, although a Haller Index can still be measured, its absolute value no longer reflects the true severity. The scientific approach would be to represent this with a negative value, but so far, this phenomenon is generally not described. This is a major flaw in the design of the Haller Index itself (Figure 1-6-3). ③ This index measures only two values: the transverse diameter of the chest and the distance from the bottom of the depression to the anterior edge of the spine. It does not take into account the height of the edges surrounding the depression. When two different patients differ only in the height of the depression's edges, their Haller Index will be exactly the same. In such cases, the Haller Index clearly cannot reflect the severity of the depression (Figure 1-6-4). ④ Additionally, for two patients with different depression areas, even if their Haller Index values are identical, the severity of their depressions differs. Here again, the Haller Index fails to accurately judge the severity between them

(Figure 1-6-5).

The widespread clinical application and high academic status of the Haller index fundamentally stem from the perceived belief in its scientific validity. However, as the above analysis reveals, the design of this index is, in fact, unscientific and in many contexts, even counter-scientific. Consequently, relying on such a metric to guide clinical practice may lead to significant complications.

Second, the measurement of the Haller index itself may be problematic [8,9]. Since this index is calculated based on specific CT scan cross-sections, and CT imaging is not continuous, sometimes with wide intervals between slices if the deepest point of the depression is missed during scanning, the Haller index will fail to reflect the true severity of the deformity. Additionally, the Haller index is influenced by the measuring physician's technique. If the selected cross-section does not accurately capture the deepest part of the depression, the measured value will likewise be unreliable. Thus, the Haller index measurement process is susceptible to both subjective and objective factors, compromising the objectivity of its results.

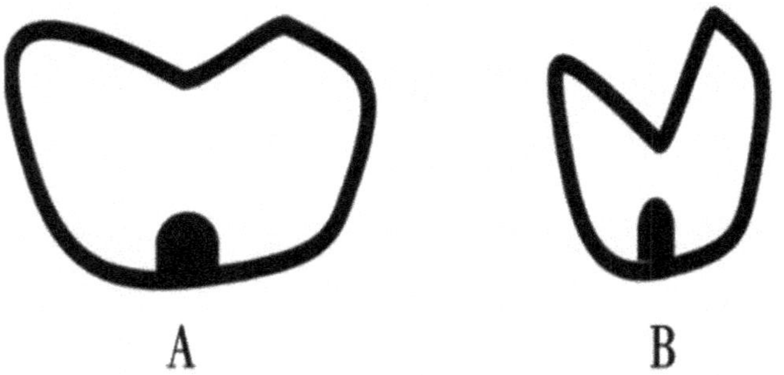

Figure 1-6-2: The Haller Index is a relative value representing the ratio of two distances, but the magnitude of this value does not necessarily reflect the actual morphological features of the deformity. When both the numerator and denominator decrease or increase simultaneously, the ratio remains unchanged, yet the actual deformity can be significantly different. Deformities A and B may have the same Haller Index, but their severity is not comparable. In such cases, the Haller Index cannot accurately represent the severity of the deformity.

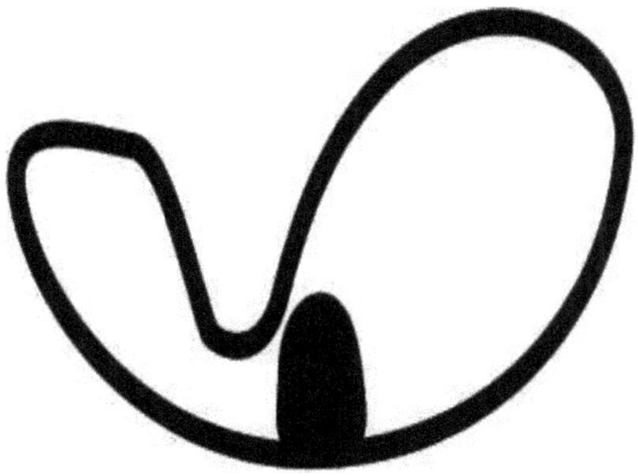

Figure 1-6-3: When the Haller Index was originally designed, it only considered typical cases of chest wall depression. However, in clinical practice, there are extreme cases, such as the one shown in the figure, where the bottom of the depression extends beyond the anterior edge of the spine, reaching below the plane of the spine's anterior margin. In such cases, the Haller Index cannot accurately reflect the severity of the depression. If this value is to be used to describe the degree of depression, it should be expressed as a negative number.

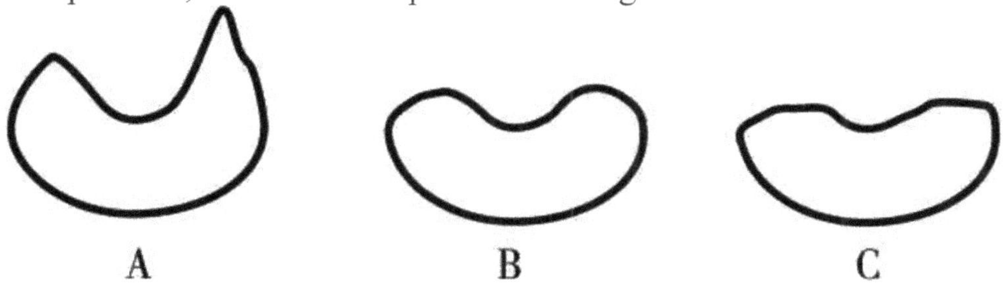

Figure 1-6-4: The Haller Index only considers the ratio of two measurements and does not take into account the specific shape of the chest wall. In the three types of depressions shown in A, B, and C, the Haller Index is exactly the same, but the severity of the deformities is completely different. At this point, using the Haller Index for comparison is meaningless.

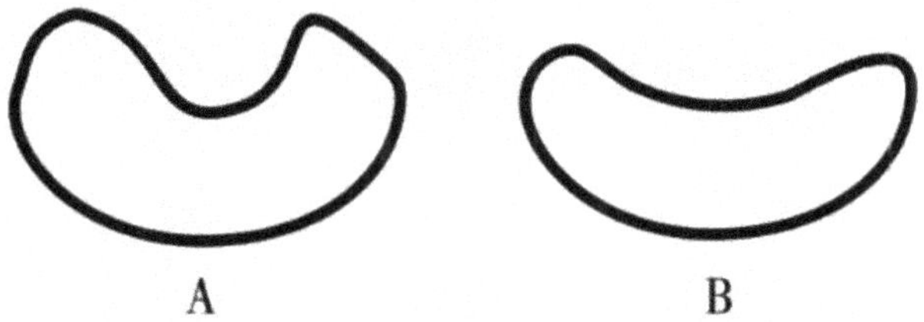

Figure 1-6-5 The Haller index only considers the relative depth of the anterior chest wall but does not account for the area of depression. When comparing deformities, A and B in the figure, the Haller index is identical, yet there is a clear visual difference between the two deformities.

Third, the numerical classification of the Haller index is inherently subjective [8,9]. This classification is merely a standard arbitrarily established by individual physicians based on their limited case experience. Failure to recognize its subjective and one-sided nature may lead to its undue glorification, thereby adversely impacting clinical practice.

From the above analysis, it can be seen that the Haller index, which appears to be very objective on the surface, is actually a subjective measure. If it is used as a gold standard to evaluate pectus excavatum and determine the need for surgery, it will lead to many practical problems. These problems mainly manifest in two aspects: ① an excessive reliance on this value, resulting in forcing every patient to undergo a CT scan. This not only delays the time needed for preoperative preparation but also increases the workload and adds to the burden on patients. ② Overreliance on this value without considering its subjective components directly affects surgical decision-making.

Objectively analyzing the Haller index, it is essentially just a parameter for assessing the degree of chest depression and should never be overly idealized. Only by understanding this index rationally can its practical value be fully realized, thereby avoiding various adverse effects caused by blind faith in it.

(3) Three-dimensional reconstruction examination

Three-dimensional reconstruction examination is an advanced diagnostic method that has emerged in clinical practice in recent years [10, 11]. This examination is performed by processing CT scan data with specialized software to ultimately produce three-dimensional images (Figure 1-6-6). These images are highly intuitive and can virtually display all structural details of the examined area, making it undoubtedly one of the most advanced diagnostic techniques available today. From the perspective of diagnostic effectiveness alone, this examination is unparalleled by any other imaging method. However, it also has inherent drawbacks. First, the imaging process takes a relatively long time and requires specialized processing before results are available, which is very inconvenient for emergency patients. for ordinary patients, if they want to obtain results quickly, this examination is also not very convenient. Second, the examination is relatively expensive, which limits its widespread use. Third, the results of the three-dimensional reconstruction often need to be viewed on specific terminals, and without the necessary equipment, accessing the results is inconvenient. Therefore, these drawbacks limit the application of three-dimensional reconstruction examinations. However, for certain special diseases, the superiority of this examination is quite evident [10, 11]. For example, in cases of complex chest wall deformities, as well as most chest wall tumors, infections, and defects, if conditions permit, it is best to perform a three-dimensional reconstruction examination. The specific advantages of this examination include: ① Clearly displaying the contours of the lesion; ② clearly showing the internal structure of the lesion; ③ Clearly demonstrating the relationship between the lesion and surrounding structures; ④ Clearly presenting the complete structure of the chest wall. The clear visualization of these structures and lesions essentially provides a holographic image of the lesion, which greatly aids in disease diagnosis. Additionally, because three-dimensional reconstruction images offer comprehensive and detailed imaging of the lesion and its surrounding structures, they allow for a certain degree of surgical simulation. This simulation is especially significant for chest wall surgery, particularly reconstructive procedures.

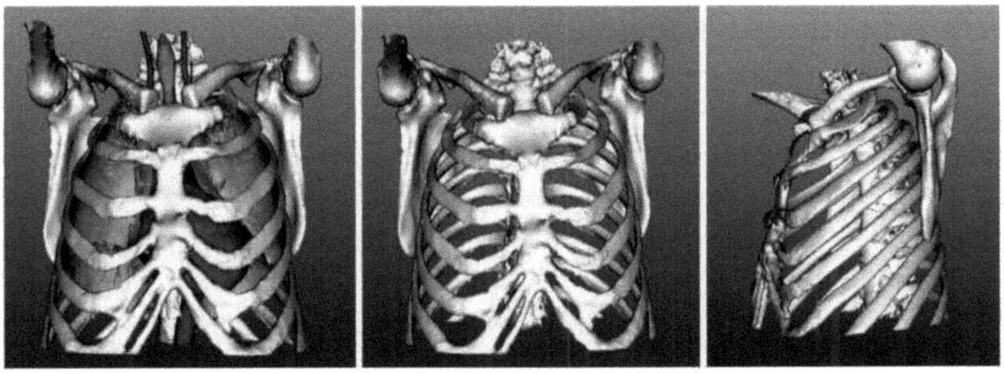

Figure 1-6-6: Three-dimensional reconstruction examination, which can clearly display information about the chest wall and various surrounding structures.

(4) Electrocardiogram (ECG) Examination

Electrocardiogram (ECG) examination is a routine and the simplest method for reflecting cardiac abnormalities. Not all chest wall surgical diseases are associated with cardiac problems. From this perspective, the ECG is not a mandatory examination. For cases that do not require surgery, the value of an ECG is limited. However, there are two situations in which an ECG examination is absolutely necessary: first, for patients suspected of having cardiac abnormalities, an ECG is essential; second, all surgical cases must undergo a routine ECG examination. This is because chest wall surgeries are performed under general anesthesia, and preoperative ECG results are required for any procedure involving general anesthesia. For the safety of the surgery,

ECG examination is indispensable.

In clinical practice within chest wall surgery, there is another situation where an ECG may be used during the bar placement in the Nuss procedure for pectus excavatum. To prevent potential injury to the heart caused by the bar, some experts recommend continuous ECG monitoring during the procedure. Changes in the ECG can serve as an indirect indicator of possible cardiac injury, enhancing intraoperative safety. However, while this approach may seem theoretically meaningful, in practice it is entirely ineffective and unnecessary. It's important to understand that very minor contact with the heart and a direct penetrating cardiac injury often show little to no distinguishable difference on an ECG. Even if a change is detected, by the time the ECG reflects cardiac damage, blood may have already begun pouring from the surgical incision. Therefore, this method lacks practical value and does not contribute meaningfully to patient safety.

(5) Echocardiography Examination

Echocardiography can provide many specialized parameters, with its primary function being the assessment of cardiac structure an aspect particularly valuable in diagnosing organic heart diseases. However, not all chest wall surgical conditions require detailed knowledge of cardiac structural features. This examination is only necessary when such abnormalities are suspected. As mentioned earlier, if a heart murmur is detected, echocardiography should be performed to rule out potential cardiac pathology [2]. Beyond such cases, routine echocardiographic examination is generally unnecessary.

Like an electrocardiogram, cardiac ultrasound is sometimes used by certain doctors during the placement of the steel bar in a Nuss procedure for pectus excavatum to monitor the heart. In such cases, transesophageal echocardiography is used in an attempt to avoid heart injury. However, this practice is largely unnecessary. Just imagine if even a thoracoscope during surgery cannot clearly detect potential injuries, how can a transesophageal ultrasound possibly guarantee a clear view? Therefore, this approach, like ECG monitoring, is ultimately a redundant measure.

(6) Ultrasound Examination

In the early days of traditional thoracic disease diagnostics, ultrasound examinations were rarely used, primarily due to the presence of air in the lungs. Over time, however, clinicians began to use ultrasound to locate and assess pleural effusions. As understanding evolved, some researchers started employing ultrasound to examine chest wall lesions. For example, ultrasound has been used to evaluate costal cartilage, rib, or sternum fractures [13,14] as well as chest wall tumors, offering information that differs from other diagnostic methods. Currently, the most commonly used clinical ultrasound is two-dimensional ultrasound. While its imaging is not very intuitive, it still provides some guidance in clinical practice. However, compared to CT or other imaging modalities, the role of ultrasound is relatively limited and cannot be used as a routine examination in clinical settings.

(7) Pulmonary Function Test

Pulmonary function testing is a controversial diagnostic procedure because the results can be influenced by many subjective factors, leading to ongoing doubts about its reliability. However, this has not seemed to affect the trust that some institutions place in this type of examination. They often treat pulmonary function testing as a mandatory preoperative examination for thoracic surgery and use its results to determine surgical indications. However, this practice is actually unscientific. If the test is done solely for surgery, does that mean severe respiratory dysfunction is an absolute contraindication for surgery? In fact, many serious chest wall conditions such as severe pectus excavatum, when accompanied by severe respiratory dysfunction, actually indicate the need for surgery and warrant early intervention, rather than being a reason to avoid surgery. Because of these issues, pulmonary function testing should never be considered a routine examination, especially for chest wall surgeries, where in many cases it is unnecessary[12].

The above provides a brief overview of the diagnostic methods for chest wall diseases. Each examination has its own characteristics and can offer relevant information from different perspectives and levels, so all have their respective roles. In clinical practice, to obtain the most appropriate and valuable information, careful consideration from multiple aspects is necessary, not only taking into account the nature of the disease but also the needs of diagnosis and treatment. Only in this way can these various examinations be best utilized and deliver their optimal effectiveness.

REFERENCES

[1] Wang, Wenlin. 2021. "Characteristics of Chest Wall Surgery Examinations." *Thoracic Deformity Surgery Experts*, August 20.

[2] Wang, Wenlin. 2015. "On Cardiac Ultrasound Examination." *Thoracic Deformity Surgery Experts*, April 3.

[3] Shelmerdine, S. C., D. Langan, J. C. Hutchinson, et al. 2018. "Chest Radiographs versus CT for the Detection of Rib Fractures in Children (DRIFT): A Diagnostic Accuracy Observational Study."

The Lancet Child & Adolescent Health 2 (11): 802–811.
[4] Weikert, T., L. A. Noordzij, J. Bremerich, et al. 2020. "Assessment of a Deep Learning Algorithm for the Detection of Rib Fractures on Whole-Body Trauma Computed Tomography." *Korean Journal of Radiology* 21 (7): 891–899.
[5] Haller, J. A., Jr., S. S. Kramer, and S. A. Lietman. 1987. "Use of CT Scans in Selection of Patients for Pectus Excavatum Surgery: A Preliminary Report." *Journal of Pediatric Surgery* 22 (10): 904–906.
[6] Zeng, Qi, Na Zhang, Maohuai Fan, et al. 2005. "Comparative Study of Nuss Procedure and Modified Ravitch Procedure." *Chinese Journal of Pediatric Surgery* 26 (8): 397–400.
[7] Nuss, D., R. J. Obermeyer, and R. E. Kelly Jr. 2016. "Pectus Excavatum from a Pediatric Surgeon's Perspective." *Annals of Cardiothoracic Surgery* 5 (5): 493–500.
[8] Wang, Wenlin. 2020a. "Funny Moment: Talking about the Haller Index." 39 Health Net, August 3.
[9] Wang, Wenlin. 2019. "Why the Haller Index Sometimes Fails to Reflect the True Degree of Depression." *Thoracic Deformity Surgery Experts*, May 24.
[10] Calloway, E. H., A. N. Chhotani, Y. Z. Lee, et al. 2011. "Three-Dimensional Computed Tomography (3-D CT) for Evaluation and Management of Children with Complex Chest Wall Anomalies: Useful Information or Just Pretty Pictures?" *Journal of Pediatric Surgery* 46 (4): 640–647.
[11] Wang, Wenlin. 2018. "Latest 3D Imaging Techniques for Pectus Excavatum." *Thoracic Deformity Surgery Experts*, January 26.
[12] Wang, Wenlin. 2020b. "Is Pulmonary Function Testing Necessary before Pectus Excavatum Surgery?" *Thoracic Deformity Surgery Experts*, March 1.
[13] Nicholson, J. A., S. T. J. Tsang, T. J. Macgillivray, et al. 2019. "What Is the Role of Ultrasound in Fracture Management? Diagnosis and Therapeutic Potential for Fractures, Delayed Unions, and Fracture-Related Infection." *Bone & Joint Research* 8 (7): 304–312.
[14] Sesia, S. B., F. Prufer, and J. Mayr. 2017. "Sternal Fracture in Children: Diagnosis by Ultrasonography." *European Journal of Pediatric Surgery Reports* 5 (1): E39–E42.

Section 7

SURGICAL INDICATIONS FOR CHEST WALL DISEASES

The primary characteristic of chest wall diseases in surgical practice is the necessity of surgical intervention, which fundamentally distinguishes them from internal medicine conditions. In recent years, with advances in technology, some non-traditional treatment methods have gradually emerged in clinical practice, and many surgical conditions no longer require traditional surgery to achieve effective treatment. On the surface, such approaches may appear to be altering the fundamental nature of surgical diseases. However, this is not actually the case. While alternative treatment methods have gradually been introduced, traditional surgical procedures remain the mainstay of treatment. Therefore, the essential nature of surgical diseases has not changed. Chest wall diseases are typical surgical conditions and likewise require surgical treatment; this is their most fundamental characteristic. However, the decision to perform surgery for such conditions is not without prerequisites. It must take into full account factors such as the nature of the disease, the need for treatment, the patient's physical condition, and available medical resources. This is what is referred to as the issue of surgical indications.

Chest wall diseases pose two types of harm to the human body: physiological and psychological. The physiological harm primarily stems from the disease's impact on the function of internal organs. This type of harm is a common characteristic shared by nearly all surgical conditions and is typically the first issue that surgical treatment aims to address. What sets chest wall diseases apart from other surgical conditions is a particularly unique form of harm: the psychological impact caused by an abnormal chest wall appearance. This type of harm is especially evident in patients with deformities. When considering only the physiological harm, the decision to proceed with surgery can follow the general principles applied in other surgical procedures, namely, assessing the severity of the disease and the patient's ability to tolerate the operation as the two main criteria for determining surgical indications. However, psychological harm is an inherently subjective experience. If one continues to rely solely on objective criteria to determine whether surgery should be performed, serious issues may arise. This highlights the fact that surgical indications in chest wall surgery are considerably more complex than those in traditional thoracic surgery. When compared directly, one can clearly see that the criteria for surgical decision-making in chest wall surgery differ significantly from those applied to more conventional thoracic conditions.

In the past, when treatment of chest wall diseases was discussed within the traditional scope of thoracic surgery, certain prevailing views often limited the development of clinical practice. For example, in the case of pectus deformity surgeries, if the patient presents no symptoms, that is, no obvious physiological impairment, most thoracic surgeons would not recommend surgery for the patient [1]. This approach follows the general principles of treating surgical diseases, but it is clearly inappropriate for the unique characteristics of chest wall conditions. Now that chest wall surgery has emerged as an independent specialty in clinical practice, it should be guided by its own distinct perspectives and principles, and the criteria for surgical indications should reflect its specific needs and considerations.

1. Surgical Indications for Thoracic Deformities

Among all five types of chest wall surgical conditions, thoracic deformities are the most unique. What makes them particularly distinct is that many of these deformities are not universally recognized as diseases, especially in cases where the deformity are relatively mild. Such deformities cause no physiological harm, and no one would typically consider them a problem, let alone a disease. However, it is often precisely these individuals who seek consultation in chest wall surgery clinics. During the consultation, they may not even acknowledge themselves as patients, yet surprisingly, they often request surgical treatment from the doctors. According to the basic principles of surgical indications for surgical diseases, such individuals would not qualify for surgery. However, in practice, it is often necessary for doctors to perform surgery on them. The reason for accommodating their requests is simple: to alleviate their psychological distress. Psychological suffering is also a form of illness; this is an essential truth that chest wall surgeons must understand.

In the past, surgical treatment of thoracic deformities has been constrained by many traditional views. Taking the most common condition, pectus excavatum, as an example, its surgical indications have been influenced by numerous factors. Existing literature has summarized the surgical indications for pectus excavatum, and many articles including so-called consensus statements and guidelines treat these summaries as mandatory rules to follow. The specific content is as follows [1]:

The surgical indications include meeting two or more of the following criteria: ①CT Haller index greater than 3.25. ② Pulmonary function tests indicating restrictive or obstructive airway disease. ③ Abnormal findings on EKG or echocardiography, such as incomplete right bundle branch block or mitral valve prolapse. ④ Progression of the deformity or the presence of clinical symptoms. ⑤ The appearance of the deformity is intolerable to the patient or their family. For a surgical procedure, establishing criteria like the above may seem rigorous and scientific. However, these standards do not withstand scrutiny. Let's start with the Haller index. Generally speaking, any indicator involving measured data is considered an objective metric. The Haller index has a standardized measurement method and is therefore an objective value. However, setting the cutoff at 3.25 is not a convincing figure, even before considering human factors that may affect the measurement. Setting this specific value as a surgical indication is, in itself, a highly subjective act. It reflects the personal opinion of one doctor being used as a standard for all practitioners. This approach lacks both scientific rigor and logical consistency and is therefore open to serious debate. Thus, no matter how objective the method or source for obtaining the Haller index may be, once a fixed number is used to determine the fate of a deformity, it plunges into the realm of subjectivity making such a value unconvincing [2]. Next, let's discuss the issue of pulmonary function parameters [3]. Pulmonary function testing is a very special examination that requires good patient cooperation. Without proper cooperation, the measured values become meaningless. Many patients with pectus excavatum are young children, and whether these children can cooperate effectively during the test is a matter worthy of discussion. For a special condition like pectus excavatum, especially considering that a significant portion of surgical patients are young children, relying on such tests as reference points inevitably raises questions about their reliability. While EKG and echocardiography indicators can be tentatively considered objective references, the assessment of deformity progression falls back into the realm of subjectivity. The progression of each deformity is not uniform; some may stabilize, others worsen, and some even improve. If doctors judge the direction of progression based solely on their own impressions, it becomes a purely subjective action with no objective basis.

Clinical symptoms themselves are the patient's subjective experience of the disease; they are purely subjective in nature. Using such symptoms alone to decide on surgery seems to conflict with the use of objective criteria. The final criterion, how the patient and their family perceive the deformity, is also inherently subjective, sharing the same nature as the other subjective indicators. Among the five criteria mentioned above, only EKG and echocardiography can be regarded as objective indicators; the other four are influenced by subjective factors. Since subjective factors are inherently human factors, and given their significant impact, it becomes very difficult to make truly objective decisions.

Moreover, the description of surgical indications specifically requires meeting "2 or more criteria 2," which further complicates and obscures these already vague standards. For example, if a patient has a very mild deformity but meets criteria 4 and 5 from the list above meaning the deformity is progressing or causing clinical symptoms, and the patient or family finds the appearance intolerable, but none of the other criteria are met, the patient feels unhappy with their appearance and strongly desires surgery. In such a case, is surgery justified? If the surgery is performed under these circumstances, it would almost certainly attract criticism based on the above criteria [4,5].

From this, it is clear that surgery for chest wall deformities is a unique type of operation; its distinctiveness lies in fully considering the special nature of these deformities. Take the example of pectus excavatum mentioned above: the patient has a mild deformity but wants surgery. Objectively speaking, this patient is not a strict "patient" in the medical sense, but rather a "normal person" dissatisfied with their body's appearance. Since they are not medically ill but simply unhappy with their appearance, if a chest wall surgeon still decides to perform surgery, then the procedure takes on an additional role, that of cosmetic surgery. The primary goal of chest wall surgery is first to treat disease, and secondly to perform reconstruction or reshaping. Both of these aims focus on addressing pathological conditions. However, once cosmetic concerns come into play, the target group becomes more complex. Chest wall appearance issues that are not classified as diseases inevitably become candidates for surgery. This situation differs from all other types of chest wall surgical diseases. In clinical practice, it is common to encounter patients with mild deformities who are not considered deformity patients by doctors but feel dissatisfied with their appearance and strongly desire surgery. From the perspective of disease, these individuals do not qualify for surgery. Yet, when cosmetic factors are involved, their desire becomes a legitimate request. Physicians should consider the patient's suffering from multiple perspectives not solely focusing on the physiological harm caused by the deformity.

When considering the surgical indications for chest wall deformities, an objective and rational approach is to evaluate two aspects of harm: 1. Whether it looks unsightly dissatisfaction with appearance that may not involve physical pain but causes psychological distress. Psychological distress is also a form of illness and requires treatment. If the patient cannot alleviate this mental suffering through other means, surgery is needed. In this case, the surgery can be either therapeutic or cosmetic. 2. Whether it causes discomfort indicating physical pain or symptoms. The presence of symptoms means the deformity is already affecting physiological function and thus requires treatment. In this situation, the surgery is therapeutic rather than cosmetic.

In summary, if a patient feels that their chest wall is unsightly or causes discomfort, surgery is needed. Conversely, if they do not feel dissatisfied with the appearance nor experience discomfort, surgery is naturally not necessary. This should be the most reasonable way to express the surgical indications for chest wall deformities. This approach places the decision-making power in the hands of the patient and their family, rather than the doctor making the final call. On the surface, this might seem to go against conventional medical logic, but upon closer examination, it actually aligns best with sound medical principles. Surgery is ultimately a decision made by the patient and their family; this is a basic truth. Throughout this process, doctors are not passive; their responsibility is to explain the objective medical condition from a professional standpoint, which does not conflict with the usual procedure for surgical decision-making in general diseases.

Among the various types of chest wall deformities, concave deformities may cause compressive symptoms. When considering surgical indications, it is often necessary to assess whether the patient experiences symptoms, that is, whether they feel discomfort. This is something doctors need to clearly communicate to patients. On the other hand, for convex deformities, since there is no compression involved, patients rarely have physical symptoms. Therefore, dissatisfaction with appearance becomes the patient's sole complaint. When encountering such patients, doctors must remain clear-headed and never assume that because these patients do not have symptoms, they are not "real" patients or don't need treatment. On the contrary, if the patient is distressed by the deformity, surgery is definitely warranted otherwise, it may lead to many problems.

When discussing the surgical indications for this special condition of chest wall deformities, it is especially important to emphasize the following specific point: ① the decision must not be influenced by traditional thoracic surgery concepts. Traditional thoracic surgery mainly deals with diseases inside the thoracic cavity, which are fundamentally different from chest wall deformities. The nature of these diseases, their harms, treatment goals, and methods all differ, so the considerations for surgical indications must be different. Chest wall surgery must have its own rules. ② Avoid absolutism. Chest wall deformities involve many subjective factors. Because of the numerous influencing factors, when considering surgical indications, each case must be analyzed specifically, avoiding rigid or absolute standards. ③ Fully consider contraindications. While performing surgery based on the patient's subjective wishes has its rationale, it is sometimes not feasible mainly due to surgical contraindications. When a patient's request exceeds the condition or technical feasibility, surgery cannot be performed. ④ Make decisions based on the individual. Each person's expectations for surgery vary, so the consideration of surgical indications should differ accordingly. When deciding on surgery, a one-size-fits-all standard cannot be applied. The patient's individual wishes must be fully considered to make a personalized decision. ⑤ Make decisions based on the specific deformity. Chest wall deformities are defined by abnormal shapes, and the appearance can vary widely. Mild deformities are often simple and feasible to operate on, but for very severe deformities, surgery is more difficult and outcomes are less ideal. If surgery is performed strictly based on the patient's wishes without considering these factors, the patient's expectations may not be met, and surgery could even fail. Thus, the unique characteristics of the deformity must be taken into account when considering surgical indications. ⑥ Make decisions based on the specific surgery. For any deformity, there is never only one surgical option, and each procedure has its limitations. When considering surgical indications, one should not focus narrowly on a single surgical method but take a comprehensive view. For example, in pectus excavatum, if only the Nuss procedure is considered, which uses a special steel bar to reshape the chest, very young patients may not tolerate it because the bar restricts chest growth. If the Nuss procedure were the only option, young patients would have no surgical indication. However, if the Wang procedure is considered, then younger patients have an opportunity for surgery and thus do have surgical indications.

2. Surgical Indications for Chest Wall Trauma

Chest wall trauma is a complex condition with a wide range of clinical presentations and severity. When considering surgery, it is necessary to fully take into account both the needs of the injury and the conditions for surgery. Because trauma cases are often urgent, doctors must make decisions within a short period of time, which places higher demands on the physicians [6].

Mild trauma can be treated conservatively, but severe trauma requires surgery. The surgical indications need to consider many specific factors: ① Whether surgery is necessary. Generally, open chest wall trauma is an absolute indication for surgery, while closed chest wall trauma requires case-by-case assessment to decide on surgery. for fractures, a single rib fracture without displacement of the fracture ends may not require surgery, but all other cases usually need surgical treatment. Sternum fractures also require consideration of the nature and extent of the fracture. If the fracture is completely detached or displaced, surgery is necessary; otherwise, it may not be. For a flail chest, surgery is definitely required once it occurs. ② Timing of surgery. Chest wall trauma is often critical; if conditions allow, emergency surgery is usually needed. For life-threatening injuries, surgery should be performed as quickly as possible. However, in some cases, if basic life support is lacking, surgery might be dangerous and the timing should be carefully assessed based on a comprehensive evaluation of the injury. ③ Surgical plan. Chest wall trauma is complex with diverse surgical methods. Emergency life-saving surgeries differ entirely from routine trauma surgeries. When considering surgical indications, the specifics of the surgical plan must be fully taken into account for the indications to be meaningful.

3. Surgical Indications for Chest Wall Tumors

The situation of chest wall tumors is also relatively complex. The general principle is that as long as surgical excision is feasible, the lesion should be removed first. However, in practice, some limitations, known as contraindications, must be considered. Surgery is generally not recommended if there are distant metastases or if the tumor locally invades vital structures. But this view is not absolute. For example, if the tumor is large and causes severe compression of the heart and lungs, seriously affecting the patient's respiratory and circulatory functions, surgical removal should be actively performed even if some contraindications exist. This essentially buys time for subsequent treatment; otherwise, the patient would have no hope of rescue.

Before performing the resection surgery, the specific surgical details must be evaluated. These details also impact the decision on surgical indications [7]. The first detail concerns the skin flap. If the tumor resection area is extensive, postoperative skin defect repair must be considered. The only method for repairing large skin defects is using skin flaps. However, obtaining a skin flap is also a surgical procedure, which directly affects the tumor surgery itself. Therefore, this must be fully considered when determining surgical indications. The second detail is the reconstruction of bony structures. Chest wall tumor surgery often requires resection of bony structures. After these structures are removed, reconstruction is necessary. Reconstruction requires special materials, and if these materials cannot be obtained or are unsatisfactory, it will affect the surgery's feasibility and must also be taken into account.

Tumor treatment has been a relatively active field in recent years, with many new methods and concepts applied clinically. Besides surgery, numerous other approaches have been proven feasible and advanced. Therefore, when considering surgery, it is necessary to make horizontal comparisons. If there are better methods available or if combining surgery with other methods can achieve better outcomes, these options should be fully considered. Of course, such considerations will inevitably influence decisions on surgical indications, but this does not negate the principles of chest wall surgery. As a newly emerging specialty, chest wall surgery should be more open to embracing new developments. This openness is not a denial of the chest wall surgery concept but rather highlights its distinctive characteristics.

4. Surgical Indications for Chest Wall Infections

Chest wall infection is a rather challenging condition to manage. The difficulty lies in the complex manifestations of the infection, which often require special methods for successful treatment. Acute infections are relatively simple to manage and can be treated with non-surgical methods. If control during the acute phase is inadequate and an abscess develops, incision and drainage are required. Clinically, the most common cases encountered are chronic infections, often secondary to incision infections following other chest surgeries. Such infections generally can only be successfully treated through reoperation and constitute an absolute indication for surgery. However, considering the particularity and difficulty of the operation, adequate preparation must be made before the operation, especially choosing the right time for the operation, which is the only way to lay the foundation for the operation [8]. In addition, since infection may also involve the reconstruction of skin and bone structures, relevant technical details also need to be considered before the operation.

5. Surgical Indications for Chest Wall Defects

Chest wall defects are inherently complex conditions involving multiple issues that require analysis based on the specific circumstances. For small primary defects that only involve local bony structures without obvious paradoxical respiration, surgery may not be necessary. However, for larger primary defects accompanied by obvious paradoxical respiration and visible surface depressions affecting appearance, surgical treatment is required. If the defect is caused by radiotherapy following breast cancer surgery, surgery is mandatory [9].

When chest wall defects involve the skin, they can cause significant inconvenience to the patient's daily life. The surgical indications in such cases require comprehensive consideration. In most situations, the decision for surgery is relatively straightforward, but in some special cases, it can be difficult to determine. For example, in cases where chest wall defects are caused by radiotherapy for breast cancer and there is also tumor recurrence or metastasis to other sites, surgery would generally be considered contraindicated according to standard principles. However, if the impact of the defect on the patient's quality of life is fully taken into account, surgery may still be necessary.

Chest wall defect surgery shares certain commonalities with surgeries for chest wall tumors and infections. If reconstruction of the skin and bony structures is required, similar technical considerations must be taken into account, which will also influence the decision regarding surgical indications.

6. Determination of Surgical Indications

Medicine is an empirical science, and the valuable experiences summarized by predecessors are worthy of learning by later generations. However, experience is often subjective, and considering the constantly evolving nature of medical science itself, the actual value of experience needs to be discounted. Many clinical diseases have specified indications, which are documented in various places, making them overwhelming. Undeniably, these regulations come from the experience of predecessors and are worth learning and referencing. However, given the subjective components and the factors of disciplinary development, blind adherence is not advisable. This should be the basic awareness every clinician must have.

In recent years, various guidelines and consensus statements have proliferated, many of which include regulations on surgical indications. However, in terms of content, these regulations can never fully escape their subjective nature. Since they are inherently subjective, they should not be used as objective standards to rigidly constrain others' actions. This means that when considering whether to perform surgery, doctors must have their own bottom line and not rely solely on so-called guidelines. It is especially important to emphasize that chest wall surgery is a brand-new discipline. Although every disease originates from traditional thoracic surgery, a new perspective is needed for understanding. When this specialty is just starting, every chest wall surgeon must embrace a spirit of reform and not be bound by traditional thoracic surgery concepts. Only when everyone approaches this specialty with a completely new mindset can chest wall surgery truly break free from the traditional framework and forge a development path that belongs entirely to itself.

REFERENCES

[1] Zeng, Qi, Na Zhang, Maohuai Fan, et al. 2005. "Comparative Study of Nuss Procedure and Modified Ravitch Procedure." *Chinese Journal of Pediatric Surgery* 26 (8): 397–400.
[2] Wang, Wenlin. 2019. "Why Does the Haller Index Sometimes Cannot Accurately Reflect the Severity of Chest Depression?" *Chest Wall Deformity Surgery Expert*, May 24.
[3] Wang, Wenlin. 2020. "Is It Necessary to Perform Pulmonary Function Tests before Funnel Chest Surgery?" *Chest Wall Deformity Surgery Expert*, March 1.
[4] Wang, Wenlin. 2015. "Questioning the Indications of the NUSS Procedure." *Chest Wall Deformity Surgery Expert*, September 12.
[5] Wang, Wenlin. 2017. "Issues Regarding the Surgical Indications of Funnel Chest." *Chest Wall Deformity Surgery Expert*, September 25.
[6] Dogrul, B. N., I. Kiliccalan, E. S. Asci, et al. 2020. "Blunt Trauma Related Chest Wall and Pulmonary Injuries: An Overview." *Chinese Journal of Traumatology* 23 (3): 125–138.
[7] Sanna, S., J. Brandolini, A. Pardolesi, et al. 2017. "Materials and Techniques in Chest Wall Reconstruction: A Review." *Journal of Visualized Surgery* 3: 95.
[8] Torto, F. L., A. Monfrecola, J. Kaciulyte, et al. 2017. "Preliminary Result with Incisional Negative Pressure Wound Therapy and Pectoralis Major Muscle Flap for Median Sternotomy Wound Infection in a High-Risk Patient Population." *International Wound Journal* 14 (6): 1335–1339.
[9] Zhang, Chuansheng, Yukun Ye, Dong Wang, et al. 1999. "Greater Omentum Pedicled Transplantation and Contralateral Breast Skin Flap Transfer to Treat Radiation Ulcers of the Chest Wall." *Chinese Journal of Thoracic and Cardiovascular Surgery* 15 (1): 29–30.

The chest wall is located on the outer surface of the chest and is a special anatomical region or can be described as a unique anatomical structure. This structure has multiple functions, which can be summarized into two main aspects: first, physiological functions; second, maintaining a specific shape [1]. Chest wall surgical diseases primarily involve structural changes, and such changes inevitably lead to functional alterations. Therefore, chest wall surgical diseases have two main impacts: first, causing problems with related physiological functions; second, causing abnormalities in the appearance of the chest wall. Both outcomes are caused by chest wall surgical diseases, so to treat the disease, intervention must address both aspects. In other words, treatment must not only restore physiological function but also restore the appearance and shape. Restoring physiological function depends on eliminating the lesion, while restoring the appearance and shape relies on reconstructive surgery. This defines the two fundamental characteristics of chest wall surgery: disease treatment and cosmetic reconstruction (Figure 1-8-1) [2,3].

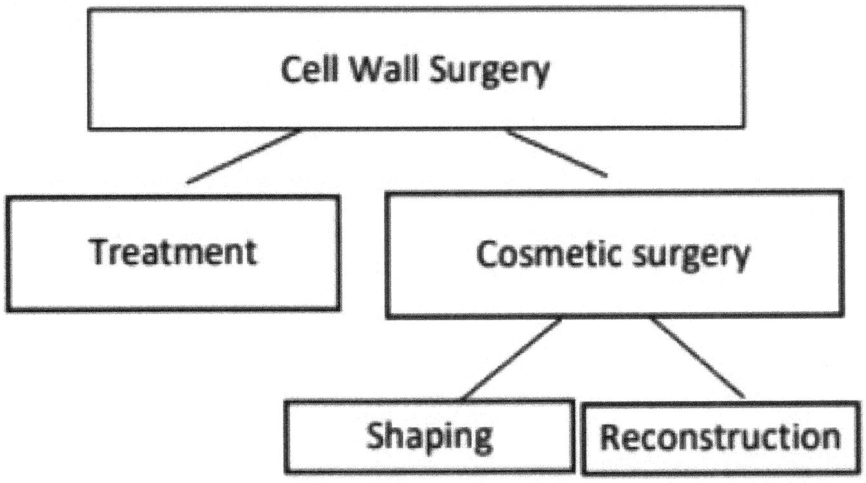

Figure 1-8-1 The nature of chest wall surgery

1. Therapeutic Nature

Chest wall diseases primarily manifest as lesions in specific areas. These lesions possess all the characteristics of surgical diseases and can include infections, deformities, trauma, defects, or even tumors. Since the lesions are clearly defined, the primary goal of treatment is to eliminate the lesion. The most direct way to achieve this is through resection of the affected tissue. However, this approach is only one option and, in certain special diseases, simple resection may not be the appropriate method.

Simple resection is suitable for diseases where the lesion itself poses serious harm. These diseases primarily include tumors and, secondly, infectious lesions. Tumors are the most appropriate for resection. Considering the particular nature of tumors, it is necessary not only to perform the resection but also to ensure that the resection is thorough. To achieve this goal, it is necessary to remove the tumor along with a certain margin of surrounding normal tissue. However, due to various objective reasons, complete resection may not always be achievable during the actual procedure [4]. For example, if the tumor is difficult to expose or has invaded important structures, only the widest possible resection can be performed rather than a complete one. In such cases, the treatment shifts from being curative to palliative. Although palliative treatment cannot completely achieve the goal of curing the disease, it can partially eliminate the harm caused by the tumor, buying time for subsequent treatments and laying a foundation. In this sense, it still falls under the scope of disease treatment.

Infectious diseases are also suitable for excision. Similar to tumor treatment, the ideal method is complete removal [5]. It is often very difficult to completely eliminate the infectious focus in terms of form, and although it is not impossible with effort, the harm caused by infectious lesions is sometimes intangible because the entire surgical field may be contaminated. In such cases, even if the lesion is removed, satisfactory results cannot be achieved without strict management measures.

Chest wall tumors and infectious lesions are suitable for excision, which is part of the treatment process. However, excision of the lesion means loss of chest wall structure. Considering the special functions of the chest wall, the missing structures need to be reconstructed. This adds more aspects to the treatment. This aspect is what will be discussed later as reconstruction [2,3].

Patients with chest wall defects are mainly characterized by the loss of chest wall structures. This loss may first involve the bony structures, and secondly, the skin and soft tissue. If there is skin and soft tissue loss, it may be accompanied by severe infection, in which case the treatment of infection becomes an additional part of the disease management. Besides treating the infection, a more important goal of treating the defect is to restore the integrity of the chest wall, which is part of the disease treatment. However, considering the appearance, another important task must also be accomplished, namely reconstruction.

Chest wall trauma is not a disease, but its outcomes are similar to those of diseases, only more acute and urgent. Therefore, it must also be treated as a disease, with a focus on curing the condition. The treatment includes thorough hemostasis, elimination of contamination, removal of necrotic tissue, and restoration of chest wall integrity [6]. The direct purpose of restoring chest wall integrity is to recover its physiological function, which belongs to the scope of disease treatment. However, there are different ways to restore integrity: it can be done without regard to appearance, or it can be done with a focus on achieving an aesthetically pleasing result. The latter clearly adds a new dimension, which is the reconstructive aspect.

Deformities, although abnormalities in the shape of the thorax, are still diseases within the scope of chest wall surgery. Therefore, the primary purpose of surgery for deformities remains treating the disease. This purpose is particularly prominent in surgeries for concave deformities. For example, in patients with severe pectus excavatum, one of the main goals of surgery targeting concavity is to relieve compression on the heart. This is part of disease treatment. There are various methods to relieve this compression. In the earliest surgeries, some surgeons completely removed the bony structures of the concave area; this was the simplest and most direct surgical method, with disease treatment as its sole goal, largely ignoring any concerns beyond curing the disease. Later on, surgeries began to address not only relieving compression but also improving the external appearance, thus adding a reconstructive aspect to the procedure. Other deformity surgeries also primarily serve the purpose of disease treatment. For example, in asphyxiating thoracic dysplasia (Jeune syndrome), the greatest harm is not the appearance but the fatal impact on respiratory and cardiac functions [7,8]. Even if surgery for such patients pays no attention to appearance, if it can restore normal cardiopulmonary function, it is considered a successful operation. The five types of chest wall surgical diseases are all real diseases; therefore, surgeries targeting any of these diseases primarily have the attribute of treating the disease. However, there are two situations that are prone to controversy. The first situation involves surgeries performed solely for cosmetic reasons when the deformity is not severe. This case seems difficult to associate with disease treatment. In fact, upon careful analysis, it still falls within the scope of disease treatment. Anyone undergoing surgery due to cosmetic concerns, even if their thoracic deformity is mild, still has a deformity that is, they still have a disease. Therefore, their surgery also possesses the attribute of disease treatment. The second situation involves individuals with a completely normal chest wall shape who undergo surgery solely to achieve a chest appearance that satisfies them. Such individuals do not have any meaningful deformity of the chest wall and therefore do not fall within the category of disease. Since it is not a disease, the surgery seemingly lacks the attribute of treating a disease. This is essentially a purely cosmetic surgery. However, from a broader perspective, since the patient has this desire, it indicates that the shape of the chest wall has become a psychological issue. A psychological issue is also a form of illness and similarly requires attention as a type of disease. If conservative methods cannot provide treatment, surgery becomes the only option. Since this too is for treating an illness, the surgery naturally also possesses the attribute of disease treatment.

Among the two situations mentioned above, the second situation is very extreme. Since chest wall corrective surgery is not a routine procedure and requires considerable cost, there are not many "healthy individuals" willing to change their chest wall shape through this method. However, such cases do occur in clinical practice. Especially some female patients may seek surgery due to various personalized demands. For these individuals, if the desire is strong, surgery can be considered. Nevertheless, it is undeniable that this situation often requires more advanced techniques, and simply relying on general chest wall deformity surgical methods makes it difficult to achieve good results. This has become a driving force for the continuous improvement of chest wall surgery techniques and also represents the direction in which chest wall surgery needs to strive.

2.The Nature of Reconstruction

Chest wall surgical diseases have a unique nature, affecting not only physiological function but also aesthetics. This requires that surgery, while treating the disease, must also take into account the postoperative appearance of the chest wall, thus giving the surgery a reconstructive attribute. Reconstructive surgery originally falls under the domain of plastic surgery, where various reconstructive techniques are already quite mature. Chest wall surgery also involves reconstructive elements. This aspect emerged alongside the development of chest wall surgery and is therefore a relatively new field. While it can draw on the mature experience of plastic surgery, it must have its own characteristics. In chest wall surgery, the goal of reconstruction is very clear: to restore the normal shape of the chest wall as much as possible. The normal shape of the chest wall is related not only to physiological function but also to aesthetic considerations, making reconstruction a particularly important part of treating chest wall surgical diseases. According to the different purposes and methods of reconstruction, the specific procedures can be divided into two types: shaping (molding) and rebuilding (reconstruction). These two fundamental operations form the complete system of reconstructive surgery [3].

(1) Shaping

Shaping surgery is designed to correct deformities of the bony structures. It involves using various specialized techniques to eliminate abnormal shapes and restore the normal contour of the chest wall. According to different surgical techniques, shaping operations can be divided into three basic types: destructive shaping, mechanical force shaping, and template shaping [9-11]. Destructive shaping achieves its goal by thoroughly damaging the deformative structures. In earlier years, chest wall deformities were almost exclusively corrected using this type of surgery. Typical examples of destructive shaping are the Ravitch procedure and the sternal turnover surgery. The principle of this type of surgery is similar to a complete overhaul of a car: the deformity is thoroughly destroyed first, followed by correction. Destructive shaping causes significant damage and is not an ideal surgical method. In the early years of chest wall deformity treatment, such surgeries were quite common. Nowadays, for some particularly severe deformities, if other surgical methods fail to achieve satisfactory results, destructive shaping must be employed. Otherwise, its use is rare. Mechanical force shaping refers to surgeries that indirectly change the deformity using special materials, with the Nuss procedure as a representative example. Template shaping is represented by the Wang procedure [12] and the Wenlin procedure [13]. Both surgeries correct deformities by using templates. Mechanical force shaping and template shaping cause significantly less trauma, so they are called minimally invasive surgeries. These two approaches are currently the mainstream surgical methods for correcting deformities.
Although there are only three basic types of shaping surgeries, there are many specific methods. Generally, using a single surgical approach can basically meet the needs of deformity correction. However, in some special deformity cases where a single surgery cannot independently complete the operation, combining different types of surgeries can often achieve unexpected and better results.

Shaping is a method designed to correct deformities of the bony structures. Besides primary thoracic deformities, it can also address secondary deformities. Secondary deformities may be caused by surgery, trauma, intrathoracic diseases, and other factors [14]. Fundamentally, the basic surgical techniques do not differ in essence. When a rib fracture occurs with displacement, resulting in local shape changes, this altered bony structure can cause a specific type of thoracic deformity, which also falls under secondary deformities. The goal of fracture surgery is to restore the normal shape of the bone, and restoring the shape equals eliminating the deformity. Therefore, fracture fixation surgery itself is also considered a shaping surgery, and in terms of its nature, it should be classified as template shaping.

Shaping surgery mainly targets the bony structures, aiming to achieve a basically normal thoracic appearance, but it does not involve detailed aesthetic considerations. If these aesthetic details are taken into account, more meticulous work is needed. Currently, the approach is quite limited, mostly involving some special treatment of the incision. Overall, the aesthetic demands of shaping surgery are not very strict; as long as a normal or near-normal shape is achieved, the surgical goal is considered met, without higher requirements. However, some patients come seeking surgery primarily for cosmetic reasons and therefore have higher expectations for shaping surgery. This adds a special attribute to shaping surgery, the cosmetic aspect. Thus, shaping can be divided into different levels: the basic level aims to restore a normal appearance, while the advanced level focuses on aesthetics, i.e., cosmetic improvement.

The goal of cosmetic improvement goes beyond general shaping and places higher demands on the surgery. These demands come from two aspects: first, the aesthetic appearance of the entire thoracic contour, and second, the cosmetic outcome of the skin incision. The aesthetic contour of the thorax must fully consider the patient's expectations. For example, some patients with a prominent sternum angle aim solely to reduce it. In such cases, a lower sternum angle represents the patient's standard of beauty. Other patients may be troubled by protruding rib arches; if surgery can successfully eliminate such defects, it also achieves a cosmetic effect. The cosmetic outcome of the skin incision involves many factors, among which it is important to make the incision as small and as hidden as possible. Additionally, during suturing, cosmetic techniques should be employed whenever possible. This represents the higher level of shaping surgery focused on aesthetics.

In actual practice, when the cosmetic aspect is considered alongside the shaping procedure, it can bring patients a pleasant surprise. However, many surgeons fail to achieve this level of care. For example, in choosing the incision, some incisions are made too casually, manifesting as arbitrary incision locations, uncontrolled lengths, and careless suturing methods. When a surgeon does not pay attention even to these basic details, it is hard to imagine they would be meticulous about the shaping of the bony structures. This inevitably affects the overall shaping outcome. Therefore, only by always keeping the cosmetic aspect in mind can the shaping results be more satisfactory and achieve better outcomes.

The emergence of cosmetic considerations may cause a shift in the nature of the surgery. As mentioned above, the treatment of chest wall surgical diseases primarily has a curative purpose. However, once cosmetic procedures are incorporated into the surgery, the target of treatment may change individuals with a normal chest wall shape who simply wish to alter their chest contour might join the ranks of surgical candidates. Superficially, cosmetic improvement appears to be the sole purpose of such surgery, but in reality, the surgery still retains its curative attribute. As noted earlier, this is a treatment of the “disease of the mind.”

(2) Reconstruction

During the treatment of chest wall diseases, many procedures involve defects in the chest wall structure. Resection of chest wall tumors and removal of infectious foci both leave defects. Chest wall defects themselves are defects, and in cases of severe chest wall trauma, large-area defects may occur. The chest wall has important physiological functions, and the performance of these functions relies on an intact structure. When defects occur, the integrity of the chest wall structure is compromised, leading to serious functional problems, which in severe cases may even threaten the patient’s life. Therefore, any disease with defects requires chest wall reconstruction. This is the most basic guarantee for treating such diseases [15].

Defects can involve bony structures as well as the skin and soft tissues. To reconstruct these structures, surgery must include two components: reconstruction of the chest wall’s bony structure and reconstruction of the skin and soft tissues. Ideal reconstruction fully restores the original structures, not only requiring the reconstructed structures to be as close to normal in shape as possible but, more importantly, to possess normal physiological function. This places very high demands on reconstructive surgery.

The essence of reconstructive surgery is to restore the original structure of the chest wall. Given that the original structure is already deficient, it is necessary to repair the defective parts using other materials. Therefore, the core issue of reconstructive surgery is the choice of materials. However, due to limitations of these materials, achieving a perfect reconstruction is very difficult. To accomplish the basic goals of reconstruction, clinicians often have to adhere to lower standards in practice.

From the perspective of reconstructing the bony structure, a lower standard of reconstruction aims to provide the chest wall with sufficient strength and rigidity while minimizing abnormal breathing, all while considering the appearance as much as possible. This type of reconstruction basically meets the needs of treating the disease and also takes into account the goal of cosmetic restoration. However, this is not an ideal reconstruction. A higher-level reconstruction should balance both aspects: achieving effective disease treatment while also obtaining a more satisfactory structure. Such a structure should have a normal shape on one hand and good functionality on the other. With continuous advancements in the development of various materials, the level of reconstruction is steadily improving. Nevertheless, there is still a long way to go to fully meet both of these requirements.

Currently, there are many materials available for clinical reconstruction, each with its own characteristics. However, not all materials can achieve perfect reconstruction results. In recent years, digital materials have appeared in clinical practice; their greatest feature is personalized design, which has made the shape of bony structures increasingly satisfactory [16]. On this basis, if the properties of these materials can be further improved to enable the reconstructed chest wall to possess more physiological functions, reconstruction surgery will become even more satisfactory.

Reconstruction of skin and soft tissue poses significant challenges. The real difficulty lies in obtaining suitable reconstruction materials. Ideally, artificial materials would be used, but such materials are still unavailable to date, making autologous materials the only viable option. However, this means that sufficient material must be harvested from other parts of the body.

This procedure may seem to conflict with the nature of reconstructive surgery. Nonetheless, to address the greater aesthetic issues caused by chest wall defects, making some aesthetic sacrifices in less visible areas does not contradict the overall reconstructive goals. In clinical practice, materials for skin and soft tissue reconstruction come from various flaps. The design and operation of these flaps require specialized knowledge and skills. This work traditionally falls under the domain of plastic surgery. If thoracic surgeons are not very familiar with these techniques, it is best to seek the assistance of plastic surgeons when performing related procedures. Overall, reconstructive surgery is also an important aspect of thoracic wall surgery, and the quality of reconstruction directly affects the success or failure of the operation. However, the reconstructive surgery in thoracic wall surgery is not the same concept as plastic surgery. The latter may pay less attention to functional issues and focus mainly on appearance, which differs significantly from thoracic wall reconstruction that combines both disease treatment and functional restoration. For example, in the treatment of pectus excavatum, plastic surgery may focus solely on correcting the depression, completely ignoring the disease aspect of pectus excavatum. Under this approach, plastic surgery might simply fill the concavity to achieve a very good appearance, but this is purely cosmetic and not curative. In fact, the presence of fillers may worsen the bony depression and increase pressure on the thoracic organs, leading to more severe disease. Similarly, in the treatment of Poland syndrome, if a patient has depression on one side of the chest wall with complete loss of soft tissue, plastic surgery often uses implants to perform breast augmentation, which can achieve a good appearance. However, such an approach can also exacerbate the chest wall depression, making it difficult to say that it is aimed at treating the disease.

Thoracic wall surgery possesses both therapeutic and reconstructive attributes; these two properties are independent yet deeply integrated. This means that within the reconstructive attribute, there is a therapeutic aspect, and within the therapeutic attribute, there is also a reconstructive aspect. Take surgery for pectus excavatum as an example: the therapeutic attribute refers to eliminating the depression's compression effects, but the depression itself is the shape that reconstructive surgery aims to correct. Therefore, the operation to remove the depression simultaneously carries reconstructive properties. Similarly, reconstructive procedures often include therapeutic elements. For instance, in Jeune syndrome, the abnormal appearance of the thorax is mainly caused by depressions on both sides of the chest wall [7,8 . When reconstructive surgery is performed to correct this deformity, it must eliminate these depressions, which are the root cause of symptoms. Hence, such surgery also has therapeutic properties.

From the above analysis, it can be seen that any thoracic wall surgery is essentially a unity of both therapeutic and reconstructive purposes, with different surgeries emphasizing one aspect over the other [2]. When the disease causes significant impairment of physiological function, the therapeutic function should take precedence; conversely, if there is no serious physiological dysfunction, greater attention should be given to reconstruction.

REFERENCES

[1] Wang, Wenlin. 2021a. "Thoracic Wall Surgery: Basic Structure and Function of the Thoracic

Wall." Jinri Toutiao, October 31.
[2] Wang, Wenlin. 2021b. "Basic Nature of Thoracic Wall Surgery." Jinri Toutiao, October 31.
[3] Wang, Wenlin. 2021c. "Thoracic Wall Surgery: Shaping and Reconstruction." Jinri Toutiao, October 31.
[4] Thomas, M., and K. R. Shen. 2017. "Primary Tumors of the Osseous Chest Wall and Their Management." *Thoracic Surgery Clinics* 27 (2): 181–193.
[5] Keum, D. Y., J. B. Kim, and C. K. Park. 2012. "Surgical Treatment of a Tuberculous Abscess of the Chest Wall." *Korean Journal of Thoracic and Cardiovascular Surgery* 45 (3): 177–182.
[6] Barata, R., C. Rodrigues, A. R. Costa, et al. 2020. "Chest Wall Trauma Surgery Review." *Revista Portuguesa de Cirurgia Cardiotorácica e Vascular* 27 (2): 83–89.
[7] Wang, Wenlin, Weiguang Long, Chunmei Chen, et al. 2021. "Surgical Treatment of Asphyxiating Thoracic Dysplasia." *Chinese Journal of Thoracic and Cardiovascular Surgery* 28 (8): 984–989.
[8] Wang, W. 2022. "Surgical Treatment of a 36-Year-Old Patient with Asphyxiating Thoracic Dysplasia." *Interactive Cardiovascular and Thoracic Surgery* 34 (1): 153–155.
[9] Wang, Wenlin. 2019a. "Three Basic Forms of Thoracic Deformity Surgery." *Thoracic Deformity Surgery Expert*, September 24.
[10] Wang, Wenlin. 2019b. "Mechanical Issues during Shaping Procedures." *Thoracic Deformity Surgery Expert*, October 6.
[11] Wang, Wenlin. 2019c. "Technical Key Points of Template Shaping." *Thoracic Deformity Surgery Expert*, October 7.
[12] Wang, W. L., C. M. Chen, W. G. Long, et al. 2018. "Wang Procedure: Novel Minimally Invasive Procedure for Pectus Excavatum Children with Low Age." *Case Reports and Images in Surgery* 1 (1): 1–2.
[13] Wang, Wenlin. 2021d. "Two Cases of Severe Pectus Excavatum Were Treated with Wenlin Procedure Today." *Thoracic Deformity Surgery Expert*, January 18.
[14] Wang, Wenlin. 2021e. "Secondary Thoracic Deformity." *Thoracic Deformity Surgery Expert*, September 21.
[15] Corkum, J. P., P. B. Garvey, D. P. Baumann, et al. 2020. "Reconstruction of Massive Chest Wall Defects: A 20-Year Experience." *Journal of Plastic, Reconstructive & Aesthetic Surgery* 73 (6): 1091–1098.
[16] Liu, Y., W. Wang, W. Long, et al. 2021. "Chest Wall Reconstruction with Digitally Designed Materials for Straight Back Syndrome with Tracheal Stenosis: A Case Report." *Annals of Translational Medicine* 9 (16): 1357.

Section 9

RISKS OF CHEST WALL SURGERY

The risks of surgery are a complex issue. When discussing surgical risks, it is first necessary to understand what risk actually means, and only then consider the magnitude of the risk. The essence of surgical risk should be understood on three levels: First, understanding the nature of surgical injury. As long as there is any injury, it should be regarded as a risk. This is the most general understanding of risk. Second, understanding the potential harm to the functions of vital organs. This is a relatively serious risk, primarily referring to severe consequences caused by injury to vital organs. Thirdly, there is the risk to life itself, which is the greatest risk of all. The three levels of risk differ in concept and severity of harm. To analyze them clearly, discussion must be conducted separately for each level. However, due to the complexity of influencing factors and the lack of unified measurement standards, it is almost impossible to thoroughly discuss them. Therefore, in the following content, the basic meaning of risk will be understood as harm, mainly referring to serious injuries. This is also what most patients and their families are concerned about. To accurately understand the risks of surgery, it is essential to recognize two fundamental characteristics of risk: first, the absoluteness of risk, and second, the relativity of risk [1]. The absoluteness of risk means that risk is ubiquitous: every surgery carries some risk. The relativity of risk indicates that risks vary in magnitude, and the presence of risk depends on certain conditions. Different conditions lead to different levels of risk. A thorough understanding of these two attributes of risk plays a positive role in conducting clinical work.

1.The Absoluteness of Risk

Every surgery has two sides: one is the attribute of curing disease, and the other is the attribute of trauma. Since trauma inevitably causes harm, this constitutes the content of risk. Therefore, as long as a surgery is performed, there will inevitably be risk. Risks are unavoidable and cannot be completely eliminated, which is why risk is absolute. The absoluteness of risk is related to certain special factors, including: ① Factors inherent to the disease itself; ② Factors related to the surgical design; ③ Factors related to medical conditions. The existence of these factors determines that risk can never be entirely eliminated, hence its absolute nature.

(1) Influence of disease-inherent factors on the absoluteness of risk

Each disease has its own characteristics, which directly or indirectly determine the magnitude of the surgical risk. The characteristics related to risk include the following aspects: the location and size of the lesion, the relationship between the lesion and surrounding structures, and the malignancy of the disease itself.

(1) The location of the lesion determines the absoluteness of the surgical risk. Lesions in certain critical areas affect the structure and function of organs. When performing surgery on these lesions, damage to the organs is unavoidable, thus constituting an absolute risk. For example, lesions in the lungs. If the lesion is extensive and requires a large-scale resection, lung function will inevitably be impaired. This damage is determined by the nature of the lesion itself, leaving no room for reversal, so the risk is absolute. The same applies to lesions in other important organs, such as the heart, brain, or major blood vessels. As long as surgery is performed in these areas, risk inevitably exists. This is a key factor determining the absolute risk of surgery. In chest wall surgery, tumors located near the central part of the anterior chest wall, if deeply invasive, may be adjacent to the heart and major blood vessels. Especially when these tumors invade these vital organs, the risk becomes an absolute risk that cannot be eliminated. The greatest harm of concave chest wall deformities is the compression of the heart and lungs. When the concavity is extremely severe, no matter what surgery is performed, it may affect the heart [2]. The specific damage may be direct injury to the heart or impact on the heart's rhythm; severe arrhythmias also carry significant risk. Therefore, the risk of such surgeries is absolute and cannot be eliminated by human factors. The lesions in asphyxiating thoracic dysplasia (Jeune syndrome) are located in multiple areas, almost all surrounding the heart. Every surgical procedure targeting these lesions may affect the heart, which determines that surgeries for this disease carry a very high risk [3,4]. Chest wall defects caused by postoperative radiotherapy for breast cancer often involve the full thickness of the chest wall, and in severe cases, may even result in a completely open thoracic cavity. Such lesions, due to their special location, are inherently very dangerous. Performing surgery in these cases is even more risky, making this risk absolute [5], and it cannot be completely eliminated by human factors. Surgery for incision infections following cardiac surgery is always considered high-risk. The fundamental reason for this understanding lies in the special location of the lesion. Because the incision is adjacent to the heart and major blood vessels, and the blood circulation in the surrounding chest wall is poor, such surgeries are considered extremely high-risk both in terms of surgical safety and surgical outcomes [6].

Although the locations of chest wall diseases are generally more superficial, the deep structures beneath are various important intrathoracic organs. This anatomical relationship determines that chest wall surgery inevitably carries risk. From this perspective, the risk of chest wall surgery is absolute. This risk does not disappear due to changes in surgical methods or techniques.

(2) The size of the lesion determines the absolute risk of surgery. Small lesions require a limited resection range, so the risk is not excessive. However, for larger lesions, the risk is absolutely present and cannot be eliminated due to subjective factors. For example, some giant tumors, even if benign, carry significant surgical risk. Such lesions can actually be seen in many locations, For example, giant tumors within the thoracic cavity that sometimes occupy the entire chest cavity. It is impossible to remove such lesions without risk. There are often large tumors on the chest wall as well. Removing these tumors requires addressing many specific issues, such as bleeding control, damage to intrathoracic organs, and postoperative chest wall reconstruction. All of these are critical concerns that directly affect the success or failure of the surgery, so the surgery carries significant risk as well.

for special conditions like thoracic deformities, the size of the lesion can be understood as the severity of the deformity. Mild deformities involve simpler surgeries and carry less risk. However, severe deformities carry absolute risks [7]. For example, surgeries for extremely severe pectus excavatum. To completely correct the deformity, the surgery itself involves multiple risks, such as the risk of surgical failure, the risk of complications, and even life-threatening dangers. These risks define such surgeries as having absolute risk.

(3) The relationship between the lesion and surrounding structures determines the absolute risk of the surgery. If there are important structures around the lesion and their relationship is not clearly defined, it will also bring absolute risk to the surgery. For example, in thoracic surgery, cancers located in the lung apex (superior sulcus tumors) involve many important structures beneath the clavicle. This area is recognized as a high-risk zone, so surgeries in this region carry absolute risk [8]. Certain chest wall tumors may also be located near this area. For example, tumors occurring in the 1 rib are situated close to these important structures, so the risk is absolutely present, and any surgical technique used for removal carries risk. Another very typical example of absolute risk in chest wall surgery is the risk associated with reoperation after a failed pectus excavatum surgery. In such patients, the chest wall is extensively adhered to the heart, and there is generally no space between the two. for these patients, no matter which surgical method is used, there is always a risk of

injuring the heart [9]. The situation for pectus excavatum surgery after heart surgery is basically the same; due to the presence of adhesions, the risk cannot be eliminated and is therefore also an absolute risk.

(4) The malignancy degree of the lesion determines the absolute risk of surgery. In chest wall surgery diseases, there are many malignant chest wall tumors. Some tumors have a very high degree of malignancy, are highly invasive, and prone to recurrence. The risk of performing surgery on such tumors goes without saying. Besides malignant tumors, some benign tumors also carry risks. For example, some large hemangiomas, although benign, can cause massive bleeding during surgery, and thus can be considered a type of malignant-like lesion in terms of risk. Naturally, surgery for these lesions carries significant risk, and this risk is absolute; it cannot be completely eliminated due to human factors.

(2) The Impact of Surgical Design on the Absoluteness of Risk

Some surgical designs inherently avoid important organs, providing good exposure without risking damage to these vital structures. Naturally, such surgeries do not carry significant risk [10]. However, some surgical designs are always centered around important organs, making exposure difficult and increasing the possibility of damaging vital structures. Such surgeries undoubtedly carry great risk [11]. As long as these surgeries are performed, risk is inevitable. This is a key manifestation of the absoluteness of risk.

The most typical example of absolute risk in chest wall surgery is the Nuss procedure [11]. Before the advent of this surgery, all operations were performed through relatively long incisions on the anterior chest wall. Although these incisions caused greater trauma, they allowed the procedure to be performed under direct vision. For a skilled surgeon, causing heart injury during such surgeries was almost unimaginable. This means that previous surgeries were relatively safe. However, after the Nuss procedure was introduced into clinical practice, because the operation must be performed close to the surface of the heart and cannot be done under direct vision, the risk of the surgery increased significantly, making risk the most prominent feature of this procedure (Figure 1-9-1). This risk is almost inseparable; no matter how skilled the surgeon is, they must face the risk whenever performing this surgery.

After the Nuss procedure was officially introduced, it quickly attracted widespread attention due to its relative simplicity, ease of operation, and especially the appealing label of being "minimally invasive." However, the risk of damaging the heart has become a critical flaw of this procedure. Many thoracic surgeons are even reluctant to perform the surgery because of this risk.

This is also the fundamental reason why the procedure has not been widely adopted. In order to minimize the risk of heart injury as much as possible, many doctors have been working on various modifications to the technique. However, all these efforts have proven to be of little effect, as no method can completely eliminate the risk. This highlights that, for a specialized procedure like the Nuss surgery, the risk of heart injury is an absolute risk as long as the surgery is performed, the risk cannot be entirely avoided.

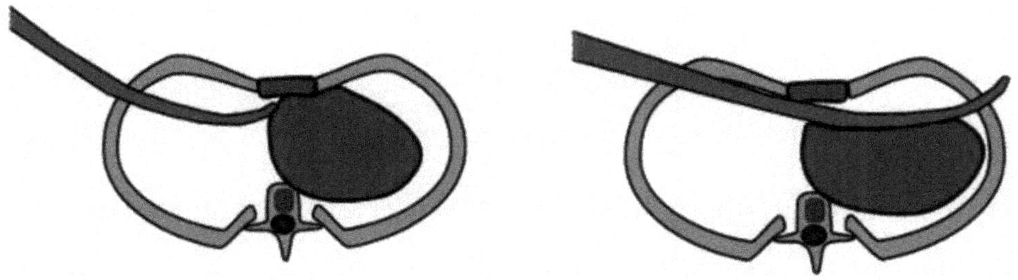

Figure 1-9-1 Risk of the Nuss Procedure

(3) The Impact of Medical Conditions on the Absoluteness of Surgical Risk

The successful completion of any surgery requires certain basic conditions as support. If these fundamental conditions are lacking, the surgical risk increases significantly. These conditions are objective and not caused by human factors, so the resulting risks are also objective and indeed absolute. As long as these conditions remain unchanged, the risks cannot be completely eliminated.

After years of development, thoracic surgery has finally entered the era of thoracoscopic surgery. Today, almost all thoracic procedures rely on the use of a thoracoscope to be completed. The excessive reliance on thoracoscopic equipment has made its quality a decisive factor in determining the level of surgical risk. If the quality is poor, it can compromise the clarity of the visual field. When operating on critical blood vessels, substandard equipment can introduce life-threatening risks. Today, many surgeons rely on thoracoscopic assistance when performing pectus excavatum (funnel chest) surgeries. If the thoracoscope is of poor quality, the surgical risks become self-evident. Therefore, the objectivity of medical conditions determines the absoluteness of the risk. Such risks cannot be eliminated simply by a surgeon's exceptional skill or performance.

In addition to standard surgical instruments and equipment, the overall medical conditions of a hospital can also introduce absolute risks. Any surgery is a complex, systematic process that involves not only the surgical procedure itself but also preoperative preparation, postoperative monitoring, rehabilitation, and more. If any part of this process goes wrong, it can affect the outcome of the surgery and introduce significant risks.

The clearest example of how medical conditions impact surgical outcomes is heart surgery. If there are issues with the level of preoperative examinations, the diagnosis may be inaccurate, which becomes the greatest risk factor. If the technology for cardiopulmonary bypass during surgery is not advanced enough to provide a safe and stable environment for the operation, the surgical risk is obvious.

Moreover, the lack of proper postoperative monitoring can cause risks to arise at any time. This clearly shows that the quality of medical conditions directly determines the success or failure of heart surgery. If the overall medical conditions are problematic, surgeries performed under such conditions carry systemic risks, that is, absolute risks.

When discussing the risks associated with medical conditions, it is important to emphasize the risk of anesthesia, which is a concern that can arise in any hospital. In clinical practice, the term "anesthesia accidents" is often mentioned, and such accidents represent absolute risks. Like surgery, anesthesia is administered by doctors, but the overall level of anesthesia care reflects the objective medical conditions of a hospital. High-quality anesthesia is associated with relatively lower risks, while lower-quality anesthesia can pose significant dangers. Therefore, the crucial fact to remember is that as long as surgery is performed regardless of the type of anesthesia used the risk of anesthesia always exists and can never be completely eliminated. This, in turn, constitutes an absolute risk of the surgery itself. The absoluteness of risk serves as a reminder that every surgery carries inherent risks. Regardless of the specialty, the disease, or who performs the procedure, risks are always present. Although chest wall surgeries are generally more superficial and carry relatively lower risks, they are not risk-free, and these risks cannot be completely eliminated by the efforts of doctors. For this reason, clinicians in their practice should approach every surgery with a cautious, "walking on thin ice" mindset. Only by doing so can the risks be minimized to the lowest possible level.

2. The Relativity of Risk

The relativity of risk refers to the varying degrees of risk that appear when comparing different situations. Although surgical risks objectively exist and can never be completely eliminated, in many cases the level of risk is relative and influenced by numerous factors.

(1) The Impact of Professional Specialization on the Relativity of Risk

In clinical practice, different specialties involve surgeries on different anatomical areas and of different natures, resulting in varying levels of risk. This risk refers to the overall risk associated with the specialty, rather than any specific surgery. Generally speaking, cardiac surgery and neurosurgery are widely recognized as high-risk procedures. Thoracic surgery, because it involves operating near major blood vessels and close to the heart and other vital structures, is also considered high-risk. In contrast, general surgery and orthopedics surgery tend to carry lower risks and are regarded as relatively safer procedures.

Chest wall surgeries involve more superficial and well-exposed areas and do not typically involve many vital organs, so they are considered relatively safe procedures. Their risks are significantly lower than those of general thoracic surgeries and even lower than those of cardiac and neurosurgeries. However, if these surgeries involve operations on deeper structures, the risks should not be underestimated. Comparing surgical risks across different specialties reflects the characteristics of each specialty and provides a general indication of surgical risk. Such comparisons effectively illustrate the relativity of risk.

(2) The Impact of a Doctor's Personal Habits on the Relativity of Risk

A doctor's habits primarily refer to their surgical techniques, which influence the choice of surgical approach. Since the surgical method itself affects the level of risk, these habits directly impact the overall surgical risk. For example, when performing pectus excavatum surgery, some doctors prefer the Nuss procedure, while others favor the Wang procedure. Clearly, the different habits of these surgeons result in different levels of risk. Even with the same surgical procedure, different operating habits can lead to varying levels of risk. Taking the Nuss procedure as an example, some surgeons prefer to use thoracoscopic assistance during the operation. This habit helps provide better visualization of the mediastinum, which theoretically can reduce risk. However, simply using thoracoscopic assistance does not necessarily guarantee that the thoracoscope will be effectively utilized. In some extreme cases, even with thoracoscopic assistance, the surgical site may remain unclear. In such situations, the risk can actually increase. On the other hand, some surgeons prefer not to use Thoracoscopy. To manage risks, these doctors develop a complete set of techniques for passing the steel bar safely. The use of these techniques can significantly improve safety and noticeably reduce risk. A surgeon's operating habits are often reflected more in the finer details of basic procedures, such as how bleeding is managed. Some doctors have a habit of immediately using hemostatic clamps when they see bleeding. This approach carries significant risk because if the clamp is applied to a vulnerable structure, it may not only fail to stop the bleeding but also cause more serious damage. Such situations can occur in any medical specialty. On the other hand, doctors with better habits will first apply pressure to the bleeding site, wait until the surgical field is clear, carefully assess the bleeding, and then take appropriate measures. This approach is far more effective at reducing risk. Overall, a doctor's operating habits are a strong reflection of their ability to manage risks. Good habits can effectively help avoid risks, while poor habits may lead to increased dangers.

(3) The Impact of a Doctor's Skill Level on the Relativity of Risk

Skill level is a relatively broad concept that can be understood as a doctor's overall ability to manage a specific surgical procedure. for the same surgery and the same operation, differences in a surgeon's skill level result in varying degrees of safety and surgical outcomes. Therefore, a doctor's skill level directly determines the level of surgical risk. [12, 13].

Take the Nuss procedure as an example: for a skilled surgeon, placing the steel bar is a basic operation with relatively low risk. However, if a doctor lacks adequate skill, they may struggle even to complete the placement of the steel bar, clearly resulting in a much higher surgical risk.

A doctor's skill impacts surgical risk in many specific ways. For example, the risk of complications, the risk of surgical failure, and even life-threatening risks are all directly related to the surgeon's expertise. Like many other surgeries, chest wall surgeries often have various potential complications. Take the Nuss procedure, for instance, where the risk of steel bar displacement is a common complication. The fundamental cause usually lies in the surgeon's skill level. If the surgeon does not fully understand the surgical principles and operates blindly, it can result in poor fixation or incorrect placement of the steel bar, making displacement much more likely. The Nuss procedure also has many other complications, such as bilateral chest wall constriction and incision infections, which are also closely related to the surgeon's skill. In clinical practice, cases of surgical failure are frequently encountered, and a careful analysis of the causes often reveals clues pointing to issues with the surgeon's technique. Technical shortcomings of the surgeon increase the risk of surgical failure. When it comes to life-threatening risks, these are even more closely tied to the surgeon's skill. For example, in the Nuss procedure, if the placement of the steel bar is not performed skillfully, accidental injury to the heart can cause immediate death. This represents the most severe risk directly resulting from a surgeon's lack of expertise.

(4) The Impact of Patient Factors on the Relativity of Risk

Besides factors related to the surgeon, the relativity of surgical risk is also influenced by the patient. During surgery, patients are generally seen as passive recipients, and it may seem that surgical risks are unrelated to them but in reality, this is not the case. In clinical practice, the choice of surgical method is often not decided solely by the doctor; sometimes, the decision-making power lies with the patient. For example, in pectus excavatum surgery, some patients may request the Nuss procedure, while others may prefer the Wang procedure. The patient's choice directly affects the level of surgical risk. Additionally, patients often make decisions about the materials and instruments used during surgery. Different materials and instruments vary in safety, which also influences surgical risk. For example, in the Nuss procedure, the steel bars used can differ: some have notched ends, while others have completely smooth edges. Because of these design differences, the surgical risks vary as well. If a patient insists on using a steel bar with notched ends, it will undoubtedly increase the risk of the surgery significantly.

The relativity of surgical risk is primarily influenced by human factors. Understanding the role of these factors is crucial for reducing surgical risks. From a doctor's perspective, this objectively requires abandoning bad habits and continuously improving their skill level [13]. For patients, the first step is to choose a good doctor. Secondly, they should cooperate with and support the doctor's work as much as possible. Only by doing so can the surgery be safer and achieve better outcomes.

In summary, the risks associated with chest wall surgery objectively exist. For thoracic surgeons, maintaining strong risk awareness at all times is essential. With this awareness comes a sense of urgency, which enables surgeons to approach every operation with utmost seriousness. At the same time, risk is relative; the level of risk can be influenced and changed by human factors. As long as chest wall surgeons continuously improve their skills, they can effectively manage and minimize risks, achieving better surgical outcomes.

REFERENCES

[1] Wang, Wenlin. 2021a. "Surgical Risk Index." *Thoracic Deformity Surgery Specialist*, July 19.

[2] Rachwan, R. J., A. K. Purpura, and B. M. Kahwash. 2018. "Sudden Cardiac Arrest in a Young Patient with Severe Pectus Excavatum." *American Journal of the Medical Sciences* 356 (6): 570–573.

[3] Wang, Wenlin, Weiguang Long, Chunmei Chen, et al. 2021. "Surgical Treatment of Asphyxiating Thoracic Dysplasia." *Chinese Journal of Thoracic and Cardiovascular Surgery* 28 (8): 984–989.

[4] Wang, W. 2022. "Surgical Treatment of a 36-Year-Old Patient with Asphyxiating Thoracic Dysplasia." *Interactive Cardiovascular and Thoracic Surgery* 34 (1): 153–155.

[5] Rouanet, P., J. M. Fabre, V. Tica, et al. 1995. "Chest Wall Reconstruction for Radionecrosis after Breast Carcinoma Therapy." *Annals of Plastic Surgery* 34 (5): 465–470.

[6] Jones, G., M. J. Jurkiewicz, J. Bostwick, et al. 1997. "Management of the Infected Median Sternotomy Wound with Muscle Flaps: The Emory 20-Year Experience." *Annals of Surgery* 225 (6): 766–778.

[7] Frantz, F. W. 2011. "Indications and Guidelines for Pectus Excavatum Repair." *Current Opinion in Pediatrics* 23 (4): 486–491.

[8] Kawai, N., T. Kawaguchi, M. Yasukawa, et al. 2017. "Less Invasive Approach to Pancoast Tumor in a Partitioned Incision." *Annals of Thoracic and Cardiovascular Surgery* 23 (3): 161–163.

[9] Wang, Wenlin. 2021b. "Risks and Outcomes of Secondary Surgery after Failed Pectus Excavatum Surgery." *Thoracic Deformity Surgery Specialist*, May 5.

[10] Wang, Wenlin. 2021c. "The Wang Procedure Is a Safe Minor Surgery." *Thoracic Deformity Surgery Specialist*, January 24.

[11] Wang, Wenlin. 2021d. "Why Does the Heart Still Get Punctured during Nuss Procedure under Thoracoscopy?" *Thoracic Deformity Surgery Specialist*, June 3.

[12] Wang, Wenlin. 2021e. "How to Make Pectus Excavatum Surgery Safer?" *Thoracic Deformity Surgery Specialist*, July 16.

[13] Wang, Wenlin. 2021f. "Safety of the Wang Procedure." *Thoracic Deformity Surgery Specialist*, April 24.

Chest wall surgery has two fundamental aspects: disease treatment and reconstruction, with reconstruction further divided into reshaping and rebuilding [1]. As introduced earlier, whether reshaping or rebuilding, the use of certain specialized materials is essential to complete the surgery; these materials form the foundation for a successful operation. Due to the need for a large number of specialized materials, chest wall surgery differs significantly from intrathoracic surgery. From one perspective, chest wall surgery is more akin to orthopedics surgery of the chest wall [2]. Because almost all chest wall diseases involve bony structures, when compared with traditional orthopedics diseases, they seem essentially similar. This represents another characteristic of chest wall diseases. From the perspective of orthopedics, nearly all surgeries involving bony structures require the use of materials. Therefore, when chest wall surgery also involves the treatment of bony structures, the issue of materials becomes a major concern for the entire discipline. This is the biggest difference between chest wall surgery and traditional thoracic surgery.

1. Reshaping Materials

Reshaping materials are primarily used in corrective surgeries for deformities, with the purpose of eliminating the abnormality. The use of these materials is often temporary; once the bone shape has been satisfactorily restored, the materials become unnecessary and need to be removed from the body.

(1) Nuss Procedure Steel Bar

The Nuss procedure is a typical example of mechanical external force reshaping. A notable feature of this surgery is the use of specialized materials to indirectly reshape the affected area [3].

It is no exaggeration to say that the surgical materials are the primary guarantee for the success of the Nuss procedure, so the materials must be meticulously designed. To date, various materials have been used clinically, with the most widely used being the standard steel bar for the Nuss procedure [4]. This type of steel bar was first used clinically and has been in continuous use ever since. Overall, it meets the basic requirements of the surgery, but its shortcomings have been increasingly recognized over time. As a result, many improved steel bars have been designed and applied in clinical practice. The Nuss procedure steel bar was specifically designed for pectus excavatum surgery and is therefore primarily limited to this operation. However, as understanding of other deformities deepened, this steel bar has also been widely used in surgeries for other deformities, playing a greater role.

(1) Classic Nuss Procedure Steel Bar

The classic Nuss procedure steel bar consists of two parts: the main steel bar and the fixation plates at both ends of the main steel bar (Figure 1-10-1) [4]. The main steel bar is a thin, strip-shaped piece of steel available in different sizes to meet various surgical needs. The edges of the middle section of the main bar are smooth and even, while both ends are rounded. Near the ends, the two edges feature serrated notches. The purpose of the serrated notch design is to facilitate the fixation of the steel bar. However, because the steel bar must be placed beneath the depressed area of the anterior chest wall by passing over the surface of the heart, the presence of the serrated notches causes significant inconvenience. These notches can not only potentially tear mediastinal structures during placement of the steel bar but also cause damage when removing the steel bar. Additionally, the presence of serrated notches makes the operation significantly more difficult. The fixation plate is a small device that fits over the main steel bar at a perpendicular angle. Once placed inside the body, because the fixation plate is positioned perpendicularly to the main steel bar, it fits precisely over the ribs. This position not only provides support to the main steel bar but also offers effective fixation. In theory, the fixation plate is a good design; however, in practical operation, this design has many issues. First, the direction of the ribs is not always parallel to the main steel bar. Since they are not parallel, the fixation plate which is perpendicular to the main steel bar cannot be perfectly perpendicular to the ribs. If the fixation plate is not perpendicular to the ribs, placing it on the rib surface will compromise the stability of the steel bar. If the steel bar is unstable, the fixation effect will be compromised, which may ultimately lead to serious complications due to poor fixation. Second, the fixation plate has a certain thickness and volume. For young pediatric patients, due to the lack of sufficient soft tissue around the incision area, the fixation plate may lie directly beneath the skin when suturing the incision, which is unfavorable for wound healing. Many patients who undergo Nuss procedures experience incision infections or poor healing, often related to the presence of this fixation plate. Third, the existence of the fixation plate prevents the incision from being very small. The fixation plate itself has a certain length, and to connect and secure it to the main steel bar, a relatively large operating space is often required. This is especially true when two or even three steel bars need to be placed, which further increases the required incision length. Therefore, it is difficult to complete the operation through a small incision. Since its introduction, the Nuss procedure has been promoted as a minimally invasive surgery, one of whose characteristics is small incisions. However, in practice, the incision for the Nuss procedure is sometimes not small. Besides the surgeon's skill, the presence of the fixation plate is a direct cause of longer incisions.

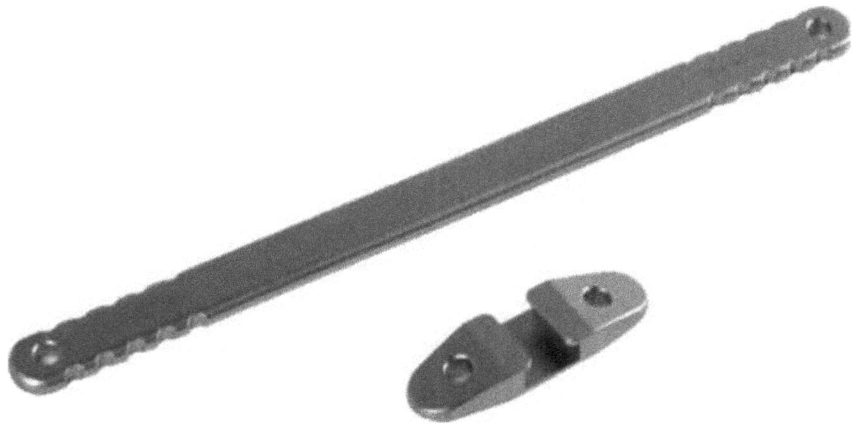

Figure1-10-1 Classic Nuss Procedure Steel Bar. The main steel bar has notches at both ends, originally designed to facilitate fixation, but these notches may cause damage when passing through the mediastinum. The short steel bar is the fixation plate, specifically used to secure the main steel bar. This design is overly idealistic and may bring various drawbacks in practical use.

(2) Improved Nuss Procedure Steel Bar

The drawbacks of the classic Nuss procedure steel bar are obvious. To eliminate these drawbacks, some improved steel bars have gradually been designed. For example, a well-known steel bar was designed by a Korean doctor, Park. This steel bar still consists of two parts: the first part is the main steel bar, and the second part is the end fixation device (Figure 1-10-2) [5]. The main steel bar completely eliminates the drawbacks of the classic Nuss procedure steel bar by adopting a fully straight edge design without the notched ends. This makes the placement and removal of the steel bar safer and easier. The end fixation device adopts a very ingenious design, consisting of two "L"-shaped fixing plates, a "T"-shaped screw, and a nut. During use, the fixing plates clamp onto the ribs, securing the steel bar firmly to the ribs. Because the "L"-shaped plates have a rectangular hole with a wide range of movement and adjustable direction, they can accommodate rib fixation from any angle. Therefore, theoretically, this

design is quite ideal. However, this type of steel plate still has issues, mainly related to the fixation devices at both ends. First, installation of these devices can sometimes be difficult. Since the fixation device is installed after the main steel plate is placed, and at that time the main steel plate may be tightly pressed against the ribs, properly securing the fixation device is not always easy. Second, sometimes the fixation effect of the plate is not satisfactory. Although the fixation plate design theoretically accounts for various fixation possibilities and should pose no problems or difficulties, the actual operating environment often prevents the fixation device from functioning perfectly. If the procedure is not performed optimally, it will affect the overall stability of the steel plate. Third, the fixation device may also negatively impact the healing of the surgical incision. The fixation device is cleverly designed, but it still has a certain thickness and size. If there isn't enough soft tissue around the patient's incision, it may hinder proper healing. Additionally, installing the fixation device requires specialized instruments, which limits the plate's widespread use.
Both the classic Nuss procedure plate and the modified Park plate consist of a main plate and fixation devices at both ends, but the fixation devices may lead to various issues. Therefore, the design of the fixation plate is the most critical issue in pectus bar procedures. However, considering the problem from a different perspective, eliminating these fixation devices and modifying the fixation method could avoid these drawbacks. Based on this reasoning, we have never used fixation plates in any of our surgeries. Instead, we developed the Wung procedure [6] for pectus excavatum and the Wenlin procedure [7] for pectus carinatum, both of which involve direct fixation of the main bar to the ribs. This design not only overcomes the disadvantages of fixation plates but also achieves superior surgical outcomes.

In addition to Park's modified plate, various specialized plates have been designed by different surgeons in clinical practice. Each of these plates features unique design innovations addressing different surgical requirements. For instance, a single-port minimally invasive plate has been developed with Beyond Park's modified plate; numerous innovative plate designs have emerged in clinical practice. Various surgeons have developed specialized plates with distinct characteristics, each incorporating unique design improvements. One notable example is a single-port surgical plate featuring an innovative T-shaped configuration - with a tapered tip at one end, a curved central body, and a perpendicular short fixation plate at the opposite end [8]. When using this specially designed plate, the surgical procedure involves inserting the tapered end through a single chest wall incision to reach the deepest point of the pectus deformity. The plate is then advanced across to the contralateral intercostal space before being rotated to elevate the depressed chest wall, followed by final fixation. This entire process requires only a single access port, hence being termed a single-port procedure. Despite its ingenious design, the technique carries significant operative risks, which has substantially limited its widespread clinical adoption.

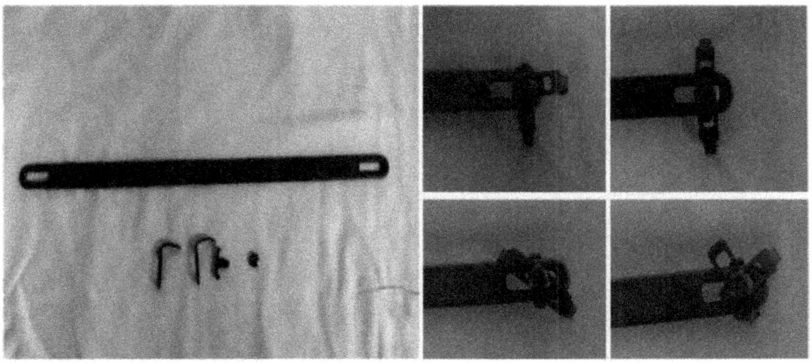

Figure 1-10-2 The modified Park plate. The smooth edges at both ends of the main plate effectively overcome the drawbacks of the classic Nuss procedure bar. The ingeniously designed fixation device allows for stable fixation in any required orientation

In addition, there is another type of steel plate in which the plate and the introducer are integrated into a single design, located at the end of the entire device. When the introducer pulls the steel plate into the bottom of the anterior chest wall depression, the introducer can be removed, and the steel plate can then be fixed directly [9]. This design is quite ingenious, especially because it eliminates the need to flip the steel plate, thereby avoiding unnecessary injuries. However, this design also has several drawbacks. First, the length of the steel plate is limited and cannot meet the needs of all surgeries for depressed deformities.

Second, the fixation devices at both ends of the steel plate are still designed vertically, and the effectiveness of this type of fixation is limited. Third, both the placement and removal of the steel plate require special equipment, which also limits the widespread use of the plate. Fourth, the curvature of the steel plate is fixed and cannot be adjusted during surgery according to shaping needs, thus limiting its shaping function; some deformities cannot be treated with this type of steel plate.

Apart from the above-mentioned designs, there are also other types of steel plates, each with its own supposedly meaningful design. However, the most widely used one remains the classic Nuss procedure steel plate. The reason why this type of steel plate is more widely accepted may be primarily due to the influence of being the first to be introduced, in addition to certain limitations in product manufacturing and sales.

(2) Wang Surgical Steel Plate

After the invention of the Wang surgical procedure, we initially used the steel plate from the Nuss procedure. During the actual operation, the plate was inserted through a small midline incision onto the surface of the bony structures of the chest wall [10]. Because there was only a single incision, the placement procedure was somewhat difficult and could potentially cause unnecessary injury. What was particularly troublesome was that removing the steel plate became even more challenging. This compelled us to come up with a more ideal design, leading to the development of a specialized steel plate. This became the steel plate we routinely used later on. The basic design concept of this steel plate was to divide a single, integrated plate into two parts, with a connecting section in the middle that could be secured with screws. During placement, each part was inserted through the central incision into the tunnels on both sides of the chest wall, and then connected and fixed in the middle. This design effectively overcame the difficulty of placing a long steel plate through a single incision. When removing the steel plate, it only requires loosening the screw in the middle, allowing both parts of the plate to be easily taken out through the midline incision. This makes the plate removal procedure extremely simple. This steel plate has several additional advantages: ① Both ends of the plate adopt a flat design without notches, making placement and removal very convenient, with no difficulties and no possibility of complications or risks ; ②The ends of the plate are designed with tongue-shaped edges, gradually narrowing and thinning at the tips. This design reduces resistance during insertion and makes removal easier ; ③The central connecting section features a special embedded design that ensures a secure connection without increasing the local thickness, which is beneficial for postoperative wound healing ; ④The connection is fixed using a single screw, making the operation extremely simple without adding complexity to its use.

From a theoretical perspective, the Wang procedure is a surgery with many advantages. However, without a specially designed steel plate, the procedure would be difficult to perform, and its benefits would not only fail to be realized but could also lead to unnecessary complications due to issues with the plate. The advent of the specially designed steel plate has not only fully demonstrated the various advantages of the original design but also brought about greater convenience. Therefore, this steel plate represents a very ideal design.

(3) Various Rib Fixation Plates

Chest wall trauma is one of the main conditions treated in chest wall surgery. Among chest wall injuries, one important category is various types of fractures Fracture surgery also falls within the scope of reconstructive procedures. The fundamental method in fracture surgery is fixation, which requires special fixation materials, and these materials also need to be introduced. Fractures involving the chest wall primarily include rib fractures, costal cartilage fractures, and sternal fractures. Currently, there are approximately three types of products used clinically for rib fractures: The first is memory alloy products, the second is titanium alloy products, and the third is the Matrix RIB system (Figure 1-10-3). The design of memory alloy products takes advantage of the shape memory properties of certain special alloys. In a low-temperature environment, the alloy becomes soft and can be shaped as needed.

Figure 1-10-3 The MatrixRIB system features different designs for the left and right sides, with varying curvatures to meet surgical needs. Additionally, it includes straight plates, which can be used for the sternum or operations on certain special areas. This material can be used not only for the fixation of rib or sternal fractures but also widely for the reconstruction of the bony structures of the chest wall, making it a valuable surgical material.

However, once the temperature rises to normal body temperature, the alloy hardens and forcibly returns to its originally designed shape. At this point, the shape is exactly the optimal form for rib fixation. This product is ingeniously designed, easy to operate, and does not require special instruments, and it has already been widely used in clinical practice. Titanium alloy products feature a clamping-type structure, using tooth-like extensions at both ends of the main plate for fixation. During the fixation process, forceps with different angles are required to clamp and secure the material. Since the forceps must be specially made, and different types are often needed during the same surgery, a large amount of surgical instrument preparation is necessary. This undoubtedly limits the use of the material. The Matrix RIB plate is similar to orthopedics plates and requires nails and screws to be directly fixed to the ribs [11]. Since the plate is designed to match the natural shape of the ribs, it better meets physiological requirements. In addition, the plate has a moderate thickness and a cross-sectional physiological curvature. This design ensures a perfect fit between the steel plate and the rib, ultimately achieving an ideal fixation effect. However, this material also has its own drawbacks, the main one being that special instruments are required to perform the surgery. This undoubtedly limits the widespread use of the material.

Costal cartilage fractures are a very special type of fracture, and there is some controversy regarding their fixation. As a result, there are currently no specially designed products for this purpose. When fixation is necessary, a commonly used method is to employ fixation plates designed for rib fractures. However, since costal cartilage is relatively brittle, special techniques are required during the fixation process.

Sternal fractures are a relatively special type of fracture. Although there are many kinds of fixation products available, none have gained widespread acceptance. The fundamental reasons can be summarized into three main aspects: ① Difficult Operational: The direction of sternal fractures is mainly transverse, which is perpendicular to the long axis of the sternum. In theory, this type of fracture should be relatively easy to fix. However, due to the uneven surface of the sternum and interference from the costal cartilage on both sides, the fixation procedure becomes quite challenging. ② Plates Are Too Thick: The steel plates currently used in clinical practice are relatively thick. Since there is little soft tissue in front of the sternum, it is difficult to adequately cover the plate. If the plate is not well covered, it may affect wound healing. ③ Unsatisfactory Outcomes: Because the sternal surface is uneven, it is hard for the fixation plate to closely conform to it. Poor conformity leads to poor fixation results.

Due to the many shortcomings of steel plates specifically designed for sternal fractures, their clinical use has not been ideal. In our clinical practice, we have found that the Matrix RIB plate is actually a very suitable alternative for sternal fractures. The specific method involves placing and securing two or three Matrix RIB plates side by side across the fracture line, which can achieve a very satisfactory fixation effect.

The development of products for fracture treatment has always been a highly active field, and in recent years, the research and development of products related to chest wall fracture surgery has continued to advance. One of the more recent trends is the use of rib fixation materials under thoracoscopic guidance, currently based on memory alloy designs. This design is quite ingenious and relatively convenient to use; however, in practical application, there are still many issues that need further improvement.

(4) Other Materials

In addition to the materials mentioned above, many other materials are also used in clinical practice for reconstructive surgery. For example, the most traditional Kirschner wires are still used in some primary-level hospitals today. As previously mentioned, chest wall surgery can be considered the orthopedics of the thoracic region. Since it shares characteristics with orthopedics, a wide range of orthopedics materials can be applied clinically. Orthopedics is an ancient discipline with extensive experience in the development of various materials. Once orthopedics concepts are applied to the development of materials for chest wall surgery, a large number of advanced materials are expected to emerge, ultimately transforming the current state of chest wall surgical materials.

2. Reconstructive Materials

Reconstructive materials are primarily used for chest wall reconstruction. In many cases involving chest wall surgical conditions, defects are often present. To repair these defects, various types of reconstructive materials are required. There are two main categories of reconstruction: One category is the reconstruction of bony structures, and the other is the reconstruction of skin and soft tissues. Correspondingly, the materials used should also fall into these two categories. At present, the clinical research and development of materials for skin and soft tissue reconstruction is not very satisfactory. Therefore, when referring to reconstructive materials, it mainly refers to materials for bony reconstruction. Reconstructive materials and shaping materials share certain similarities but also have significant differences. The main distinctions are as follows: ① the purposes of use are different. Shaping materials are used to correct the shape of bony structures and serve a supportive role. Reconstructive materials, on the other hand, are used to replace bony structures and play a direct, structural role. The fundamental purposes of the two functions are different.

Leading to differences in the various properties of the materials. ② the physical properties of the materials are different. Shaping materials are used to alter the shape of bones, so they must possess high hardness and strength. Reconstructive materials, on the other hand, are only required to restore the normal shape and function of the chest wall, so their hardness and strength do not need to be as high as those of shaping materials. ③ the shapes of the materials are different. Shaping materials are used to modify bony structures, functioning similarly to a "tool." Such materials do not need to match the shape of normal human bony structures. However, the goal of reconstruction is to replace normal structures with materials, so their shape must closely resemble that of the natural structure as much as possible. ④ the final purpose of the materials is different. The mission of shaping materials is to restore the shape of bony structures. Once this goal is achieved, their role is complete. Therefore, in most cases, such materials need to be surgically removed afterward. In contrast, the mission of reconstructive materials is to serve as a permanent part of the body's structure. This role is lifelong, so reconstructive materials should not be removed. From the above comparison, it is clear that reconstructive materials are a very specialized type of surgical material. An ideal reconstructive material should not only possess a normal structure but also closely resemble the original in terms of performance and function; this represents the highest standard for reconstructive materials. However, due to limitations in manufacturing processes and other practical constraints, achieving such materials is not easy. In fact, many reconstructive materials currently used in clinical practice fall far short of these standards, which undoubtedly affects surgical outcomes. Nevertheless, in order to carry out surgery under existing conditions and provide patients with the most basic level of treatment, these materials still have to be used.

(1) Digital Materials

Digital materials are a special concept proposed by us [12,13]. The core technology of such materials is digital processing. Because digital processing is involved in every step of the material's fabrication process, we refer to them as "digital materials."

The process of obtaining digital materials requires specific steps (Figure 1-10-

4). First, imaging examinations are conducted on the patient to collect data on both the lesion site and the normal chest wall. Second, based on the collected data, a three-dimensional simulation of the lesion and the entire chest wall is created. Third, the surgical resection range is designed on the 3D image. Fourth, according to the planned resection range, the shape and size of the

Data Collection	Conduct CT and other examinations to obtain data in specific formats.
Image Simulation	Simulate a 3D image of the lesion and surrounding structures based on the data.
Surgical Simulation	Simulate the surgical resection on the 3D image to determine the location and extent of the area that needs reconstruction.
Material Design	Design the shape and size of the material.
Material Manufacturing	Fabricate the material using different processes

Figure 1-10-4 Main Steps for Obtaining Digital Materials

Among the overall steps, the first four are basically fixed and are mainly completed through collaboration between doctors and engineers. The fifth step varies depending on the manufacturer. Some manufacturers obtain materials through 3D printing technology; thus, such materials are also called 3D printed materials [14]. Other manufacturers use CNC machining to process the materials, and these materials are referred to as custom-made materials (Figure 1-10-5). Regardless of the processing method used, all these materials possess the attributes of digital materials and are therefore considered digital materials.

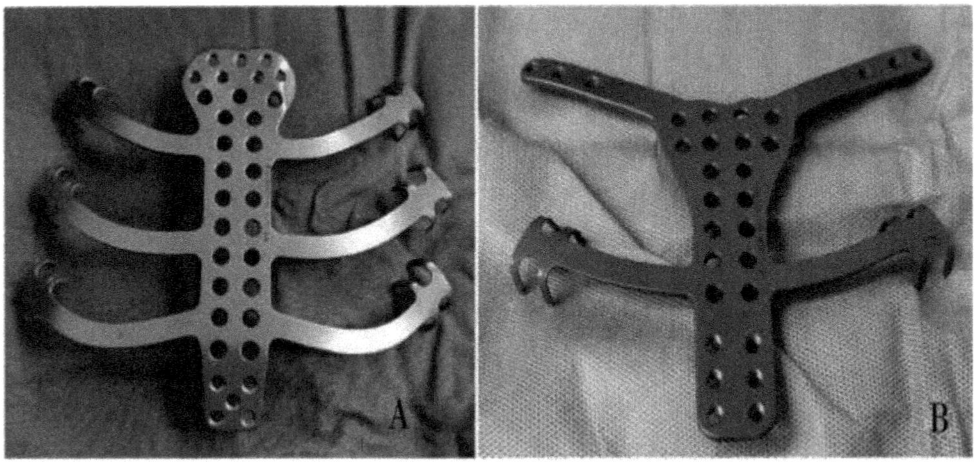

Figure 1-10-5 Customized materials, which are designed and fabricated according to the lesion and the actual surgical requirements. Ideal materials can have the advantage of personalized design, but the materials actually produced often find it difficult to fully meet the surgical needs. Achieving true personalization remains a significant challenge.

The greatest advantage of digital materials is personalized design. Since the data come directly from the patient's lesion, and the final material is precisely fabricated based on that data, the material has distinctive personalized characteristics that can maximally meet the needs of the surgery. However, digital materials also have inherent drawbacks. These drawbacks include: ① the fabrication process is complicated and time-consuming. Digital materials are not off-the-shelf; they can only begin to be made after the patient is admitted, and generally require several working days to complete. The long fabrication time often causes significant inconvenience to clinical workflow. ② the process requires full involvement of the physician. From data acquisition to the successful final design of the material, every step requires the doctor's participation, which consumes a large amount of the physician's effort. ③ Although the design is strictly personalized, due to the difficulty in establishing professional tacit understanding between engineers and clinicians, the fabricated product often cannot fully meet surgical needs, greatly diminishing the advantages of personalization.

Digital materials, as a new concept in clinical practice, were originally considered relatively ideal reconstructive materials. However, various shortcomings have limited their widespread use. To overcome the disadvantages of digital materials, some other types of materials have gradually gained attention. Currently, the materials under development are mainly standardized components, designed with the original intention of creating ready-made parts that can be temporarily assembled during surgery according to reconstruction needs. This approach can address some of the difficulties encountered in acquiring digital materials, and if designed properly, can meet the personalized needs of surgery. However, no matter how perfectly the materials are designed, it is still difficult to achieve complete personalization Additionally, because these modular materials need to be assembled intraoperatively, surgery time may be extended. Besides newly developed materials, the functions of some existing materials continue to be explored, For example, MatrixRIB, whose reconstructive advantages have been increasingly recognized.

(2) Matrix RIB

The original design intention of Matrix RIB was for rib fracture fixation. However, because its shape closely resembles ribs, and it has sufficient length and a reasonable curvature, along with good elasticity, it can also be used for reconstructive surgery of rib defects. Currently, there are no other reconstructive materials clinically available that resemble ribs in shape, making Matrix RIB the only choice. Theoretically, digital materials can be used for reconstruction at all sites, but considering the various shortcomings in the processing of digital materials, such materials are not suitable for rib reconstruction.

In addition to rib reconstruction, Matrix RIB can also be used for sternal reconstruction. Although this reconstruction cannot restore the appearance of the sternum, it can maintain the functional integrity of the thoracic cage. If Matrix RIB is designed properly, very satisfactory results can be achieved, with outcomes comparable to or even better than the standardized materials mentioned above.

(3) Other Materials

Apart from the two types of materials mentioned above, a large number of other materials have been used clinically. These include acrylic glass, bone cement, titanium mesh, and various patches. The common characteristic of these materials is that they only focus on defect reconstruction without considering the shape and function of the bony structures within the defect. Because of this, various shortcomings are obvious, and these materials have gradually been replaced when more reasonable alternatives become available.

In theory, reconstructive surgery is a highly demanding procedure because its goal is to restore normal anatomical structures. However, in actual practice, due to limitations of available materials, reconstructive surgeries often fall short of ideal outcomes. Although the emergence of digital materials has significantly improved the quality of reconstructive surgery, there is still a long way to go before fully achieving the goal of restoring normal structures.

REFERENCES

[1] Wang, Wenlin. 2021a. "Basic Nature of Chest Wall Surgery." *Today's Headlines*, October 31.

[2] Wang, Wenlin. 2021b. "Related Issues of Chest Wall Tumors." *Today's Headlines*, October 31.

[3] Wang, Wenlin. 2019a. "Three Basic Forms of Thoracic Deformity Surgery." *Thoracic Deformity Surgery Expert*, September 24.

[4] Nuss, D., R. J. Obermeyer, and R. E. Kelly. 2016. "Nuss Bar Procedure: Past, Present, and Future." *Annals of Cardiothoracic Surgery* 5 (5): 422–433.

[5] Yoo, G., J. Shin, E. Y. Rha, et al. 2020. "Quadrangular Fixation of Pectus Bars to Prevent Displacement in Nuss Procedure." *Thoracic and Cardiovascular Surgery* 68 (1): 80–84.

[6] Wang, Wenlin. 2021c. "Safety of the Wing Procedure." *Thoracic Deformity Surgery Expert*, April 24.

[7] Wang, Wenlin. 2021d. "Two Severe Pectus Carinatum Women Surgeries Today." *Thoracic Deformity Surgery Expert*, January 18.

[8] Tao, Qilin, Bing Jia, Xiangang Yan, et al. 2016. "Single-Incision Modified Nuss Procedure for Correction of Pediatric Pectus Excavatum." *Chinese Journal of Minimally Invasive Surgery* 16 (2): 127–130.

[9] Li, Guoqing, Ju Mei, Fangbao Ding, et al. 2013. "Preliminary Clinical Experience with the Newly Improved NUSS Procedure." *Chinese Journal of Pediatric Surgery* 34 (7): 493–496.

[10] Wang, W. L., C. M. Chen, W. G. Long, et al. 2018. "Wang Procedure: Novel Minimally Invasive Procedure for Pectus Excavatum in Young Children." *Case Reports and Images in Surgery* 1 (1): 1–2.

[11] Ramponi, F., G. T. Meredith, C. Bendinelli, et al. 2012. "Operative Management of Flail Chest with Anatomical Locking Plates (MatrixRib)." *ANZ Journal of Surgery* 82 (9): 658–659.

[12] Wang, Wenlin. 2019b. "Broad and Narrow Definitions of Digital Materials." *Thoracic Deformity Surgery Expert*, November 23.

[13] Liu, Y., W. Wang, W. Long, et al. 2021. "Chest Wall Reconstruction with Digitally Designed Materials for Straight Back Syndrome with Tracheal Stenosis: A Case Report." *Annals of Translational Medicine* 9 (16): 1357.

[14] Wang, L., L. Huang, X. Li, et al. 2019. "Three-Dimensional Printing PEEK Implant: A Novel Choice for Reconstruction of Chest Wall Defect." *Annals of Thoracic Surgery* 107 (3): 921–928.

Surgery is an invasive treatment method. While it aims to achieve therapeutic goals, it also inevitably causes some degree of tissue damage. Although such damage is harmful to the human body, a certain extent of trauma is an unavoidable and therefore justifiable cost of surgery. In addition to acceptable surgical trauma, additional or unintended injuries may occur in clinical practice; these are referred to as complications. Chest wall surgery primarily involves operations on the chest wall itself. If all procedures were limited strictly to the chest wall, the types and frequency of complications would be minimal. However, because chest wall surgery often involves structures within the thoracic cavity, complications related to intrathoracic organs frequently occur. This is a relatively distinct characteristic of chest wall surgical procedures.

1. Bleeding

Bleeding is the most common complication. According to the severity of bleeding, it can be divided into: Massive bleeding, Moderate bleeding, Minor bleeding. Massive bleeding generally refers to a large volume of blood loss occurring in a short period of time. It mainly occurs when the heart or major blood vessels are injured. Chest wall surgery primarily involves operations on the chest wall, and generally does not affect the heart or major blood vessels. However, some special procedures may involve these structures. For example, in the Nuss procedure for pectus excavatum, the placement of the steel bar is performed over the surface of the heart. If the procedure is not done carefully, it may lead to massive bleeding. This is considered the most serious complication in chest wall surgery [1]. In most Nuss procedures, such complications can be avoided by paying close attention to operative details. However, some special cases remain exceptions such as extremely severe pectus excavatum, failed previous Nuss surgeries, and pectus excavatum following cardiac surgery. These patients are considered high-risk, with a significantly increased chance of cardiac injury [2,3]. In addition to the Nuss procedure, other chest wall surgeries may also cause massive bleeding. For instance, during resection of large, highly vascularized chest wall tumors, massive bleeding can occur. Moreover, some tumors located in special regions of the chest wall may invade major blood vessels. For example, tumors in the upper chest wall may involve the subclavian vessels. If surgical handling is not adequate, this may also lead to massive bleeding [4].

Among the many blood vessels in the chest wall itself, the larger one is the internal thoracic artery. Injury to this vessel can also lead to a considerable amount of bleeding [5]. This situation can occur in various types of surgeries. For example, during a Nuss procedure performed via the extra-pleural approach, placement of the steel bar may damage this artery. In a typical Nuss procedure, repeated flipping or adjustment of the steel bar may also injure this vessel. Additionally, during sternal turnover procedures or certain chest wall tumor resections, the internal thoracic artery may be damaged, leading to bleeding.

Although injury to the internal thoracic artery is not as catastrophic as cardiac rupture, it can still result in a large loss of blood volume within a short period, leading to serious consequences. This type of bleeding is also classified as massive bleeding.

Moderate bleeding is mostly caused by bleeding from smaller blood vessels, such as the intercostal arteries. This type of bleeding tends to be slower, involves a smaller volume of blood, and may stop on its own, thus it usually does not develop into massive bleeding. Minor bleeding is mostly due to oozing in the surgical field or brief bleeding from tiny vessels. Such minor bleeding is not particularly harmful and can be regarded as a common and acceptable cost of any surgical procedure.

The three levels of bleeding massive, moderate, and minor can be defined using artificial standards to help differentiate them. However, such artificially defined standards are inherently subjective, and subjective measures are difficult to qualify as scientific. Therefore, it is best not to establish rigid definitions. Even so, most people have a clear understanding of the amount of bleeding that can result from something like cardiac rupture. Having this awareness is essentially sufficient, as it at least provides a realistic sense of the potential danger involved.

2. Pleural Effusion

When a significant amount of fluid accumulates in the pleural cavity, it is referred to as pleural effusion. Pleural effusion can have multiple sources. After chest wall surgery, the most common type is bloody effusion, which is primarily related to exudation from the surgical field. The blood may originate from the intercostal vessels or from the surgical incision. The bleeding can be either active or old/clotted. Active bleeding may result in continuous hemothorax (blood in the pleural cavity), and if not addressed, can lead to serious consequences. In contrast, old/clotted blood can often resolve after drainage and typically does not pose a serious threat.

Almost every type of chest wall surgery can potentially result in bloody pleural effusion. To prevent adverse postoperative effects, the best approach is to place a closed thoracic drainage system during the operation. For older patients, such drainage tubes are especially necessary.

In addition to bloody effusion, some patients may develop pleural effusions of other types after surgery. These effusions may be caused by irritation from the implanted steel plate or may result from a postoperative pleural reaction. The volume of effusion in such cases is generally small and typically resolves after aspiration or drainage.

Chest wall infection surgeries are relatively unique. If the infection is not well controlled, purulent effusion may occur postoperatively. This type of effusion is more harmful, and drainage alone is often insufficient to achieve good results. Further intervention is usually required.

In addition to the types of effusion mentioned above, chest wall surgery can also lead to chylothorax. Although the exact mechanism is unclear, the outcome is well-defined: the fluid accumulated in the pleural cavity in such cases originates from the lymphatic system and has distinct characteristics.

3. Pneumothorax

Pneumothorax primarily refers to the presence of air within the pleural cavity. The air has two main sources: one is lung injury, and the other is air entering the chest cavity through the surgical incision during the procedure. Although chest wall surgical procedures are performed on the chest wall, they can sometimes cause lung injuries this is actually not uncommon. For example, during the placement of the steel bar in pectus excavatum surgery, the introducer or the steel bar may pass through lung tissue, resulting in direct lung injury [6]. In some secondary surgeries for pectus excavatum, due to extensive adhesions within the thoracic cavity, lung tissue may also be injured during the process of freeing these adhesions [6]. In certain chest wall tumor or infection surgeries, where the lung tissue may be adherent to the lesion, lung damage can also occur during resection. Additionally, in reconstructive surgeries for chest wall collapse secondary to empyema, the lung is highly susceptible to injury during pleural decortication. Pneumothorax is generally present following such procedures. Apart from pneumothorax caused by direct lung injury, the most common clinical source of pneumothorax is air entering through the surgical incision that is, residual air left in the pleural cavity during the procedure. This can occur in nearly all chest wall surgeries. for some operations that require entry into the thoracic cavity, postoperative pneumothorax is easy to understand. However, in certain special procedures such as the Wenlin procedure, which appears not to involve entering the thoracic cavity and is therefore assumed unlikely to cause pneumothorax this is not actually the case. This is because, during the placement of the steel guiding wire, the procedure involves repeatedly crossing over the upper and lower borders of the ribs, which creates opportunities for air to enter the pleural cavity and cause a pneumothorax.

The most effective way to prevent pneumothorax is to place a closed thoracic drainage system. However, in many chest wall surgeries, due to various concerns about potential drawbacks, surgeons are often reluctant to place such drainage tubes. This hesitation is the fundamental reason why many patients develop pneumothorax after surgery.

The management of pneumothorax is relatively straightforward; in most cases, the placement of a closed thoracic drainage system is sufficient to effectively eliminate it. However, if the lung tissue is severely damaged, especially in the presence of a large airway leak, closed thoracic drainage alone may not be enough to control the pneumothorax. In such cases, direct surgical repair of the lung injury is necessary; otherwise, it is nearly impossible to resolve the pneumothorax.

4. Subcutaneous Emphysema

Subcutaneous emphysema mainly occurs when gas enters the subcutaneous tissue through specific pathways. The gas may originate from within the pleural cavity or from an open drainage tube. A necessary precondition for the formation of subcutaneous emphysema is excessively high air pressure. It can occur in cases of tension pneumothorax or in pediatric patients who experience intense crying after surgery. When air continuously enters the subcutaneous tissue through a certain pathway, subcutaneous emphysema will develop. While subcutaneous emphysema itself is generally not seriously harmful and can be quickly resolved with appropriate treatment, its underlying cause is often more significant. If the cause is not addressed, it may lead to more serious consequences.

5. Intrathoracic Infection

Intrathoracic infections have become quite rare in recent years, largely due to improvements in sterile surgical techniques and the effective use of antibiotics. However, such infections still occasionally occur. In the early stages, they may present as pleuritis, and in more severe cases, can develop into empyema. This type of complication can arise after any chest wall surgery. In procedures involving infected lesions of the chest wall which are inherently infectious surgeries the risk increases significantly if the infection spreads into the thoracic cavity during lesion resection.

6. Injury to Intrathoracic Organs

Although chest wall surgery is performed on the body surface, the underlying lesions may involve deeper structures, potentially leading to injury of intrathoracic structures. These injuries may include damage to the heart, lungs, trachea, esophagus, thoracic duct, and other structures.

Cardiac injury is extremely dangerous and has been described earlier. Lung injury was also previously discussed, mainly referring to damage that occurs during the placement of the steel bar or during the separation of adhesions [6]. Once lung tissue is injured, it may result in two major complications: bleeding and air leakage. If left untreated, these can lead to more serious consequences. Due to their deep anatomical location, injuries to the trachea, esophagus, and thoracic duct are relatively rare. However, in some severe chest wall conditions, these structures may become involved, making such injuries possible.

7. Atelectasis

There are multiple causes of atelectasis following chest wall surgery. It may be related to compression from implanted materials, lung tissue becoming trapped in a gap [6], or delayed postoperative expectancy. The primary manifestation of atelectasis is the collapse of lung tissue. The most immediate consequence is impaired breathing. If the lung cannot re-expand over time, it may lead to localized necrosis and infection.

8. Impairment of Respiratory Function

The maintenance of respiratory function involves many contributing factors, and the role of the chest wall aside from the lungs should not be overlooked. After most chest wall surgeries, respiratory function is inevitably impaired due to factors such as postoperative pain. However, this is not the main cause of impaired respiratory function. In addition to pain, there are many other factors that affect respiratory function. For example, the restrictive effect of the steel plate on the thoracic cage during reconstructive surgery. When most of the bony structures of the chest wall are unable to move effectively due to the presence of the steel plate, respiratory function will inevitably be affected. Furthermore, respiratory function may also be impaired due to direct compression of the lung tissue. In some surgeries for protruding-type deformities, steel plates are used to apply pressure on the protruding chest wall. If this pressure is too excessive, it may directly restrict lung expansion, thereby affecting respiratory function. In addition, if pulmonary inflammation occurs postoperatively, it can also impair respiratory function.

There is another particularly unique situation, which arises from the direct destruction of chest wall function. In surgeries for tumors, infections, or defects, one of the key components is chest wall reconstruction. If the reconstruction is unsatisfactory or not performed at all it may compromise the integrity of the chest wall, thereby affecting respiratory function. Similarly, in trauma patients, if a flail chest occurs and is not properly stabilized, respiratory function will also be adversely affected.

9. Impairment of Cardiac Function

Impairment of cardiac function can be observed after chest wall surgery, with compression being the most common cause. In some surgeries for protruding-type deformities, if the anterior chest wall is overcorrected, it may result in direct compression of the heart, potentially leading to postoperative cardiac insufficiency. Generally, routine pectus carinatum surgeries do not cause this type of complication. However, if the compression is excessively severe, it can still lead to cardiac compression. Cardiac compression can also occur during the Nuss procedure. Generally speaking, the steel bar used in the Nuss procedure is intended to eliminate compression and therefore should not cause further cardiac compression. However, if the steel bar is improperly positioned or fails to adequately elevate the chest wall, it may lie across the surface of the heart and cause significant compression. This condition is often not detected by the surgeon but can lead to cardiac dysfunction. On CT cross-sectional images, this kind of compression is usually quite evident. Another situation arises in surgeries for asphyxiating thoracic dystrophy, where patients already have compromised cardiac function. In such cases, excessive compression can further impair heart function, and in severe instances, may even result in cardiac failure.

10. Cardiac Arrhythmia

Cardiac arrhythmia is a common complication in chest wall surgery and is mainly related to irritation of the heart. In the treatment of pectus excavatum using the Nuss procedure, since the placement of the steel bar is performed over the surface of the heart, the introducer or the steel bar passing through the chest may induce arrhythmia. Mild cases may present as transient premature beats, while severe cases can cause ventricular fibrillation, leading to serious consequences. Because heart rhythm changes often occur during the passage process, some surgeons use these changes as an indirect indicator of whether the heart has been injured. This practice is very dangerous and has limited significance.

11. Delayed Wound Healing

If a surgical incision does not heal within a certain period, it is considered delayed wound healing. This is a common complication in clinical practice and can occur after almost any type of chest wall surgery (Figure 1-11-1). There are many causes of delayed healing, with the most common reasons as follows: ① Infection, Infection is the most common cause. Once an incision becomes infected, the healing process is affected. Not only can the skin fail to close properly, but the wound may also reopen and discharge purulent secretions. This represents the most severe form of delayed healing, commonly referred to as wound infection. ② Blood circulation, Adequate blood supply is essential for wound healing. If blood circulation is poor, the incision cannot receive sufficient nutrients, local resistance decreases, and ultimately healing may be impaired. ③ Artificial materials, in chest wall surgery, shaping or reconstructive materials are commonly used. Since these materials are foreign bodies, if they remain within the incision and are not adequately covered by soft tissue, they can also lead to delayed wound healing. ④ Local incision exudation, for an incision to heal properly, the two sides must be closely apposed. If there is exudate within the incision, the two sides will separate, which negatively affects healing. Incision exudate can come from direct fluid leakage or from fat liquefaction. Incomplete hemostasis during wound closure can also lead to fluid accumulation inside the incision. The presence of these fluids all hinders the healing process. ⑤ Skin damage, If the skin around the incision site is severely injured or has a significant defect, it will directly affect skin healing and similarly lead to delayed wound healing. ⑥ Suturing technique, Wound healing is also related to the suturing technique used on the incision. Poor skin alignment or inversion of the local skin edges can lead to delayed healing. ⑦ Systemic factors can also cause delayed wound healing. For example, severe malnutrition and serious chronic wasting diseases can both negatively affect incision healing.

12. Complications Related to Plastic Surgery

Chest wall surgery has two fundamental attributes: one is treatment of disease, and the other is reconstruction. From the reconstructive perspective, surgery can be further divided into shaping procedures and reconstructive procedures. These two types of surgery are not entirely independent but may be associated with specific complications. To better understand these complications, the following section will introduce them separately.

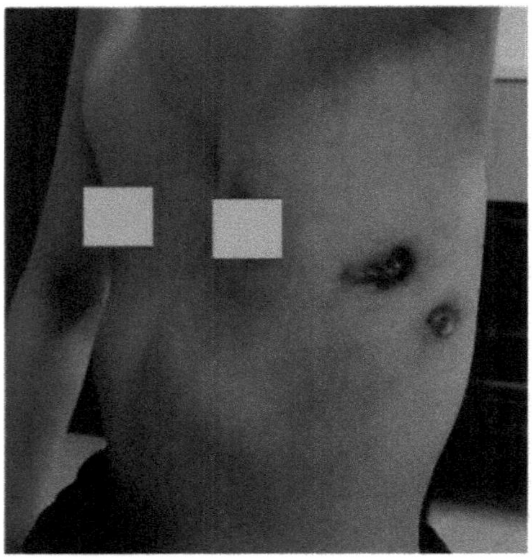

Figure 1-11-1 Delayed Wound Healing. Because a steel plate is present beneath the deep surface of the incision, once delayed healing occurs, management is often very difficult. In severe cases, it may even be necessary to remove the steel plate prematurely.

(1) Rib Fractures

Rib fractures are a relatively common complication, mainly occurring during chest wall deformity shaping surgeries, such as the Nuss procedure. Since the steel bar must be placed at a specific location to lift the depressed chest wall, if the depression is too severe, the bone too hard, or the rib supporting the steel bar too fragile, rib fractures may occur. Especially in surgeries for young and middle-aged patients with pectus excavatum, if excessive force is applied to flip the steel bar against strong resistance, rib fractures may occur. Similarly, in surgeries for protrusion-type deformities, uneven or excessively concentrated stress distribution can also lead to rib fractures. This situation is commonly seen in patients who have fewer steel bars implanted or whose bars are fixed at only one site. In shaping surgeries, the ribs are the load-bearing structures for the steel plates. Once a rib fracture occurs, the entire shaping procedure will fail. Therefore, to ensure the steel plate functions effectively, it is essential to minimize the occurrence of rib fractures as much as possible.

(2) Exposure of Materials

Chest wall surgery often requires the use of artificial materials. Sometimes, these materials may become exposed outside the body through the incision or a skin wound, causing serious consequences (Figure 1-11-2). This situation is related to the following factors: ① Incision infection, when an incision becomes infected, it may rupture, causing tissue liquefaction and necrosis, which easily leads to the exposure of implanted materials. ② Material rejection, during the use of artificial materials, the body may sometimes reject the material, leading to severe local reactions. This not only affects healing but can also cause the material to become exposed through the incision. ③ Skin abrasion, if the material does not fit snugly against the chest wall during surgery and causes a local protrusion, it may gradually abrade the skin and eventually become exposed on the body surface. ④ Postoperative accidental injury, If the patient experiences a fall or collision after surgery, and the impact occurs at the site of the implanted material, it may cause local skin rupture and material exposure. Material exposure is a relatively serious complication. If infection occurs, the material often has to be removed. If there is no infection, direct suturing after local treatment can often achieve satisfactory results.

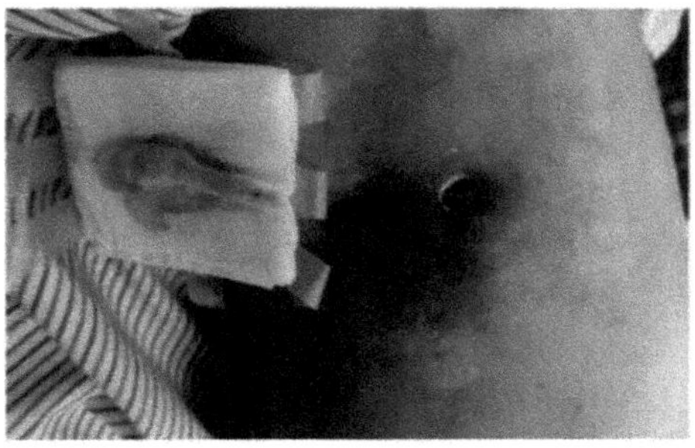

Figure 1-11-2 Steel plate exposed on the body surface. When wound healing problems occur, local soft tissue may undergo necrosis and ulceration, eventually causing the deep steel plate to become exposed on the body surface.

(3) Displacement of the Steel Plate

In chest wall deformity shaping surgeries, the position of the steel plate is crucial. Once displacement occurs, the shaping effect will be directly affected, and in severe cases, it may lead to surgical failure (Figure 1-11-3) [7]. This situation is most commonly seen in the Nuss procedure. When the steel plate slides from the deepest part of the depression toward one side, the depression may return to its original shape under its own stress, causing the anterior chest wall deformity to reappear. This situation can also occur in surgeries for protrusion-type deformities. If the protruding area is small and uneven, the steel plate may slide sideways from this location, ultimately leading to surgical failure. Steel plate displacement is a relatively common complication. Its occurrence is related not only to the deformity itself but also mainly to the surgeon’s technique. The key to preventing displacement lies in the method of steel plate placement and fixation. If the plate is properly positioned and securely fixed, displacement generally does not occur.

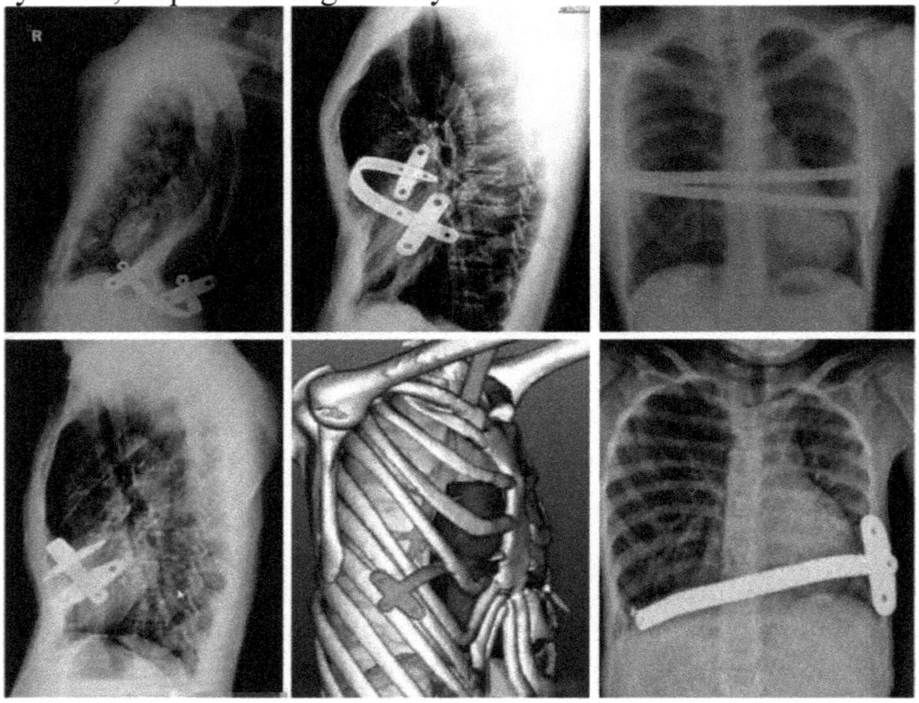

Figure 1-11-3 Various forms of steel plate displacement. Once steel plate displacement occurs, the plate can no longer function effectively on one hand, it leads to recurrence of the deformity, and on the other, it may cause additional injury due to the displacement itself.

(4) Material Fracture

In shaping surgeries, material fracture may sometimes occur. This can happen either during surgical preparation or during the operation itself. Fractures are mainly related to improper handling by the surgeon, although spontaneous fracture is also possible (Figure 1-11-4). If the fracture occurs before surgery and there are no replacement materials available, it may delay or prevent the procedure from proceeding. If it happens during surgery, it can potentially lead to surgical failure.

(5) Organ Injury Caused by Materials

During the placement of materials, there is a risk of injuring intrathoracic organs, which can have adverse effects. In the Nuss procedure, aside from the

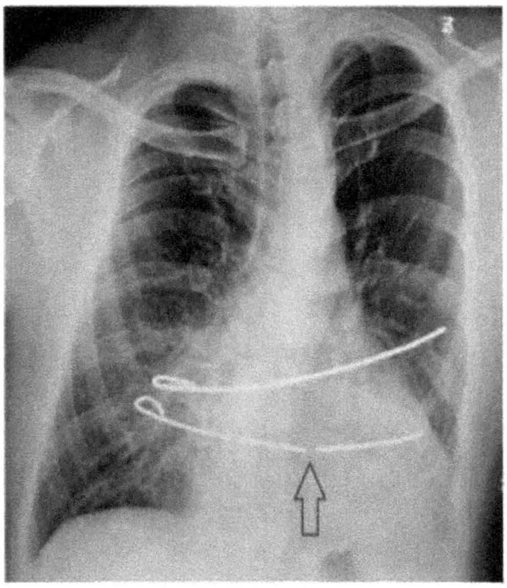

previously mentioned possibility of lung injury, there is another type of injury caused by the notched ends of the steel plate. Since the plate must pass through the mediastinum, the notches may tear nearby structures along the way, sometimes resulting in serious consequences. In addition, once the steel plate is inserted into the thoracic cavity, significant adhesions often form around it. When the steel plate adheres to lung tissue, the lungs may suffer considerable damage (Figure 1-11-5).

Figure 1-11-4 Fracture of Fixation Material

(6) Sharp-Angled Deformity

Sharp-angled deformity is a very unusual type of deformity. It can occur independently or as a complication following certain chest wall deformity surgeries, and it is considered a serious complication [8]. In the Nuss procedure for pectus excavatum, if the steel bar is positioned on one side of the depression rather than at its deepest point, the depressed chest wall may shift entirely toward that side. This causes the edge of the depression to rise sharply, forming a sharp-angled protrusion, known as a sharp-angled deformity (Figure 1-11-6). Once this complication occurs, it not only indicates a complete surgical failure but also worsens the deformity, making correction significantly more difficult.

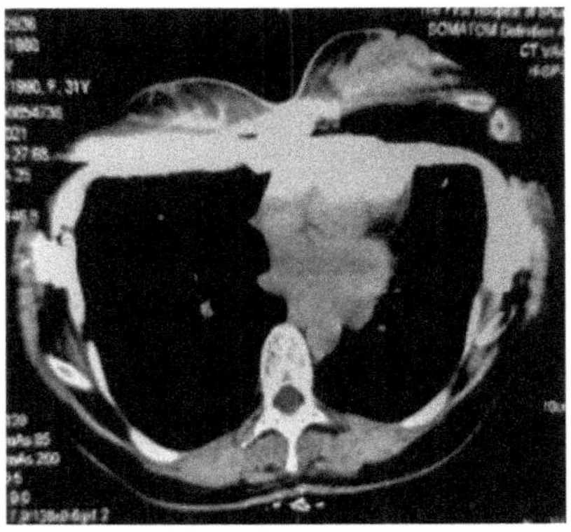

Figure 1-11-5 Lung tissue injury caused by steel plate

(7) Overcorrection

This is a very common complication and can occur in the correction of any type of deformity. In the Nuss procedure for pectus excavatum, if the curvature of the steel bar is too great, it may cause the anterior chest wall to bulge outward, resulting in a protrusion deformity. This is the most common form of overcorrection. In surgeries for protrusion-type deformities, if the compression is too excessive, a depression may appear at the midline of the anterior chest wall, forming a deformity that is completely opposite to the original [9]. This situation also occurs frequently. Transforming one deformity into its complete opposite may technically count as a correction, but it often becomes a new source of regret. This is a complication that should be avoided as much as possible.

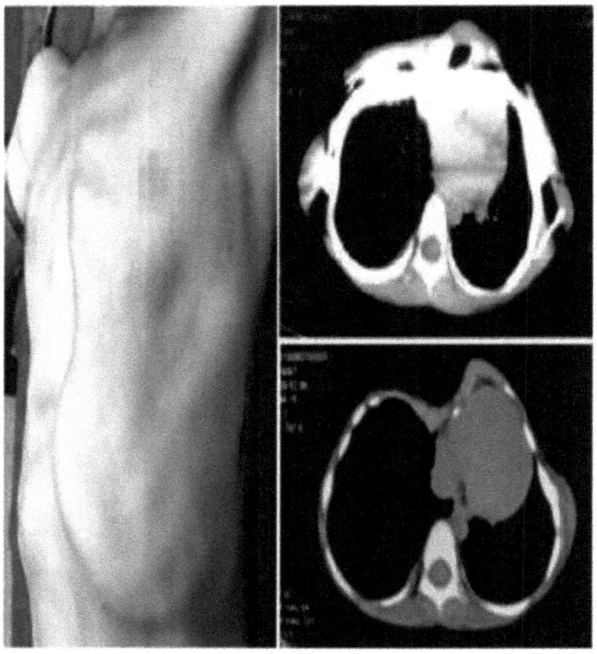

Figure 1-11-6 Sharp-Angled Deformity.
Due to improper placement of the steel plate, the depressed chest wall changes shape, with one edge rising sharply to form a sharp-angled deformity. The appearance of this deformity signifies surgical failure. To perform a second corrective surgery, special treatment targeting the sharp-angled deformity is required

(8) Shaping Failure

In various types of shaping surgeries, almost every complication that occurs can result in shaping failure. Therefore, strictly speaking, shaping failure is not a single, specific complication. It is mentioned here in order to collectively discuss all other causes that may lead to the failure of shaping outcomes.

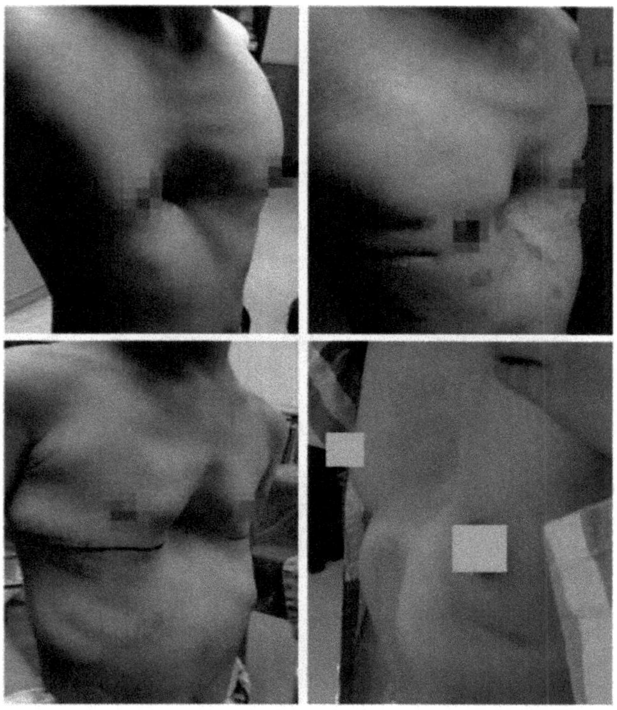

Figure 1-11-7 Shaping Failure. The chest wall fails to return to a normal shape, which may present as a recurrence of the original deformity or as a new deformity. Even outcomes with partial improvement can be considered shaping failures. Only those shaping surgeries that completely eliminate the deformity can be regarded as successful.

The purpose of shaping is to eliminate the deformity and achieve a normal chest wall contour. If this goal is not met, it can be considered a surgical failure (Figure 1-11-7) [3]. Surgical failure is related to many factors, and all of the aforementioned complications can lead to failure. However, more often, it is directly caused by the surgeon's technique. If the surgeon's technique is flawed, the surgery will encounter problems and cannot yield a satisfactory outcome, resulting in a failed operation. Surgical failure often leads to serious consequences, as it may create an even more severe new deformity. Such deformities are often extremely challenging, with high surgical risk and great difficulty, and even with tremendous effort, it is difficult to achieve a satisfactory result. Therefore, for shaping surgeries, surgical failure should be considered the most serious complication.

(9) Flap Necrosis

In shaping surgeries, reconstruction is an important aspect. Reconstruction can involve bony structures or skin and soft tissue. The latter is mainly achieved through various types of skin flaps. After flap transplantation, ensuring flap survival requires consideration of many factors — including blood circulation, infection, fixation, and mechanical forces. Each of these factors can impact flap viability, and in severe cases, may lead to flap necrosis. Once flap necrosis occurs, the surgery will result in complete failure [10].

In summary, chest wall surgery can involve a wide range of complications. Although some of these complications may be related to intrathoracic organs, the majority are associated with the inherent characteristics of the chest wall itself. In clinical practice, it is essential to fully understand the nature of chest wall surgery and to master the necessary surgical techniques in order to eliminate complications and ensure the ultimate success of the operation.

REFERENCES

[1] Wang, Wenlin. 2021a. "Risks Associated with the Nuss Procedure." *Chest Wall Deformity Surgery Expert*, April 25.

[2] Wang, Wenlin. 2021b. "Risks and Outcomes of Secondary Surgery after Failed Pectus Excavatum Operations." *Chest Wall Deformity Surgery Expert*, May 5.

[3] Wang, Wenlin. 2016. "Clinical Analysis of 39 Cases of Secondary Pectus Excavatum Surgery." *Chinese Journal of Clinical Thoracic and Cardiovascular Surgery* 23 (10): 1026–1028.

[4] Wang, Wenlin. 2020. "Third Surgery for Chest Wall Tumors at the Apex of the Thorax." *Chest Wall Deformity Surgery Expert*, November 7.

[5] Wang, Wenlin. 2019. "Potential Injury to Internal Thoracic Artery during NUSS Procedure." *Chest Wall Deformity Surgery Expert*, October 9.

[6] Wang, Wenlin. 2021c. "Possible Lung Injury Caused by the Nuss Procedure." *Chest Wall Deformity Surgery Expert*, August 23.

[7] Wang, Wenlin. 2014. "How to Handle Steel Plate Displacement after Nuss Procedure?" *Chest Wall Deformity Surgery Expert*, August 13.

[8] Wang, Wenlin. 2021d. "Sharp-Angled Deformity." *Chest Wall Deformity Surgery Expert*, August 18.

[9] Wang, Wenlin. 2018. "Overcorrection in Pectus Carinatum Surgery: Resulting Pectus Excavatum Deformity." *Chest Wall Deformity Surgery Expert*, May 29.

[10] Wang, Maosheng. 2008. "Prevention of Flap Necrosis and Subcutaneous Fluid Accumulation after Radical Mastectomy." *Chinese Journal of General Surgery* 17 (5): 515–516.

Chest wall surgery has two fundamental characteristics: one is treatment of disease, and the other is cosmetic shaping [1]. These are also the basic goals of the surgery. The evaluation of surgical outcomes essentially depends on whether these goals have been achieved in other words, whether the disease has been cured and whether the appearance of the chest wall has been restored to normal. This is the core of assessing the surgical outcome. Among the five types of chest wall diseases, although all involve both therapeutic and cosmetic goals, different diseases place emphasis on different aspects. For example, in the case of chest wall tumors, patients may prioritize disease treatment more. Similarly, patients with chest wall infections tend to focus more on treatment. However, for patients with chest wall deformities, the emphasis may be more on cosmetic correction. Due to the varying nature of the diseases, the surgical focus and evaluation standards naturally differ. Furthermore, the evaluation of surgical outcomes is essentially a subjective process. As such, it is influenced by many human factors, and achieving complete objectivity and fairness is almost impossible. However, the evaluation of surgical outcomes is an ongoing process every surgery is followed by some form of assessment. There is self-evaluation by the surgeon, peer evaluation by colleagues, and feedback from patients and their families. When so many people may be involved in the evaluation process, it becomes increasingly complex. To ensure that the evaluation is as fair and objective as possible, the process must be carefully designed so that it gains broad acceptance and accurately reflects the true outcomes of the surgery.

1. Evaluation of Therapeutic Outcomes

From a therapeutic perspective, evaluating surgical outcomes requires analysis based on different types of diseases. for tumor patients, surgery is only considered successful if the tumor is completely removed. of course, this success must also include proper healing of the surgical incision and the absence of complications during the perioperative period. for malignant tumors, the ideal outcome is no recurrence of the lesion. In the case of chest wall infections, the expected result of surgery is the elimination of the infected area and proper healing of the chest wall skin incision. These outcomes represent the basic expectations of patients. When these expectations are met, the surgery is considered successful in the patient's view. Chest wall trauma surgery must be analyzed in two situations. If the trauma is not too severe, the patient's expectations regarding treatment may not be very high. However, if the trauma is extremely serious and even life-threatening, the patient will place great importance on the therapeutic outcome. In cases of chest wall defects, if only the bony structure is missing and physiological function is not affected, the treatment goal may not be emphasized. But if the defect involves the skin, then treatment becomes the primary concern for the patient. The situation for deformity patients is more complex except for some cases of severe depression-type deformities, most patients are not concerned about the therapeutic aspect. This shows that patients with different types of chest wall diseases evaluate surgical outcomes from different perspectives. To evaluate from a therapeutic perspective, it is essential to consider the characteristics of each specific disease and to carefully understand the patient's needs. Only in this way can the evaluation come as close as possible to reflecting the true outcome.

2. Evaluation of Cosmetic Outcomes

From a cosmetic standpoint, evaluating the outcomes of chest wall surgery also presents many challenges. for patients with tumors or infections, cosmetic results can be almost entirely disregarded. for patients with severe trauma, cosmetic outcomes are often also overlooked. Similarly, for defect patients involving skin loss, cosmetic concerns are usually secondary.

In contrast, patients with deformities are the ones who value cosmetic results the most. The purpose of cosmetic surgery is to reshape or reconstruct the appearance of the chest wall in order to achieve an appearance as close to normal as possible. In this sense, the evaluation of cosmetic outcomes is essentially an assessment of chest wall appearance the closer it looks to normal, the better the cosmetic result [2]. Cosmetic procedures include two types of surgeries: reconstruction and reshaping [3]. Reconstructive surgery typically refers to the restoration of chest wall structures after the removal of lesions in patients with tumors, infections, or defects. Since these patients are usually more concerned about the therapeutic outcome, reconstructive procedures are often considered secondary and, in most cases, receive less attention. Therefore, when discussing cosmetic outcomes, such cases are not the main focus. Reshaping refers to the corrective surgeries for chest wall deformities, where patients place the highest value on the postoperative appearance of the chest. Hence, these cases are best suited for evaluating cosmetic outcomes from a shaping perspective. To better assess reshaping results, two types of indicators can be used: one is a relatively objective indicator, such as imaging examinations, and the other is a more subjective measure, which involves direct visual assessment of appearance.

(1) Objective Evaluation

Radiological imaging is a relatively objective method of evaluation. There are various techniques available, but to most accurately reflect the shaping outcome of the bony structure, the ideal method is three-dimensional reconstruction. With this technology, all bony structures and surrounding visceral tissues can be clearly visualized. This type of imaging is the most intuitive and comprehensive, making the quality of the result immediately apparent. Even patients with no medical knowledge can easily understand the outcome. This allows both the patient and the surgeon to reach a consensus more easily, making the evaluation relatively objective. However, there is one important consideration: the difference between the shape of the bony structure and the appearance of the chest wall. Patients and their families often care more about the external appearance of the chest wall rather than the shape of the internal bones. Therefore, even if the bony structure is corrected perfectly, a dissatisfying appearance can still undermine the patient's trust in the imaging results. It is evident that while 3D reconstruction provides convenience for evaluation, it also presents certain challenges. However, overall, having a visual representation of the thoracic structure serves as a tangible standard. This makes it relatively easier for doctors and patients to reach a consensus. That said, 3D reconstruction imaging is not yet widely available, and many institutions lack access to this technology, which undoubtedly affects the evaluation of outcomes. If 3D reconstruction is not feasible, standard CT or X-ray imaging can be used instead. However, these methods are less intuitive and require professional expertise to interpret. Most patients and their families cannot understand the results of such examinations, making it difficult for doctors and patients to find common ground based on imaging alone.

(2) Subjective Evaluation

When radiological imaging is not available, the evaluation of surgical outcomes can only be performed through subjective methods [4]. Subjective evaluation involves a direct assessment of the external appearance. In theory, if the external appearance of the chest wall closely resembles a normal shape, it is relatively easy for both the doctor and the patient to reach an agreement, with little disagreement about the outcome. Evaluations made under such circumstances are the most satisfactory. However, the most subjectively influenced cases are those where the surgical results are unsatisfactory. The doctor may believe that there has been a significant improvement in the deformity, while the patient and their family may have higher expectations and feel disappointed with the outcome. This leads to disagreements, and at such times, it is very difficult to reach a unified evaluation.

If the outcome of chest wall deformity correction is evaluated based on the appearance of the chest wall, then the only tool we rely on is the human eye. Since different eyes belong to different individuals, there will inevitably be different evaluations. As mentioned earlier, when the reshaping result is nearly perfect, meaning it closely resembles a normal chest wall, the observations made by different people are generally similar, with little disagreement. However, when the appearance falls short of the normal standard, differences in opinion emerge [5,6]. Situations that may lead to such discrepancies include the following:

First, incomplete correction of the deformity. When a deformity is not fully corrected, there are often very obvious signs. In such cases, the result is easily noticeable, as the appearance of the chest wall does not reach a normal standard. There may be some degree of improvement, but the deformity has not been completely resolved. Take pectus excavatum surgery as an example: if the depression is only reduced but not completely eliminated, the correction is incomplete. The same applies to pectus carinatum if the protrusion still remains after surgery and has not been fully flattened, it also constitutes incomplete correction. Opinions on incomplete correction vary. Some strict observers may regard it as a surgical failure, while more lenient individuals may consider it partially effective. This type of result is, in fact, the most likely to cause disputes between the surgeon and the patient.

Second, overcorrection. Correction is intended to eliminate a specific type of deformity. However, if the procedure is overdone during the operation, it may lead to the opposite result. For example, a deformity that was originally a depression may result in a protrusion after surgery; or a protruding deformity may turn into a depression postoperatively. Such situations can potentially occur in almost all types of surgeries. Overcorrection is generally considered an undesirable outcome and should be avoided whenever possible. However, in pursuit of better long-term results, intentional overcorrection is sometimes necessary, mainly due to the delayed shaping effect that can occur after surgery. Sometimes, in order to prevent postoperative recurrence of the deformity, intentional overcorrection is performed. If done deliberately, such results are usually temporary and may actually lead to better long-term outcomes. However, aside from these planned cases, if irreversible overcorrection occurs, it becomes a sign of surgical failure. Patients may sometimes express dissatisfaction with overcorrected results, which is understandable. In such cases, especially when overcorrection is intentional, it is essential that the doctor properly explains the reasoning to the patient otherwise, it may cause confusion or disputes.

Third, replacing one deformity with another. The goal of surgery is to eliminate the deformity, but in some special cases, while the original deformity is corrected, a new deformity appears. This situation is similar to overcorrection but not exactly the same. In overcorrection, the result is a complete reversal of the original deformity, and the deformity still appears in the same location. However, in this scenario, the new deformity has no relation to the original one and arises in a different area. For example, this commonly occurs in Nuss procedures, where the depression originally lies in the center of the anterior chest wall, but due to pressure from both ends of the steel bar, a new depression develops in the lateral chest wall. This is essentially replacing one form of pectus excavatum with a new one. Such a deformity is referred to as secondary saddle chest. Another scenario may occur in cases of complex (combined-type) chest wall deformities: if the surgeon corrects only one part of the deformity while neglecting the other, the uncorrected deformity may worsen, resulting in the combined deformity transforming into a more severe, single-type deformity For example, if a patient initially presents with a combination of upper chest protrusion and lower chest depression, and the surgeon only corrects the protrusion by flattening the upper chest wall, the depression in the lower chest may become more pronounced. This can ultimately result in a very severe case of pectus excavatum. In essence, the patient's complex deformity has been converted into a severe single-type deformity. On the surface, replacing one deformity with another may appear to be a treatment of the original deformity, On the surface, replacing one deformity with another may appear to be a treatment for the original deformity, as it eliminates the primary condition. However, the new deformity may be just as harmful as the original one. As a result, many patients may dispute this outcome, and some may even consider such a result to be a surgical failure.

Fourth, local imperfections. The correction of a deformity typically focuses on addressing the main deformity, and it is impossible to handle every aspect perfectly. In other words, small local defects are unlikely to be meticulously corrected. This is a common characteristic of chest wall deformity reshaping surgeries and is entirely normal in surgical practice. For example, many patients with pectus excavatum may experience anterior protrusion of the costal arch after surgery. This type of protrusion is seen in many cases postoperatively and can be considered the most common imperfection following this procedure. If this imperfection is not addressed, it does not indicate surgical failure in the treatment of pectus excavatum. In general, the more complex the deformity, the more likely it is that residual imperfections will remain. For example, thoracic insufficiency syndrome surgery is considered the most complex and demanding procedure among all chest wall deformity surgeries. There are many different surgical techniques for this condition, each with its own drawbacks or imperfections. If one fails to appreciate the overall reshaping outcome and instead focuses solely on these minor flaws, it can lead to a misjudgment of the surgical results. Overall, when it comes to local imperfections, it's important to understand the difference between reshaping surgery and cosmetic surgery. Reshaping surgery is not the same as aesthetic surgery, and therefore, minor local defects are not considered problems in the context of reshaping procedures. However, if a patient is concerned about these imperfections and the surgeon fails to provide proper explanation, it can lead to conflict and dissatisfaction.

Fifth, surgical scar. The evaluation of reshaping outcomes is a visual assessment. Since it is based on appearance, it inevitably involves visible details, one of the most obvious being the surgical scar. The longer and more noticeable the scar, the more it can negatively affect the overall evaluation. Conversely, if the scar is short, small, and well-hidden, patients are generally more satisfied and more likely to give a positive evaluation. The issue of scarring is influenced by many factors: patient-related factors, the nature of the condition, the choice of surgical approach, and of course, the surgeon's technical skill. If noticeable scarring occurs due to certain objective factors, it may still impact the patient's perception of the surgical outcome. Sixth, worsening of the deformity. Doctors are not deities, but ordinary human beings of flesh and blood, so every surgery carries the possibility of failure. In the previously mentioned situations, the deformity was at least partially improved. However, there is another scenario where, after surgery, the patient's deformity not only fails to improve but actually becomes more complex and severe. Such cases are not uncommon. At the root of it, the responsibility lies with the surgeon. Worsening deformity is an outcome that no one wants to face. Even the most defensive surgeon eager to protect their reputation must acknowledge the reality of failure when confronted with postoperative deformity worsening. For this reason, both doctors and patients usually reach a rare consensus: such a result is clearly considered a surgical failure. But understandably, patients are often extremely unwilling to accept this outcome.

Seven, Death. No matter how unsatisfactory a deformity correction may be even if it worsens there is usually an opportunity for remediation. However, there is one outcome that offers no chance for remedy: the patient's death. Such tragedies occasionally occur during the Nuss procedure for pectus excavatum. Undoubtedly, this remains a consequence of suboptimal surgical technique. When this occurs, the patient no longer has any opportunity to evaluate the surgical outcome.

Eight, Occurrence of other complications. The assessment of the shaping outcome is generally based on the premise that there are no significant complications. The various situations mentioned above are, in fact, all considered complications, and once they occur, they will certainly affect the evaluation of the results. In addition to these complications, other clinical complications may also arise. When complications occur, regardless of how the chest wall appears externally, the final evaluation will inevitably be affected. For example, complications such as incision infections. Although such complications may seem minor, they can lead to prolonged wound healing, and in severe cases, the patient may even have to undergo premature removal of the steel plate. The suffering caused by these complications is easy to imagine. When faced with such issues, even if the chest wall appearance is nearly perfect, it is difficult for the patient to give a favorable evaluation of the outcome. Especially when the steel plate has to be removed earlier than planned, the surgical results are directly affected, making it absolutely impossible for the patient to provide a positive assessment.

In summary, aside from outright surgical failure or patient death, whenever the outcome of surgery is unsatisfactory, disagreements between doctors and patients are inevitable; this is one of the most common situations in clinical practice. For doctors, no matter how guilty they may feel internally, they tend to present a more forgiving attitude toward their own work on the surface and may offer a relatively positive evaluation. Especially when facing potential disputes, it is understandable that doctors try to defend themselves, often leading to assessments that are more favorable than the actual outcome. On the other hand, the perspectives of patients and their families are usually quite different. Having spent money and endured suffering, patients naturally hope for a good result. If they are met with disappointment, there is a strong tendency to magnify their dissatisfaction, leading to conflict. Generally, patients and their families share the same viewpoint, but due to various complex factors, differences of opinion may also arise. Some parents, in an effort to comfort their children, may reluctantly accept the reality and show tolerance toward the outcome. However, there are also more critical parents who, despite the child being relatively satisfied with the results, will scrutinize every detail ultimately leading to disagreements even within the family.

(3) Evaluation System

When everyone has differing opinions about the outcome, evaluation becomes difficult. In order to eliminate disagreements and establish a universally accepted evaluation standard, many authors have attempted to design relevant frameworks to gain broader acceptance. However, achieving such a goal is very difficult.

In order for the evaluation of surgical outcomes to be accepted by everyone, the opinions of all parties must be fully considered, which means that many detailed criteria must be established. However, for the specific task of evaluating surgical results, the more complex the process becomes, the less accurate the outcome may be, potentially leading to counterproductive results.

As mentioned above, real disagreements often arise when the results are unsatisfactory. At such times, the evaluations are made by different individuals, and since they are human, subjectivity is inevitable. Subjective judgments carry a great deal of uncertainty. For such cases, if one insists on using overly complex and highly detailed criteria for evaluation, the results may become even more distorted. Therefore, the most rational evaluation approach is simplification—using the most straightforward methods possible. The simpler the method, the less interference from subjective factors, which in turn increases objectivity and makes the evaluation more reliable.

According to the above principle, we have designed a special evaluation method that takes into account the opinions of the doctor, the patient, and the family members, assigning equal weight to each party's input. The final evaluation is then based on the combined score [7]. The specific method is as follows:

Each of the three parties rates the outcome of the shaping surgery: Very satisfied – 3 points, basically satisfied – 2 points, and not satisfied – 1 point. The scores from all three parties are then added together to obtain a total score, based on which the final evaluation is made: 8~9 points: Satisfied – appearance has basically returned to normal; 5~7 points: Basically satisfied, appearance has significantly improved; 3~4 points: Not satisfied: no change or worsening of appearance.

This method fully integrates the opinions of all three parties, with a fair and equal distribution of weight, making it more accurate and scientific. As a result, the outcome is more likely to be accepted by everyone. We have consistently used this method for evaluation in clinical practice, and the results have been generally recognized by doctors, patients, and their families.

Like other subjective actions, when there is a lack of objective standards, a compromise-based evaluation method is generally acceptable to all parties. This approach takes into account the opinions of the doctor, the patient, and the family members, and is designed to eliminate disagreements [4] However, whether it is the doctor, the patient, or the family, when each reflects on the surgical outcome in their heart if not influenced by any special motive, they will arrive at an assessment that is closest to the truth. Such an evaluation comes closest to the essence of the matter and represents a relatively objective result For example, when it comes to the quality of a surgery, doctors are usually very clear in their own minds. At such times, the doctor has an internal, invisible standard. Though it cannot be seen or touched, it is highly objective. The same applies to patients and their families. In order to treat the deformity, patients often make great sacrifices and naturally have high expectations. These expectations may influence the evaluation, but they do not necessarily reflect the person's true inner thoughts especially when disputes arise and the patient hopes to seek compensation through certain channels, which may take them further away from their true assessment. Nevertheless, it cannot be denied that everyone has an objective standard in their heart. People tend to use the simplest and most intuitive way to judge the outcome of a surgery that is the most objective measure, though most are unwilling to reveal it openly. In summary, chest wall surgery involves two main surgical goals.

The therapeutic goal is influenced by many factors and lacks a unified standard, making it difficult to reach a consistent evaluation. The aesthetic goal is also affected by various factors, and it is nearly impossible to evaluate the shaping outcome for every type of condition. However, for chest wall deformities of this specific type of chest wall surgical disease, if the evaluation is based on the shaping outcome, certain special evaluation systems can be applied. Although such systems are not entirely objective, they take into full account the opinions of the relevant parties and can ultimately form a relatively fair evaluation framework.

REFERENCES

[1] Wang, Wenlin. 2021a. “The Fundamental Nature of Chest Wall Surgery.” *Toutiao Today*, October 31.

[2] Wang, Wenlin. 2013. “Evaluation Criteria for Chest Wall Deformity Surgery.” *Chest Wall Deformity Surgery Expert*, September 9.

[3] Wang, Wenlin. 2021b. “Chest Wall Surgery: Shaping and Reconstruction.” *Toutiao Today*, October 31.

[4] Wang, Wenlin. 2017. “Evaluation Standards for Chest Wall Deformity Surgery Outcomes.” *Chest Wall Deformity Surgery Expert*, November 25.

[5] Wang, Wenlin. 2021c. “Five Types of Outcomes in Chest Wall Deformity Surgery.” *Chest Wall Deformity Surgery Expert*, September 22.

[6] Wang, Wenlin. 2019. “The Consequences of Failed Pectus Excavatum Surgery.” *Chest Wall Deformity Surgery Expert*, November 18.

[7] Wang, Wenlin, Chunmei Chen, Weiguang Long, et al. 2015. “Experience in the Treatment of Pectus Excavatum in Elderly Patients.” *Journal of Practical Medicine* 31 (Suppl 7): 311–312.

Chest wall surgery, like all other surgical procedures, is an invasive form of treatment. During this process, the human body undergoes an extraordinary impact not only physical but also psychological. Many patients may not appear seriously ill before surgery, but after undergoing the procedure, they become patients in the absolute sense. Once the treatment is complete, the patient must emerge from the treatment process and restore themselves to a state of health. This transition is extremely important. To ensure that this transition proceeds smoothly, appropriate efforts must be made. These efforts constitute what we call rehabilitation. It is thus evident that rehabilitation is a comprehensive concept. It is the sum of a series of efforts and measures that help patients recover both physically and psychologically to a normal state.
Chest wall diseases are relatively unique, and so are the surgeries required to treat them. Therefore, postoperative rehabilitation also involves several distinctive requirements. Based on the characteristics of chest wall surgery, the entire postoperative rehabilitation process can be divided into three stages [1]: Stage One: From the end of the surgery to the time of hospital discharge. Stage Two: The three-month period after hospital discharge. Stage Three: From three months post-discharge to the time the steel bar is removed. In each of these three stages, the patient's overall condition is different, the primary challenges vary, and the content and methods of rehabilitation are also different.

1. Rehabilitation in the First Stage

The first stage of rehabilitation essentially corresponds to the perioperative rehabilitation period, and its primary goal is to ensure that the patient is discharged smoothly. To achieve this, the following specific rehabilitation measures need to be implemented: Provide psychological comfort, alleviate early-stage pain, ensure proper wound healing, prevent early postoperative complications, encourage appropriate physical activity

(1) Psychological Comfort

Surgical operations are a tremendous shock to any patient, leaving both their body and mind in a very vulnerable and unique state. Therefore, psychological comfort becomes essential. Such comfort helps relieve fear and anxiety enabling patients to positively engage in their recovery process. This is especially important for patients with malignant, chronic, or serious illnesses, who often carry a heavy psychological burden before surgery. Postoperative reassurance acts like a healing remedy, helping them recover emotionally and face life and rehabilitation with optimism.

For patients with chest wall deformities, psychological issues are common [2]. Completing the surgery can feel like removing a deep-rooted mental burden, bringing a great deal of emotional relief. However, some patients may not be able to let go of their psychological distress so quickly. In such cases, ongoing reassurance is very beneficial.

Patients with other chest wall conditions may also face postoperative emotional challenges. For example, those with chest wall tumors, especially malignant ones, often worry about the effectiveness of the surgery. These patients not only need comfort but also it is necessary to encourage patients and help them build confidence to face further treatment. Patients with chest wall infections or defects often have a long history of illness, and some may have undergone more than one surgery. These patients are often filled with doubts about the surgical outcome and worry about the possibility of failure. They too need psychological reassurance. Trauma patients usually have extraordinary trauma histories; even after the surgery is completed, they may still remain in a state of shock or fear. Such patients require even more patient and careful emotional support.

When a patient's psychological burden is relieved, their mood improves, and they are more likely to actively cooperate with the doctor's guidance. This results in faster and higher-quality recovery. If psychological support is neglected, some patients may fall into a true mental crisis. Even if their physical pain is resolved by surgery, they may continue to suffer from psychological distress. This demonstrates that psychological comfort is of vital importance, and precisely because it is so important, it must be taken seriously.

(2) Pain Management

Chest wall surgery is performed on the body surface, an area rich in sensory nerve distribution. Therefore, postoperative pain is one of the most common complaints. Among different incision types, median incisions generally cause less pain, while lateral chest wall incisions result in more noticeable pain, possibly due to differences in nerve endings distribution. Among various surgical procedures, deformity correction surgery, which involves extensive manipulation of bony structures, tends to cause more significant postoperative pain. Other types of chest wall surgeries usually result in less severe pain. However, pain affects not only the patient's subjective comfort but also critical functions such as respiratory movement, coughing, sputum clearance, and overall activity level, which are vital for recovery. Therefore, pain must be effectively managed.

To reduce pain, analgesic interventions can begin during surgery. Before closing the incision, local anesthetic infiltration can be used for pain relief and may produce good results. Postoperative analgesia can include continuous intravenous analgesia, as-needed medications, and other methods.

Pain is a highly subjective experience and is strongly influenced by psychological factors [3]. Individuals with strong willpower tend to have a higher pain tolerance, while those who are mentally weaker may struggle to cope with pain. Moreover, pain perception can be heavily affected by suggestion. If other patients or family members describe postoperative sensations in a fearful or exaggerated manner, patients are more likely to internalize these impressions and experience similar levels of pain. Therefore, pain management must include both pharmacological and psychological approaches. Alongside medication, patients should be comforted and encouraged, and positive, reassuring information should be conveyed to avoid fear-based influence. This dual approach is often highly effective. It is crucial not to use painkillers indiscriminately, as improper use can lead to addiction, resulting in serious consequences.

(3) Incision Healing

To complete the tasks of the first stage of recovery, the surgical incision must heal well, which is the main focus during this stage. Incision healing is influenced by many factors beyond intraoperative technique, including:[4]: ① The environment around the incision ; ② Blood supply to the incision area ; ③ Presence of exudate (discharge) ; ④ Any mechanical trauma or impact ; ⑤ Use of antibiotics ; ⑥ Timing of suture removal.

The healing of a surgical incision objectively requires a clean, dry, and physiologically suitable surrounding environment, which is primarily maintained through proper dressing and bandaging. Timely and sterile dressing changes are fundamental to incision healing. If this is not done well, problems will arise. Key factors affecting healing include: Blood supply to the incision area, mainly determined by intraoperative handling. However, postoperative factors like prolonged pressure or tightly wrapped dressings can reduce local blood flow. Infrared therapy can be used postoperatively to improve circulation by increasing local temperature. Fluid accumulation or exudate around the incision can also hinder healing if not properly drained. Mechanical trauma (e.g., bumping the wound) before complete healing can cause the incision to open, disrupting recovery. Although chest wall incisions are often sterile, most chest wall surgeries involve the use of implanted materials, which are foreign bodies and may require antibiotic use to prevent infection. Lack or improper use of antibiotics can impair healing. Lastly, the timing of suture removal matters: removing stitches too early can lead to incision dehiscence, while delayed removal usually does not affect healing adversely

In addition to the above factors, many other elements can affect wound healing, such as: Skin edge alignment of the incision, foreign bodies inside the wound, The patient's overall nutritional status, these all play a role in the healing process. It's clear that incision healing is highly susceptible to various influences. Therefore, to promote proper healing, every step must be carefully managed by eliminating adverse factors and creating favorable conditions to ensure the incision heals well in the shortest possible time.

(4) Prevention of Complications

The early postoperative period is the time when complications are most likely to occur, and preventing complications is a critical task during the first stage of recovery. Chest wall surgery can result in various complications, and in many cases, the root cause of these complications lies in the surgical procedure itself, rather than in the postoperative care. Therefore, strictly speaking, the focus of postoperative recovery during this phase is not about completely preventing complications, but rather about minimizing their occurrence as much as possible.

There are many types of thoracic wall diseases, and the postoperative complications vary for each type. Therefore, the content of postoperative rehabilitation also differs. for patients with chest wall deformities, since steel plates are commonly used during surgery for correction, preventing displacement of the steel plate becomes the most critical aspect of postoperative recovery. Specific measures include [5] : ① Avoid vigorous physical activity. The main target of chest wall deformity correction is the bony structure, which is altered during surgery and fixed or supported by a steel plate. This fixation is not very rigid. To ensure stability, patients must rest adequately during the early postoperative phase and avoid early or intense physical activity. Excessive movement may lead to displacement of the steel plate and associated complications. ② Lie flat as much as possible and avoid side-lying positions. In deformity correction surgeries, steel plates are generally placed symmetrically on the anterior chest wall. This specific placement requires the patient to lie flat during early recovery. In the supine position, the force on the plate is evenly distributed, minimizing the risk of movement. However, lying on one side causes uneven force distribution and may result in the plate shifting to the opposite side, leading to recurrence of the deformity. With regard to sleeping positions, adults and adolescents can usually control this, but young children may have difficulty staying flat. If occasional side-lying is unavoidable, efforts should be made to reduce it. Additionally, when holding infants or young children during early recovery, caregivers should be cautious of the holding posture to avoid affecting the steel plate's position. ③ Crying should be minimized as much as possible. When infants or young children cry, the chest wall moves vigorously. Such intense movements are detrimental to both the bony structures of the chest wall and the fixation of the steel plate. Therefore, it is essential to avoid crying episodes as much as possible during the postoperative recovery period. ④ Avoid collisions as much as possible. In the early postoperative period, the position of the steel plate is not firmly fixed and has low resistance to external impact. During this time, mechanical collisions should be avoided as much as possible, as they can not only cause the steel plate to shift but may also lead to other serious consequences.

In addition to complications related to the position of the steel plate, various other complications may also occur after chest wall deformity surgery. These include pneumothorax, pleural effusion, and atelectasis, all of which can negatively affect recovery. In clinical practice, careful observation and effective preventive measures should be taken to minimize the occurrence of such complications.

Apart from chest wall deformities, surgeries for other chest wall conditions can also lead to various associated complications. Once these complications occur they can severely affect the recovery process. Therefore, preventing or minimizing the occurrence of such complications is also a key component of postoperative rehabilitation for these surgeries.

(5) Appropriate Physical Activity

Any surgical procedure is a form of trauma to the body, and to recover from it as quickly as possible, physical activity must begin at an appropriate time after the operation. This activity represents a transition from a pathological to a healthy state. The importance of such activity lies in the following aspects [6]:① Boosting Confidence and Accelerating Recovery: After thoracic wall surgery, once the disease has been treated, appropriate movement instils confidence in the patient, which helps promote overall postoperative recovery. ② Improving Blood Circulation and Laying a Foundation for Recovery: Moderate activity enhances blood circulation not only around the incision site and surgical area but also throughout the entire body which greatly benefits recovery. ③ Increasing Physical Tolerance and Helping to Reduce or Eliminate Pain: Early movement may initially cause discomfort, but it strengthens the body's pain tolerance and helps alleviate subsequent pain. Patients who avoid movement out of fear of pain may experience prolonged discomfort, which negatively affects recovery. ④ Reducing Complications: Although thoracic wall surgery is localized, it still impacts the chest, where vital organs are located. Surgery inevitably affects respiratory and circulatory functions. Prolonged bed rest increases the risk of pulmonary and other complications. Early, appropriate movement significantly reduces this risk. ⑤ Shortening Recovery Time and Helping the Body Return to Health Sooner: The goal of rehabilitation is to restore normal activity. The sooner a patient begins moving, the faster recovery occurs. Conversely, a lack of activity delays or even prevents recovery.

Postoperative physical activity plays a vital role in patient recovery. However, it must follow certain basic principles: ① Avoid getting out of bed before anesthesia fully wears off: Thoracic wall surgeries are typically performed under general anesthesia. While generally safe, the effects of anesthesia can last for some time. During this period, the body is still in a vulnerable state, and premature movement may lead to complications. ② Be cautious with movement before drainage tubes are removed: Closed drainage tubes are often placed after thoracic surgery and may remain for an extended period. Movement with these tubes in place is inconvenient and risky. Patients must be especially careful to protect the tubes to prevent accidental dislodgement or injury. ③ Activity must be gradual and progressive avoid sudden or intense movement: In the early postoperative phase, patients are physically weak. Intense activity at this stage is not only detrimental to recovery but may also cause unnecessary pain or lead to complications. Activity should be increased step by step as the patient's condition improves.

In the first stage after surgery, the patient has just undergone the trauma of the operation, with unstable vital signs and extreme physical weakness. While rehabilitation during this period is essential, it must be approached with the right methods and intensity. Only by doing so can the recovery process be accelerated and a solid foundation laid for the next phases of rehabilitation.

2. Second Stage of Rehabilitation

The second stage of rehabilitation following thoracic wall surgery is a transitional period, marking the shift from the perioperative stage to complete recovery. The patient’s discharge from the hospital indicates the end of the perioperative period and the beginning of this second phase, which continues until full recovery is achieved. It's important to note that "recovery" in thoracic surgery differs from that in general surgery. While healing of the incision is often seen as the endpoint in other procedures, thoracic wall surgery involves remodeling of bony structures, which requires a longer healing time. Generally, the three months following surgery are considered the period for bone healing. During this time, the main goal of rehabilitation is to help the patient recover from the effects of surgery, restore strength, and return to a normal state as quickly as possible. To achieve this, attention must be paid to the following aspects: ① Adequate nutritional intake to support healing and energy needs. ② Sufficient rest to aid physical recovery. ; ③ Scientific and moderate exercise to regain physical function without stressing the surgical area. ; ④Prevention of complications through careful observation and adherence to medical guidance.

Nutritional supplementation is a crucial aspect of recovery. After undergoing surgery, the body experiences significant stress and consumes a large amount of energy. At the same time, proper nutrition is essential for the healing process. Therefore, ensuring adequate nutrition after surgery is absolutely necessary. Rest is equally important. Proper rest provides a solid foundation for recovery. Patients should not rush back to work immediately after discharge, as doing so may hinder the healing process. Exercise is also very important. There are many benefits to moderate physical activity. Appropriate exercise can shorten the recovery period, improve overall physical fitness, and help the body return to a healthy state more quickly. The final point to keep in mind is the prevention of complications. After discharge, while the incision may appear to have healed on the surface, that does not mean the body has fully recovered. Many internal structures may still be in the process of healing. If the patient engages in intense physical activity or suffers an accidental injury during this time, it could not only slow down recovery but also lead to various complications. Therefore, extra care and caution are still necessary during this stage.

3. Third Stage of Recovery

After completing the first two stages of recovery, the patient enters the third stage. By this point, the surgical incision has fully healed, the bone structures have completely recovered, and the shape of the chest wall has stabilized marking a state of complete recovery in the true sense. For most types of chest wall surgeries, recovery during this stage mainly involves functional exercises within the patient's capacity to enhance physical strength and overall well-being.

At this stage, although the bony structure in patients with chest wall deformities has already been shaped, its form is still not stable. If exposed to external force, the shape can easily and rapidly change. Therefore, this stage serves as a consolidation period for the skeletal form. Only by going through this stabilization process can the thoracic structure become permanently set, ensuring that the deformity does not recur at this stage, the focus of recovery is relatively limited, mainly aimed at improving physical fitness, maintaining the function of the implanted steel plate, and providing support for its shaping effect. There are two key precautions during this phase: ① Avoid injury: Any external force or trauma may affect the already shaped chest structure or cause displacement of the steel plate ; ② Refrain from bodybuilding: Intense strength training or muscle building exercises should be avoided temporarily, as they may interfere with the positioning and shaping function of the steel plate.

After chest wall deformity surgery, patients finally emerge from the shadow of the deformity and often have a strong desire for social acceptance. One way to gain such recognition is by participating in group activities or sports. These activities are beneficial for helping patients overcome psychological trauma. However, if the exercises are too intense, they can lead to injury. Since steel plates are implanted inside the body, severe injury could result in even more serious consequences, which would be highly detrimental to recovery. Therefore, any physical activity must be approached with extreme caution to prevent potential tragedies.

Patients with chest wall deformities often have high expectations for their chest appearance. After surgery, many actively engage in bodybuilding activities, hoping to achieve a better physique. However, bodybuilding can also pose problems. Its goal is to enhance the shape of the chest muscles, which appears harmless from the outside. Yet, one must consider the future removal of the implanted steel plates. If the muscles become overly thick, it can make the removal surgery much more difficult. In such cases, the original incision often needs to be extended, resulting in a longer scar. Ironically, while bodybuilding aims to improve appearance, the resulting scarring becomes an unavoidable cost of that effort. Moreover, bodybuilding involves intense physical activity. If not done carefully, it can lead to displacement of the steel plates, ultimately affecting the surgical outcome. Therefore, postoperative bodybuilding is not an ideal choice. Patients who wish to pursue it are advised to wait until after the steel plates have been removed, when bodybuilding can truly yield positive and lasting results.

In summary, postoperative rehabilitation following chest wall surgery is a critical process that must be implemented based on the characteristics of different diseases and surgical procedures. Scientific rehabilitation helps consolidate the treatment outcome and enables patients to recover as soon as possible. If rehabilitation is handled carelessly or unscientifically, it can not only delay recovery but may also lead to unnecessary complications or even surgical failure. Therefore, postoperative rehabilitation must be taken seriously. Only with proper attention can the best possible results be achieved.

REFERENCES

[1] Wang, Wenlin. 2021a. "Rehabilitation Issues after Thoracic Wall Surgery." *Thoracic Deformity Surgery Specialist*, November 2.

[2] Wang, Wenlin. 2021b. "Psychological Issues and Mental Disorders in Patients with Pectus Carinatum." *Thoracic Deformity Surgery Specialist*, April 28.

[3] Wang, Wenlin. 2017. "Subjectivity and Objectivity of Postoperative Pain." *Thoracic Deformity Surgery Specialist*, June 17.

[4] Wang, Wenlin. 2021c. "Factors Affecting Wound Healing after Thoracic Wall Surgery." *Toutiao Today*, November 2.

[5] Wang, Wenlin. 2021d. "After Thoracic Wall Surgery: Preventing the Occurrence of Complications." *Toutiao Today*, November 2.

[6] Wang, Wenlin. 2021e. "Postoperative Rehabilitation: The Importance of Early Mobilization." *Toutiao Today*, November 2.

THE PRINCIPLE OF MINIMALISM AND THORACIC WALL SURGERY

The principle of minimalism is both a belief and a habit. It requires that one's thinking and actions follow the principle of simplification to the greatest extent possible. Although minimalism may not be accepted by everyone, it represents an objective law that aligns with the direction of nearly all technological advancements.

Looking back at the history of surgical technique development, many concepts and procedures have evolved in the direction of simplification. In the early days, many surgical techniques were quite complex. This complexity manifested in two main aspects: first, the techniques themselves were intricate and difficult for doctors to master; second, the procedures were technically demanding, making it hard for most surgeons to perform them effectively. Such complexity limited the advancement of the specialty. However, with continuous technological progress, every type of surgery has been moving toward simplification. This trend marks the maturity of the technique and represents the inevitable direction of its development [1].

The development of thoracic wall surgery also reflects the trend toward simplification. Take pectus excavatum surgery as an example: in the early days, open surgery was quite complex, requiring complete destruction of the deformity details followed by reshaping all anatomical components. To complete such a surgery, doctors had to put in a tremendous amount of effort. Later, the internal turnover procedure emerged. Although this surgery still involved many steps, it was significantly simplified. This procedure no longer needed to address every deformity detail but treated the affected chest wall as a whole for correction. The number of operational steps clearly decreased, and the specific details were fully simplified, making it widely adopted. Subsequently, the Nuss procedure was introduced, which was clearly simpler than all previous surgeries [2]. The fundamental reason for the strong vitality of this procedure is that it follows the natural trend of surgical development and perfectly embodies the minimalist principle. Following this direction, it is easy to imagine that the next stage of pectus excavatum treatment must be a procedure even simpler than the Nuss procedure. Thus, the Wang procedure came into the spotlight and immediately attracted great attention. The Wang procedure involves direct manipulation of the depression deformity under direct vision. Since the depression can be eliminated simply by lifting, the surgery is simplified to the extreme, further embodying the essence of the minimalist principle [3].

Each disease requires increasingly in-depth and detailed research. However, within a large discipline like thoracic surgery, due to various objective limitations, it is impossible to conduct comprehensive research on every single disease. This leads to the demand for more refined development, which is also the fundamental reason why many surgical disciplines evolve into subspecialties.

The transition from the broad field of general thoracic surgery to the more focused study of thoracic wall diseases thoracic wall surgery is a typical example of reductionism and a manifestation of simplification. Therefore, it is also a direct interpretation of the minimalist principle. Thoracic wall surgery is a brand-new discipline. As the field gradually takes shape, it actively absorbs the most advanced technologies and concepts, progressively forming its own distinctive features. Among these features, many aspects reflect the influence of the minimalist principle. This principle is not only embedded in the fundamental concepts, but also in the surgical principles and specific operational details. The minimalist principle has become the true essence of this discipline.

1.Conceptual Minimalism

The issue of ideology is a major concern in any discipline, as it guides all aspects of its work. Since the emergence of thoracic wall surgery, the principle of minimalism has consciously become its most important guiding ideology. In clinical practice, examinations strive to be minimalist, preoperative preparation aims for minimalism, intraoperative setup seeks simplicity, surgical procedures are simplified, postoperative monitoring is kept minimal, and recovery protocols are streamlined. This minimalist ideology has gradually integrated into every aspect of thoracic wall surgery and become the soul of its operations. Such a mindset clearly differs from that of traditional thoracic surgery. However, it may be precisely this approach that showcases the discipline's strengths and lays a solid foundation for its future development.

2. Surgical Principles of Minimalism

Strictly speaking, traditional thoracic wall surgeries are not truly thoracic wall surgical procedures, because those operations were designed by thoracic surgeons or doctors from other specialties. For example, the Nuss procedure was developed by a pediatric surgeon and existed many years before the thoracic wall surgery field became independent. Therefore, such a procedure should not be considered a thoracic wall surgery. After the emergence of thoracic wall surgery, a modified technique targeting the Nuss procedure was developed, this is the Wung procedure [4]. The emergence of this procedure perfectly embodies the principle of minimalism. Its most distinctive feature is the complete simplification of the steel plate fixation method, which later became known as the Wang technique.

Due to its simplicity, ease of operation, firm effectiveness, and ability to be performed through very small incisions, this technique quickly gained nationwide popularity upon its introduction and has now become the mainstream method for steel plate fixation. The transition from the Nuss procedure to the Wung procedure mainly involved the simplification of the fixation principle; this is the soul of the Wang procedure.

Thoracic wall surgery also introduced another specialized procedure, the Wenlin procedure designed specifically for correcting protrusion deformities [5,6]. This surgery is considered an improvement upon the earlier Abramson procedure [7]. Since the Abramson procedure was developed before the formal establishment of thoracic wall surgery, it similarly cannot be regarded as a typical thoracic wall surgical procedure. The greatest drawback of the Abramson procedure lies in its method of steel plate fixation. It uses the same specialized steel plate as the Nuss procedure for pectus excavatum. During fixation, a short fixation plate must first be attached to the ribs, and only then can the main steel plate be secured to the short plate. This approach is technically challenging, the fixation is often unreliable, and it requires relatively large incisions. All of these are significant shortcomings in what should be a minimally invasive procedure. The Wenlin procedure, however, adopts a completely different fixation principle. It eliminates the use of the short fixation plate and instead fixes the main steel plate directly to the ribs. This shifts the fixation from an indirect to a direct method and dramatically improves the surgical outcome. As a result, all of the defects associated with the Abramson procedure are resolved. In the evolution from the Abramson procedure to the Wenlin procedure, the simplification of surgical principles became the key to surgical advancement.

3. Simplification of Surgical Techniques

After the emergence of thoracic wall surgery, the overall appearance of surgical procedures underwent a complete transformation. In addition to the simplification of concepts and surgical principles, the specific techniques themselves also evolved toward minimalism. This development is reflected in almost all technical improvements. Take the Nuss procedure for pectus excavatum as an example from skin incision to skin closure, all procedural details have been significantly simplified, thoroughly transforming the operation. The simplification of techniques is demonstrated in the following aspects: ① Wang Technique for Fixing the Steel Plate: In the standard Nuss procedure, steel wires are typically placed after the steel plate is inserted. Due to the presence of the plate in the incision at that point, wire placement becomes difficult and carries a risk of piercing lung tissue. To simplify this, we place guiding wires before the steel plate is inserted. This avoids interference during the operation and ensures safety. With these changes, wire placement becomes safer, simpler, and provides excellent fixation results. ② Placement of the Introducer: In the standard Nuss technique, the introducer is placed under thoracoscopic guidance a process that is time-consuming, labor-intensive, and condition-specific. To thoroughly simplify this step, we use direct penetration to place the introducer, abandoning Thoracoscopy. This approach is not only safe and accurate, but also greatly simplifies the procedure. ③ Insertion of the Steel Plate: After placing the introducer, the standard Nuss method uses a thick strap to tie the steel plate to the introducer's end, then pulls it across the mediastinum to the base of the depression. This method is cumbersome and, due to the non-smooth connection between the plate and the introducer, can damage surrounding structures during pulling. To improve this, we use a special guiding tube to insert the steel plate indirectly. Specifically: First, thread the guiding tube through the introducer, drag the guiding tube across the mediastinum, then use the guiding tube to pull the steel plate into the desired position. Although this adds one more step, the presence of the guiding tube makes the operation smoother, simpler, and safer.

Apart from the example of the Nuss procedure, the operative techniques of almost all other clinical surgeries are also evolving toward minimalism. These surgeries include not only those for thoracic deformities, but also procedures for chest wall tumors, defects, infections, and trauma. The simplification of surgical techniques not only points the way forward for technical advancement but also provides strong motivation for continued progress.

4. Conceptual Minimalism

In clinical practice of thoracic wall surgery, aside from the minimalism in concepts, surgical principles, and techniques, several other ideas related to the minimalist principle have also been introduced. These additions have further enriched the theoretical system of minimalism in thoracic wall surgery

(1) Tubeless Technique

The Tubeless technique is a surgical concept proposed by Professor He Jianxing. Broadly speaking, it falls under the category of Enhanced Recovery After Surgery [1,8]. This technique advocates for tubeless management during thoracic surgery, aiming to eliminate the use of various drainage tubes as much as possible. Although this concept originally emerged in thoracic surgery, with the advent of thoracic wall surgery, a large number of thoracic wall procedures became suitable for applying this technique. As a result, thoracic wall surgery has become the best practitioner of the Tubeless technique. The core of the Tubeless technique lies in the non-use of various drainage tubes, which perfectly embodies the essence of the principle of minimalism.

In traditional thoracic surgery, procedures typically require general anesthesia, which in turn necessitates endotracheal intubation. To ensure perioperative safety, various so-called "life channels" must be established: First, venous catheterization ensures rapid fluid replacement in emergencies and allows monitoring of venous pressure. Second, arterial catheterization is used for real-time blood pressure monitoring. Third, urinary catheterization facilitates smooth urination and enables monitoring of urine output. In addition to these life-support tubes, closed thoracic drainage tubes are also standard in thoracic surgery. These tubes have long been considered essential in traditional thoracic surgical practices. The absence of any one of these was previously deemed highly unsafe even contrary to established medical norms. Clearly, the presence of these tubes makes perioperative management quite complex. However, for a long time, the negative impact of this complexity was not fully recognized in clinical practice. Under certain influences, even more tubes and procedures were added, inevitably leading to further drawbacks. With the introduction of the Tubeless technique, a profound shift occurred in clinical thinking. More and more practitioners began to realize that many operations previously thought indispensable could, in fact, be omitted. As long as the technical design is sound, these so-called "life tubes" can be removed in the era of truly tubeless surgery.

For the vast majority of thoracic surgeons, the full implementation of Tubeless technology still requires time. This is mainly due to the specific requirements of thoracic surgery and personal habits. However, in the case of thoracic wall surgery, the conditions for applying the Tubeless technique are uniquely favorable. Firstly, thoracic wall surgeries generally have shorter operation times, making it possible to avoid the use of conventional tracheal intubation (Fig. 1-14-1) and urinary catheters. Since the procedures are performed on the chest wall and are relatively safe, arterial and venous catheterization can also be omitted. Secondly, because these surgeries rarely involve entering the thoracic cavity, there is often no need to place a closed thoracic drainage tube. These features of thoracic wall surgery allow the Tubeless technique to integrate seamlessly, yielding highly satisfactory outcomes.

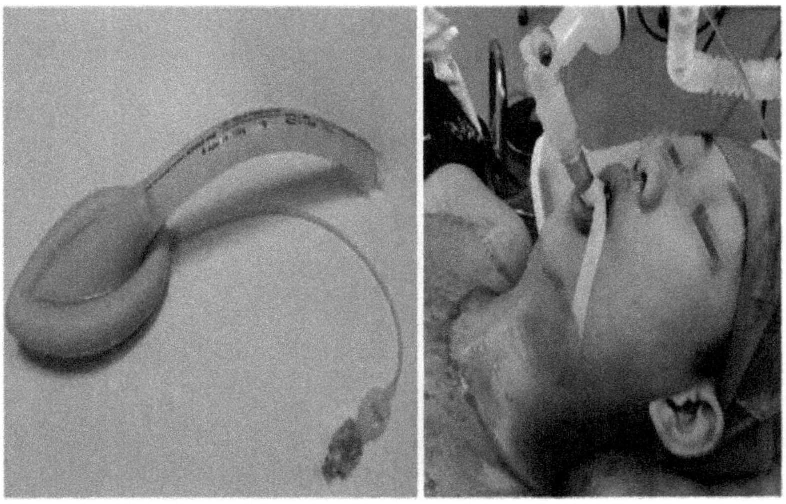

Figure 1-14-1: The most critical step in Tubeless technology, oxygen delivery via laryngeal mask.

The widespread application of Tubeless technology in thoracic wall surgery is a perfect embodiment of the principle of minimalism. With many procedures omitted, perioperative operations become extremely simple, significantly improving the quality of patient recovery and greatly shortening recovery time. The overall medical experience for patients is substantially enhanced.

(2) Clean Surgery

Clean surgery is a minimalist surgical concept that we have proposed. Just like the Tubeless technique, the introduction of this concept is a perfect embodiment of the minimalist principle [9]. The term "clean" here is no different from its meaning in everyday life, its core meaning is tidiness. One of the basic requirements of tidiness is the avoidance of complexity, or in other words, keeping things to a minimum. This clearly aligns perfectly with the demands of the minimalist principle.

Clean surgery must be understood from different dimensions and levels. It fundamentally includes three basic dimensions (Figures 1-14-2, 1-14-3, 1-14-4): Clean surgical field, Clean operating table, Clean operating room [10]. Only when cleanliness is achieved in all three dimensions can the most thorough cleanliness and the most complete minimalism be truly realized.

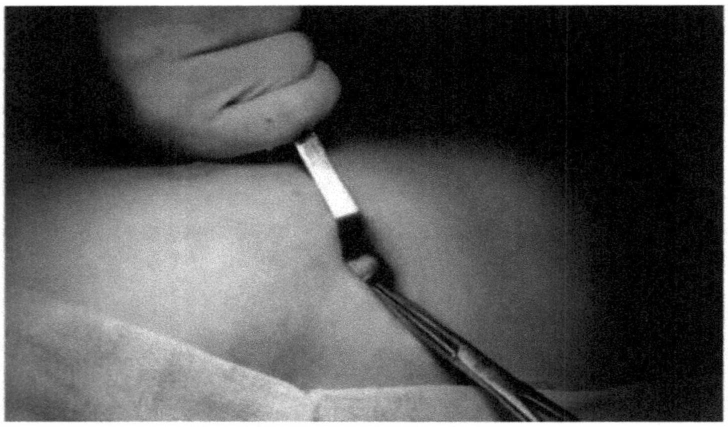
Figure 1-14-2 Clean Surgical Field

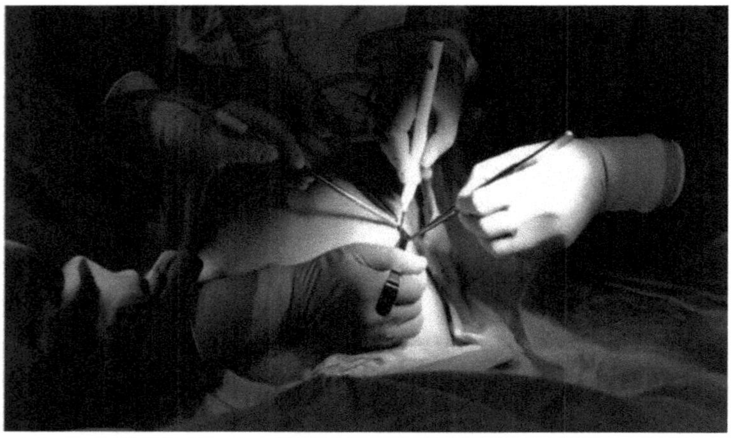
Figure 1-14-3 Clean Operating Table

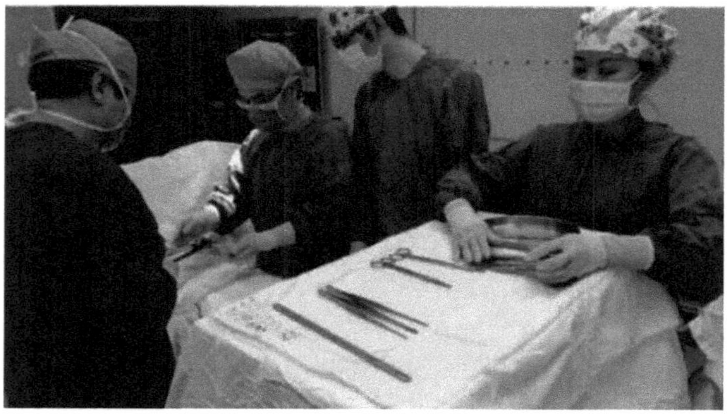
Figure 1-14-4 Clean Operating Room

The cleanliness of the surgical field represents the most fundamental level of sterility. It requires that the operative area remains free from excessive materials, tubes, instruments, and dressings. Everything must be organized in a clear and layered manner, with even visible bleeding kept to a minimum. Achieving this standard demands a high level of skill from the surgeon; this is the most basic form of minimalism and a fundamental requirement for all surgeons. A clean operating table reflects an even higher level of cleanliness. This requires the surgeon not only to have excellent technical skills but also strong situational control and more importantly, a deep understanding of minimalism. If the operating table is cluttered with various tubes and instruments, cleanliness is impossible. Cleanliness not only implies order but also necessitates a reduction in content. When the operating table becomes clean, the overall surgical procedure is inevitably simplified, allowing the principle of minimalism to be further embodied. The cleanliness of the operating room may seem unrelated to the surgeon's actions, but in reality, this is not the case. Nowadays, many operating rooms are becoming increasingly chaotic, with a wide array of auxiliary devices and instruments appearing, making the environment more and more crowded. This situation is not primarily the fault of others, the main responsibility lies with the surgeon. If a surgeon can ensure that their procedure avoids the use of unnecessary devices, a higher level of cleanliness can be achieved. This level of cleanliness is undoubtedly more advanced and better reflects the essence of the minimalist principle.

In general, surgical procedures, achieving cleanliness across all three dimensions is not easy. However, in thoracic wall surgery, clean operations can be well accomplished. In terms of the surgical field, many procedures can be performed with virtually no visible bleeding. When even the naked eye cannot detect any bleeding in the operative field, the surgery can be considered truly clean and such procedures are often the simplest. From the instrumentation perspective, many thoracic wall surgeries require only a minimal number of instruments. When no special tools are needed, the operating table remains very clean. Looking at the entire operating room, because no special equipment or excess tubing is required, and in many cases even thoracoscopes are unnecessary, the room appears extremely tidy achieving cleanliness in the third dimension. Thus, cleanliness in thoracic wall surgery is not an unattainable ideal, but a practical reality from the outset perfectly embodying the principle of minimalism.

Understanding "clean surgery" from different dimensions is merely a superficial, quantitative perspective not a deep comprehension. The true essence of clean surgery must be grasped through varying levels of mastery. We categorize all clean surgeries into four levels of realm [11]: Primary Level, Lower-Intermediate Level, Intermediate Level, Highest Level. Interpreting clean surgery through these levels allows for a more precise depiction of its true essence.

The primary level of clean surgery can be understood as sensory cleanliness. This refers to cleanliness that is visible and tangible a reduction in physical mess or contamination. For example, a clean surgical field, a tidy operating table, and a sterile operating room all fall under this basic level of cleanliness.

The secondary intermediate level of clean surgery can be understood as cleanliness in operation. While sensory cleanliness is static, surgery is a dynamic process of a series of actions. Therefore, a more advanced form of cleanliness arises from the details of these actions. Every surgery has specific steps, and different surgeons may perform them differently. Some surgeons operate with clarity an efficiency, while others are messy and imprecise. Both may complete the surgery successfully, but the impression they leave is vastly different. Operational cleanliness refers to procedures that are simple, precise, and free of unnecessary movements. This level of cleanliness is clearly more refined than sensory cleanliness, representing a higher understanding of clean surgery.

The intermediate level of clean surgery can be understood as cleanliness in surgical principles. For treating the same disease, there may be multiple surgical approaches. Some procedures are complex, difficult to perform, and require various instruments and materials. Such surgeries cannot be considered clean. In contrast, another method might use entirely different principles, drastically reducing and simplifying the steps involved. From a theoretical standpoint, this kind of surgery appears much cleaner. The principle behind a surgery determines its quality, its procedural content, and the required technical details. Cleanliness at the level of principles is undoubtedly of great importance. It represents a higher realm of cleanliness, and at the same time, a higher level of minimalism.

The highest level of clean surgery can be understood as conceptual cleanliness. This reflects the excellent quality and disciplined thinking of a surgeon. Conceptual cleanliness is the purest embodiment of the minimalist principle; it represents minimalism at the level of treatment philosophy, and it is the ultimate form of cleanliness. for a surgeon, only by thoroughly embracing minimalism in their mindset can they truly achieve the highest realm of clean surgery. Thoracic wall surgery incorporates many techniques that embody the concept of clean surgery. From a sensory perspective, many existing procedures strive for visible cleanliness not only in themselves but also in comparison to other thoracic surgeries. From the operational content perspective, many procedures are being simplified as much as possible. For example, although the standard Nuss procedure is already relatively simple, it can be designed to be even more streamlined, making it a surgery with minimal procedural steps that reflects cleanliness in operation. In terms of surgical principles, many procedures are becoming increasingly simplified. The Wang procedure for treating pectus excavatum is a vivid example of this. Similar principles can be found in the treatment of other conditions as well, indicating that the design concepts in thoracic wall surgery are evolving toward greater simplicity. Conceptual cleanliness is arguably the most distinctive feature of thoracic wall surgery. Since the establishment of this specialty, all its underlying concepts have reflected the essence of clean surgery. This also represents the most profound impact that the principle of minimalism has had on the field.

The concept of "clean surgery" represents a profound reflection and realization about surgical techniques. Throughout the history of surgical development, every technique has been evolving toward a cleaner and more refined form. During this process, some “less clean” techniques may emerge, but such methods are often short-lived and cannot endure over time. Only truly clean techniques align with the trends and direction of technical advancement, meet the demands of the minimalist principle, possess real vitality, and are capable of genuine, lasting development.

Thoracic wall surgery, as a completely new clinical specialty, has been influenced by numerous advanced concepts from the very beginning. Under the guidance of these ideas, thoracic wall surgery has not only actively embraced concepts such as Tubeless techniques and clean surgery, but has also carried out substantial innovations in many specific techniques. As a result, the essence of the principle of minimalism has been most perfectly embodied in the development of thoracic wall surgery. It not only aligns with the natural course of development but also provides momentum for the further advancement of thoracic wall surgery. Under the guidance of the principle of minimalism, thoracic wall surgery is destined to become increasingly refined and achieve comprehensive progress more streamlined, making it a surgery with minimal procedural steps that reflects cleanliness in operation. In terms of surgical

principles, many procedures are becoming increasingly simplified. The Wang procedure for treating pectus excavatum is a vivid example of this. Similar principles can be found in the treatment of other conditions as well, indicating that the design concepts in thoracic wall surgery are evolving toward greater simplicity. Conceptual cleanliness is arguably the most distinctive feature of thoracic wall surgery. Since the establishment of this specialty, all its underlying concepts have reflected the essence of clean surgery. This also represents the most profound impact that the principle of minimalism has had on the field.
The concept of "clean surgery" represents a profound reflection and realization about surgical techniques. Throughout the history of surgical development, every technique has been evolving toward a cleaner and more refined form. During this process, some "less clean" techniques may emerge, but such methods are often short-lived and cannot endure over time. Only truly clean techniques align with the trends and direction of technical advancement, meet the demands of the minimalist principle, possess real vitality, and are capable of genuine, lasting development.

The concept of "clean surgery" represents a profound reflection and realization about surgical techniques. Throughout the history of surgical development, every technique has been evolving toward a cleaner and more refined form. During this process, some "less clean" techniques may emerge, but such methods are often short-lived and cannot endure over time. Only truly clean techniques align with the trends and direction of technical advancement, meet the demands of the minimalist principle, possess real vitality, and are capable of genuine, lasting development.

Thoracic wall surgery, as a completely new clinical specialty, has been influenced by numerous advanced concepts from the very beginning. Under the guidance of these ideas, thoracic wall surgery has not only actively embraced concepts such as Tubeless techniques and clean surgery, but has also carried out substantial innovations in many specific techniques. As a result, the essence of the principle of minimalism has been most perfectly embodied in the development of thoracic wall surgery. It not only aligns with the natural course of development but also provides momentum for the further advancement of thoracic wall surgery. Under the guidance of the principle of minimalism, thoracic wall surgery is destined to become increasingly refined and achieve comprehensive progress.

REFERENCES

[1] Wang Wenlin. Professor He Jianxing's Surgical Philosophy: Tubeless Surgery and the Principle of Minimalism. Specialist in Thoracic Deformity Surgery, 2020-02-19.
[2] Schwabegger A. H. Pectus Excavatum Repair from a Plastic Surgeon's Perspective. Annals of Cardiothoracic Surgery, 2016, 5(5): 501–512.
[3] Wang W. L., Chen C. M., Long W. G., et al. Wang Procedure: Novel Minimally Invasive Procedure for Pectus Excavatum in Young Children. Case Reports and Images in Surgery, 2018, 1(1): 1–2.
[4] Wang Wenlin. The Safety of the Wing Procedure. Specialist in Thoracic Deformity Surgery, 2021-04-24.
[5] Wang W. L. Minimally Invasive Surgical Technique for Barrel Chest. Surgical Case Reports, 2018, 1(2): 1–2.
[6] Wang Wenlin. The Minimalist Principle and Wenlin Chest Surgery. Specialist in Thoracic Deformity Surgery, 2018-12-15.
[7] Abramson H., Aragone X., Blanco J. B., et al. Minimally Invasive Repair of Pectus Carinatum and How to Deal with Complications. Journal of Visualized Surgery, 2016(2): 64.
[8] Wang Wenlin. Tubeless Surgery for Thoracic Deformity and the Minimalist Principle. Specialist in Thoracic Deformity Surgery, 2018-11-25.
[9] Wang Wenlin. Clean Surgery: Bleedingless Surgery and Tubeless Surgery. Specialist in Thoracic Deformity Surgery, 2019-01-19.
[10] Wang Wenlin. The Three Dimensions of Clean Surgery. Specialist in Thoracic Deformity Surgery, 2019-01-24.
[11] Wang Wenlin. The Four Realms of Clean Surgery. Specialist in Thoracic Deformity Surgery, 2019-01-26.

Thoracic surgery is an ancient specialty and currently one of the major disciplines in clinical practice. Many hospitals have very strong thoracic surgery departments with highly renowned experts. Logically speaking, such a powerful specialty should be comprehensively developed, with excellence in every aspect. But unfortunately, in recent years, the development of this specialty has deviated from its intended path. A large amount of human and material resources have been concentrated on the treatment of intrathoracic diseases, while thoracic wall diseases have been neglected. This situation clearly does not align with the status of a major clinical specialty. The lack of attention given to thoracic wall diseases hinders their treatment and research, which is an abnormal state of affairs. The reasons for this situation are multifaceted—some are objective, but more are subjective, that is, related to human factors. When human factors excessively permeate clinical practice, such an outcome becomes inevitable. As most professionals focus their work on intrathoracic diseases, that field naturally experiences rapid development, as evidenced by many of its current achievements. However, thoracic wall diseases, though overlooked by many, cannot remain neglected forever. Because patients will not simply disappear, and the incidence of thoracic wall diseases remains quite high. Faced with such significant treatment demand, physicians' neglect can only be temporary. When the majority of practitioners turn a blind eye to these patients, there will inevitably be a few who recognize the opportunity—thus, thoracic wall surgery emerged. In this sense, the deviation in the development of thoracic surgery has, in fact, provided thoracic wall surgery with a unique opportunity for growth and laid the foundation for it to eventually become an independent specialty[1].

From the developmental process of thoracic wall surgery, it has gone through two distinct stages: the first stage was as a sub-specialty of thoracic surgery, and the second stage has been its evolution into an independent new specialty. At different stages, thoracic wall surgery has exhibited different characteristics, and its relationship with thoracic surgery has also varied accordingly. Properly understanding the relationship between the two is of great guiding significance for advancing the work of thoracic wall surgery.

1. Sub-specialty Stage

Thoracic wall surgery did not come into existence inherently, nor was its concept casually proposed. Based on the experience of establishing and developing the first thoracic wall surgery department, there was no guiding philosophy at the outset, only a focus on thoracic deformities. At that time, such work could only be carried out within the framework of thoracic surgery and did not even qualify as a sub-specialty. As surgical procedures for thoracic deformities gradually became more mature, patients with other thoracic wall conditions such as tumors and infections also began to receive attention. It was at this point that the distinct characteristics of thoracic wall surgery began to emerge. The major difference from traditional thoracic surgery was a greater focus and precision, with more prominent and defined features. Once these distinctive qualities were established, they drew increasing attention not only from medical peers but also from patients, leading to a growing number of individuals seeking treatment. When the number of thoracic wall disease patients exceeded that of other types of thoracic surgery patients, the time had come to establish a true subspecialty. Within the broader framework of thoracic surgery, thoracic wall surgery began to be systematically developed [2,3]. At this stage, although thoracic wall surgery had its own distinguishing features, it was still considered a part of thoracic surgery. All the diseases treated were those traditionally classified under the thoracic surgery umbrella. While treatment methods were continually improving, they largely followed the conventional techniques of thoracic surgery. If one were to distinguish thoracic wall surgery from general thoracic surgery at this point, the main difference would be a greater focus or narrower specialization. Thoracic surgery provided the platform for thoracic wall surgery supplying patient sources, techniques, and personnel so thoracic wall surgery was entirely encompassed within thoracic surgery. In essence, during the subspecialty phase, thoracic wall surgery was merely a small branch of thoracic surgery. If it had any uniqueness, it was mainly in the types of conditions treated, rather than in the techniques used. However, this phase held significant importance because it signaled that some people had recognized the opportunity within the field. They began to move forward and would eventually achieve remarkable success.

2. Independent Specialty Stage

From a subspecialty to a new specialty, thoracic wall surgery has gradually emerged from the shadow of traditional thoracic surgery, presenting itself in clinical practice with a completely new identity [4,5]. Over time, through continued development and refinement, its theoretical system has gradually taken shape, its concepts have evolved, and its techniques have advanced. All of these changes mark a fundamental distinction from traditional thoracic surgery, signifying its full independence as a separate discipline.

(1) Clarification of the Discipline's Positioning

An independent thoracic wall surgery discipline positions itself specifically for the treatment of thoracic wall diseases. This positioning is entirely different from that of traditional thoracic surgery. The establishment of such a position inevitably impacts the identity of thoracic surgery itself. Within the same medical institution, the emergence of thoracic wall surgery essentially negates the previous scope of thoracic surgery. As a result, thoracic surgery would no longer include the treatment of thoracic wall diseases and would instead focus solely on intrathoracic conditions precisely the direction most thoracic surgery departments in hospitals have pursued. In the early days of clinical practice, such a division might have caused some friction. However, against the backdrop of thoracic surgery having largely deviated toward a “deformed” developmental path where most surgeons concentrate on intrathoracic conditions the clear distinction of thoracic wall surgery not only failed to create a sense of crisis but actually helped relieve thoracic surgeons of peripheral burdens. This became a true win-win situation. The separation of these two "brothers" did not result in conflict but in mutual satisfaction. Such positioning was both timely and necessary.

(2) Improved the Theoretical System of the Discipline

Before the emergence of thoracic wall surgery, certain theoretical concepts had already appeared, but they existed independently without being organically connected, let alone forming a complete theoretical system. After thoracic wall surgery was established, theoretical research began to develop, and a systematic theoretical framework gradually took shape. It unified previously scattered ideas and concepts into a comprehensive and coherent system. The establishment of this theoretical system laid a solid foundation for the clinical practice of thoracic wall surgery.

(3) Introduction of New Concepts

Thoracic wall surgery itself is an entirely new concept, and accordingly, a large number of new related concepts have gradually been introduced. These include the concept of thoracic wall surgical diseases, the distinction between thoracic wall deformities and thoracic cage deformities, the concept of pre-shaping, delayed shaping, and digital materials. All of these are new ideas that emerged only after the development of thoracic wall surgery. The introduction of these concepts has not only enriched and improved the theoretical framework of thoracic wall surgery, but also provided theoretical guidance for the further advancement of clinical practice.

(4) Standardization of the Scope of Inclusion

During the subspecialty phase, the scope of thoracic wall surgery was not standardized; it might have focused more on deformities or tumors. However, once established as an independent department, it became necessary to consider issues of operation and development. The most practical concern at that point is patient inclusion. Clearly defining the scope of inclusion is the prerequisite for effective patient management. The five basic thoracic wall diseases were designated by referencing the inclusion criteria used in general surgical specialties. This regulation is both scientific and practical, providing a solid foundation for the clinical practice of thoracic wall surgery [6].

In the actual operation process, for a new specialty like thoracic wall surgery, conflicts with other traditional specialties are inevitable. It is essential to carefully coordinate these relationships to avoid unnecessary disputes. For example, spinal surgery and breast surgery also involve thoracic wall diseases. To handle these relationships well, the first step is to clearly define the specialty's areas of expertise; secondly, to avoid overstepping boundaries, self-awareness can help minimize conflicts. Additionally, it is necessary to manage the relationship with plastic surgery properly. Plastic surgery is also a relatively new specialty, covering almost everybody's area, and often intersects with other clinical specialties. Since nearly every thoracic wall disease may involve plastic surgery, their relationship needs careful handling. Some hospitals have pediatric surgery departments performing thoracic deformity surgeries, which inevitably conflicts with thoracic wall surgery work. Thoracic wall surgery is a comprehensive department, and the age range of patients it treats should not be limited; therefore, it should also include children or young patients with thoracic deformities. Overlapping responsibilities cause conflicts, which must be properly managed to benefit the specialty's development.

fortunately, after the emergence of thoracic wall surgery, the patient inclusion criteria for this specialty were clearly defined, and disputes with other specialties regarding patient admission were properly resolved. This has paved the way for the healthy development of the specialty.

(5) Invention of New Techniques

After the independence of thoracic wall surgery, specialists have had more focus and energy to dedicate to the study of thoracic wall diseases. This concentrated effort inevitably leads to greater achievements. One such achievement is the invention of new techniques and methods. While this is something that could happen in any specialty even within traditional thoracic surgery if attention were given to thoracic wall diseases the undeniable fact is that since the independence of thoracic wall surgery, related technological development has been advancing rapidly. A large number of results have been developed, fully demonstrating the strong vitality of this emerging field.

(6) Lateral Development

The process of chest wall surgery becoming an independent discipline is one of inheritance and development. The theories and experience of traditional thoracic surgery form the foundation for chest wall surgery's existence. The true purpose of disciplinary independence is development, which involves not only the vertical advancement of existing theories but also cross-disciplinary lateral development. Vertical development means deepening the original theories and techniques, while lateral development involves exploring entirely new fields. There are two notable areas of lateral development: First is orthopedics, and second is plastic surgery [7]. The skeleton is the fundamental structural framework of the chest wall, forming its main body; therefore, any chest wall surgical disease involves skeletal pathology. This basic characteristic closely aligns chest wall surgery with orthopedics, to the extent that chest wall surgery can even be called "chest wall orthopedics." Such a title is not possible in traditional thoracic surgery and provides valuable reference and guidance for new techniques and concepts in chest wall surgery. The second area of lateral development is plastic surgery. Chest wall surgery has two fundamental attributes: disease treatment and reconstruction. Although the reconstruction is limited to the chest wall, it overlaps with plastic surgery. Chest wall surgery traditionally adopts a relatively conservative reconstructive approach and pays less attention to certain details. Applying plastic surgery principles to chest wall surgery would significantly improve reconstructive outcomes. Furthermore, in previous chest wall surgeries, operations such as flap transplantation or transfer traditionally the domain of plastic surgery were often done in collaboration. With the development of chest wall surgery, these procedures will increasingly be performed by chest wall surgeons themselves, marking another aspect of lateral development toward plastic surgery.

Cross-disciplinary lateral development has provided new fields and new perspectives for the development of chest wall surgery and has become a powerful catalyst for the growth of the discipline. This cross-disciplinary development has clearly become a distinctive feature and hallmark of chest wall surgery.

(7) Establishment of New Clinical Departments

After gradually becoming independent, chest wall surgery will show many obvious signs, among which the most fundamental is the establishment of an independent departmental structure. This independent structure includes separate ward units, independent medical teams, and dedicated nursing staff. Only when chest wall surgery can operate healthily like other mature specialized departments can its independence become a reality.

In summary, every clinical specialty has its distinctive characteristics, which arise not only from theory but, more importantly, from clinical practice. Only when all clinical work is carried out in an organized and focused manner around the new specialty can true independence be achieved. Chest wall surgery has undergone a long and arduous process from nothing to its current state. Even today, it is still immature and continues to advance through exploration. However, as a newly emerging field, once chest wall surgery appears in clinical practice, its progress cannot be stopped. This is both a requirement for the development of the discipline and an inevitable path for the advancement of traditional thoracic surgery.

3. Differences Between Independent Chest Wall Surgery and Thoracic Surgery

Chest wall surgery originated from thoracic surgery, but after becoming independent, it has acquired new connotations, resulting in clear distinctions between chest wall surgery and thoracic surgery. These differences are reflected in the following aspects:

(1) Nature of the Surgery

Traditional thoracic surgery focuses solely on treating the disease; as long as this goal is achieved, other considerations can be disregarded. However, in chest wall surgery, since the primary work is performed on the body surface, every procedure involves concerns about appearance. Thus, an additional important attribute arises: reconstruction. Reconstruction and disease treatment are fundamentally different types of surgery. Treatment involves destruction removing the diseased structures whereas reconstruction involves shaping or rebuilding. Essentially, these two types of surgery are almost completely contradictory. Traditional surgery does not need to consider how to resolve this contradiction extensively, but chest wall surgery must balance the two to achieve the best surgical outcome. This unique nature places higher demands on chest wall surgical procedures.

(2) The Concept of Minimally Invasive Surgery

The concept of minimally invasive surgery is widely promoted in modern surgical fields. Traditional thoracic surgery has fully entered the era of minimally invasive techniques. As a newly emerging specialty, chest wall surgery also consistently emphasizes the idea of minimally invasive procedures. However, the concept of minimally invasive surgery in thoracic surgery differs from that in chest wall surgery. In thoracic surgery, minimally invasive mainly refers to smaller incisions, primarily reducing the trauma caused by the incision itself, but the trauma inside the thoracic cavity remains unchanged. From this perspective, thoracic surgery's minimally invasive approach is somewhat one-sided, not fully comprehensive. Chest wall surgery's minimally invasive approach also starts with smaller incisions. However, this form of minimal invasion does not represent the entirety of trauma, because besides the incision, other parts of the chest wall inevitably experience trauma, which is difficult to avoid. Thus, minimally invasive surgery in chest wall procedures is likewise partial and incomplete. This incompleteness is especially evident in major disease surgeries within chest wall surgery. Among the five main disease categories in chest wall surgery, the concept of minimally invasive surgery can only be fully realized in deformity correction surgeries. for almost all other surgeries, achieving further minimal invasiveness is not possible. This represents the biggest difference in trauma considerations between chest wall surgery and traditional thoracic surgery.

However, a large trauma is not a flaw of the surgery itself, but is determined by the nature of the procedure. For example, in chest wall tumor surgery, no matter how much the trauma is minimized, extensive removal of structures on the chest wall cannot be avoided. Such an operation is unavoidable, and therefore the trauma cannot be very small. The same applies to chest wall defects, infections, and trauma. The nature of these diseases dictates that the surgery can only be completed through operations causing relatively large trauma, and it is impossible to accomplish them with overly minimally invasive techniques.

(3) Use of Thoracoscopy

Modern thoracic surgery can be described as thoracoscopic surgery. A thoracoscopic a device used to observe structures inside the thoracic cavity. The application of this device can greatly reduce the size of the chest wall incision.

However, thoracoscopic surgery is not equivalent to minimally invasive surgery. This distinction is evident in thoracic surgeries and is even clearer in chest wall surgeries. For example, in the Nuss procedure, most surgeons use a thoracoscope. Like ordinary thoracic surgeries, the use of a thoracoscope indeed allow the surgery to be completed through very small incisions. However, if the surgery can still be completed through small incisions without using a thoracoscope, and even with fewer incisions, then thoracoscopic surgery cannot be considered minimally invasive surgery. Chest wall diseases are located on the body surface, making exposure convenient and allowing surgery to be performed under direct vision. The thoracoscope is designed to facilitate the observation of structures inside the thoracic cavity. If chest wall surgery must be performed through a thoracoscope, it seems to be going in the wrong direction. This is a particularly important issue to be aware of during the development of the specialty. In pursuit of so-called minimally invasive surgery, some mistakenly equate minimally invasive surgery with thoracoscopic surgery. This approach essentially complicates the simplest surgeries and does not conform to the fundamental principles of surgery. If this is considered the direction of surgical development, it will mislead the path. Fortunately, as chest wall surgery has developed to date, thoracoscopes have not found a significant role in various chest wall surgeries. This trend is sure to continue and will become one of the distinguishing features of chest wall surgery compared to thoracic surgery.

(4) Instruments and Materials

A clear difference between chest wall surgery and thoracic surgery lies in the nature of the operations. Chest wall surgery involves procedures on bony structures, requiring a large number of materials that serve two main functions: shaping and reconstruction. Shaping materials are relatively rigid, primarily consisting of various shaping steel plates. With technological improvements, various modified products have gradually emerged. Reconstruction materials are diverse and represent one of the most active research areas in chest wall surgery today. Recently, digital materials have gained attention and are expected to become the most important materials for chest wall reconstruction. However, since such materials require longer design and processing times, more convenient materials are still needed in clinical practice as substitutes.

Thoracic surgery is increasingly developing towards greater precision, fundamentally supported by the research and development of various instruments and materials. Currently, two main types of materials are primarily needed in clinical practice: one is the instruments required for thoracoscopic procedures, and the other is the materials needed at the surgical site. The rapid development of both has directly propelled thoracic surgery to a higher level. In terms of instruments, the most important tool in thoracic surgery is the thoracoscope, with its development pinnacle being the robot. Various signs indicate that more and more advanced and expensive instruments are being continuously introduced into clinical thoracic surgery today. Chest wall surgery, however, mostly involves procedures performed under direct vision and does not require highly specialized instruments. The vast majority of chest wall surgeries can be completed using general surgical instruments. While the rapid development of surgical instruments raises the technological content of surgeries and seems to be the direction of surgical advancement, a potential issue must be noted. Instrument development requires investment; the deeper the research, the higher the instrument costs, which increases the overall cost of surgery. When surgical costs become unaffordable for society, the use of high-level instruments will inevitably limit the advancement of clinical techniques. This, on the contrary, hinders the progress of clinical technology. Take general thoracic surgery as an example: before the era of Thoracoscopy, many doctors could easily perform thoracic surgeries. However, once Thoracoscopy developed, the difficulty of performing surgeries increased significantly, and the number of surgeons proficient in these procedures noticeably declined. At the stage of robotic surgery, the difficulty and threshold became even higher. If related access standards are established in the future, the vast majority of thoracic surgeons would lose their qualifications to perform surgeries. This is obviously detrimental to the development of thoracic surgical techniques. In contrast, such a situation cannot exist in chest wall surgery. Since it does not require specialized instruments, the costs of instrument development and usage will not be too high. This enables many hospitals, especially primary care hospitals, to have the conditions to perform chest wall surgeries, which undoubtedly will become a true driving force for the advancement of the discipline.

(5) Surgical Risks

Thoracic surgery involves some vital organs, especially the heart and great vessels. Injury to these structures can cause extremely serious consequences. The risk further increases during thoracoscopic procedures. In contrast, chest wall surgery is performed on the body surface, with easy exposure and direct operation, so the risks are generally lower. This is very favorable for the promotion of the technique. However, some surgeries have inherent risks, such as the Nuss procedure. During this surgery, the steel bar needs to be placed at the deepest part of the depression, and much of the operation is performed under Thoracoscopy. for thoracic surgeons who frequently use Thoracoscopy, this should have been a simple procedure. However, almost all cases of heart injury have occurred under thoracoscopic guidance. The reason is quite simple: when passing close to the surface of the heart, the thoracoscope often cannot visualize the area. The purpose of using the thoracoscope is to obtain a good view; the more dangerous the operation, the more it requires good visualization and thoracoscopic assistance. But in reality, precisely at the moments when the thoracoscope is most needed, it is often absent. This causes the most dangerous operations to become blind procedures, making accidents almost inevitable. This has become the greatest risk of the surgery. Therefore, thoracic wall surgery has consistently advocated for a return to basic principles and techniques. Returning to simplicity does not mean technological regression; on the contrary, it represents the most fundamental respect for the technique itself. When thoracic wall surgeons earnestly perform their surgeries under direct vision, the surgical risks can be minimized to the lowest level.

(6) Surgical Difficulty

Intrathoracic surgery performed under Thoracoscopy first requires mastery of various thoracoscopic techniques, making the learning curve relatively long and the surgical procedures more difficult. In contrast, chest wall surgery is completed under direct vision without the need for special instrumental assistance. The operations are straightforward and can be performed once the basic surgical principles are understood, so the difficulty is generally lower.

However, whether it is intrathoracic surgery or chest wall surgery, there are both simple and complex procedures. For simple surgeries, chest wall operations may be easier. But for complex surgeries, sometimes chest wall procedures can be more complicated. For example, surgeries for asphyxiating thoracic dysplasia and extremely severe chest wall deformities are great challenges to surgeons' skills, and their difficulty is no less than that of any intrathoracic surgery.

4. Inevitable Connection

The independence of chest wall surgery essentially represents a complete rejection of traditional thoracic surgery. However, no matter how much the discipline overturns tradition, the inherent connection between chest wall surgery and thoracic surgery cannot be severed. This connection is reflected in the following aspects:

(1) Chest wall surgery cannot be completed independently of intrathoracic operations.

Many chest wall surgeries involve intrathoracic operations. For example, the most common Nuss procedure requires placing a steel bar through the thoracic cavity. Such an operation cannot be completed without involving the chest cavity. Similarly, although the Wenlin procedure for pectus carinatum appears not to involve the thoracic cavity on the surface, it actually does because the operation of passing fixation wires around the ribs essentially enters the chest cavity. Although the Wang procedure does not enter the thoracic cavity, there have been occasional cases of pleural injury causing pneumothorax, which can be considered indirect damage to intrathoracic structures.

Apart from deformities, other diseases have a greater impact on the thoracic cavity. For example, chest wall tumors can directly invade intrathoracic structures. Chest wall defects, trauma, and infections may also affect intrathoracic structures. From the perspective of intrathoracic diseases, these diseases are not always confined to the thoracic cavity; many can involve the chest wall, such as tumors, trauma, and infections. More broadly, all thoracic surgeries require incisions through the chest wall to be performed. Therefore, although chest wall surgery and thoracic surgery have become distinct specialties, they remain intricately connected and inseparable, maintaining a natural link at all times.

(2) Combined Surgery

Chest wall diseases and intrathoracic diseases are inherently interconnected and cannot be separated. Therefore, in many cases, combined surgeries are often required. For example, in chest wall tumor surgeries, some tumors have extensive invasion, directly involving the lungs or mediastinal structures, making it impossible to limit the surgery to the chest wall alone. In other cases, chest wall tumors coexist with lung or mediastinal tumors, necessitating surgeries for both the chest wall and intrathoracic tumors. Similarly, chest wall infections often extend through the entire chest wall and involve intrathoracic structures, requiring simultaneous surgical intervention. Intrathoracic lesions combined with deformities are also common, usually isolated conditions. For instance, pectus excavatum with pulmonary bullae or funnel chest combined with congenital heart disease these cases generally require simultaneous surgery. Traumatic cases are even more common; many chest wall injuries are accompanied by intrathoracic injuries, and if surgery is performed, both intrathoracic and chest wall structures must be addressed concurrently.

(3) Connection with Auxiliary Procedures

Both chest wall surgery and thoracic surgery share some common procedures that cannot be exclusive to one specialty. For example, closed chest drainage is a fundamental operation in thoracic surgery and is used after almost every surgery. It is also frequently applied in non-surgical management of certain special intrathoracic diseases. In chest wall surgery, although the disease is limited to the chest wall, pleural effusion and pneumothorax may occur, so this procedure is also commonly used. Another procedure that both specialties must inevitably handle is the management of chest wall incisions. Thoracic surgery requires making and suturing chest wall incisions, and chest wall surgery similarly requires incision and suturing. These two specialties were originally one; even when fully independent, their connections cannot be completely severed.

In summary, nothing remains static; everything is constantly evolving. With continuous advancements in clinical theories and techniques, traditional surgical specialties inevitably face challenges. Thoracic surgery, as an established clinical specialty, has developed over many years. Great achievements have already been made, and it is precisely because of these successes that the development of subspecialties has become possible. Chest wall surgery, having separated from thoracic surgery, has begun the journey of subspecialty development, which will elevate the treatment of chest wall diseases to a new level. However, no specialty exists in isolation; even seemingly unrelated fields are intricately connected. Therefore, it is absolutely impossible for chest wall surgery to completely break away from thoracic surgery and become fully independent. Only by properly managing the relationship between the two can they make good use of each other's excellent research achievements and experience, advance together, and develop harmoniously.

REFERENCES

[1] Wang, Wenlin. 2019a. "The Birth of the Concept of Chest Wall Surgery." *Expert on Thoracic Deformity Surgery*, November 13.

[2] Jiang, R., and L. Liao. 2019. "Wenlin Wang: A 'Weird Doctor' Defying the Matthew Effect." *Journal of Thoracic Disease* 11 (7): E90–E95.

[3] Wang, Wenlin. 2019b. "The Development Process of Chest Wall Surgery." *Expert on Thoracic Deformity Surgery*, November 1.

[4] Wang, Wenlin. 2019c. "The Inevitable Path for the Development of Chinese Chest Wall Surgery." *Expert on Thoracic Deformity Surgery*, February 16.

[5] Wang, Wenlin. 2018a. "The Path to Independence: The Breakup between Chest Wall Surgery and Thoracic Surgery." *Expert on Thoracic Deformity Surgery*, August 17.

[6] Wang, Wenlin. 2018b. “Research Contents of Chest Wall Surgery (1).” *Expert on Thoracic Deformity Surgery*, August 11.
[7] Wang, Wenlin. 2021. “The Relationship between Chest Wall Surgery and Other Specialties.” *Today’s Headlines*, November 2.

Section 16

BASIC QUALITIES OF A CHEST WALL SURGEON

A professional doctor must treat special patients and solve specialized problems, and thus must possess specialized knowledge. Different specialties have different knowledge structures. This knowledge is reflected in every detail of clinical work from the approach to disease management and fundamental principles, to specific operative techniques, clearly showcasing the uniqueness of each specialty. Professional tasks require professionals to carry them out, and professionals must have professional competence. This professional competence is the fundamental guarantee for accomplishing specialized work. There are many specialties in clinical medicine, and each specialty requires professionals with corresponding specialized qualities. Take thoracic surgery, for example: this specialty places specific demands on every thoracic surgeon. In the era of open surgery, thoracic surgical work mainly involved conventional thoracotomies. Because it dealt with vital organs such as the heart, lungs, esophagus, and major blood vessels, thoracic surgeons had to be thoroughly familiar with a vast amount of knowledge related to these anatomical structures. This formed the most distinctive difference between thoracic surgeons and other specialists, making a certain level of professional competence essential.

In the era of minimally invasive surgery especially when thoracoscopic techniques became standard thoracic surgeons were required to master Thoracoscopy proficiently. These skills are unique to thoracic surgeons and clearly reflect the defining characteristics of the specialty in the modern, minimally invasive surgical era.

Thoracic wall surgery originated from traditional thoracic surgery, and thoracic wall surgeons are first and foremost thoracic surgeons thus, they must possess all the qualities expected of a thoracic surgeon. However, if thoracic wall surgery were merely a part of thoracic surgery, then its so-called independence would be meaningless. When thoracic wall surgery emerges as an independent specialty in clinical practice, such independence must represent a development based on inheritance. In other words, it both inherits the characteristics of traditional thoracic surgery and adds new content. This kind of independence is similar to the development of subspecialties within traditional orthopedics. For example, when spinal surgery became an independent specialty separated from orthopedics, it added neurosurgical components in addition to retaining the basics of orthopedics. As a result, spinal surgery acquired elements not found in traditional orthopedics. Similarly, when plastic surgery split from orthopedics, it incorporated elements of cosmetic medicine, gradually evolving content that had no relation to conventional orthopedics. These examples illustrate that the independence of a subspecialty is not simply a division of disciplines it is a process of inheritance and advancement, with its growth precisely involving new elements the original specialty could not possess.

After becoming fully independent, thoracic wall surgery added new elements to the foundation of traditional thoracic surgery. These new elements primarily include three aspects: Orthopedics content, Plastic surgery content, and Cosmetic surgery content. These three components were not part of traditional thoracic surgery but are critically important to thoracic wall surgery. This clearly shows that thoracic wall surgeons must possess specialized qualities in order to fulfill the dual mission of inheritance and innovation.

1. A Thoracic Wall Surgeon Should First Be an Excellent Thoracic Surgeon

Before thoracic wall surgery became an independent specialty, it could only be considered a part of thoracic surgery or one of its subspecialties. Since it was only a subspecialty, it did not necessarily attract attention from everyone. In the era of open surgery, many thoracic surgeons paid attention to chest wall diseases, and mastering the skills to treat such conditions was considered a basic competence for thoracic surgeons. However, with the advancement of thoracoscopic techniques, traditional thoracic surgery seems to have deviated from its original path, leading to a significant decline in the number of doctors focusing on chest wall diseases. The result of this distorted development is that many well-known doctors now only perform lung or esophageal surgeries, and are almost incapable of performing other types of operations. In principle, any surgeon who excels in a specific procedure deserves equal recognition and is a true expert. However, in reality, various biases exist particularly when it comes to the treatment of chest wall diseases. Although many doctors are renowned as thoracic surgery experts, they never perform chest wall surgery and, in fact, may not even know how to perform such procedures. If such doctors are considered thoracic surgery experts, it would likely be unconvincing to many. In clinical practice, some astonishing phenomena are often observed. For example, the Nuss procedure, one of the most common chest wall surgeries, is one that a significant proportion of thoracic surgeons are either unable or unwilling to perform [1]. Since traditional thoracic surgery includes chest wall surgery, and thoracic diseases encompass conditions affecting the chest wall, a thoracic surgery expert must be proficient in the Nuss procedure. Whether a doctor who dares not perform the Nuss procedure can truly be called a thoracic surgery expert is open to debate. This indirectly proves an important point: to become an excellent chest wall surgeon, one must first be an excellent thoracic surgeon. This is the most basic requirement the specialty demands of its practitioners. From the perspective of actual clinical needs, such a requirement is entirely reasonable. It's important to understand that the majority of chest wall surgeries involve thoracic surgical techniques, and without these as a foundation, chest wall surgery cannot advance at all. Therefore, thoracic surgical competence is a fundamental quality that every chest wall surgeon must possess. These qualities are reflected in the following aspects:

First, a chest wall surgeon must be well-versed in the fundamental knowledge of thoracic surgery. The chest wall is located on the outer surface of the thorax and may appear, on the surface, to be independent from intrathoracic structures. However, functionally, it forms an integrated whole, as these structures directly contribute to the function of the thoracic organs. For example, in respiratory function, the chest wall plays a crucial role. When chest wall diseases occur, the structural abnormalities can impair respiratory function. As a result, patients may not only experience localized symptoms in the chest wall but also develop symptoms due to compromised breathing. This intrinsic link between the chest wall and the thoracic organs makes them inseparable as a functional unit. Therefore, in order to thoroughly understand the diseases of this specialty, a chest wall surgeon must master the core theories of thoracic surgery. Only then can one be considered a qualified chest wall surgeon.

Second, a chest wall surgeon must be proficient in the fundamental operative skills of thoracic surgery. Chest wall surgery and thoracic surgery share many common issues that require similar techniques. For example, managing pneumothorax and pleural effusion though these are among the most basic procedures in thoracic surgery they are also encountered in chest wall surgical procedures. Therefore, in order to competently carry out clinical work within the field of chest wall surgery, a surgeon must have a firm grasp of these essential operative skills.

Third, a chest wall surgeon must be proficient in treating common thoracic surgical diseases. Chest wall conditions often involve intrathoracic structures, and during surgical treatment, it is necessary to address thoracic cavity diseases simultaneously. In some special cases, chest wall diseases may be accompanied by intrathoracic pathologies. For example, flat chest combined with pulmonary bullae [2], pectus excavatum with pulmonary adenocystic tumors [3], or pectus excavatum associated with congenital heart disease [4]. These situations require that both the chest wall deformity and the intrathoracic condition be treated concurrently. Therefore, being proficient in the treatment methods of thoracic surgical diseases is of great significance for ensuring the optimal treatment of chest wall disorders.

Fourth, chest wall surgeons must be proficient in emergency rescue techniques for thoracic surgical conditions. During surgeries for chest wall disorders, two types of emergencies involving intrathoracic structures may occur: one involves accidental injuries during the procedure, such as rupture of the heart or major blood vessels; the other involves injuries to intrathoracic structures associated with chest wall trauma. The first type of situation is commonly seen in various trans-thoracic chest wall surgeries, such as procedures for pectus excavatum. If an accident occurs during the placement of the steel bar, emergency thoracostomy may be required. Such procedures fall under the category of traditional thoracic surgical emergency management. The second type typically occurs in cases of severe chest trauma, where both the chest wall and intrathoracic structures are damaged. In these cases, simultaneous treatment is necessary, which also falls under the domain of thoracic emergency care. For a chest wall surgeon, lacking the basic skills to handle such emergencies during surgery can lead to disastrous consequences, making it impossible to ensure even basic surgical safety.

According to the current development status of thoracic surgery, a thoracic surgeon can still be considered qualified—and even achieve considerable reputation—without having any knowledge of chest wall surgery. However, for a chest wall surgeon, if they do not possess the fundamental qualities required of a thoracic surgeon, it is almost impossible to continue progressing.

2. A Chest Wall Surgeon Should Also Be A Good Orthopedics Surgeon.

The chest wall surgery specialty includes five fundamental types of diseases, and the treatment of each one involves the bony structures of the chest wall. Chest wall deformities are themselves deformities of the bony structure; the key and most challenging part of chest wall trauma surgery is managing injuries to the bones; chest wall defects mainly concern defects in the bony structure; and one of the main focuses in the surgical treatment of chest wall tumors and infections is the reconstruction of the chest wall's bony structure. Every disease in chest wall surgery is closely related to the chest wall bones, so it is no exaggeration to say that chest wall surgery is essentially chest wall orthopedics [5]. Precisely because of this positioning, if chest wall surgery differs from traditional thoracic surgery in any way, the first difference is the inclusion of orthopedics elements. In traditional thoracic surgery, chest wall diseases have also received corresponding treatment, and the treatment process likewise involved orthopedics aspects. However, the significance of chest wall surgery becoming an independent specialty lies in its emphasis on these new orthopedics components. It can be envisioned that when a chest wall surgeon is able to skillfully apply orthopedics expertise to handle fractures, bone tumors, bone defects, bone deformities, and bone infections, the final outcomes will inevitably be more effective and more professional than when a thoracic surgeon uses conventional techniques to address them. This clearly shows that a chest wall surgeon must not only be a competent thoracic surgeon but also a competent orthopedic surgeon. Possessing such qualities will enable chest wall surgeons to perform their work with greater precision and depth.

3. A Chest Wall Surgeon Should Be A Good Plastic Surgeon

Chest wall diseases are located on the body surface, and one of their most prominent characteristics is their impact on the appearance of the chest wall. This kind of impact does not exist with intrathoracic diseases. Precisely because of this feature, there is an objective requirement for chest wall surgeons to place special emphasis on the appearance of the chest wall. In many cases, the alteration in appearance is the patient's only complaint, making it sometimes the sole aspect that the surgeon needs to focus on. Appearance-related matters fall within the scope of plastic surgery. All five types of chest wall diseases involve issues related to appearance, which naturally creates an overlap with the work of plastic surgery. One of the major harms of thoracic deformities is the abnormal appearance they cause. Restoring the chest wall to a normal shape has always been a key objective for plastic surgeons. In the past, plastic surgery has consistently dealt with the treatment of thoracic deformities, such as pectus excavatum and Poland syndrome; these have long fallen under the domain of plastic surgery. Chest wall trauma involves injuries to both the bony structures and soft tissues of the chest wall, and treating such injuries also includes elements of plastic surgery. For diseases such as chest wall tumors, defects, and infections, one of the main aspects of surgery is reconstruction not only of the bony structures but also of soft tissue and skin. These tasks clearly fall within the scope of plastic surgery. Although the work of plastic surgery is fundamentally different from that of chest wall surgery, it is undeniable that certain principles and techniques from plastic surgery are precisely what chest wall surgery needs to draw upon. Therefore, for a chest wall surgeon to perform surgeries to perfection, it is essential to master basic plastic surgery techniques. With such skills, many procedures can be executed much more effectively. Without specific plastic surgery techniques such as those involving flaps many operations would be impossible to carry out.

4. A Chest Wall Surgeon Should Also Be A Good Aesthetic Surgeon

Although chest wall diseases are generally considered common conditions, their location on the body surface makes patients more concerned about aesthetics than the average patient. This places higher demands on chest wall surgeons. These requirements are reflected not only in the overall appearance of the chest wall, but also in aesthetic-related details such as the size, location, direction of the incision, and the suturing technique all of which are areas of particular concern to patients. for chest wall surgeons to earn the trust of their patients and increase patient satisfaction, they must make a dedicated effort in handling these aspects carefully [6]. The basic skills of plastic surgery can significantly improve the appearance outcomes of chest wall surgery, but they may not necessarily meet the standards of cosmetic surgery. To achieve more aesthetically pleasing results, chest wall surgeons must acquire certain techniques from the field of cosmetic surgery. Mastery of such techniques can lead to a qualitative leap in surgical quality. Without attention to this aspect, the quality of the surgery may inevitably have flaws. As people's living standards continue to rise, the emphasis on cosmetic outcomes in chest wall surgery will grow steadily, placing higher demands on the qualifications of chest wall surgeons.

Chest wall surgeons must possess extensive interdisciplinary knowledge.

Chest wall surgeons originate from thoracic surgery. In order to achieve professional development, they need to master extensive knowledge and skills from thoracic surgery, orthopedics, plastic surgery, and cosmetic surgery. Specialized knowledge is the fundamental guarantee for chest wall surgeons to perform their duties. However, having only specialized knowledge is often not enough; chest wall surgeons also need knowledge beyond their own specialty.

The first type of knowledge beyond one's specialty is mechanical knowledge. Almost all chest wall surgery diseases involve issues related to the thoracic cage and spine, and at the core of these issues are mechanical principles [7,8]. For example, the relationship between chest wall deformities and scoliosis, the pathogenesis of pectus excavatum and pectus carinatum, the mechanisms of various deformity correction surgeries, and thoracic reconstruction surgeries all are directly related to mechanical principles. If a surgeon can master these relationships and principles, surgeries can generally proceed smoothly. On the contrary, without basic knowledge of mechanics, serious problems may arise during surgery. Numerous clinical cases support this viewpoint. For example, the principle of the Nuss procedure was not specifically studied by doctors around the world for a long time. Without understanding the surgical principles, operations tend to be performed in an extremely arbitrary manner. Before the concept of chest wall surgery was introduced, this procedure was carried out by thoracic surgeons, pediatric surgeons, and even orthopedic surgeons. When a surgeon steps onto the operating table without even understanding the fundamental principles, the outcome is easy to imagine. We have encountered a large number of patients with failed surgeries in clinical practice. Upon analyzing the reasons for these failures, nearly all were related to the surgeon's lack of understanding of the fundamental principles. On the surface, the Nuss procedure does not appear to be a simple or singular action; it is a complex and integrated operation. Without a professional mechanical perspective to examine this procedure, it is difficult to grasp its essence. In physics, one of the most commonly used analytical methods is decomposition: forces can be decomposed, and movements can also be decomposed. When the principle of the Nuss procedure is analyzed using this method, the problem quickly becomes much simpler. In 2014, we were the first to conduct an in-depth analysis of the principles behind this procedure and ultimately discovered that its essence is equivalent to the most basic principle of the lever [9]. This marked the first time the underlying mechanism of the Nuss procedure was explained more than ten years after its introduction. During all those years, surgeons around the world had been performing the operation without understanding its fundamental principle. Countless patients have suffered the pain of surgical failure due to doctors performing procedures blindly. However, after the underlying principle was clarified, the quality of the surgery improved significantly, the success rate greatly increased, and the number of failed cases noticeably declined. There are many more examples of the importance of biomechanics such as the principles behind the Wenlin procedure, template shaping, and pre-shaping all of which are based on fundamental mechanical principles. Mastery of these principles plays a crucial role in ensuring the successful completion of surgery. In fact, almost every well-known surgical method in chest wall surgery is grounded in biomechanics. Without understanding these foundations, it is nearly impossible to achieve perfection in surgery.

The primary focus of thoracic surgery is operations within the thoracic cavity. When thoracoscopic surgery began to be used in clinical practice, intrathoracic operations almost became synonymous with thoracic surgery in many people's minds. These surgeries typically involve two fundamental actions: resection and repair, and rarely go beyond these. Such procedures generally do not involve traditional mechanical principles. This is one of the most fundamental differences between thoracic surgery and chest wall surgery. For a chest wall surgeon to be competent in all aspects of their specialty, they must shift away from the conventional mindset of thoracic surgeons and acquire a solid foundation in biomechanics.

The second type of non-specialized knowledge required is psychological knowledge. Chest wall diseases are located on the surface of the chest and pose two fundamental types of harm: physiological and psychological. While physiological harm is the domain of medical expertise, the psychological impact is often overlooked by doctors. For chest wall surgeons, many of their patients experience psychological issues [10], which requires them to possess strong knowledge of psychology. This knowledge not only helps patients overcome psychological distress but also allows clinical practice to better meet patients' overall needs.

Traditional thoracic surgery also involves external appearance to some extent. However, even for past chest wall conditions such as chest wall tumors or chest wall trauma thoracic surgeons rarely considered the aesthetic outcome. As for intrathoracic diseases, since they generally do not involve appearance, most thoracic surgeons focus primarily on curing the disease without considering aesthetic concerns. Ignoring appearance issues can lead to overlooking the psychological impact they may have on patients. In contrast, chest wall surgeons' different appearance is a central concern for them. Therefore, they must learn to understand the patient's psychology and ultimately meet the patient's needs on a psychological level.

The third type of knowledge outside the professional domain is aesthetic knowledge. This kind of knowledge is relatively abstract, yet very practical. Chest wall surgery involves the appearance of the chest wall, and different patients have different standards when it comes to judging beauty. For example, a high sternal angle is something that most people would not consider a disease or a defect. However, some individuals are extremely concerned about it and may have specific surgical requests. Similar demands are often made in cases involving other deformities or shapes as well. The doctor's responsibility is to respect each individual's right to aesthetic preference. This is similar to procedures like breast augmentation or rhinoplasty. Since the work of a chest wall surgeon carries elements of plastic and cosmetic surgery, their approach to such patients' needs should also shift accordingly. In other words, the surgeon should consider the patient's desires from an aesthetic perspective, not just from a medical or disease-centered viewpoint. With this mindset, many tasks become easier. Otherwise, failing to adopt this perspective may lead to difficulties in the surgeon's practice.

5. The Essential Virtues A Chest Wall Surgeon Must Possess

In fact, doctors in any specialty whether in thoracic surgery, orthopedics, or spinal surgery should possess strong moral character, professional ethics, and a dedicated work ethic. However, due to the influence of certain negative practices, it is almost impossible for all doctors in established traditional specialties to uphold such high standards of conduct. These undesirable habits inevitably affect emerging specialties as well. Since chest wall surgery is a relatively new clinical field, it is crucial to eliminate the influence of these bad habits from the very beginning. Ensuring that all practitioners in this field maintain good character and professional integrity will play a vital role in promoting the healthy and sustainable development of the specialty.

(1) Pioneering Spirit

Chest wall surgery has only recently emerged in clinical practice, and all aspects of the field must start from scratch. Since there are no existing experiences to draw upon, every task must progress through exploration. At this stage, what is most needed is a pioneering spirit, one that does not fear difficulties, dares to move forward, and constantly summarizes experiences to help the specialty mature. Without such a pioneering spirit, chest wall surgery will inevitably remain dependent on traditional thoracic surgery, making complete independence and gradual maturity impossible.

(2) Fighting Spirit

As a newly established specialty, chest wall surgery is bound to face numerous difficulties from patient intake and surgical implementation to the enforcement of various regulations and protocols. At such a time, professionals in the field must possess a strong fighting spirit, be courageous in facing challenges, continuously overcome obstacles, and actively drive the development of the discipline.

(3) Pragmatic Spirit

Chest wall surgery is an entirely new endeavor. Many insightful individuals have made tremendous contributions to its development. However, as a new specialty, its foundation is not yet solid and requires a substantial amount of groundwork to ensure its establishment and sustainability. Therefore, it is essential for all chest wall surgeons to work with an unwaveringly pragmatic spirit. Only by taking each step with solid, down-to-earth effort can a strong foundation be laid for the specialty's long-term advancement.

(4) Craftsmanship Spirit

Craftsmanship spirit is embodied in the relentless pursuit of technical excellence. Like all surgical specialties, chest wall surgery is centered around operations. Surgery, at its core, is a craft that is fundamentally about skill and technique. Striving for perfection in technique is the most essential requirement for any surgeon. Without solid technical skills, everything else becomes meaningless. Therefore, for a chest wall surgeon, having a strong craftsmanship spirit is not optional, it is absolutely essential.

(5) Critical Thinking Spirit

The very establishment of chest wall surgery is itself the result of a critique of traditional thoracic surgery. Therefore, critical thinking is one of the most essential qualities a chest wall surgeon should possess. Rational criticism enables practitioners to break free from the constraints of tradition, step into new fields, and achieve true professional independence and advancement. Without a spirit of critique, it is impossible to break away from outdated customs, and the meaningful development of chest wall surgery would be extremely difficult.

6. Chest Wall Surgeons Must Eliminate Unethical Practices

Many bad habits have become prevalent in clinical practice, and these unhealthy practices are found in nearly every medical specialty. Chest wall surgeons are not exclusively newly recruited young doctors; most of them come from traditional thoracic surgery backgrounds. Even the new recruits, during their training phase, are likely to be influenced by these entrenched bad habits. Such habits have long affected traditional surgical fields, and if they infiltrate the newly emerging specialty of chest wall surgery from the very beginning, they could severely hinder its development. Therefore, eliminating these negative practices at the early stage of the specialty is of great significance. It lays a solid ethical and professional foundation, ensuring that chest wall surgery grows with integrity, innovation, and a commitment to the highest standards of patient care.

(1) Eliminate Academic Vanity

Academic vanity is a bad habit that exists in every medical specialty. Its typical manifestation is the exaggerated boasting of academic achievements and accomplishments. This kind of behavior can cause extremely negative consequences if left unchecked, it may lead to unhealthy competition, create a culture of exaggeration, and seriously hinder the development of the discipline.

As a newly emerging specialty, chest wall surgery involves a great deal of pioneering work. If individuals begin to flaunt and exaggerate every single contribution as a major breakthrough, it will create an atmosphere of confusion and chaos in the field. Such a scene does not represent the prosperity of a discipline, but rather its downfall and sorrow. Therefore, this bad habit must be eliminated from the very beginning to ensure that chest wall surgery grows on a foundation of truth, humility, and meaningful progress.

(2) Eliminate underworld-like behavior

The academic community can often resemble a vast underworld-like arena. In recent years, such undercurrents have become increasingly pervasive, infiltrating every traditional medical specialty and every corner of the professional landscape. As a newly emerging field, chest wall surgery is not immune to these influences and is inevitably touched by some of these underworld-like tendencies. These tendencies may include cliquish behavior, status jockeying, excessive politicking, and prioritizing personal gain over academic integrity. Though subtle at times, their presence can severely compromise the academic purity and developmental direction of a specialty still in its infancy. Recognizing this vulnerability, chest wall surgeons must remain especially vigilant, resisting the temptation to engage in such practices and instead fostering a culture of integrity, professionalism, and scientific discipline from the outset. Many signs indicate that certain "underworld-style individuals" have already brought such undesirable tendencies into this emerging specialty. For example, in the early stages of the discipline's development, various professional organizations for chest wall surgery were established. These organizations were originally intended to promote the advancement of chest wall surgery, but traces of underworld-like behavior were evident throughout their formation and operation. Such phenomena are highly abnormal yet unfortunately widespread. When underworld influences become too deeply entrenched, they inevitably hinder the development of the discipline. This makes such tendencies a particularly harmful habit that must be eliminated. During the development of the China Chest Wall Surgery Alliance, similar issues once arose. However, once the problems were identified, they were quickly addressed and corrected. This timely intervention helped to pave the way for the healthy, nationwide development of chest wall surgery.

(3) Abandoning Self-Interest and Opportunism

The pursuit of personal gain is a deeply ingrained and widespread vice. It becomes especially serious when many of a clinician's direct interests become tied to specific external elements. Nowadays, the most prominent among these are SCI publications, research grants, and funded projects. While these elements are not inherently contradictory to the conduct of clinical work, once rigidly mandated, they tend to give rise to numerous absurd practices. This not only leads to a massive waste of social resources, but also drains the time and energy of physicians. From the very day of its inception, chest wall surgery must draw a clear line against such unhealthy trends. What this field truly requires is a spirit of pragmatism, a down-to-earth entrepreneurial mindset, and solid technical competence not hollow academic papers. It does not need fabricated "consensus statements" or "clinical guidelines," nor the self-important interpretations from so-called experts. Eliminating the pursuit of personal gain is a task that chest wall surgery must take on from the very beginning of its development.

In summary, thoracic wall surgery, as a brand-new clinical specialty, although closely connected to traditional thoracic surgery in many ways, takes on a new developmental direction and growth space once it fully branches out. Surgeons in this specialty must, due to professional demands, establish new concepts, learn new techniques, continuously enrich their theoretical knowledge, and cultivate a unique set of skills to attain the highest level of professional excellence. Furthermore, thoracic wall surgeons must always distance themselves from various negative habits. Only by doing so can they continue to grow in maturity and ultimately achieve true success.

REFERENCES

[1] Wenlin Wang. Pectus Excavatum Surgery in the Eyes of a Thoracic Surgeon. Expert in Thoracic Deformity Surgery, 2020-04-11.

[2] Wenlin Wang. Single-Stage Surgery for Flat Chest Combined with Pulmonary Bullae. Expert in Thoracic Deformity Surgery, 2020-06-29.

[3] Wenlin Wang. Surgical Issues in Congenital Pulmonary Airway Malformation Combined with Pectus Excavatum. Expert in Thoracic Deformity Surgery, 2020-10-17.

[4] Wenlin Wang. Successful Single-Stage Surgery for Congenital Heart Disease Combined with Pectus Excavatum and Pulmonary Cyst. Expert in Thoracic Deformity Surgery, 2013-12-20.

[5] Wenlin Wang. The Relationship Between Thoracic Wall Surgery and Other Specialties. Toutiao Today, 2021-11-02.

[6] Wenlin Wang. Incision Aesthetics and Scar Cosmesis. Expert in Thoracic Deformity Surgery, 2020-03-15.

[7] Wenlin Wang. Delayed Remodeling: A Master Sculptor's Concept of Mechanics. Expert in Thoracic Deformity Surgery, 2019-10-04.

[8] Wenlin Wang. Mechanical Changes After Thoracic Deformity Surgery. Expert in Thoracic Deformity Surgery, 2018-10-22.

[9] Wenlin Wang. Depression of the Lateral Chest Wall After Nuss Surgery. Expert in Thoracic

Deformity Surgery, 2014-08-12.
[10] Wenlin Wang. Psychological and Mental Illness in Patients with Pectus Carinatum(Pigeon Chest). Expert in Thoracic Deformity Surgery, 2021-04-28.

CHAPTER 2
PART 1

CHEST WALL DEFORMITIES

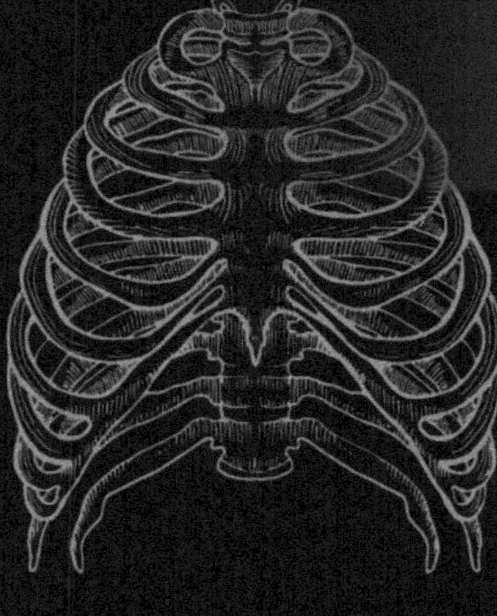

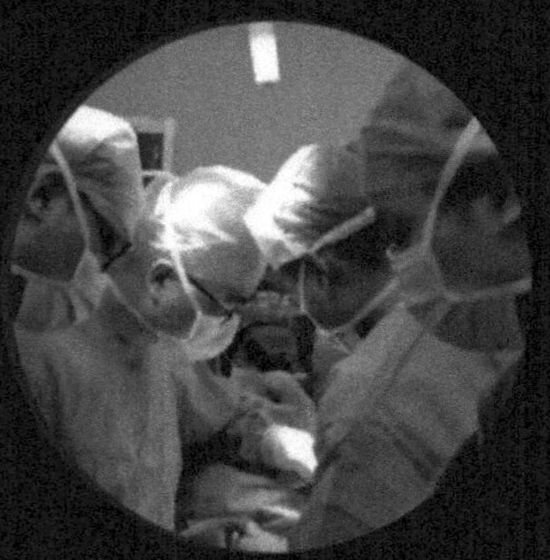

Chest wall deformity is one of the five major diseases in chest wall surgery, and it is also a common condition [1]. As previously introduced, chest wall deformity is a broad concept. Any abnormal appearance of the chest wall can be considered a chest wall deformity. Such conditions include not only abnormalities in the shape of bony structures but also appearance abnormalities caused by other structural anomalies. For example, in cases of chest wall tumors or chest wall abscesses, the external appearance of the chest wall may show significant abnormalities, which can also be regarded as deformities. In some non-pathological situations such as abnormally hypertrophied muscles due to bodybuilding or appearance changes caused by excessive obesity, these changes may also be considered deformities. Another scenario involves asymmetrical development of the soft tissues on both sides of the chest wall, resulting in an imbalanced overall appearance. Although not traditionally classified as a disease, such conditions differ from the normal chest wall appearance and therefore, strictly speaking, also fall under the category of deformities. It can be seen that in its broad sense, chest wall deformity covers a wide range and is difficult to define clearly. It is not only easily confused with other chest wall surgical diseases but may also lead to disagreement or controversy. In order to better understand this condition, it is necessary to narrow down its definition. Generally, when we refer to "chest wall deformity," it specifically means abnormality in the shape of the bony structure of the chest wall. This bony structure is defined as the thoracic cage, so in essence, it refers to what is known as a thoracic deformity. This is the narrow definition of chest wall deformity [1]. Establishing this definition makes the concept clearer and facilitates clinical work. Therefore, in this book, we usually refer to chest wall deformity as thoracic deformity to avoid conceptual confusion and ensure clarity.

1. The Nature of Thoracic Deformity

Thoracic deformity is one of the major diseases treated in chest wall surgery, and it is significantly different from other types of diseases. A deformity is primarily understood as a structural abnormality, which is the most basic and general recognition of the condition. However, to scientifically define what qualifies as a “deformity,” it is first necessary to clearly define what constitutes a normal structure. Without a precise understanding of the normal anatomical form, it is impossible to accurately identify or interpret what constitutes an abnormal or deformed structure. In other words, defining deformity begins with defining normality. Only when the standards of normal chest wall structure are established can deviations from it be scientifically and clinically recognized as deformities.

(1) Normal Structure, Variation, and Deformity

Human anatomy is the science that studies the normal structure of the human body. It defines the essential physical characteristics of body structures and organs through a scientific framework. These definitions are based on statistical analysis of large volumes of data. The term "normal structure" refers to the anatomical forms that are shared by the vast majority of individuals in the population. Such structures are supported by relatively consistent data in terms of shape, size, location, and internal composition. In other words, a structure is considered "normal" if it aligns with the common pattern observed in most people, as established through rigorous anatomical studies and measurements. If a certain structure does not exactly match the normal one, but its parameters are relatively close to the standard data and the differences are not significant, this difference is referred to as (variation) [2]. Mutation can be considered a mild abnormality in shape and is not within the scope of disease. However, if it exceeds the range of general variations, it constitutes a type with an extremely low incidence statistically. Such a type may even have abnormalities in physiological function, which is referred to as a deformity(abnormality) [2].

The thorax is not an independent anatomical structure, but rather a complex organic whole composed of various specific structures arranged according to certain rules. Each of these individual structures has its own so-called normal shape and internal configuration. Take ribs, for example, each rib has a relatively fixed shape, but in clinical practice, it is impossible for every individual's rib to be exactly the same, which is actually what is referred to as variation. If the mutation is too severe, it becomes a deformity, and such a deformity does not necessarily constitute a thoracic deformity. Thoracic deformity refers to an abnormal shape that appears when the thorax is considered as a whole or as an independent structure. Before the deformity appears, it may merely present as a variation of the thorax. For most people, the shape of the thorax is similar, which is referred to as the normal shape. If the shape of an individual's thorax slightly differs from the normal shape, it is referred to as a variation. Mutation is not a disease, nor is it a deformity. Generally, it has no clinical symptoms and does not require treatment. If the structure changes drastically and deviates significantly from the normal shape,

it is no longer a mutation but a deformity.
The progression from normal structure to variation and then to deformity is a gradual process without clear boundaries, and therefore, there is no objective standard for judging variations and deformities. Imaging examinations can serve as a reference for judgment, but they are not absolute. In most cases, the determination relies on the patient's own perception and the doctor's experience.

(2) Local structural abnormalities and overall shape abnormalities

In studying thoracic deformities, it is necessary to clarify the relationship between local structural abnormalities and overall shape abnormalities. To clarify this relationship, research is required on two levels: on one hand, the relationship between the structure and shape of the thorax should be studied from a macro perspective; on the other hand, the relationship between the structure and shape of the thoracic components should be studied from a micro perspective. Research on two levels will help to comprehensively understand the essential characteristics of thoracic deformities. There are three basic relationships between the local structure and overall shape of thoracic deformity:

(1)The composition structure is abnormal, but the overall shape is normal.

The basic components of the thorax are the costal cartilages, ribs, and sternum. The spine also contributes to the structure of the thorax, but since spinal diseases fall under the category of spinal surgery, they will not be discussed here. The shapes of the three basic components are generally similar in most patients, but variations and deformities are possible. For example, cervical ribs [3], lumbar rib variations [4], or rib bifurcations [5], and fusion deformities [6], all differ from normal structures. These anomalies themselves are not clinically significant in most cases, but since these structures are involved in forming the thorax, they may affect the shape of the thorax. Because the overall shape of the thorax does not necessarily depend on the shape of its components, the overall shape of the thorax may not change even if there are issues with the shape of the components. Structural abnormalities of the thoracic components are generally discovered during physical examinations. Since they do not affect the body's function or alter the appearance of the thorax, theoretically, such abnormalities do not require treatment. However, in past clinical work in thoracic surgery, some doctors have performed surgical treatment on such structures. The rationale behind this approach is open to discussion.

(2) The composition structure is normal, but the overall shape is abnormal.
There are only three types of components that make up the thorax, but the specific structures are quite numerous. If each structural individual shape is upright. If there are some imperfections within the normal range, these imperfections may accumulate and result in an additive effect, ultimately leading to an abnormal overall shape of the thorax. At this point, it is difficult to find problems on specific costal cartilages, ribs, or sternum, yet the appearance of the thorax has already significantly deviated from its normal shape, becoming a factual deformity. This type of deformity can be seen in barrel chest, flat chest, or certain types of pectus carinatum; large concave deformities can also have such a condition. Since there are no obvious abnormalities in the local structure, correcting deformities only requires consideration of the overall shape without needing to address the local structure. Therefore, the surgery is relatively simple, and satisfactory results are generally attainable.

(3) Abnormal component structure, abnormal overall shape
If there is a significant abnormality in the structural components, it is more likely to cause an overall abnormality in the shape of the thorax. This condition is the most common in clinical settings and is a relatively common type of deformity. During clinical examination or intraoperative exploration of this deformity, obvious local abnormalities can generally be detected. Such abnormalities often relate to the success or failure of the surgery. If not properly addressed, they will affect the surgical outcome. The overall abnormal appearance of a patient with pectus excavatum is a depression, and the severe local changes often occur at the deepest part of the depression. The structure here is obviously abnormal, typically manifesting as localized thickening and enlargement of the bony structure, forming an inward protrusion towards the spinal side. The most critical procedure when treating this deformity is addressing the protrusion. However, some indirect corrective surgeries, such as the Nuss procedure, do not directly address this [7]. If not handled, it may affect the placement of the steel plate, ultimately leading to surgical failure. Additionally, the consequence of untreated delays is the recurrence of depression. The management of visible local deformities is sometimes equally important. Unlike the Nuss procedure, the Wang procedure directly targets the most severe local deformity at the bottom of the depression. After direct correction is applied, it is then fixed in place, which significantly improves the orthopedics effect and eliminates the possibility of deformity recurrence [8]. The thoracic deformity in patients with asphyxiating thoracic dystrophy (Jeune syndrome) is obvious, but the local lesions are more severe. There can be severe

deformities at the contact points between the ribs and the costal cartilage, and in previous surgeries, almost no treatment was directed at local deformities. This is bound to affect the long-term outcome. The Wenlin surgery primarily addresses local deformities, and after this treatment, the overall growth direction of the ribs and costal cartilage changes, fundamentally eliminating the source of the lesion, thus achieving a relatively ideal therapeutic effect [9].

(3) Structural abnormalities and quantitative abnormalities

The thoracic cage is composed of multiple different entities, and abnormalities in these entities can manifest in two aspects: one is an abnormality in the structure itself, and the other is an abnormality in the number of structures. Structural abnormalities mainly refer to variations and deformities, while numerical abnormalities refer to the difference between the actual and normal quantities. A decrease in quantity can manifest in two forms: one is deficiency, and the other is fusion. Absence most commonly occurs with rib absence, which can involve a reduction in the number of ribs. Absence can also occur in the costal cartilage. The sternum can be partially absent, often occurring with other deformities. Fusion often occurs in the costal cartilage and ribs, and after fusion, it can also lead to a reduction in the number of structures. In addition to a decrease in quantity, the number of structural entities may also be greater than normal. For example, 13 rib anomalies, where the patient has one more pair of ribs than normal [10]. The increase in quantity can also manifest as the appearance of ectopic structures, such as lumbar ribs and cervical ribs, all of which increase the total number of ribs. Whether structural and quantitative abnormalities are ultimately meaningful depends on their impact on the appearance and physiological function of the thorax. If the impact is significant, it is clinically significant and requires intervention, otherwise it is not necessary.

(4) Structural Abnormalities and Shape Abnormalities

In general descriptions of deformities, there is no clear distinction made between structural abnormalities and shape abnormalities, but in fact, there is an essential difference between the two. The emphasis of structural abnormalities is on the anomalies in the spatial position, arrangement order, and number of components. Abnormal shape emphasizes only the appearance, without concern for the internal structure. On the surface, the two seem to be completely different concepts, but in reality, they are closely related. Any structural anomaly will manifest as an abnormal shape. Even if the overall appearance is not abnormal, the shape of its internal components will still be abnormal. From another perspective, any anomaly in shape will have an anomaly in internal structure. Shape anomalies are an inevitable result of structural anomalies and are also their external characteristics. This indicates that abnormal shape and structural anomaly are actually two different ways of describing deformities. Although they are presented from different perspectives, the facts they reflect are exactly the same. Therefore, in our discussion of deformities, no strict distinction is made. Generally speaking, anatomical descriptions of deformities also involve abnormalities in two aspects. Due to their close relationship, no clear distinction is made.

(5) Relativity of Abnormal Shapes

Any deformity is an abnormality of shape. However, the assessment of abnormal shapes is a subjective process. Since subjectivity cannot be absolute, an objective standard cannot exist, and therefore, the judgment of deformity must be relative [11]. This means that the same deformity will be perceived differently by different people. Some consider it a deformity, while others do not; some think it is a severe deformity, while others are not concerned. Precisely because of this relativity, it is necessary to view deformities with flexibility in clinical work. The fact that must be remembered is that a doctor's own opinion is not absolute and may also be one-sided. This fact has significant guiding implications for the diagnosis of deformities, particularly in determining surgical indications. Under the premise of providing reasonable advice, doctors must listen to the opinions of patients and their families as much as possible. If the patient and their family are dissatisfied with the appearance of the chest wall and consider it a deformity, it should be regarded as a deformity. On the other hand, if the patient and their family are not concerned about the appearance of the chest wall, it is best not to worry excessively on behalf of the patient. On the surface, this approach may seem to lack principle, but in reality, it is the most practical principle. It is important to understand that there has never been an objective standard for the perception of deformities. Since there is no standard, if doctors always use their own opinions or feelings as the measure, it is itself a manifestation of a lack of principles. When doctors give the decision-making power to patients and their families, it greatly benefits the conduct of clinical work. Otherwise, it may not only cause trouble at work but also lead to various disputes.

(6) Deformities and Other Diseases

Deformity is defined as an abnormality in shape and appearance, and in clinical practice, almost every disease can manifest abnormalities in shape and appearance. For example, a tumor is characterized by the growth of new tissue, which often grows towards the surface of the body, causing changes in the local and overall appearance of the chest wall. In the early stages of chest wall infection, localized redness and swelling may occur. In later stages, abscesses or even necrosis and ulceration of the local skin may develop, all of which can lead to abnormalities in appearance. When a defect occurs, there is a varying degree of loss in different parts of the chest wall structure, which inevitably affects the appearance of the chest wall. In various categories of chest wall trauma, chest wall external various degrees of abnormalities may appear during observation. It can be seen that if the issue of appearance is simply regarded as a deformity, the definition of deformity will become biased. In fact, there is an essential difference between deformities and other lesions, which lies at the substructural level. This means that the tissue and cellular structure of deformities is basically normal, whereas the tissue and cellular structures of all other thoracic surgical diseases exhibit significant pathological changes. This is the most fundamental difference between deformities and other diseases.

2. Pathogenesis of Thoracic Deformity

The primary issue with thoracic deformities is the abnormal shape of the bony structure. The medical community has yet to reach a consensus on the causes of this type of deformity. In fact, for the vast majority of deformities, the causes are difficult to determine clearly. For example, in the case of pectus excavatum, some people will unthinkingly say it is related to calcium deficiency, while others believe it is associated with malnutrition. These claims are actually not scientifically valid. The occurrence of deformities is related to many factors, including congenital factors and acquired factors. Congenital factors can sometimes be identified clearly, but more often they are unclear. Acquired factors are relatively clear, but there are also cases that are unclear. The pathogenic factors of the deformity are unclear, and the pathogenic mechanism is even more complex, making it difficult to have a specific explanation. However, since the change is in the shape of the bone, the most common pathogenesis of deformity is clear, involving no more than two basic mechanisms: first, changes in bone structure, and second, the effect of external forces [12,13]. Various factors can lead to changes in the bony structure of the thorax, including nutritional factors, pathological factors, and other environmental factors. Their ultimate effect is to alter the internal structure of the bones, changing their physical properties and laying the foundation for changes in shape. External forces can originate from multiple sources and may impact the bony structure of the thorax in various forms. The most common external force is mechanical force, which comes from the direct traction or compression of objects. For example, the impact of the heart against the anterior chest wall is the most common mechanical force. This external force plays a decisive role in the formation process of certain types of pectorals (Figure 2-1-1) [14]. For example, the traction effect of the diaphragm after congenital diaphragmatic hernia surgery is also a form of mechanical force. This force can directly act on the anterior chest wall, leading to localized indentation deformities [15]. Mechanical external forces can also be seen in the formation process of some congenital malformations. For example, the pectus excavatum deformity in a single identical twin brother is most likely caused by the compression from the twin brother. This is a typical case of a deformity caused by mechanical external force. Another type of external force is an implicit external force, which does not have a specific object but truly exists. This external force comes from the negative pressure within the thoracic cavity. pressure. When the negative pressure value inside the thoracic cavity becomes too large, a significant pressure difference occurs on both sides of the chest wall, potentially causing the chest wall to shift in position and resulting in deformity. This condition can be seen in children with severe asthma [16], as well as in children who have undergone surgery for congenital diaphragmatic hernia and pulmonary cystadenoma [17]. In both of these surgical procedures, the volume of the thoracic cavity suddenly increases, and the lung tissue is unable to promptly fill the enlarged space within the thoracic cavity. As a result, the negative pressure increases, ultimately leading to deformity. Overall, the etiology and pathogenesis of thoracic deformities are quite complex, making it difficult to thoroughly understand them. From a therapeutic perspective, treatment targeting the cause or mechanism is, of course, the ideal approach. However, in many cases where the cause and mechanism are unclear, treatment must resort to some generalized methods. This approach will certainly have problems, but it is a last resort. However, in cases where the cause and mechanism of the disease are unclear, arbitrary treatment based on imagination will not only fail to achieve good therapeutic effects but may also delay the condition and lead to serious consequences. The most common example in this regard is the misuse of calcium supplements and vitamin D. Many people attribute all thoracic deformities to calcium deficiency and indiscriminately administer calcium supplementation to patients, which is undoubtedly an irresponsible practice.

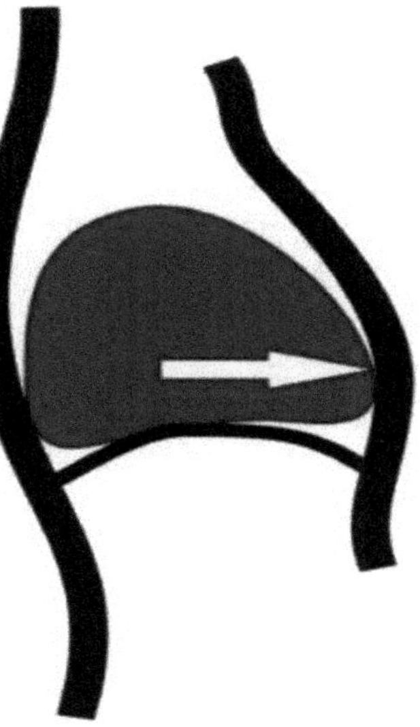

Figure 2-1-1 Mechanism of Pectus Carinatum formation: The heart is located deep behind the anterior chest wall and slightly to the left. Under normal circumstances, there is some contact between the heart and the anterior chest wall. Because the chest wall is normally strong enough, this contact does not cause it to protrude. However, if for some reason the chest wall is relatively weak or thin, the impact from the heart's pulsations may cause the chest wall to bulge outward, ultimately leading to the development of pectus carinatum (pigeon chest).

3. Mechanism of Harm of Thoracic Deformities

Any structural abnormality in the human body may eventually lead to functional abnormalities. In addition to affecting function, abnormalities in chest wall structure also have an impact on appearance. This is determined by the properties of the special structure of the chest wall. Essentially, whether in terms of functionality or appearance, there are two forms of hazards: direct hazards and indirect hazards. From a functional perspective, direct harm often manifests as compression or even erosion of adjacent vital organs, which is the most common form of harm. For example, the compression of the heart and lungs by the anterior chest wall in patients with pectus excavatum is the most common direct harm. The direct consequence of the harm is the impact on cardiopulmonary function, which manifests as various related symptoms and signs. Indirect harm is a secondary type of harm, such as the impact of pectus excavatum on the shape of the spine, primarily resulting from changes in the forces applied to both sides of the spine [18]. Such harm is more insidious, and without in-depth research, it is difficult to identify its causal relationship.

Thoracic deformities generally pose risks to the spine; not only pectus excavatum, but various deformities can actually cause such harm. Due to the hidden dangers, no thoracic surgeon has conducted research on its potential mechanisms for a long time. Spinal surgeons have conducted in-depth research on the mechanism of scoliosis, but have not similarly focused on its relationship with thoracic deformity. The revelation of this relationship began with our research. We were the first to discover the causal relationship between pectus excavatum and scoliosis, and then found the prevalence of the relationship between thoracic deformity and scoliosis (Figure 2-1-2, 2-1-3) [19]. This provides theoretical guidance for the development of related clinical work.

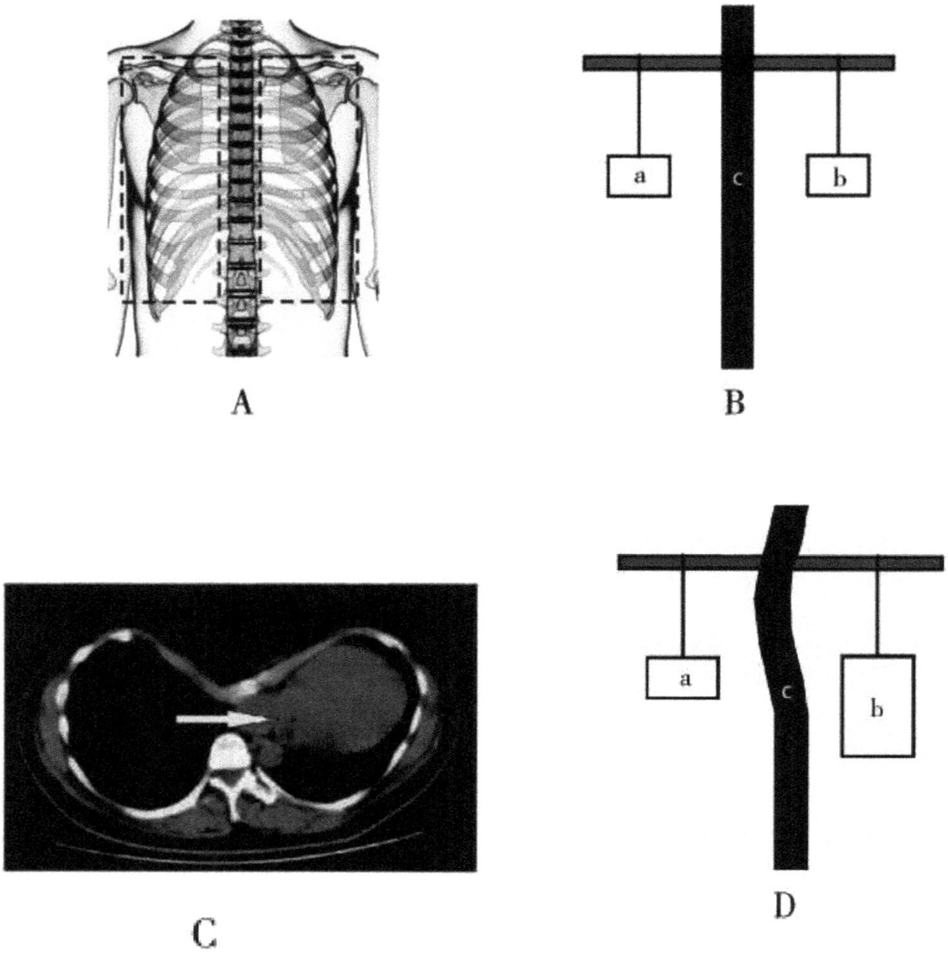

Figure 2-1-2 Mechanism of Scoliosis Caused by Pectus Excavatum, (A, B) Under physiological conditions, the spine is the main load-bearing structure of the human torso. All the weight of the torso is directly or indirectly loaded onto the spine. Normally, the forces on both sides of the spine are evenly and symmetrically distributed, so lateral deviation does not occur. (C, D) When a depression appears in the anterior chest wall, as seen in pectus excavatum, the heart is pushed toward the left thoracic cavity. This displacement of the heart pulls the entire mediastinum toward the left through the great vessels. Since both lungs are connected to the mediastinum via the hilum, the weight of the

lungs also shifts toward the left when the mediastinum is displaced. This results in asymmetric loading on both sides of the spine, which in turn causes the spine to bend. In most cases, the spine curves toward the left. However, the direction of curvature can be influenced by other factors, such as obstruction by the heart, so the actual direction of spinal curvature must be analyzed based on the specific situation. Regardless of these influencing factors, spinal curvature will inevitably develop over time. This is a common complication seen in the later stages of pectus excavatum. Once spinal curvature appears, it indicates that the anterior chest wall depression is already severe and that surgery should be considered promptly. If surgery is not performed, not only will the deformity remain uncorrected, but the scoliosis may also worsen. Since correcting spinal curvature comes at a much greater cost, early surgical intervention is recommended to avoid unnecessary complications.

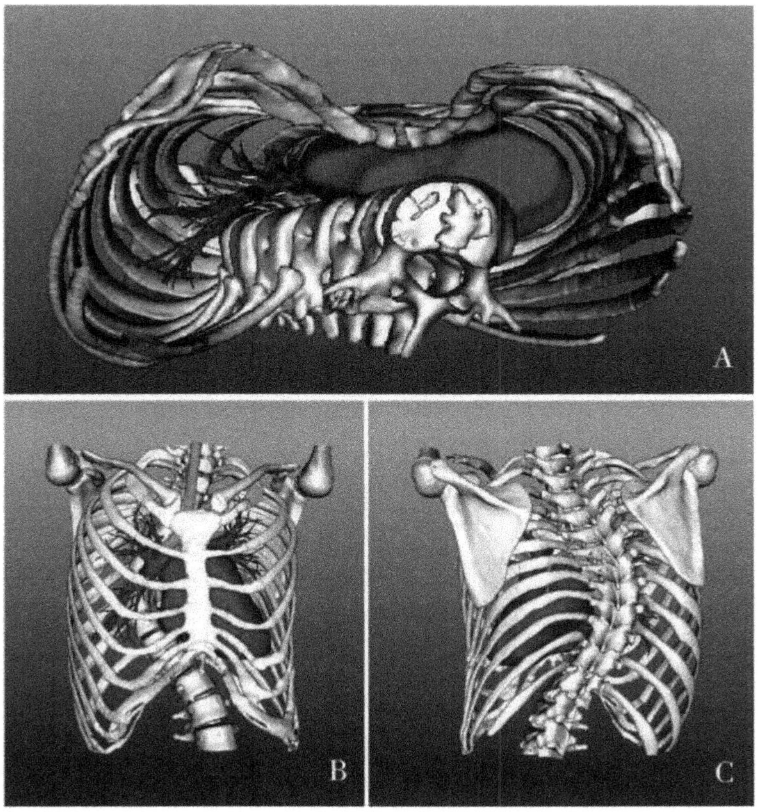

Figure 2-1-3 Case of Scoliosis Caused by Pectus Excavatum (A) The anterior chest wall is sunken, causing the heart to be pushed to the left side. The mediastinal structures also shift to the left, resulting in uneven force distribution on both sides of the spine, leading to scoliosis. (B) The heart is located at the left edge of the spine, and its intrinsic positive pressure pushes the spine in the opposite direction, further worsening the spinal curvature. (C) The spine shows a pronounced curvature.

The impact of thoracic deformities on shape includes both direct and indirect harm. The direct harm is mainly caused by obvious abnormalities in the structure itself. For example, both pectus carinatum and pectus excavatum are caused by abnormalities in local structures, which directly lead to an abnormal overall appearance. This is the most common impact of thoracic deformities. Some structural abnormalities affect the shape of the thorax through indirect mechanisms. For example, the fusion or absence of ribs, if not too severe, generally does not cause abnormalities in the overall shape of the thorax. However, these factors can, in turn, affect the overall shape of the thorax through abnormalities in the shape of the spine, which is an indirect hazard. Indirect harm can be seen in patients with thoracic dysplasia syndrome and Poland syndrome, where the patient may develop scoliosis due to uneven forces on both sides of the spine or direct loss of support. The scoliosis, in turn, affects the shape of the thorax. This is an example of indirect harm. This harm can also appear in cases after thoracic deformity surgery. Some patients experience pain on one side of the chest wall after surgery and prefer to adopt a protective posture, which often leads to scoliosis. Scoliosis can affect the shape of the thoracic cage, potentially leading to surgical failure. This is also an example of indirect harm. The direct harm of thoracic deformities is more likely to attract the attention of clinicians, whereas the indirect harm is often overlooked due to its unique concealment, thus requiring more attention.

4. Clinical Manifestations of Thoracic Deformities

The chest wall is located on the body surface and is a very special area. The hazards of thoracic deformities have been detailed, including two basic aspects: one is the impact on appearance, and the other is the impact on function [20]. The impact of appearance is related to psychological perception, and therefore it affects the psychological aspect. The impact on function is an objective impact, belonging to the physiological aspect of impact. Psychological effects may have no symptoms, but physiological effects can have obvious symptoms. Thoracic deformities, while having both physiological and psychological harm, do not necessarily manifest simultaneously. This means that the patient may not care about their appearance, or they may be extremely concerned about it. The clinical symptoms of patients may not always manifest; some patients exhibit extremely obvious symptoms, while others may not have any symptoms at all. Thoracic deformities generally do not present with local symptoms; their symptoms mainly manifest through changes in the function of thoracic organs. The most common symptoms are related to the respiratory system, followed by cardiovascular symptoms, and occasionally, digestive system symptoms may occur. This symptom, along with the characteristic of being distinct from the

lesion, constitutes a notable feature of the clinical presentation of thoracic deformity. The presence of this particular feature is precisely what maintains the intricate connection between chest wall surgery and thoracic surgery. The thoracic wall surgery department wants to be completely independent, but it always remains connected to thoracic surgery.
The characteristics of thoracic deformity symptoms pose specific requirements for clinical diagnosis. Since the symptoms are not specific, when symptoms appear, two possibilities should be considered simultaneously: in addition to diagnosing thoracic deformity, the possibility of concurrent intrathoracic disease should also be considered. This situation is actually not uncommon. If the latter is not considered, it may lead to missed diagnoses.
When analyzing the symptoms of thoracic deformities, it is essential to clarify that there is no strict correlation between the severity of the deformity and the symptoms. Some patients may have extremely severe deformities but exhibit no symptoms or only mild symptoms, while other patients may have less severe deformities yet experience extremely severe symptoms. When assessing the severity of a patient's deformity, it is necessary to approach it from two aspects: both the appearance of the deformity and the clinical manifestations must be considered. Only by doing so can a more objective evaluation be made. Additionally, the impact of psychological factors on patients must also be fully considered. A mental condition is also an illness. Even if there is no obvious deformity, if a patient is constantly distressed about the appearance of their chest, this mental condition also requires treatment. Considering that the root of the heart disease lies in the appearance of the thorax, the only treatment at this time is to change the shape of the thorax.

5. Surgery for Thoracic Deformities

There are various thoracic wall surgical diseases, and each disease's surgery will have its own characteristics. Although thoracic deformity is a benign condition, it still has the characteristics of a disease, so the primary purpose of surgery should be to treat the disease. However, due to its location on the body surface, aesthetic considerations cannot be ignored, thus it also includes attributes of plastic and cosmetic surgery. The nature of the surgery and other related issues have been clearly explained in the general discussion. This chapter will provide a detailed introduction to the technical issues of surgery, which will be the focus of this chapter.
Surgery for thoracic deformities is the first procedure initiated in chest wall surgery. Traditionally, this surgery was performed by two types of specialists: thoracic surgeons and pediatric surgeons. Due to differences in professional habits and philosophies, the treatments from two different specialties

There are bound to be differences in treatment methods. Thoracic wall surgery originated from thoracic surgery, and many of its concepts are closer to thoracic surgery. The undeniable fact is that there are differences between thoracic surgery and pediatric surgery compared to chest wall surgery in many aspects. When chest wall deformity surgery is performed by a specialized thoracic surgeon, it inherently has its own characteristics. This characteristic is reflected in the following aspects:

(1) The issue of concepts

When thoracic surgeons consider chest wall deformities, they first recognize its two most fundamental harms, a perspective that differs from doctors in other specialties. With different perspectives, the starting point for solving problems varies. Thoracic surgeons and pediatric surgeons may focus more on the treatment of diseases, while the focus of thoracic wall surgeons includes both objectives: treating the disease and performing reshaping or even cosmetic procedures [21]. The differences in treatment philosophies determine the variations in surgical methods, and the final outcomes will inevitably differ as well. The same kind of deformity, if only for the purpose of treatment, can disregard many factors unrelated to the treatment. For example, incisions and injuries can be disregarded. However, when considering factors related to cosmetic or plastic surgery, the surgical methods will vary significantly.

(2) The issue of methods

The surgical treatment of the chest wall encompasses attributes of both orthopedics and plastic surgery, providing a wide range of advanced interdisciplinary techniques for the treatment of thoracic deformities [22]. This kind of technique has never been available in either thoracic surgery or pediatric surgery, which makes the advantages of chest wall surgery particularly evident.

(3) The issue of using Thoracoscopy

Thoracoscopy is an important device used for the treatment of diseases within the thoracic cavity. In today's thoracic surgery, the thoracoscope has become standard equipment, and almost no operation can be performed without this device. When performing thoracic deformity surgery, thoracic surgeons are often influenced by concepts and habits, and many times cannot do without the thoracoscope. Pediatric surgeons, influenced by thoracic surgery concepts, often use Thoracoscopy during surgeries. The use of Thoracoscopy can occasionally facilitate thoracic deformity surgery, but more often it causes complications. When treating thoracic deformities, thoracic surgeons always adhere to professional standards and do not blindly use Thoracoscopy. This principle lays the foundation for better promotion of surgical techniques for thoracic deformities.

(4) Issues with minimally invasive procedures

Trauma is a very complex concept, and measuring the extent of trauma is not a simple task. Therefore, when clinicians frequently describe a certain surgery as minimally invasive, its accuracy is questionable. In fact, minimally invasive is only a relative concept. When it comes to thoracic deformity surgery, it only holds practical significance when compared to traditional open surgery. In the past, when discussing the treatment of thoracic deformities, it was generally believed that we had entered the era of minimally invasive surgery, and non-minimally invasive surgery had become a sign of outdated technology. Compared to open surgery, numerous popular procedures can be considered minimally invasive surgeries. However, thoracic deformities are a large group of diseases. In addition to the most common simple deformities, there are also many complex deformities. These deformity surgeries are impossible to complete the correction through a simple so-called minimally invasive surgery. At this point, if one blindly pursues minimally invasive techniques, it will inevitably limit the treatment of deformities [23]. Therefore, as long as there is a demand, surgeries with greater trauma are also justified. If the concept of minimally invasive techniques is always used to constrain deformity correction, one will be helpless when faced with complex deformities. This approach is neither scientific nor reasonable.

(5) Issues with the Use of Nuss Procedure

For a long time, clinicians' understanding of thoracic deformities has almost entirely come from one disease, namely pectus excavatum. Precisely because of this, the surgery for treating pectus excavatum has naturally become the hallmark procedure for correcting thoracic deformities. Nuss surgery is the first widely recognized effective procedure, and since its inception, it has been regarded as the standard surgical method for treating pectus excavatum. As there is no better surgical alternative, this procedure has been gradually acknowledged and elevated to a state of reverence or even complete myth, so much so that even when discussing the treatment of other deformities, many people still cannot forget the Nuss procedure. Rational thinking tells everyone that any surgery has its own scope of application, its own indications, and cannot be universally applicable. Nuss Surgery is clearly the same. Even for deformities like pectus excavatum, the Nuss procedure is not a panacea. Therefore, when such a procedure is used for the treatment of other deformities, the outcome is predictable [24].

Clinically, tragedies of abusing the Nuss procedure are often encountered. Not only is the deformity not treated, but it can also lead to more severe deformities. This shows that, when performing surgery for thoracic deformities, it is essential to flexibly choose the surgical method based on the characteristics of the deformity, rather than blindly fixating on the Nuss procedure. In the dictionary of thoracic surgeons, besides the Nuss procedure, there are actually many other surgical options available. This is also one of the distinctive features that differentiate chest wall surgery from surgeries in other specialties.

6. Treatment Outcomes for Thoracic Deformities

Thoracic deformity refers to an abnormality in the shape of the bony structure of the thorax. The ideal treatment outcome should aim to eliminate the deformity and restore its normal shape. However, due to the unique nature of deformity surgeries, achieving such outcomes is not easy. This resulted in three other effects: improvement, no effect, and deterioration. Improvement and ineffectiveness are outcomes that are relatively easy to understand, while deterioration often comes as a surprise. However, in clinical practice, situations that worsen the deformity are often encountered. The main reason is often directly related to the doctor's skills. Overall, some classify treatment outcomes into two categories: success and failure [25]. A surgery is considered successful if it can completely eliminate the deformity. Conversely, if the criteria for success have not been met, meaning the thorax has not returned to its normal shape, even if there is improvement, the surgery cannot be considered successful. When a surgery is ultimately classified as a failed operation, the loss suffered by the patient will be difficult to measure. This is an important manifestation of the special nature of thoracic wall surgery, and it also places exceptionally stringent demands on the skills of thoracic wall surgeons.

REFERENCES

[1] Wang, Wenlin. 2018. "Content of Research in Thoracic Wall Surgery (Part 1)." *Expert in Thoracic Deformity Surgery*, August 11.

[2] Kachlík, D., V. Varga, V. Bača, et al. 2020. "Variant Anatomy and Its Terminology." *Medicina (Kaunas)* 56 (12): 713.

[3] da Silva, E. R., M. B. Dalio, et al. 2021. "Surgical Treatment of Cervical Rib-Associated Arterial Thoracic Outlet Syndrome." *Jornal Vascular Brasileiro* 20: e20200106.

[4] Carmaco, C. R. 2016. "Lumbar Rib Causing Chronic Pain after Minor Thoracic Injury." *Pain Medicine* 17 (11): 2149–2151.

[5] Kumar, N., A. Guru, J. Patil, et al. 2013. "Additional Circular Intercostal Space Created by Bifurcation of the Left 3rd Rib and Its Costal Cartilage: A Case Report." *Journal of Medical Case Reports* 7: 6.

[6] Dunlay, R. P., K. B. Jones, and S. L. Weinstein. 2007. "Scoliosis Caused by Rib Fusion Following Thoracostomy for Tracheoesophageal Fistula: Case Report." *Iowa Orthopaedic Journal* 27: 95–98.
[7] Wang, Wenlin. 2021a. "Nuss Surgery's Most Distinctive Features." *Expert in Thoracic Deformity Surgery*, July 13.
[8] Wang, W. L., C. M. Chen, W. G. Long, et al. 2018. "Wang Procedure: A Novel Minimally Invasive Procedure for Young Children with Pectus Excavatum." *Case Reports and Images in Surgery* 1 (1): 1–2.
[9] Wang, W. 2022. "Surgical Treatment of a 36-Year-Old Patient with Asphyxiating Thoracic Dysplasia." *Interactive Cardiovascular and Thoracic Surgery* 34 (1): 153–155.
[10] Hatti, R. B., A. H. Nyamagoudar, T. G. R. Patil, et al. 2020. "Thirteen Ribs and Long Gap Esophageal Atresia: The Embryological Hypothesis for Exploration." *African Journal of Paediatric Surgery* 17 (3–4): 99–103.
[11] Wang, Wenlin. n.d. "Subjective Feelings and Objective Standards."
[12] Wang, Wenlin, Chunmei Chen, Weiguang Long, et al. 2015a. "Preliminary Exploration of the 'Thoracic Defect Hypothesis' in the Pathogenesis of Pectus Excavatum." *Journal of Practical Medicine* 31 (Suppl): 200–201.
[13] Wang, Wenlin, Weiguang Long, Chunmei Chen, et al. 2015b. "Analysis of the Pathogenesis of Pectus Carinatum." *Journal of Practical Medicine* 31 (Suppl): 313–314.
[14] Wang, Wenlin. 2017. "The Pathogenesis of Pectus Carinatum and Metabolic Diseases." *Expert in Thoracic Deformity Surgery*, August 30.
[15] Wang, Wenlin. 2020a. "The Mechanism of Funnel Chest Formation after Surgery for Congenital Diaphragmatic Hernia." *Expert in Thoracic Deformity Surgery*, November 24.
[16] Wang, Wenlin. 2021b. "Why Can Asthma Cause Pectus Excavatum?" *Expert in Thoracic Deformity Surgery*, June 30.
[17] Wang, Wenlin. 2020b. "Postoperative Pectus Excavatum after Pulmonary Cystadenoma." *Thoracic Deformity Surgery Specialist*, October 24.
[18] Wang, Wenlin. 2021c. "Another Severe Harm of Pectus Excavatum: Scoliosis." *Expert in Thoracic Deformity Surgery*, May 12.
[19] Wang, Wenlin. 2017b. "Thoracic Deformities and Scoliosis: Mechanical Principles." *Expert in Thoracic Deformity Surgery*, September 30.
[20] Wang, Wenlin. 2020c. "Another Harm of Thoracic Deformity." *Expert in Thoracic Deformity Surgery*, March 27.
[21] Wang, Wenlin. 2021d. "Basic Nature of Thoracic Wall Surgery." *Today's Headlines*, October 31.
[22] Wang, Wenlin. 2021e. "The Relationship between Chest Wall Surgery and Other Specialties." *Today's Headlines*, November 2.
[23] Wang, Wenlin. 2021f. "Thoracic Deformity: Minimally Invasive Surgery and Open Surgery." *Expert in Thoracic Deformity Surgery*, May 4.
[24] Wang, Wenlin. 2021g. "The Painful Lesson of Wang Wenlin: Nuss Surgery Is Not a Cure-All." *Expert in Chest Deformity Surgery*, October 5.
[25] Wang, Wenlin. 2021h. "Five Outcomes of Thoracic Deformity Surgery." *Expert in Thoracic Deformity Surgery*, September 22.

In various clinical surgery textbooks and thoracic surgery specialized books, there are only four types of thoracic deformities mentioned: pectus excavatum (funnel chest), pectus carinatum (pigeon chest), flat chest, and barrel chest. The impression given to many doctors seems to be that apart from these few types of deformities, there will not be any other kinds of deformities. In reality, the shape of the thorax is much more complex, and a variety of unusual deformities may be encountered in clinical practice. If the diagnosis of these deformities is made using the existing four names, it is difficult to achieve a satisfactory result. If the diagnosis is unsatisfactory, the characteristics of the deformity may not be recognized, ultimately affecting the treatment of the deformity. Many patients have suffered surgical failures due to inaccurate diagnoses. This is a significant regret in the field of thoracic deformity treatment. In our past work, we encountered a large number of unusual deformities, which in terms of shape and structure are completely different from those described in textbooks. In order to more accurately understand and treat these deformities, we have given them new names [1-8]. The abnormal naming highlights its own characteristics, making it more convenient for the development of clinical work. However, for each type of deformity, naming is an independent task, and it is difficult to discern their interconnections from the deformity names themselves. To better elucidate this connection, we have systematically classified various deformities from a holistic perspective. The development of naming and classification work not only clarifies the characteristics of each deformity but also reveals the connections between them. This has played a positive role in further understanding deformities and directly guiding diagnosis and treatment work.

1. Naming of New Deformities

The essence of deformity lies in its abnormal morphology. Anyone familiar with the concept of malformation knows that once the morphology becomes abnormal, it cannot develop in a standardized or predetermined direction. The very concept of malformation implies that the specific shape will be unpredictable. However, the past naming of four types of deformities was evidently an idealized or standardized approach. This method itself contradicts the variable nature of deformities, thus there are many issues with the naming itself. In clinical practice, we have encountered many new deformities; some of these are mistakenly identified as previously named deformities, while others lack an appropriate name. This situation has significantly impacted clinical work. In order to eliminate adverse effects, we have named a large number of deformities. These deformities include: groove chest, saddle chest, Wenlin chest, flat pigeon chest, lateral chest wall depression deformity, localized protrusion deformity, rib arch deformity, and xiphoid process deformity, etc [1-8]. A brief description of the characteristics of these new deformities is provided below.

(1) Groove-shaped chest

A groove-shaped chest is a very special deformity that was previously always considered as funnel chest, and its characteristic is also a depression in the anterior chest wall. Depression (Fig. 2 – 2 - 1). However, the indentation of a groove-shaped chest is completely different from that of a funnel chest [1]. The reason pectus excavatum is named "funnel chest" is that its appearance resembles a funnel. The depression of pectus excavatum is a "pit" in the anterior chest wall, with a centrally sunken area surrounded by relatively higher edges. This type of depression is generally located near the middle of the anterior chest wall. A sulcus chest also features a depression in the anterior chest wall, but it's a distinct "groove" rather than a "pit". This groove is a transverse depression at the lower part of the anterior chest wall. Both types of deformities have depressions, but their characteristics are different. If this distinction is not recognized, it is easy to cause treatment errors. There are often cases of surgical failure for a groove-shaped chest on the clinical bed. These patients were misdiagnosed with pectus excavatum and treated with the Nuss procedure, which easily fails due to the lack of a structural basis necessary for the Nuss procedure to be effective [10]. When the treatment of a disease fails due to its naming, it indicates that the naming is inappropriate and needs to be changed [5]. The indentation of the sulcus-shaped chest is groove-like. To distinguish it from a funnel chest, we have introduced a new designation, sulcus-shaped chest. After completing this naming process, we designed a surgery targeting the characteristics of the deformity, achieving good results.

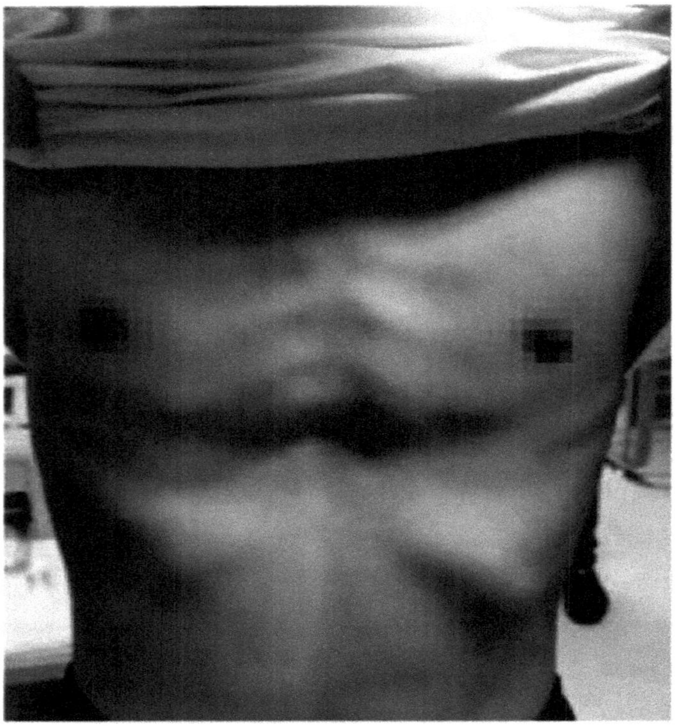

Figure 2 – 2 - 1 appearance of trench-like chest wall. This deformity is a type of depression deformity, but it is clearly different from the "pit" of pectus excavatum. This deformity is a distinct "groove," and therefore, a more accurate term would be "groove chest" rather than pectus excavatum. The purpose of this naming is to facilitate surgery, especially when the Nuss procedure is regarded as the standard surgical method for treating pectus excavatum. It is essential to have a targeted naming to avoid surgical failure when treating deformities such as sulcus chest.

(2) Saddle Chest

Saddle chest is another new deformity. No one has ever paid attention to this kind of deformity in the past. Characterized by bilateral depressions on the lower chest wall, with a normal midline. This type of deformity can be regarded as a combined form of bilateral chest wall depression deformity, due to the absence of this characteristic receives attention, thus often regarded as a complex type of deformity, and there is a lack of treatment approaches. In fact, this deformity is not uncommon and has distinct characteristics. Considering the deformed appearance resembles a saddle, we name it saddle thorax (Fig. 2 – 2 - 2) [2]. The depression of a saddle chest is not comparable to the depression of a funnel chest. The sides are concave, while the central part can be regarded as a relative protrusion. This protrusion is completely different from the protrusion seen in pectus carinatum. Therefore, the surgery cannot draw on procedures for pectus excavatum or pectus carinatum and must be specifically designed based on the characteristics of the deformity. Only in this way can good treatment results be achieved.

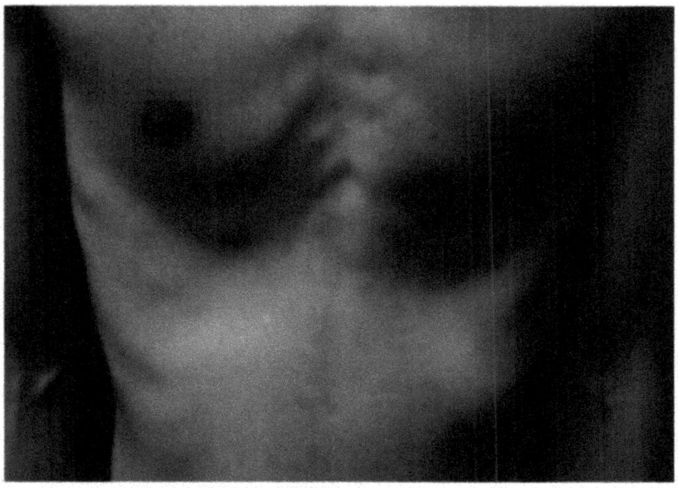

Figure 2 – 2 - 2 Saddle-shaped chest wall appearance. This type of deformity is actually a composite deformity, formed by the concave deformities of the two lateral chest walls. The central area is not elevated above the normal chest wall plane, so it cannot be considered a pectus carinatum, and certainly not pectus excavatum. This deformity resembles a saddle; hence, it is named saddle chest.

(3) Wenlin Chest

Wenlin chest is a rare thoracic deformity, previously always considered a type of pectus carinatum, occasionally referred to as pigeon breast or pigeon chest [12,13], which are highly inaccurate names. The names in foreign literature are confused, with multiple naming conventions. Confusing naming can affect treatment. We began focusing on this deformity early on due to the fundamental challenge of surgery. In order to more profoundly reveal the nature of deformities and provide guidance for surgical treatment, we have proposed a new nomenclature [3].

Wenlin, the nature of the chest is a complex deformity, with both protrusion and depression, which is different from any previous form of single deformity (Figure 2-2-3). Wenlin. The protrusion of the chest shows a significant difference compared to the protrusion of an ordinary chicken breast. The protrusion of a pigeon chest can be located in all parts of the anterior chest wall, with varying size and degree. Apart from the protrusion, another distinct feature is the central depression, with its center located on the body of the sternum. Due to both protrusions and indentations involving the sternum, the sternum exhibits characteristic changes, becoming overall thickened with a cross-section in the shape of an "S". Overall, the chest of Wenlin shows distinct visual characteristics. Since it is not a single deformity, it cannot be regarded as either pectus carinatum or pectus excavatum. In the past, we have encountered multiple cases of surgical failure in clinical practice where these patients were treated as having isolated pectus carinatum or pectus excavatum. The surgery cannot be successful due to the failure to address the merger deformities.

Wenlin, While the chest has both protrusions and depressions, its significant characteristic is that this composite deformity is not a simple addition of protrusions and depressions, but rather an extremely special deformity [3,14]. The effective method for general compound deformities is recognized as the sandwich surgery. The specific procedure involves using a steel plate to first push up the indentation from the bottom, and then flattening the protrusion from the raised surface. This is equivalent to performing both pectus excavatum surgery and pectus carinatum surgery simultaneously. However, for Wenlin's chest, a simple sandwich surgery cannot address the treatment of the two deformities due to the inherent uniqueness of the sternum. Due to the thickening of the sternum and its inherently abnormal rigidity, local reshaping is almost impossible to achieve through indirect methods. Therefore, to achieve satisfactory results, it is necessary to perform a special surgery for correction, as the typical sandwich surgery clearly lacks the capability for treatment.

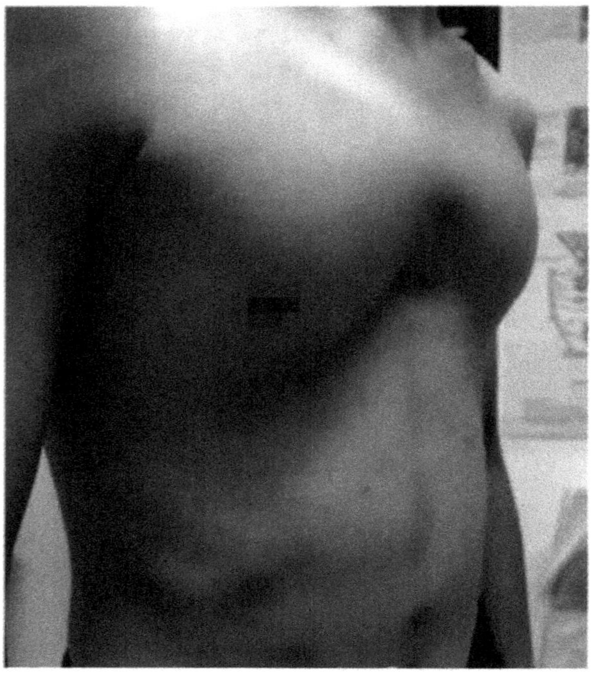

Figure 2 – 2 - 3 Wenlin-Appearance of the chest wall. This is a very special deformity. General thoracic surgeons do not prioritize deformities and rarely encounter such deformities. Pediatric surgeons may encounter this, but because the deformity often only exhibits typical characteristics in adulthood, they do not often see many typical patients. When two doctors who mainly specialize in treating thoracic deformities have limited exposure to this deformity, their basic understanding of it will be lacking. This will undoubtedly affect the treatment of the deformity. In fact, the pathological features of this deformity are very distinctive, making it an independent deformity unrelated to general pectus carinatum, and thus it requires a separate naming. When a more appropriate name could not be found, we had to use the very simple name Wenlin. In our subsequent work, we found that we had made the right decision.

(4) Pectus Carinatum

The condition of a flat chicken breast is somewhat similar to Wenlin chest, but it is not the same deformity. The characteristic of pectus carinatum is primarily a pronounced protrusion deformity of the anterior chest wall, while simultaneously there is a noticeable depression in the central region amid the overall protrusion (Figure 2-2-4) [5]. This is also a combination of two types of deformities, but it is not simply a sum of pectus excavatum and pectus carinatum. Because of this, the surgery has become more complicated. If treatment is performed using a simple sandwich technique, it is difficult to achieve good results. This indicates that this deformity cannot be considered a typical compound deformity. In order to better understand and treat this deformity, we have named it, that is, flat chest deformity, and subsequently, we specially designed a surgical procedure for it, achieving satisfactory results.

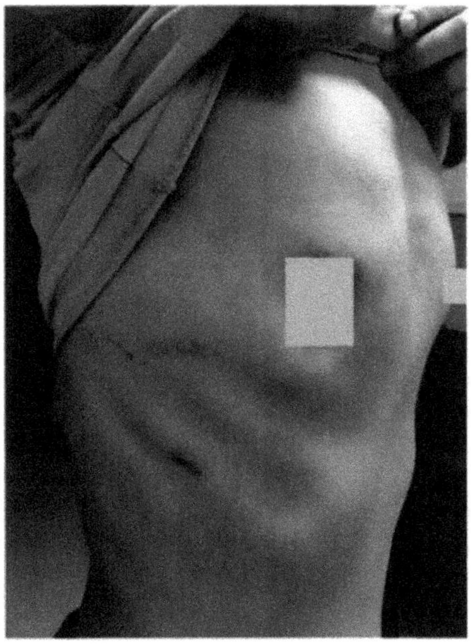

Figure 2 – 2 - 4 Appearance of the chest wall with pectus carinatum. This deformity is also a very unique deformity. It looks like a pectus carinatum, but there is a depression in the middle. Thus, we named it pectus excavatum.

(5) Deformity of the lateral chest wall depression

Lateral chest wall depression is also a type of depression deformity, but this deformity cannot be referred to as pectus excavatum (Figure 2 – 2 – 5). Pectus excavatum depression is located near the midline, typically involving the sternum. The deformity of the lateral chest wall depression is located on one side of the chest wall, involves only the ribs, and is unrelated to the sternum, with the sternum maintaining a normal shape. Such deformities were formerly also known as funnel chest, but it is clearly not a typical deformity. If the Nuss procedure is used to treat this deformity, it is difficult to achieve satisfactory results because it is hard to find a fulcrum for the steel plate on the concave side. This deformity is distinct, especially differing significantly from the depression seen in pectus excavatum, in order to better understand and treat this deformity, we have given it a specific name [4]. On this basis, we have also specially designed the surgical method, achieving excellent therapeutic results.

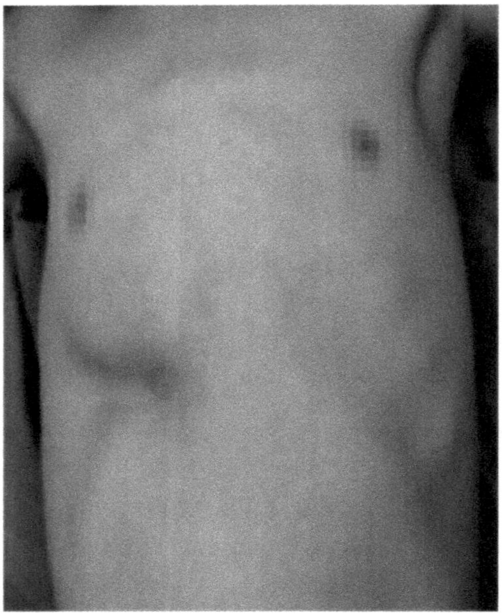

Figure 2 – 2 - 5 Appearance of the chest wall with pectus excavatum. Mediastinal deformity is a type of concave deformity, but it is clearly different from pectus excavatum. The depression of pectus excavatum is located in the center or slightly off-center, while the depression in this case is completely located on the lateral chest wall and has no relation to the central sternum. Therefore, it cannot be considered a pectus excavatum and requires a separate designation.

(6) Limitation of Protrusion Deformity

All of the above deformities vary in form and nature, but they share a common characteristic: they are not deformities of a certain local area, but deformities over a larger range. These malformations can affect multiple adjacent structures, so they can also be described as malformations of multiple structures. In addition to these deformities, there is a special type of protruding deformity in clinical practice. This deformity is confined to a small area of the chest wall, with the surrounding structures being completely normal. Due to its prominent protrusion significantly affecting the appearance of the thorax, it is also categorized as a deformity, but it is clearly not a typical pigeon chest. To highlight its fundamental characteristics, we also named it as limited bulging deformity [15]. Because it is a localized protrusion, its clinical manifestations and treatment methods differ from other deformities, thereby further highlighting the value of its nomenclature.

(7) Rib arch deformity

Costal arch deformity is a thoroughly overlooked malformation that no one has paid attention to before (Figure 2 –2-6). This deformity can exist independently or in combination with various other deformities. Since no one paid attention, no author has addressed it. Even when pectus excavatum is addressed, treatment often focuses solely on the pectus excavatum itself, with few addressing the deformity of the costal arch. for older patients, since the anterior chest wall is an integrated structure with considerable mechanical strength, if only the depression is treated, the costal arch will lift as the depressed chest wall moves

forward, ultimately resulting in more severe protrusion. This will undoubtedly affect Surgical outcomes. It is evident that rib arch deformities should not be considered part of other deformities but should be viewed as an independent deformity requiring special treatment.
In fact, independent rib arch deformities are also quite common. Such deformities are unrelated to other deformities and may manifest as local protrusions and depressions. We propose the concept of rib arch deformity, not essentially to name it, but to draw attention to it. Based on an in-depth study of the pathological structure of this deformity, we have classified it and designed surgical approaches. These procedures not only correct rib arch deformities that are combined with other anomalies, but also provide satisfactory treatment for isolated rib arch deformities [8].

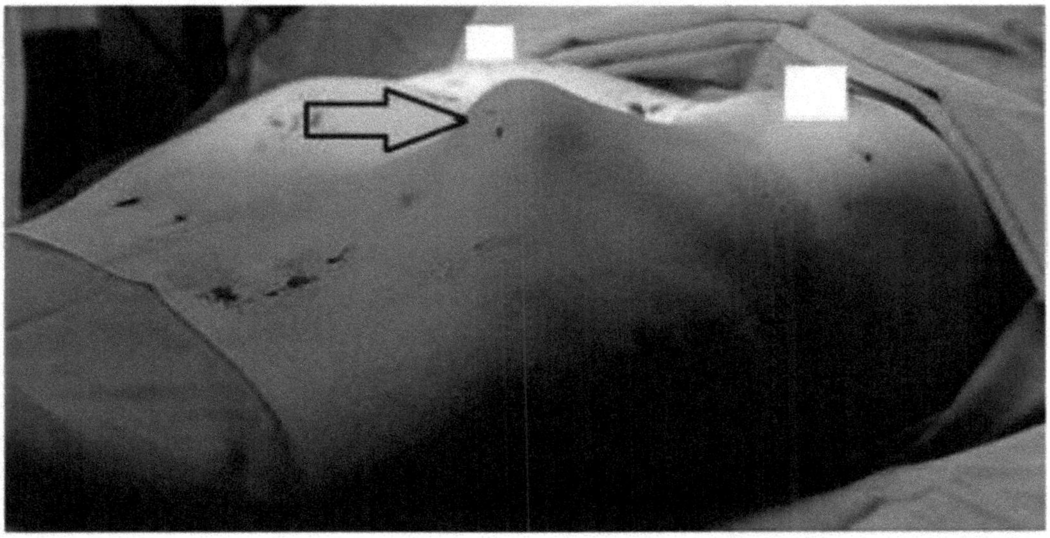

Figure 2 – 2 - 6 Appearance of rib arch deformity. This deformity can manifest in various types, can exist independently, or can be combined with other deformities.

(8) Xiphoid Process Deformity

Among the structures of the thorax, the xiphoid process is the one most easily overlooked, and its shape generally does not attract attention. However, in clinical practice, deformities of the xiphoid process can also occur, and such deformities can lead to various problems, so it is necessary to pay attention to them. Just like rib arch deformities, we did not name it; instead, we meticulously observed the deformity and based on this, we classified it [7. These efforts have played a positive role in the treatment of the deformity.
Deformity naming is an important and serious task, as its significance lies in

drawing attention to the characteristics of certain deformities and facilitating more in-depth research on them. However, the term "malformation" has its limitations, as general naming conventions struggle to fully and profoundly reflect the essential characteristics of malformations. In order to eliminate these limitations as much as possible, additional work is needed to compensate. Thus, another important task emerged, which is the overall classification of deformities.

2. Classification of Deformities

In the early years, there was limited research on deformities, and clinical work on various deformities was conducted quite independently, making it difficult to examine from a macro perspective. Examine various types of deformities. In recent years, as research on deformities has continued to deepen, the intrinsic connections between deformities have been continuously discovered. At this point, some commonalities naturally emerge, providing the possibility for more detailed naming or classification. Before observing the characteristics of various deformities, there is one task that must be completed in advance, which is to establish observation standards. With such standards, it is possible to compare various deformities and identify the underlying patterns. The observational standard we identified is the surface of the chest wall in a normal human body. This is the most scientific and the most easily recognized standard or measure.

Once the standard is found, all deformities can be compared to this standard, naturally categorizing them into two major types: the first type being deformities below the reference plane, and the second type being deformities above the reference plane. The former is a depression-type deformity, while the latter is a protrusion-type deformity. This classification connects all deformities with a unified standard, quickly establishing their intrinsic connections.

After deformities are divided into two major types, different deformed individuals can be arranged clearly in sequence, thus establishing a comprehensive classification system. This is the classification of deformities as a whole (Figure 2 – 2 - 7, Figure 2 – 2 - 8) [9].

The overall classification method first uses the normal anterior chest wall plane as a standard and divides the deformity into two basic types, namely type I and type II. Type I refers to a type that is below the standard plane, whereas Type II is the opposite, referring to a type that is above the standard plane. Based on the different characteristics of various deformities of the anterior chest wall, type I is further divided into seven subtypes: I-a, I-b, I-c, I-d, I-e, I-f, and I-g. Type II is divided into four subtypes: II-a, II-b, II-c, and II-d.

Type- I-a is a deformity where the depression is located at the center of the anterior chest wall, corresponding to symmetric pectus excavatum. Type I-b is a deformity where the depression deviates from the midline but also involves the sternum, equivalent to asymmetrical pectus excavatum. Type I-c is a deformity where the depression is completely located on one side of the chest wall, corresponding to a lateral chest wall depression deformity, and is unrelated to the sternum. Type I-d is characterized by the complete collapse of one side of the chest wall, with the opposite chest wall being normal or exhibiting secondary changes, corresponding to unilateral thoracic hypoplasia syndrome. Type I-e is a deformity where the depression is located at the lower level of the anterior chest wall. The depression is situated on both sides of the lower chest wall, with the middle chest wall being normal and not protruding, resembling a saddle chest. I-f type is a transverse groove-shaped depression located at the lower part of the anterior chest wall, corresponding to a groove-shaped chest. I-g type is a general depression of the entire anterior chest wall, equivalent to a flat chest.

Type–IIa is a deformity with protrusion located at the midline of the anterior chest wall, corresponding to the symmetrical type of pectus carinatum. Type II-b is a deformity characterized by a protrusion deviating from the midline, equivalent to an asymmetrical pectus carinatum. Type II-c is characterized by a protrusion located on the upper anterior chest wall, with a relatively concave area directly below, corresponding to a Wenlin chest. Type II-d is a deformity characterized by a protrusion of the entire anterior chest wall, similar to a barrel chest. In the overall classification system, the population originally classified under the funnel chest has been divided into two subtypes: I-a type and I-b type. The Poland syndrome, due to its non-uniform deformity manifestations, no longer exists as a separate category. Part of it is merged into the I-a type, and another part is merged into the I-b type. A small number of patients are excluded from the overall classification system due to complex deformities. The patients originally classified with pectus carinatum are divided into two subtypes: II-a type and II-b type. The Wenlin chest is specifically categorized into the II-c type, forming its own independent type.

It is particularly important to explain the distinction between flat chest and barrel chest. Since the anterior chest wall itself does not have any localized protrusion or depression, it is difficult to associate it with general deformities. By overall classification, the two types of deformities are categorized into Type I and Type II deformities, respectively, and their essential pathological changes are uncovered, laying the foundation for their treatment.

The holistic classification method has many advantages: ① Inclusivity. This classification method is an open classification system, under which, according to the same standard, all types of deformities can be incorporated into this system. This system not only encompasses all existing deformities but also remains open to new deformities that may arise in the future, ready to incorporate them into the system at any time. ② Generalization: This system provides a high-level summary of the characteristics of all thoracic deformities, clearly highlighting the two most fundamental features. This not only facilitates the understanding of the deformities but also enhances their treatment. ③Scientific nature. This system adopts scientific standards, recognized scales, and reasonable methods, thus demonstrating a high level of scientific rigor both in theory and practice. ④ Practicality. This system closely focuses on the two main characteristics of deformities, providing a strong reference for surgeries. This leads to all thoracic deformity surgeries being classified into two basic types: concave deformity surgeries and convex deformity surgeries. The classification of surgical types directly provides the most effective solutions for the treatment of various deformities. For example, within this system, all I-type deformities are concave deformities, and concave deformities can be treated using roughly two methods, namely the Nuss procedure and the Wang procedure. Therefore, regardless of how complex the deformity is, whether it is type I-a, type I-b, or type I-g, these two surgical procedures can be used to complete the treatment. The overall classification method not only categorizes various deformities in an orderly manner but also proposes solutions for the treatment of various deformities. From both diagnostic and treatment perspectives, this classification method is very practical[10-15].

The comprehensive classification method not only organizes different deformities into a systematic structure but also proposes clear treatment pathways. From both diagnostic and therapeutic perspectives, this classification method is highly practical.

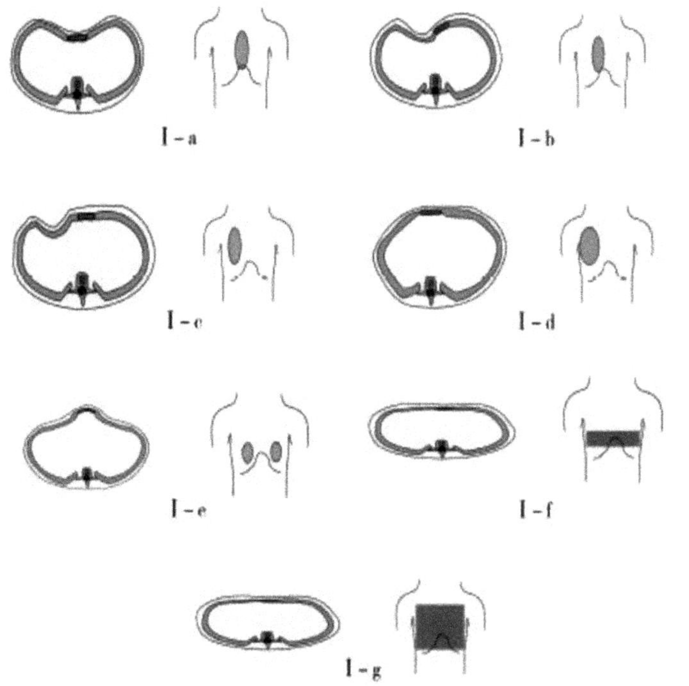

Figure 2 – 2 - 7 Overall Classification Diagram (Type I). This type of deformity is classified as a concave deformity, and various deformities can be grouped under this category. The depression is an intrinsic structural feature, which not only helps to discover the internal connections of various deformities but also aids in the treatment of similar deformities.

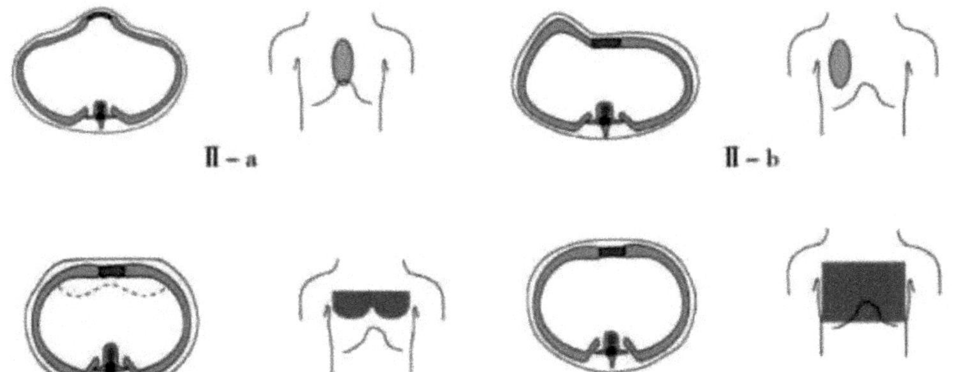

Figure 2-2-8 Overall Classification Diagram (Type II). This type of deformity is a protuberant deformity. By understanding the characteristic feature of protuberance, the intrinsic connections among various deformities can be discovered, which also aids in their treatment.

3. Practical Applications of Overall Classification

For any method of classifying diseases, practicality is always the true essence. No matter how grand in theory, if it is not practical, such a classification is meaningless. Therefore, when designing classification methods, in addition to fully considering their various inherent attributes, it is crucial to focus on their application issues.

The comprehensive classification of thoracic deformities is the latest classification method in the field of deformities. This method has many advantages, among which practicality is one of its distinct features. However, having practicality and effectively using this method are two different things. To fully realize its practicality, it needs to be explored from a clinical perspective[10-15].

Firstly, fully establish the connection between the overall classification method and the naming method. Distorted traditional nomenclature has deeply rooted itself in people's minds, and replacing it with a new classification system will involve a process of adjustment. But time will make unfamiliar things become familiar, and as time goes by, the new system will gradually be accepted by people. In this process, it is necessary to align the names from the two systems, understand their intrinsic connections, and master the naming conventions. This approach not only avoids hindering the understanding of anomalies but also aids in recognizing anomalies from a more updated perspective, ultimately facilitating the diagnosis and treatment of anomalies.

Second, grasp the main characteristics and perform proper deformity classification. The purpose of classification is, on one hand, to standardize abnormal concepts, and on the other hand, to guide the implementation of clinical work. When encountering a patient with a deformity, the first step is to identify the main characteristic of the deformity, whether it is a depression or a protrusion, and categorize it into these two main types. Subsequently, classify it into various subtypes according to the detailed characteristics of the deformity. Following this procedure in carrying out work not only allows for a more precise understanding of deformities but also aids in their diagnosis and treatment.

Third, be adept at identifying anomalies and effectively expanding classifications. In recent years, although research on deformities has made tremendous progress, it is merely the beginning, and this momentum will not stop. As relevant research progresses, new deformities will be discovered. After the appearance of a new deformity, a new name must be assigned. Since the overall classification method is an open classification system, new deformities can be added to this system at any time, ultimately making the classification complete and more comprehensive, and the classification system itself will also be well expanded.

Fourth, be adept at decomposing anomalies and ensure proper classification and supplementation. The overall classification method divides deformities into two categories, which can almost encompass all deformities. However, in clinical practice, many deformities are quite complex, and their pathological changes are not singular. In other words, there are both depressions and protrusions. For such deformities, an overall classification approach seems difficult to be effective. However, this is merely a superficial phenomenon. In fact, this complex malformation precisely provides an opportunity for the overall classification method to play a role. The two main types of overall classification are depression and protrusion, and no matter how complex a deformity is, it only falls under these two basic characteristics. The complexity of malformations is merely due to the complex combination of concavities and protrusions. The two basic pathological changes objectively exist at all times, which are precisely the two major characteristics that the overall classification method firmly grasps. Therefore, as long as one conducts an in-depth study and careful observation of complex deformities, the existence of two basic types of deformities can be discovered, thereby allowing for correct classification and naming.

REFERENCES

[1] Wang, Wenlin. 2016. "The Naming and Morphological Characteristics of Gutter Chest." *Journal of Practical Medicine* 32 (2): 335–336.

[2] Wang, Wenlin. 2017. "The Naming and Morphological Features of Saddle Chest." *Journal of Practical Medicine* 33 (Suppl): 380–381.

[3] Wang, Wenlin. 2019a. "Wenlin Chest and Wenlin Surgery." *Expert in Thoracic Deformity Surgery*, June 22.

[4] Wang, Wenlin. 2015. "The Naming of Localized Depression of the Lateral Thoracic Wall." *Journal of Practical Medicine* 31 (Suppl): 196.

[5] Wang, Wenlin. 2019b. "The Naming of Flat Pectus Carinatum: A Special Type of Thoracic Deformity." *Expert in Thoracic Deformity Surgery*, May 23.

[6] Wang, Wenlin. 2021a. "The Uniqueness of Surgery Determines the Naming of Deformities." *Expert in Thoracic Deformity Surgery*, June 11.

[7] Wang, Wenlin. 2019c. "The Basic Concept of Xiphoid Deformity." *Expert in Thoracic Deformity Surgery*, February 17.

[8] Wang, W. L. 2018. "Minimally Invasive Operation for Costal Arch Deformity." *Surgical Case Reports* 1 (2): 1–3.

[9] Wang, Wenlin, Chunmei Chen, Xuejun Li, et al. 2018. "Comprehensive Classification System for Thoracic Deformities." *Chinese Journal of Clinical Thoracic and Cardiovascular Surgery* 25 (11): 981–985.

[10] Wang, Wenlin. 2018. "Today's Surgery: Revision Surgery for Failed Gutter Chest Repair." *Expert in Thoracic Deformity Surgery*, December 26.
[11] Shang, Ziyin, Xianlun Duan, Peng Zhang, et al. 2012. "Surgical Treatment of Pediatric Funnel Chest with Spherical Pectus Carinatum." *Chinese Journal of Pediatric Surgery* 33 (2): 148–149.
[12] Lester, C. W. 1953. "Pigeon Breast (Pectus Carinatum) and Other Protrusion Deformities of the Chest of Developmental Origin." *Annals of Surgery* 137 (4): 482–489.
[13] Lester, C. W. 1954. "Pigeon Breast, Funnel Chest, and Other Congenital Deformities of the Chest." *Journal of the American Medical Association* 156 (11): 1063–1067.
[14] Wang, Wenlin. 2021b. "The Uniqueness of the Wenlin Chest." *Expert in Thoracic Deformity Surgery*, June 10.
[15] Wang, Wenlin. 2021c. "Local Protrusion Deformity of the Thoracic Wall." *Expert in Thoracic Deformity Surgery*, October 6.

Section 3

NATURE OF THORACIC DEFORMITY SURGERIES

Thoracic deformities are a narrow category of chest wall deformities and represent an important condition in chest wall surgery. Since they fall under chest wall surgery, such operations inherently have two fundamental attributes: therapeutic and cosmetic [1]. For most thoracic deformities, physiological harm is not the primary concern; instead, cosmetic correction is the main goal of the surgery. From a broader perspective, even if the deformity does not present obvious symptoms, it still falls within the scope of disease. Therefore, cosmetic surgery in this context still retains therapeutic properties; the therapeutic and cosmetic aspects are integrated, though with a greater emphasis on the cosmetic.

The cosmetic aspect can be divided into two forms: reshaping and reconstruction [2]. Reconstruction mainly refers to surgeries performed for primary and secondary defects, while reshaping specifically refers to corrective surgeries for thoracic deformities.

The essence of thoracic deformity lies in the change in the shape of the bony structure of the thoracic cage, and the result of this change differs significantly from the normal shape. To treat such structural deformities, specific methods must be used to alter the shape and ultimately restore it to normal. We refer to these methods as reshaping, which essentially means remolding the shape of the thoracic cage. Based on their fundamental nature, reshaping surgeries can be categorized into three basic types [3]: destructive reshaping, mechanical force reshaping, and template reshaping. These three types of surgeries differ in their basic principles and operational techniques, and each has its own distinct characteristics.

1.Destructive Reshaping

Destructive reshaping is a relatively common surgical method and was once a popular approach in the early treatment of thoracic deformities. On the surface, destructive reshaping appears highly invasive, seemingly contradicting the core idea of reshaping which is to restore normal form whereas destruction implies damaging the basic structure. Although the two objectives seem fundamentally opposed, their essence is actually aligned. Destructive reshaping targets the deformity of the thoracic cage, meaning the abnormal bony structure in the affected area. Without removing or altering the abnormal structure, it is impossible to replace it with a normal form. In a broad sense, all deformity surgeries are essentially a rejection or destruction of the pathological structure.

In this context, destructive reshaping refers primarily to the method of operation, not the outcome, and therefore does not conflict with the intention of reshaping. Specifically, destructive reshaping involves directly operating on the abnormal, diseased area to alter its structure and form, with the ultimate goal of restoring the normal shape of the thoracic cage.

Thoracic deformity is a pathological change of the bony structure, and such structural abnormalities are extremely rigid, making shape correction quite difficult. If conventional methods cannot alter the shape, then it becomes necessary to use strong destructive force to break down the deformed structure in order to enable reshaping. To achieve this, at least three fundamental procedures must be performed: incision, transection, and resection. All of these procedures are notably destructive in nature. Once these operations are completed, the basic structure of the deformity is dismantled, laying the groundwork for the reconstruction of a new thoracic cage. Laying the foundation for reconstructing the shape of the thoracic cage. From this, it is clear that destructive reshaping is not merely about destruction; more importantly, it is about reconstruction. That is the true ultimate goal of the surgery. This approach is comparable to a major overhaul of a car thorough, comprehensive repair and restoration

In the early years of thoracic deformity surgery, due to the lack of ideal treatment methods, many procedures had the characteristics of destructive reshaping. For example, in the case of pectus excavatum surgery, the early approach involved simply removing the costal cartilages. This attempt was essentially a destructive procedure. The removal of structural components is the most thorough form of destruction. On this basis, if reshaping of the remaining structural elements is carried out, it becomes a standard destructive reshaping surgery. The earliest surgeries focused more on destruction without proper reshaping, and thus were not ideal. Later, the Ravitch procedure clearly represented a step forward. During this surgery, the most severely affected areas are first treated with destructive methods such as wedge-shaped incisions or transections and the most severely diseased sections are directly removed. After these destructive steps, all related structures are rearranged, repositioned, and fixed in place to achieve the desired shape which becomes the most important aspect of the reshaping process. Clearly, the Ravitch procedure is a representative example of destructive reshaping surgery [4]. The sternal turnover procedure may appear not to involve the destruction of the local deformity structure, but from a broader perspective, it can be considered a form of overall deformity destruction [5]. At the moment the depressed anterior chest wall is flipped, the most complete destruction is essentially achieved. At the same time, this maneuver eliminates the sunken appearance, thus fulfilling the function of reshaping as well. This means that destruction and reshaping occur simultaneously, making this procedure both the most complete form of destruction and the most comprehensive reshaping. It is a typical destructive surgery. However, because it does not involve direct destruction of the detailed local deformities, the procedure lacks the thoroughness of a "major overhaul." As a result, the internal turnover procedure often fails to achieve the most ideal reshaping outcome. After the surgery, obvious localized deformities may still be present, with a prominent bulge replacing the previous depression. Although chest wall compression is relieved, the deformity remains, merely in a different form. This procedure strongly emphasizes its therapeutic value, but its cosmetic outcome is less than optimal, and therefore it is not considered a perfect surgery. For a long time, this procedure coexisted with the Ravitch technique, but was used less frequently due to its notable shortcomings.

For the special category of destructive reshaping surgeries, both destruction and reshaping are indispensable elements. Without thoroughly eliminating the pathological structure, it is impossible to achieve satisfactory reshaping. This unique nature gives these surgeries several distinct characteristics: First, due to the highly destructive nature of the procedure itself, the surgical trauma is usually significant. Before the advent of minimally invasive surgery, surgical trauma was not a major concern; the sole purpose of surgery was to eliminate bony deformities and restore normal shape. As long as the patient could endure the trauma, very few paid attention to the damage caused by the procedure itself. This mindset provided the foundation for the existence and acceptance of destructive reshaping. Second, because destruction often requires operations over a relatively wide area, such surgeries typically involve large incisions. A large incision means a large scar, which inevitably affects the aesthetic appearance of the skin post-surgery. The goal of thoracic deformity surgery is to eliminate the deformity and make the chest wall appear more aesthetically pleasing. If the postoperative scar is too prominent, it can undermine the cosmetic success of the reshaping effort.

Both the Ravitch procedure and the sternal turnover procedure involve significant surgical trauma and often result in prominent postoperative scars. In the early days of such surgeries, trauma and scarring were seen as inevitable costs, and few questioned their necessity. However, as more advanced surgical techniques emerged, these issues began to draw attention and were soon recognized as shortcomings of the procedures. As a result, such surgeries were eventually given a somewhat unfavorable label: open surgery.

The concept of open surgery only emerged after the idea of minimally invasive surgery was introduced. As the concept of minimally invasive techniques swept across the globe, open surgery came to be seen as outdated. In the context of surgeries for thoracic deformities a special type of condition destructive reshaping gradually came to be viewed as an obsolete option due to issues like trauma and large incisions. As a result, this technique has largely fallen out of use, and nowadays, it is rarely performed.

However, from the perspective of basic surgical principles, there is no fundamental flaw in the concept of destroying pathological structures and reshaping them. The reason these procedures have been questioned lies in the methods of execution, not in the principles themselves. For surgeries like the sternal turnover procedure and the Ravitch procedure, if achieving the surgical goal requires large incisions and significant trauma, then skepticism is inevitable. However, if under the same guiding principles, it becomes possible to accomplish destruction and reshaping through reasonable techniques, involving smaller incisions and simpler operations, then such a surgery could be considered an ideal form of destructive reshaping.

2. Mechanical force Reshaping

The essential characteristic of destructive reshaping is destruction. Since destruction is involved, the integrity of the thoracic cage is inevitably affected meaning that the connections between various parts are disrupted. The disruption or removal of connections between diseased structures lays the foundation for rebuilding a normal structure. This is the fundamental process of reshaping after destruction. However, if one does not thoroughly destroy the deformed structure, but instead reshapes directly on top of the existing form, this should theoretically also be feasible. Putting this theory into practice gives rise to another type of reshaping surgery: mechanical force reshaping [3].

The biggest difference between mechanical force reshaping and destructive reshaping is that the latter involves destructive procedures performed on the deformed, pathological structures, while the former does not. Instead, mechanical force reshaping relies on the application of external force to the affected area using special materials, ultimately altering the shape of the deformity. In this type of surgery, the structural integrity of the thoracic cage remains intact, which clearly distinguishes it from destructive reshaping.

In mechanical force reshaping, there is no need to directly operate on the deformed area. Instead, the procedure is performed by applying external force, typically with the help of special materials. This characteristic transforms the surgery from direct reshaping to indirect reshaping. Due to the use of specialized materials, indirect reshaping gains new advantages such as the ability to make incisions away from the deformity site, which opens up the possibility for minimally invasive surgery.

The Nuss procedure is a prime example of mechanical force reshaping. For pectus excavatum, a specific type of thoracic deformity, the most severely affected area is typically located at the base of the depression, usually near the sternum. While destructive reshaping involves directly operating on the deformed area, the Nuss procedure avoids this by performing the surgical intervention on the lateral chest wall instead [6]. After completing the operation on the lateral chest wall, mechanical force is applied at that site, and a specially designed steel bar is used to indirectly reshape the central deformity of the anterior chest wall. Thanks to the involvement of this custom steel bar, direct destructive intervention on the deformity is avoided. This not only results in smaller incisions and less trauma, but also makes the incisions more discreet, greatly enhancing postoperative cosmetic outcomes.

Mechanical force reshaping has many advantages, especially when compared with destructive reshaping, where these benefits become even more apparent. However, like any surgical procedure, this type of surgery is not without flaws and certainly not perfect. The drawbacks include:

Inaccurate Operation: In mechanical force reshaping, the surgical site is not located directly at the site of the deformity but rather at a distance from it. Since direct manipulation is not performed, the deformity cannot be precisely addressed, which may lead to various issues. Take pectus excavatum as an example the most severe deformity is located at the deepest point of the depression, where bony structures often undergo hyperplasia, fusion, and distortion, eventually forming an inward bulge that protrudes toward the interior of the body. Proper handling of this area is critical to the success of the surgery. In destructive reshaping, this structure is directly addressed, whereas in mechanical force reshaping, it is often neglected. Once the large anterior chest wall depression is elevated, the central deformity remains untreated, which may cause several problems: First, it may affect the placement of the steel bar. From an orthopedics standpoint, the optimal position for the bar is at the lowest point of the depression. However, due to the inward bulge, this area cannot provide adequate support for the bar, and as a result, the bar is often placed beside the bulge, where the surface is sloped and unstable for bar placement. Second, it may lead to bar displacement. If the inward bulge at the base of the depression is not removed, the bar cannot remain stable. Once external forces are applied, the bar may shift, compromising its supporting function. If support is inadequate, the surgical outcome will eventually fail. Third, it may cause relapse of the deformity after bar removal. While the bar is in place, the depression typically doesn't recur due to the support it provides. However, once the bar is removed, the persistent inward bulge may lead to a rapid return of the depression, resulting in deformity recurrence. As seen above, since mechanical force reshaping involves only indirect manipulation using special materials, it is difficult to ensure precise correction of the affected area. This lack of precision in reshaping may lead to a variety of practical complications.

Unstable Operation: In mechanical force reshaping, the surgical operation is performed at a site distant from the actual deformity. Because direct manipulation of the affected area is not possible, it becomes difficult to ensure a stable outcome. For example, in the Nuss procedure, the most critical step is to place the steel bar at the deepest point of the depression and to secure it firmly in that position to ensure effective reshaping. However, due to the inability to directly secure the bar at that specific location, it can easily shift to another position effectively resulting in bar displacement. Once displacement occurs, the surgical correction fails. for any surgery, stability of the operation is a key factor for success. In mechanical force reshaping, the lack of guaranteed stability during the procedure can lead to numerous problems.

Suboptimal Results: Thoracic deformities are not only reflected in the overall shape of the chest, but also in localized pathological areas. The goal of surgery is reshaping, and that includes not just the general external appearance, but also the correction of local deformities, which is equally important. However, mechanical force reshaping often focuses only on the overall appearance, while neglecting finer structural details. From the standpoint of overall aesthetics, this lack of attention to detail can negatively affect the surgical outcome. On a deeper level, since the correction of local deformities often determines the success or failure of the entire operation, ignoring them may ultimately compromise the effectiveness of the overall reshaping. This drawback is particularly evident in the Nuss procedure, and is a notable limitation of mechanical force reshaping.

Surgical Risk: The inaccuracy of mechanical force reshaping not only affects the effectiveness of the procedure, but may also endanger surrounding organs. If those organs are critical, the consequences can be severe. In pectus excavatum, the depression directly compresses the heart, and since the operation cannot be performed under direct vision, cardiac injury becomes the greatest risk. Every year, there are patients who die as a result of undergoing the Nuss procedure. At the root of this danger lies the fact that mechanical force reshaping is an indirect method. Its indirect nature leads to inaccuracy and also prevents direct visualization. Performing imprecise procedures on vital organs without direct vision is, in itself, a disregard for risk and when risk is not taken seriously, danger becomes inevitable.

Prone to Complications: Although performing the operation away from the deformity site has certain advantages, it can also lead to new complications at the surgical site. In the Nuss procedure, the actual surgical field, the lateral chest wall, is often the source of complications. For example, local compression of the ribs may cause depression deformities of the lateral chest wall. Additionally, the curved steel bar may restrict the development of the ribs in the lateral chest wall, which is another inherent complication of this type of surgery. Furthermore, considering that indirect reshaping requires the use of special materials, there is a risk of material-related complications as well.

Increased Surgical Difficulty: Destructive reshaping is performed under direct visualization, making it relatively straightforward for any surgeon with basic surgical training. In contrast, mechanical force reshaping is an indirect procedure, and in most cases, it cannot be performed under direct vision. Even with the assistance of a thoracoscope, it still cannot compare to the clarity of direct exposure. The difficulty of performing surgery without direct visualization is evident. Therefore, although many claim that the Nuss procedure is simple, this is not entirely accurate. In reality, for many specific cases such as adult pectus excavatum, asymmetric deformities, or large-area depressions the surgical difficulty is quite high. The primary reason for this increased complexity lies in the indirect nature of mechanical force reshaping.

Requirement for Special Conditions: Destructive surgeries do not require special materials and can therefore be widely performed. In contrast, mechanical force reshaping relies on specialized materials to complete the procedure, which places unique demands on surgical conditions. Take the Nuss procedure for example, without custom-designed steel bars and instruments, the surgery cannot be carried out. Furthermore, considering that many surgeons depend on thoracoscopic assistance, if a surgeon is not proficient in thoracoscopic techniques, the procedure becomes impossible to perform.

In summary, the evolution from destructive reshaping to mechanical force reshaping represents a fundamental shift in the nature of the surgery. The trauma is significantly reduced, the incisions are more aesthetically pleasing, and the procedures are more readily accepted by patients. However, this transition has also introduced many practical challenges, and as such, this type of surgery still has notable shortcomings that require further improvement.

3. Template Reshaping

Template reshaping is a special surgical concept proposed by us, inspired by similar processes found in everyday life. For example, operations like photocopying or the use of molds in manufacturing served as sources of inspiration. Based on these observations, the concept of template reshaping was eventually developed.

The basic idea of template reshaping is to first design a template based on the shape of a normal chest wall, then closely align and securely fix the deformed chest wall to this template, so that the chest wall eventually takes on the same shape as the template [7]. Since the template is pre-designed to match the form of a normal thoracic structure, the corrected chest wall will, in theory, also attain the normal shape of the thorax.

Reshaping is a process that requires work to be done, and thus involves the application of external force. Just like in destructive reshaping and mechanical force reshaping, template reshaping also relies on external force but its purpose and effect differ significantly from those of the other two methods. In destructive reshaping, external force is applied to destroy the pathological structure. In mechanical force reshaping, it is used to indirectly alter the shape of the deformity. However, in template reshaping, an external force is applied to press the deformed chest wall as closely as possible against the template. This use of force is clearly different from the other two approaches. Under the action of external force, when all details and local areas of the chest wall are closely fitted to and merged with the template, the goal of reshaping is achieved. Since template reshaping uses the appearance of a normal chest wall as the reference or template, the theoretical outcome of the reshaping should be the most ideal in the actual surgical process, if the operational details are designed more precisely, and local trauma is minimized while ensuring more aesthetically pleasing incisions, the outcome is bound to be highly effective.

We have designed two types of template reshaping surgeries: the Wenlin procedure [8] and the Wang procedure [8,9]. The Wenlin procedure is designed for protrusive deformities, while the Wang procedure targets depressive deformities. In the Wenlin procedure, a specially shaped template steel plate is first created based on the appearance of a normal chest wall. Then, the protruding bony structures are flattened so that all parts are closely pressed against the steel plate and securely fixed, ultimately achieving the reshaping goal. In the Wang procedure, similarly, a template steel plate is designed according to the normal chest wall's shape, and the sunken chest wall is elevated and tightly fixed to the plate to complete the reshaping.

By observing the operational details of the two procedures, one can see that although they correct different types of deformities and use different specific techniques, their essence is the same. The core principles of both procedures involve two key steps: First, to design an ideal steel plate template; Second, to securely fix the deformed chest wall to the template. This approach is essentially similar to the principles of printing or casting. Since the reshaping is done with reference to a normal anatomical template, it is theoretically the most ideal surgical method.

Template reshaping has distinct characteristics and clear advantages. However, this type of surgery also has its own limitations, which are reflected in the following aspects: ① Limited reshaping range: Since the material used for reshaping is still a long, narrow steel plate, the final reshaping effect is mainly focused on a narrow linear area. If the chest wall structure is not very rigid, the reshaping range becomes quite restricted. For patients with a small deformity area, this limitation is not very noticeable. But for those with a larger deformity, it becomes difficult to achieve complete and ideal reshaping as per the theoretical model. The only effective solution to this problem is to increase the number of reshaping plates. However, adding more plates leads to increased cost and more complex procedures, which is clearly a major drawback of template reshaping. ② Fixation strength issue:

In cases of severe localized deformities, if the chest wall structure is too rigid, it may require tremendous force to fix the chest wall tightly to the steel plate. However, applying too much force may result in local structural fractures, either of the bony structures or the fixing wires. Regardless of what breaks, any structural failure will negatively affect the surgical outcome. ③ Incision placement tissue:

When the fixation area is wide and involves multiple locations, surgical access becomes more demanding, requiring careful planning of incision position and number. If proper exposure cannot be achieved, the effectiveness of the procedure will be compromised. On the other hand, making too many or poorly placed incisions just to complete fixation can negatively affect the cosmetic outcome. Therefore, incision design can become a critical flaw in template reshaping surgery.

Template reshaping is a cleverly designed minimally invasive surgery that offers advantages not found in other procedures. However, due to its unique surgical requirements, it is essential to carefully design the procedural details. If attention is not paid to these critical details, it may negatively affect the reshaping outcome, ultimately leading to numerous complications.

From destructive reshaping, to mechanical force reshaping, and finally to template reshaping, the concept of reshaping has undergone a fundamental transformation, with continuous improvements in technique. Due to differences in the time of emergence and the technologies used, it may create the impression that template reshaping is superior to the other two procedures. In reality, however, the quality of a surgical method is not an absolute concept; the most important factor is whether it is appropriate for a specific type of deformity. This relates to the concept of surgical indications. For a deformity that is well-suited to a particular type of procedure, that surgery may indeed be the ideal choice. But if the procedure is not suitable for a certain deformity, then even template reshaping is not a good option. Therefore, simply comparing which surgery is better is meaningless. The key is to choose the appropriate method based on the characteristics of the deformity. Take pectus excavatum as an example: for children with softer bone tissue and localized depressions, the Wang procedure, a typical template reshaping surgery, may be a suitable choice. However, for patients with rigid bones and a wide range of depression, this procedure is not ideal. In such cases, the Nuss procedure, a classic example of mechanical force reshaping, shows clear advantages. Choosing the appropriate surgical method based on the characteristics of the deformity is a basic skill every thoracic wall surgeon should possess. If one selects a procedure mechanically without tailoring it to the patient's condition, it will inevitably affect the surgical outcome. In most cases, the three types of reshaping surgeries are relatively independent techniques, each with fundamental differences. However, from a broader perspective, these three procedures also share intrinsic connections. For example, the destructive element is not exclusive to destructive reshaping; it is also present in the other two methods. Whether in mechanical force reshaping or template reshaping, there are elements of destruction involved. Similarly, the template reshaping concept appears in destructive reshaping as well during the reshaping of structures after destruction, template-like materials are often used, representing another form of template reshaping. In mechanical force reshaping, although the shape of the steel plate may not be an exact match to the target shape, it still closely resembles it in many cases, thus performing a partial template function. Therefore, although the three basic procedures differ in form, they are internally connected. A deep understanding of these connections not only helps in fully grasping the essence of reshaping, but also aids in performing complex deformity surgeries more effectively.

In the process of reshaping various deformities, a special technique is often used known as pre-reshaping. The essence of this technique is destructive reshaping, and its purpose is to disrupt the original structure, altering its shape or mechanical properties to lay the foundation for proper reshaping. In clinical practice, there is a special type of pectus excavatum in which one edge appears as a severely protruding, sharp-angled deformity. This type of deformity cannot be corrected using the Nuss procedure; the Wang procedure becomes the only viable option [10]. However, when performing the Wang procedure in such cases, if template reshaping is done directly, the sharp-angled deformity creates significant challenges and negatively affects the final outcome. To simplify the operation, pre-reshaping is often carried out first; in other words, destructive reshaping is applied to the localized deformity. After this step, local stress is completely released, the reshaping becomes significantly easier, and the Wang procedure can be performed smoothly. In this process, two fundamentally different reshaping methods destructive reshaping and template reshaping are combined, resulting in a much more ideal outcome than using a single method alone. In surgeries for complex deformities, where different types of structural issues coexist, a single surgical approach often fails to achieve satisfactory results. In such cases, it is common to combine reshaping methods with different properties. When the strengths of each technique are fully utilized, optimal outcomes can be achieved.

In summary, surgical reshaping of thoracic deformities can be categorized into three distinct types, each with its own unique characteristics. However, these methods are not entirely independent — they share intrinsic connections. During the reshaping of deformities, it is essential to choose the surgical approach based on the specific characteristics of the deformity. Only by doing so can the surgery achieve a successful outcome.

REFERENCES

[1] Wang, Wenlin. 2021a. "The Fundamental Nature of Thoracic Wall Surgery." *Toutiao (Jinri Toutiao)*, October 31.

[2] Wang, Wenlin. 2021b. "Thoracic Wall Surgery: Reshaping and Reconstruction." *Toutiao (Jinri Toutiao)*, October 31.

[3] Wang, Wenlin. 2019. "The Three Basic Forms of Thoracic Deformity Surgery." *Thoracic Deformity Surgery Expert*, September 24.

[4] Nasr, A., A. Fecteau, and P. W. Wales. 2010. "Comparison of the Nuss and the Ravitch Procedure for Pectus Excavatum Repair: A Meta-Analysis." *Journal of Pediatric Surgery* 45 (5): 880–886.

[5] Liu, T., H. Liu, and Y. Li. 2014. "Comparison of the Nuss and Sternal Turnover Procedures for Primary Repair of Pectus Excavatum." *Asian Journal of Surgery* 37 (1): 30–34.

[6] Wang, Wenlin. 2021c. "Common Complications of the Nuss Procedure: Secondary Saddle Chest." *Thoracic Deformity Surgery Expert*, May 17.

[7] Wang, Wenlin. 2019b. "Technical Essentials of Template Reshaping." *Thoracic Deformity Surgery Expert*, October 7.

[8] Wang, Wenlin. 2018. "The Wang Procedure and the Wenlin Procedure." *Thoracic Deformity Surgery Expert*, October 11.

[9] Wang, Wenlin. 2020. "Working Principle of the Wang Procedure." *Thoracic Deformity Surgery Expert*, September 22.

[10] Wang, Wenlin. 2021d. "Surgical Issues of Sharp-Angled Deformities." *Thoracic Deformity Surgery Expert*, September 8.

Section 4

PECTUS EXCAVATUM

Pectus excavatum is a common thoracic deformity. Estimates of its incidence vary among authors, ranging from 0.1% to 0.8% [1]. Upon closer examination, even an incidence rate of 0.1% represents a very high number of cases higher than almost any other thoracic surgical disease. Among patients hospitalized in thoracic wall surgery departments today, pectus excavatum remains the most common type of deformity and also the most maturely treated. In earlier years, there were no effective treatment methods for pectus excavatum, resulting in unsatisfactory outcomes and limited attention to the condition. In 1998, with the introduction of the Nuss procedure, the treatment of pectus excavatum underwent a true revolution [2]. The surgery became simpler and the outcomes more satisfactory, bringing great hope to patients with pectus excavatum and sparking widespread enthusiasm among doctors. Many thoracic surgeons, pediatric surgeons, orthopedics surgeons, and even plastic surgeons began to engage in the treatment of pectus excavatum. As doctors began paying more attention to the condition, so too did patients and their families. This surge in interest propelled the treatment of pectus excavatum to new heights, leading to the development of numerous new surgical techniques and concepts. These advancements not only improved the treatment of pectus excavatum itself but also benefited the treatment of other deformities, even directly contributing to the emergence of thoracic wall surgery as a specialized field. It is evident that among all thoracic wall diseases, pectus excavatum is an extremely important condition that warrants serious study and attention.

1. Pathogenesis

The pathogenesis of pectus excavatum is a very complex issue. Many have studied it, but there is still no unified explanation [3]. Some people assume that pectus excavatum is related to calcium deficiency or a lack of certain nutrients. However, this view is completely unfounded, and blindly supplementing calcium or other nutrients does not help eliminate the chest depression. Earlier theories suggested that the depression might be caused by abnormal fibrous traction at the base of the inner chest wall. However, subsequent thoracoscopic observations did not reveal any abnormal fibrous tissue, leading to a rejection of that hypothesis. However, in certain specialized surgeries particularly when an incision is made below the xiphoid process to mobilize the posterior aspect of the sternum fibrous traction from the diaphragm can be clearly observed.

These fibers are located exactly at the base of the depression in pectus excavatum. Due to the significant tension they exert, they are considered a likely culprit behind the chest depression. Thus, the theory of fibrous traction is currently regarded as the most probable pathogenesis. In addition, pectus excavatum often occurs in multiple members of the same family, showing a clear hereditary tendency, which supports the possibility of a genetic cause [4,5]. Genetic-level evidence can be found, but the specific mechanism by which it leads to the chest wall depression remains unclear. Cases of pectus excavatum caused by genetic factors are classified as congenital pectus excavatum, but not all congenital cases are due to heredity. In some monozygotic (identical) twins, one individual may develop pectus excavatum while the other does not [6]. This phenomenon clearly challenges the genetic hypothesis, but upon closer analysis, it suggests another possible cause is mechanical compression. For two individuals sharing a confined space, this is almost the only reasonable explanation.

In addition to the possibilities mentioned above, there are various other theories regarding the pathogenesis of pectus excavatum. These theories attempt to explain the depression of the anterior chest wall from different perspectives, but most remain speculative and lack solid evidence. However, some cases of pectus excavatum do have a clear cause for example, those secondary to trauma or surgery. Since the causative factors are well-defined in such cases, the mechanism of onset can be more easily explained.

There is a relatively common disease in newborns known as pulmonary cystadenoma. Some doctors perform cystadenoma resection surgery shortly after the infant is born. Since the cystadenoma itself occupies a relatively large volume, and a portion of healthy lung tissue must also be removed during the resection, a significant loss of intrathoracic tissue occurs after surgery. Although the volume of the thoracic cavity does not decrease, the remaining lung tissue cannot immediately expand to fully fill the residual cavity. This leads to a marked increase in negative pressure within the chest cavity. Under normal physiological conditions, there is a balanced pressure difference between the two sides of the chest wall, which plays a vital role in maintaining the normal shape of the chest wall. However, when the negative intrathoracic pressure increases significantly, a pronounced pressure difference may develop across the chest wall. If the chest wall has sufficient hardness, that is, mechanical strength, this pressure difference will not affect its shape. However, in young infants, the chest wall near the xiphoid process lacks midline structural support and is very weak. Under the influence of the trans-thoracic pressure

gradient, it is easy for a depression to form, resulting in pectus excavatum. This explains the mechanism by which pectus excavatum may develop after such surgeries [7].
Another congenital condition is congenital diaphragmatic hernia (CDH), which is characterized by abdominal organs herniating into the chest cavity through a defect in the diaphragm. Since this condition severely affects the infant's physiological function, surgical intervention is necessary. During surgery, the first step is to return the herniated abdominal organs to the abdominal cavity, followed by suturing the diaphragmatic defect. After the abdominal organs are repositioned, the remaining lung tissue cannot immediately expand to fill the residual thoracic space. This result is very similar to what happens after pulmonary cystadenoma surgery, leading to a significant increase in negative pressure within the chest cavity. In addition to this, because the diaphragm needs to be repaired, if the diaphragm is under tension, the muscle fibers may directly exert a pulling force on the anterior chest wall. These two mechanisms increased intrathoracic negative pressure and mechanical traction from the diaphragm can both lead to a depression in the anterior chest wall, ultimately resulting in pectus excavatum [8].

Pectus excavatum secondary to surgery can also be seen after median sternotomy performed for cardiac surgery. The occurrence of this deformity is believed to be associated with two main factors: Inadequate sternal fixation, and mediastinal adhesions causing traction postoperatively. The interaction between these two factors directly contributes to the depression of the anterior chest wall [9].

In clinical practice, pectus excavatum can also be secondary to trauma. This condition typically occurs after extensive chest wall injuries, where the chest wall first becomes softened, followed by malunited healing, ultimately resulting in a depression of the chest wall. During this process, fibrous tissue proliferation within the thoracic cavity is considered a potential pathogenic factor [10]. This mechanism is similar to that of chronic empyema-induced chest wall collapse, where fibrous tissue directly connects to the chest wall, and when massively proliferated, exerts significant traction, eventually leading to depression [11].
In all of the above mechanisms behind the formation of secondary pectus excavatum, two important factors are consistently present: Weakness of the chest wall structure, and the action of external forces. The pathogenesis of secondary pectus excavatum is very clear. Although the exact cause of primary pectus excavatum remains unknown, it is very likely to be similar to that of the secondary form. In other words, regardless of the origin of the deformity, the

underlying mechanism leading to the depression is likely essentially the same [12].

2. Pathological Characteristics

(1) Gross Structure

The main pathological change in pectus excavatum is the depression of the bony structure of the anterior chest wall. In the past, no further distinction was made regarding the nature of all depressions that were simply classified as pectus excavatum. During the era of open surgery, this classification posed no issue. However, with the advent of minimally invasive surgery especially after the introduction of the Nuss procedure the location of the depression began to significantly influence surgical outcomes. As a result, it became necessary to classify chest wall deformities more precisely. In other words, not all depressions should be indiscriminately labeled as pectus excavatum. Strictly speaking, the reason this deformity is called "pectus excavatum" is not merely due to the presence of a depression, but because the appearance of the depression resembles a funnel. Most people are familiar with the shape of a funnel. When used to describe a chest wall depression, it refers (Figure 2–4–1): The typical appearance of the chest wall in a patient with pectus excavatum the anterior chest wall presents as a "pit" rather than other types of depressions.

The main pathological change in pectus excavatum is the depression of the bony structure of the anterior chest wall. In the past, no further distinction was made regarding the nature of all depressions that were simply classified as pectus excavatum. During the era of open surgery, this classification posed no issue. However, with the advent of minimally invasive surgery especially after the introduction of the Nuss procedure the location of the depression began to significantly influence surgical outcomes.

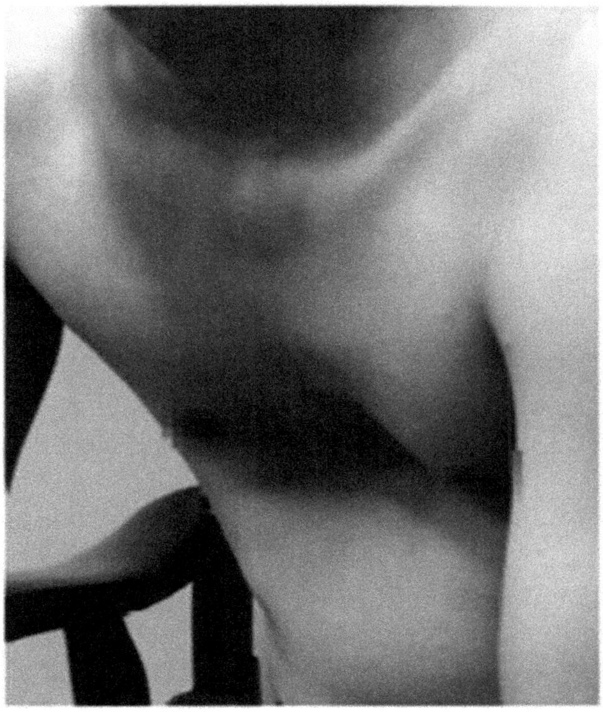

Figure 2–4–1: The typical appearance of the chest wall in a patient with pectus excavatum the anterior chest wall presents as a "pit" rather than other types of depressions.

As a result, it became necessary to classify chest wall deformities more precisely. In other words, not all depressions should be indiscriminately labeled as pectus excavatum. Strictly speaking, the reason this deformity is called "pectus excavatum" is not merely due to the presence of a depression, but because the appearance of the depression resembles a funnel. Most people are familiar with the shape of a funnel.

(Figure 2– 4–2): ① the depression must be located on the anterior chest wall. The anatomical range of the chest wall is extensive. In addition to the anterior chest wall, it includes the lateral chest wall and, anatomically speaking, even the back. Any area of the chest wall can exhibit protrusions or depressions. However, based on the historical and conventional understanding of pectus excavatum, only depressions on the anterior chest wall are classified as pectus excavatum. Depressions on the lateral chest wall or back do not qualify as pectus excavatum. ② the depression must involve the sternum. The anterior chest wall broadly includes the sternum in the center, flanked by costal cartilages and ribs on both sides. In general, pectus excavatum is located centrally. Even in asymmetric types, it is never completely confined to one side of the chest wall. A shared feature of all types is involvement of the sternum. If the depression does not affect the sternum, it is instead a lateral chest wall deformity, which should not be classified as pectus excavatum. ③ the depression must resemble a "pit." Emphasizing the "pit" shape helps uphold the fundamental concept of a "funnel," from which the condition derives its name. This classification is not merely semantic, but has direct implications for the choice of surgical technique. A "pit" is, by definition, a depression with a defined base and surrounding edges, where the edges are typically fully enclosed without any openings. Such a structure resembles a funnel and represents the classic form of pectus excavatum. The most typical cases are often located near the xiphoid process. In some instances, the lowest point of the depression is situated below the xiphoid, where the edge appears incomplete or open at the bottom. However, this interpretation is incorrect, because the boundary can consist not only of bony structures, but also of muscle or soft tissue. If the abdominal wall is considered the lower edge of the depression, then the border becomes fully enclosed, and the structure still qualifies as a standard funnel-shaped depression.

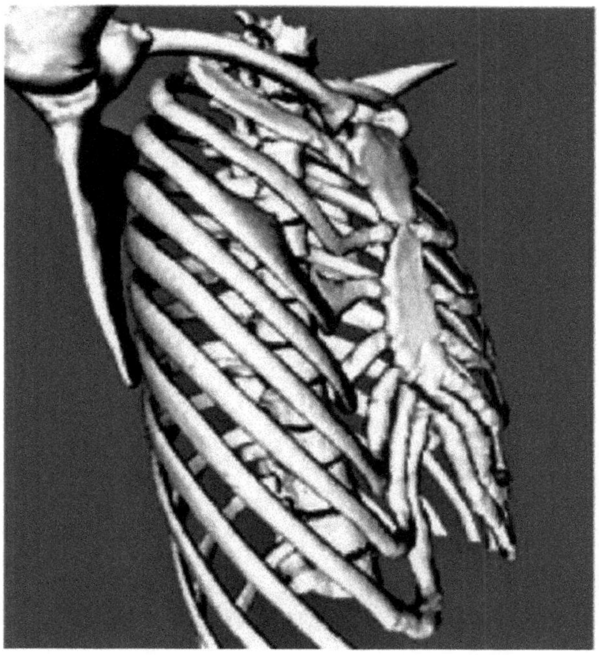

Figure 2–4–2: Pathological features of pectus excavatum. Depression of the anterior chest wall involving the sternum, forming a "pit" of various shapes.

(2) Gross Classification

Pectus excavatum shares common features in its general morphology, but there are significant differences among individuals. Based on variations in individual morphology, pectus excavatum can be classified into the following types (Figure 2-4-3):

(1) Typical Pectus Excavatum [1]: Typical pectus excavatum is a symmetrically depressed deformity located at the midline of the anterior chest wall. The depression is generally situated lower down, near the lower end of the sternum or around the xiphoid process. In some cases of low-lying deformities, the base of the depression may extend below the xiphoid process. This is the most common type of pectus excavatum.

(2) Asymmetrical Pectus Excavatum [14]: This type of deformity can be understood in two different ways. In the narrow sense, asymmetrical pectus excavatum refers to depressions located on one side of the chest wall, with the base of the depression formed by ribs or costal cartilage. The sternum is involved but tilted, positioned on the sloped side of the depression. This is a commonly seen variant. In the broader sense, there are two additional forms of asymmetrical pectus excavatum (see Fig. 2-4-4): In the first case, the depression appears similar to symmetrical pectus excavatum centrally located, with the sternum forming the base and symmetrical side edges but the underlying bone structure is clearly asymmetric. Physical examination may reveal thick and rigid bone structures on one side, while the other side is thin and flexible. This is a form of latent skeletal asymmetry and is considered part of the broader definition of asymmetrical pectus excavatum. In the second case, although the depression is centrally located, the edges on both sides are visibly asymmetric, one side being higher and the other lower. This type also falls under the category of asymmetrical pectus excavatum. The concept of broadly defined

asymmetrical pectus excavatum represents a more precise understanding of the deformity and holds significant clinical importance in guiding its surgical treatment.

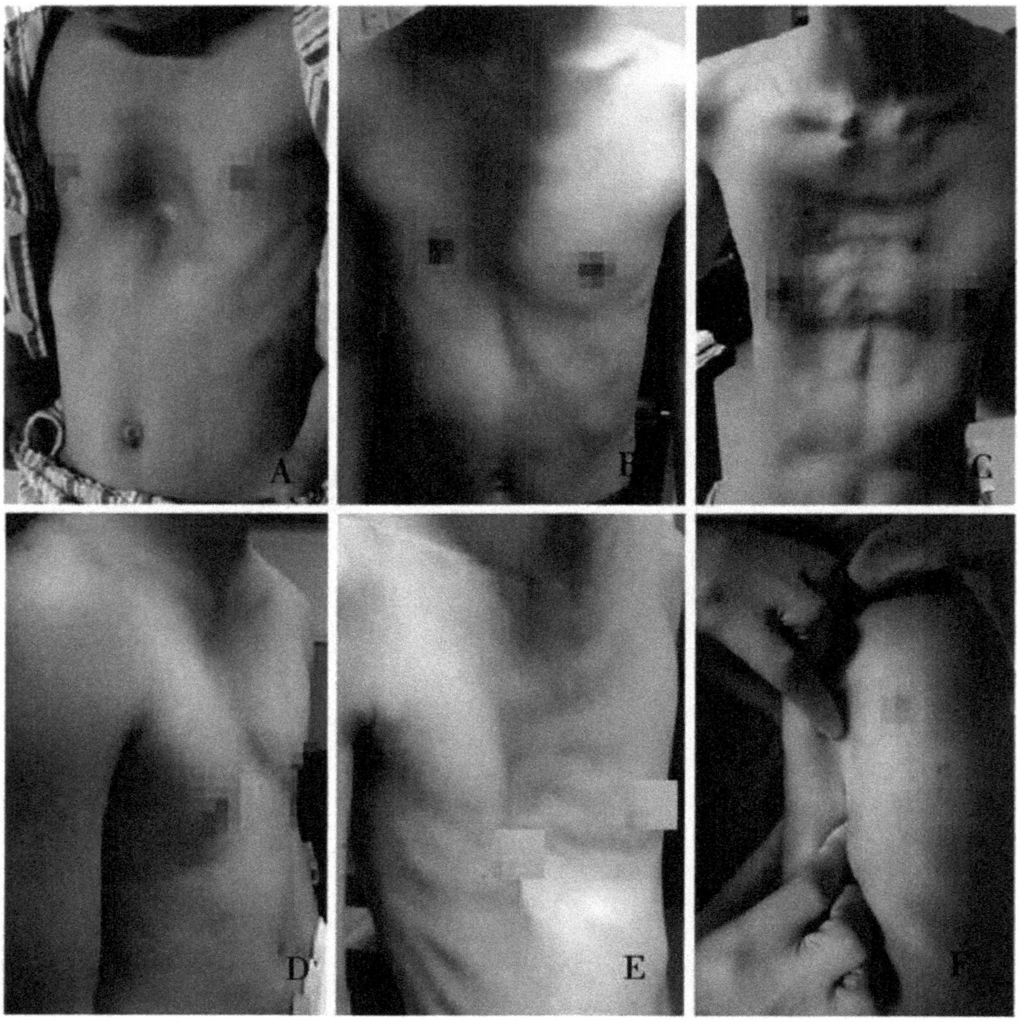

Figure 2-4-3: Various Types of Pectus Excavatum. (A. Typical pectus excavatum; B. Asymmetrical pectus excavatum; C. Extensive pectus excavatum; D. High-positioned pectus excavatum; E. Grand canyon-type pectus excavatum; F. Pectus excavatum with angular deformity at the margin)

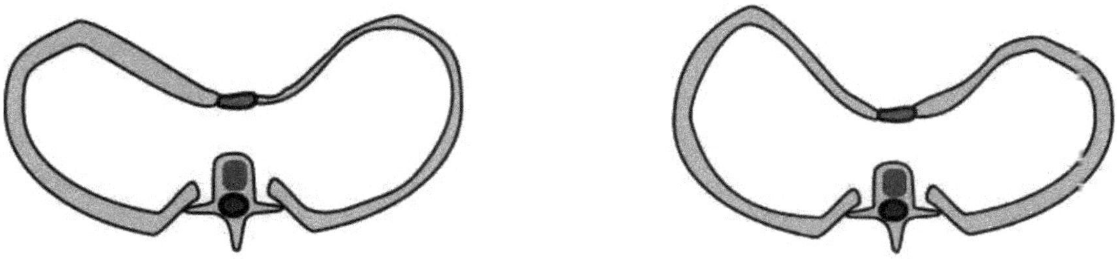

Figure 2-4-4: Two Broad Categories of Asymmetrical Pectus Excavatum (A. The appearance is approximately symmetrical, but there is a significant difference in bone structure between the left and right sides; B. The depression is centrally located, but the edges on both sides are at different heights; thus, it also falls under the category of asymmetry.)

(3) Large-area Pectus Excavatum [15]: This type of deformity is characterized by a wide-ranging and extensive depression, often involving most of the anterior chest wall, without a specific boundary. In terms of severity, the depth of the depression varies, but the height of the edges is generally not very prominent. Using the Haller index alone to evaluate this deformity, the index value is often quite high, yet the actual depression may not be very deep. This may result in a falsely elevated Haller index, creating a misleading impression of the severity of the deformity.

(4) High-position pectus excavatum [16]. In this type of deformity, the depression is generally located higher on the chest wall. The base of the depression may lie at the body of the sternum or at higher-positioned ribs or costal cartilages. The deep part of a high-position pectus excavatum typically corresponds to the base of the heart, where the major blood vessels enter and exit the heart. If the depression is severe, it is more likely to affect cardiac function.

(5) Grand Canyon-type pectus excavatum [17]. This deformity is characterized by a large surface area and extensive range, making it an extremely severe type of pectus excavatum. The depression appears as a longitudinal groove that extends from the upper chest wall all the way down to the abdominal wall. It may be centrally located but is more often oblique. The depth of the depression is significant, resulting in a highly pronounced and severe external deformity.

(6) Pectus excavatum with angular deformity [18]. This type of deformity features sharply angled edges or a sharply pointed depression extending either toward the body surface or deep into the thoracic cavity. It is an extremely severe form of deformity that requires specialized corrective techniques.

Apart from the typical pectus excavatum, the other five types represent relatively special forms. Each has distinct characteristics and differs significantly in shape from the typical presentation. However, since all of these types share the three fundamental features of pectus excavatum, they are still classified within its scope.

(3) Overall Classification

Pectus excavatum is an ancient condition with a long history of naming. If viewed alone and only in terms of its own treatment, current structural studies are sufficient. However, when thoracic deformities are considered as a broader group especially when analyzing multiple types together pectus excavatum must be seen as one member among many. To better illustrate the relationships among different deformities, we proposed a new system: the Overall Classification of Thoracic Deformities [19]. In this system: Type I-a: Depression located in the center of the anterior chest wall equivalent to typical pectus excavatum. Type I-b: Depression deviated from the midline but still involving the sternum equivalent to asymmetric pectus excavatum. This classification connects pectus excavatum to other depression-type deformities and contrasts it clearly with protrusion-type deformities, providing valuable insight for diagnosis and treatment.

(4) Structural Characteristics

The above discussions describe pectus excavatum (PE) from various perspectives, but these descriptions remain incomplete as they primarily address general morphological features, that is, the external shape without exploring the specific structural characteristics of the chest wall. In fact, PE is associated with distinct structural changes in the thoracic wall, which directly impact surgical outcomes and therefore merit serious attention. When a chest wall depression occurs in PE, some suggest that the local ribs and costal cartilages are elongated, or that their growth rate exceeds that of normal structures, a hypothesis proposed as a potential cause of the deformity. Structurally, it is true that these ribs and cartilages are longer than average. However, interpreting this lengthening as the cause of PE is controversial. The debate centers on whether this elongation is the primary cause or a secondary adaptation.

The true relationship between cause and effect remains unclear. If an external factor leads to the formation of the depression, then the elongation of the ribs and costal cartilages is more likely a result rather than a cause. Regardless of the underlying mechanism, the fact remains that the ribs and costal cartilages in such cases are objectively longer than normal, a pathological change that is clearly evident in this type of deformity.

From a structural perspective, the lower part of the sternum, ribs, and costal cartilages may all exhibit related abnormalities. The more severe and localized the depression, the more pronounced these structural changes tend to be. Specific pathological changes may include localized twisting, thickening, fusion, or even absence of tissue. In symmetrical pectus excavatum, the deformity is typically limited to the area near the base of the depression, mainly involving the lower sternum and adjacent costal cartilages. In asymmetrical cases, where the depression is located toward the lateral chest wall, the deepest point often includes the ribs and costal cartilages, which may show severe structural changes. In the most extreme cases, a sharp-angled deformity may occur where the depression projects as a sharp angle toward the mediastinum or thoracic cavity representing one of the most severe forms of pectus excavatum. Based on the definition of pectus excavatum, the sternum is a structure that must be involved, and thus pathological changes in the sternum are always present. In symmetrical pectus excavatum, the sternum lies at the deepest point of the depression, typically near the lower end of the sternum. Since it is connected to the xiphoid process, this junction can exhibit specific configurations, generally in one of the following three forms [1] (Figure 2-4-5): ① the sternum itself is curved, forming the base of the depression, with the xiphoid process extending directly from the lower end of the sternum, projecting outward toward the anterior chest wall. ② the sternum is not significantly curved, but the lower end of the sternum forms an angle with the xiphoid process, which together form the bottom of the depression. In this case, the xiphoid may protrude toward the anterior chest wall. ③ the sternum continues directly into the xiphoid process, with the tip of the xiphoid forming the deepest part of the depression. The relationship between the sternum and xiphoid is crucial, as the characteristics of this region directly affect surgical procedures and outcomes, making preoperative assessment essential. In asymmetrical pectus excavatum, although the sternum is still involved, it does not form the base of the depression. The sternum is often tilted and misaligned with the main plane of the chest, resulting in a twisted or distorted appearance.

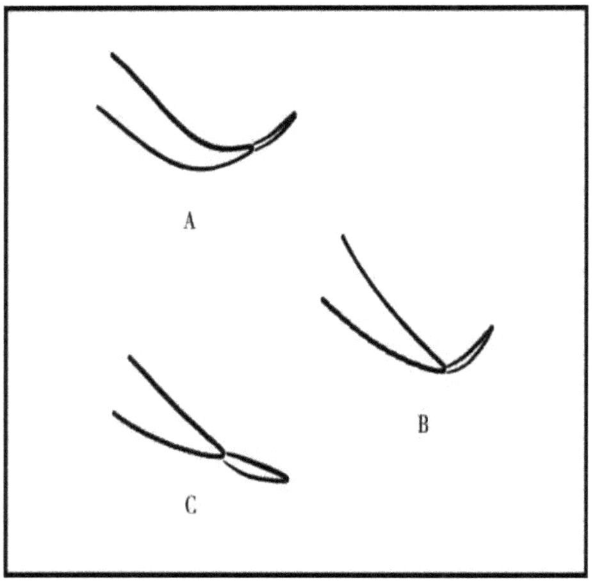

Figure 2-4-5. Three basic structural configurations at the base of pectus excavatum: A. The lower end of the sternum forms the deepest point of the depression. B. The lower sternum and the xiphoid process form an angle, together constituting the bottom of the depression. The xiphoid process is a direct continuation of the lower sternum, and its tip forms the deepest point of the pectus excavatum.

In the overall morphology of pectus excavatum, two key areas require particular attention: the base of the depression and its edges. Regardless of which structure constitutes the base, various pathological changes may be present.

When viewed from the thoracic cavity, the base of the depression can exhibit different structural features: In some cases, the base is broad and gently sloped. In others, the base is narrow and pointed, forming a sharp, angular depression. Additionally, prominent bony overgrowths may occasionally appear at the base. These pathological alterations are objectively present and can significantly impact the outcome of surgery. Therefore, they must be carefully evaluated and addressed during the operative procedure.

In most cases of pectus excavatum, the edges of the depression do not protrude beyond the chest wall surface and typically remain level with the surrounding thoracic wall. However, in certain patients, the edges of the depression may protrude outward, forming a noticeable bulge. When this occurs, it creates a composite deformity, which significantly complicates the treatment process.

The most severe example of this condition is the sharp-angled (angular) deformity, which often appears along one edge of the depression [18]. In such cases, the Nuss procedure becomes contraindicated, and the Wang procedure becomes the only viable surgical option.

As mentioned earlier, a sharp-angled deformity is not limited to protruding abnormalities; it can also occur at the base of deep depressions in severe pectus excavatum cases [20]. Therefore, once this deformity appears whether it presents as a depression or a protrusion it is considered the most severe form of chest wall abnormality (Figure 2-4-6).

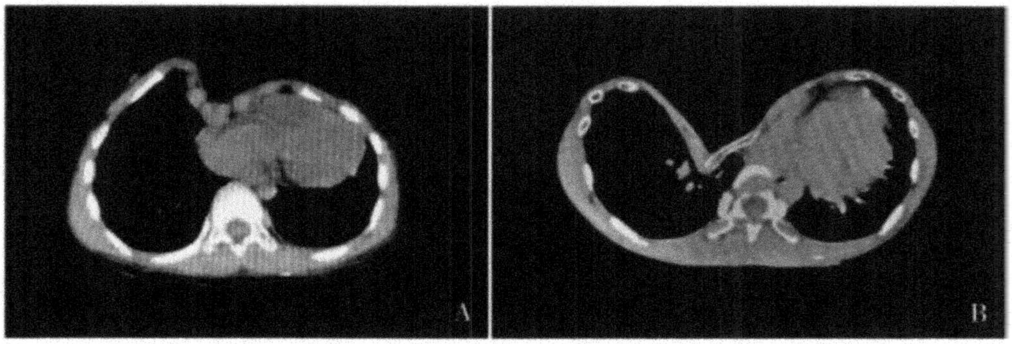

Figure 2-4-6 Sharp-Angled Deformities (A) The edge of the depression protrudes outward in a sharp-angled manner. (B) The base of the depression protrudes inward toward the thoracic cavity in a sharp-angled manner. Both types of deformities cannot be corrected by direct mechanical force reshaping alone. Successful treatment requires appropriate pre-reshaping techniques or even destructive reshaping methods.

(5) Classification by Severity

When discussing the pathological structure of pectus excavatum, in addition to the aforementioned aspects, it is also necessary to pay attention to the issue of severity. In order to establish an objective standard, some people use the Haller index for classification [21]. This is a commonly used method. However, as long as human factors are involved, subjectivity is inevitable, so it can only serve as a reference and should not be overly relied upon. In addition to its subjectivity, the Haller index has two situations it cannot handle (Figure 2-4-7): The first is the case of an infinitely large Haller index [17, 22]; The second is the case of a negative value [23]. Both situations are extremely severe, and although they are not common, it is precisely in these critical cases where the Haller index is expected to demonstrate its value that the index becomes powerless.

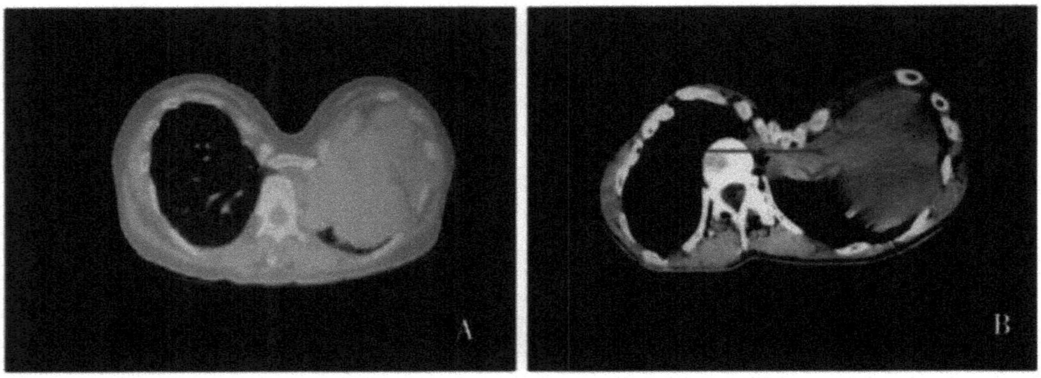

Figure 2-4-7 Two types of deformities where the Haller index fails to reflect the degree of depression:(A) Haller index is infinitely large in this case, the value is meaningless; (B) Haller index is negative and the depression is extremely severe. If the Haller index alone is used as a reference, it is difficult to obtain an accurate understanding.

To eliminate the inherent limitations of the Haller index, we have developed a simpler and more practical method for evaluating the severity of pectus excavatum, which does not rely on the Haller index at all. For ease of application, this method has been named the Wenlin Evaluation Method. It classifies pectus excavatum into four severity levels: mild, moderate, severe, and extremely severe. The specific steps are as follows (Figure 2-4-8): On the patient's CT cross-sectional image, draw a straight line connecting the highest points of the anterior chest wall. From the anterior border of the spine, draw a perpendicular line to this connecting line. Divide the perpendicular line into three equal parts. Then, determine the severity of the depression based on the location of the deepest point of the depression: If the deepest point lies within the upper one-third 1/3 of the perpendicular line it is classified as mild pectus excavate the deepest point lies within the middle one-third 1/3 it is classified as moderate pectus excavate the deepest point lies within the lower one-third 1/3 it is classified as severe pectus excavate the deepest point extends beyond the anterior edge of the spine, intruding deeper than the spine itself it is classified as extremely severe pectus excavatum, which represents the most serious form of the deformity.

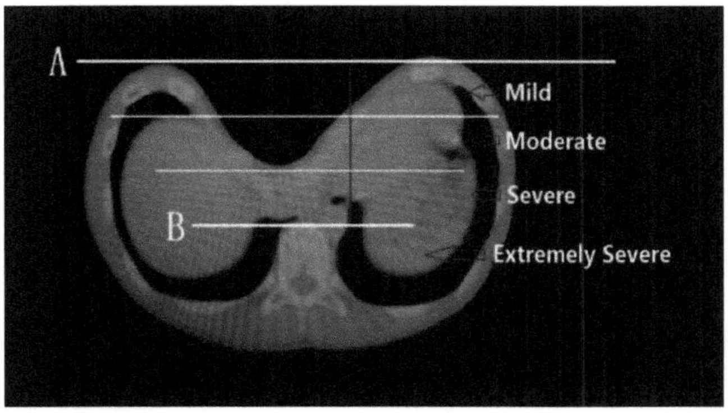

Figure 2-4-8 Wenlin Evaluation Method for Assessing the Severity of Pectus Excavatum (A. The plane of the highest points at the edge of the depression; B. The plane of the anterior border of the spine). The area between A and B is divided into three equal parts, and the deformity is classified into four severity levels: mild, moderate, severe, and extremely severe based on the location of the deepest point of the depression. This evaluation method does not require specific measurements or calculations. A rough assessment can be made visually, making it a practical and easy-to-use tool in clinical settings.

To compare the Wenlin evaluation method with the severity classification based on the Haller index, we measured the Haller index at the relevant regions in our method. The results are as follows: The Haller index corresponding to the upper 1/3 of the section is approximately 3.37. The Haller index corresponding to the lower 1/3 is approximately 6.74. According to the conventional Haller index classification: A Haller index less than 3.2 is considered mild, 3.2 ~ 3.5 is considered moderate, Greater than 3.5 is considered severe [1] This standard differs significantly from the measured Haller indices in our method. Such discrepancies can be regarded as different interpretations of severity between the two approaches. Considering that the Haller index cannot accurately represent the severity of all types of depressions, we believe the Wenlin evaluation method to be more reasonable. To quantify the Wenlin evaluation method, we have defined the Wenlin Index [24], calculated as: Wenlin Index = Depth of Depression ÷ Distance from Anterior Vertebral Line to the Plane of Depression Edge. The classification based on the Wenlin Index is: Less than 0.33 Mild, 0.33 ~ 0.67 Moderate, 0.68 ~ 1.0 Severe, Greater than 1.0 Extremely Severe, the proposal of the Wenlin Index provides a more practical and reliable reference for evaluating the severity of pectus excavatum.

3. Hazards

The primary hazards of pectus excavatum (funnel chest) lie in two main areas: psychological and physiological [1]. The psychological harm mainly stems from the abnormal appearance. Many patients develop a sense of inferiority due to the deformity, which can lead to a series of mental health issues. The physiological harm primarily arises from compression of intrathoracic organs, particularly the heart and lungs. In early stages, these organs generally do not show functional abnormalities due to their robust functional reserves. However, prolonged compression over time may gradually lead to symptoms. Another significant physiological impact is on the spine. Many patients develop spinal scoliosis as a result of pectus excavatum [25]. In addition to these more obvious effects, pectus excavatum may also affect other bodily functions, such as digestive function. Many children with the condition exhibit indigestion and body emaciation, which may also be related to the underlying deformity.

The hazards of pectus excavatum generally worsen with age. In early childhood, the condition may have little to no impact. However, as age increases, the depth and extent of the chest depression tend to worsen, with the changes becoming more pronounced during puberty. After puberty, due to bone calcification, the bony structures in the affected area of the chest wall become more rigid and pronounced, making the deformity itself more severe. This progression can lead to increasingly serious effects on the patient's health and well-being.

When discussing the dangers of pectus excavatum, one specific form must not be overlooked — malignant pectus excavatum. In most cases, when a depression forms in the anterior chest wall, the heart is displaced toward the left thoracic cavity, resulting in lateral compression. Although this compression does affect the heart, its impact on cardiac function is typically minor.

However, if the depression directly presses against the heart without any leftward displacement, the consequences can be very severe. This condition is referred to as malignant pectus excavatum [26] (Figure 2-4-9). Patients with this condition may experience early onset of cardiac dysfunction, with prominent symptoms, making early surgical intervention essential.

There is also a secondary form of malignant pectus excavatum, commonly seen in patients who develop the condition after cardiac surgery or as a recurrence after open surgical correction of pectus excavatum. In such cases, severe adhesions cause the heart to become firmly attached to the anterior chest wall, preventing any lateral displacement. As a result, the depression exerts direct pressure on the heart, significantly impairing cardiac function. These patients often exhibit symptoms more readily, further emphasizing the need for timely surgical treatment (Figure 2-4-10).

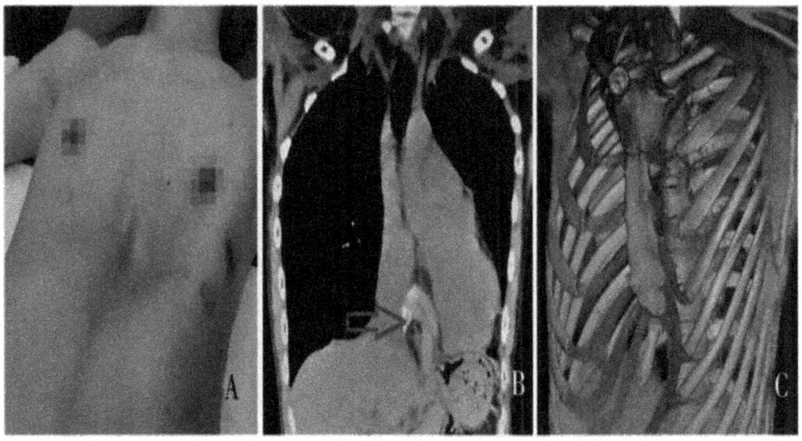

Figure 2-4-9 Malignant Pectus Excavatum. The heart is unable to escape the compression from the anterior chest wall, resulting in early cardiac dysfunction and early onset of symptoms in the patient.A. External appearance of the patient's anterior chest wall, showing an asymmetric pectus excavatum, with the depression skewed to the left and extremely deep. The deepest point of the depression overlaps with the cardiac silhouette, causing direct compression of the heart; the heart has not shifted to the left. 3D reconstruction of the anterior chest wall.

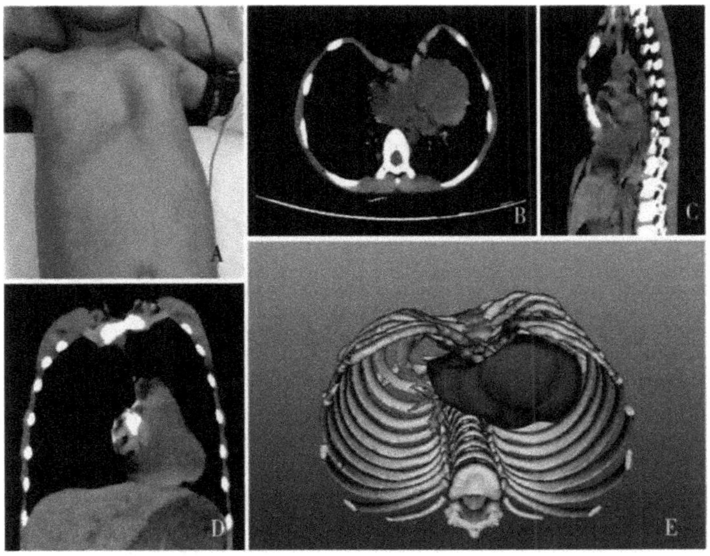

Figure 2-4-10 Secondary Malignant Pectus Excavatum (Post-Congenital Heart Disease Surgery) A. Postoperative appearance of the anterior chest wall following congenital heart disease surgery, showing significant depression, with a surgical scar at the bottom of the depression. B. CT axial view: the depression base is adherent to the heart, causing cardiac compression; the heart cannot evade the pressure. C. CT sagittal view: the anterior chest wall is clearly sunken, with the depression base compressing the heart. D. CT coronal view: the deepest point of the depression overlaps with the cardiac silhouette, the heart cannot shift left, and the depression directly compresses the heart. E. 3D reconstruction: the anterior chest wall directly compresses the heart, resulting in obvious cardiac deformation.

4. Clinical Manifestations

The symptoms of pectus excavatum are mainly related to its associated complications, as previously described, involving both physiological and psychological aspects [1]. Physiological complications primarily stem from impaired organ function and may present with various symptoms: Respiratory system: Symptoms often include chest tightness and shortness of breath, which worsen with physical activity. In severe deformities, symptoms may occur even during minimal activity or at rest. When associated with other respiratory conditions, coughing and sputum production may also be present. Circulatory system: Symptoms may include palpitations, heart fluttering, and chest pain in the anterior thoracic region. Digestive system (occasionally involved): Symptoms such as loss of appetite and indigestion may occur. In addition to the above complications, pectus excavatum can also be associated with scoliosis. This is frequently seen in patients with severe depression of the chest wall or in those who have had the condition for many years. Scoliosis may present with other related symptoms.

Psychological complications are often overlooked but can be significant. These issues typically emerge after the onset of puberty and present in various forms, ranging from mild anxiety to complex psychological disorders. Common manifestations include: Low self-esteem, social withdrawal, with some patients developing complete social isolation. In more severe cases, patients may show signs of autism-like behavior or clinical depression. If left untreated, these psychological impacts may progress into serious mental health conditions, making early recognition and intervention essential.

Patients with pectus excavatum often avoid standing upright with chest out and head held high. The underlying reasons are as follows [1]: ① When the patient stands upright, the pressure on the heart from the anterior chest wall increases, leading to significant discomfort. As a protective reflex, patients instinctively adopt a bent-forward or hunched posture, which helps relieve the pressure and makes them feel more comfortable (Figure 2-4-11).② In the upright posture, the chest wall depression becomes more visible, which patients may find unacceptable. As a result, they often adjust their posture deliberately to conceal the chest deformity and avoid embarrassment.

Figure 2-4-11 Mechanism of forward Bending and Hunching in Patients with Pectus Excavatum. (A) When standing upright with the chest out and head held high, the depression directly compresses the heart, impairing cardiac function and causing discomfort. (B) When bending forward or hunching, the pressure in front of the heart is relieved, making the patient feel more comfortable. As a result, the patient naturally adopts this more comfortable posture.

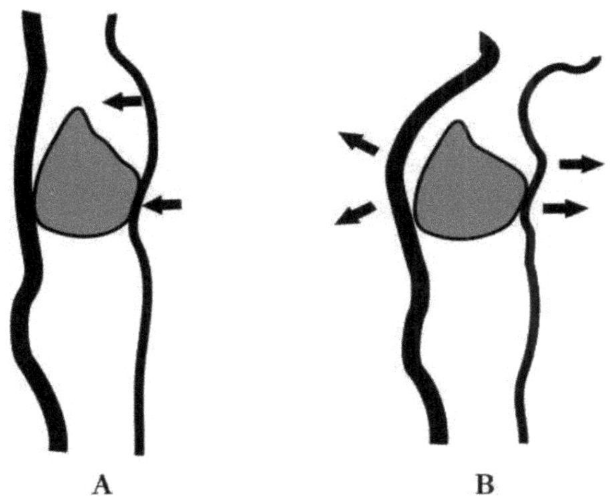

In addition to the abnormal postures mentioned above, patients with pectus excavatum often exhibit specific sleeping positions. They typically prefer to sleep in a lateral or prone position and tend to avoid lying on their back. This is because when lying supine, the anterior chest wall exerts the greatest pressure on the heart, leading to significant discomfort. As a result, patients consciously choose alternative sleeping positions to relieve this pressure and improve comfort (see Figure 2-4-12) [1].

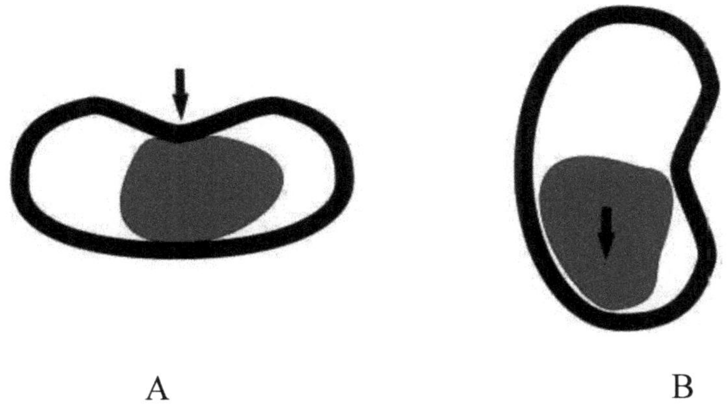

Figure 2–4-12 Mechanism behind side-lying preference in patients with pectus excavatum: (A) When lying supine, the anterior chest wall depression compresses the heart, causing discomfort for the patient. (B) In the left lateral position, the heart avoids the pressure from the depression, making the patient feel more comfortable. Therefore, patients prefer this position.

Through extensive clinical observation, we have found that the vast majority of patients with pectus excavatum exhibit three distinct clinical manifestations: kyphosis (hunchback posture), side-lying sleep position, and scoliosis. These three signs are unique to pectus excavatum and are not present in other deformities. To highlight their specificity, we have named this group of symptoms the (Wenlin Triad) [27].

The most characteristic sign of pectus excavatum is a depression of the anterior chest wall, which can vary in location. The depth and extent of the depression can range from mild to severe and from small to extensive. It may be symmetrical or asymmetrical. Due to direct compression of the heart by the depression, cardiac pulsations are visible on the anterior chest wall in most patients. The cardiac border is often displaced to the left, and in some cases, a systolic murmur can be heard during auscultation. Significant scoliosis may also be present.

4. Examination

There are numerous examination methods available for pectus excavatum, and a wide variety of tests have been used clinically. However, it must be clearly understood that pectus excavatum is a surface deformity, and therefore the most important diagnostic tool is the physician's eye, rather than any specific instrument. Imaging examinations can provide some auxiliary support, but they are not essential. Some individuals undergo certain tests such as CT scans simply to obtain specific values like the Haller Index. This approach is questionable [1], because the Haller Index is not a mandatory parameter. Recommending an examination solely to obtain a numerical value lacks sufficient justification. Likewise, calculating the Wenlin Index also requires a CT scan, but just like the Haller Index, it is not a necessary test. CT scans should only be considered when there is a suspicion of additional thoracic pathology. In addition, if a cardiac murmur is heard during auscultation, cardiac structural evaluation is needed to rule out any underlying heart condition.

5.Diagnosis and Differential Diagnosis

The diagnosis of pectus excavatum is relatively simple. As long as there is a clear depression on the anterior chest wall, and the depression involves the sternum, presenting a clear "pit" appearance, the diagnosis can be confirmed. When making a diagnosis, it is necessary to differentiate it from other depression deformities that do not look like a "pit"[1]. Grooved chest is a groove-like depression running horizontally in the lower part of the anterior chest wall, which is significantly different from the depression of pectus excavatum. The lesion of the lateral chest wall depression deformity is located on the lateral chest wall and does not involve the sternum. The difference from pectus excavatum lies mainly in the location of the depression. A flat chest can be regarded as a "depression" of the entire anterior chest wall. This so-called "depression" does not actually exist as a "pit" and is therefore easy to distinguish from pectus excavatum. In addition to simple depression deformities, depression also exists in many special deformities, which need to be differentiated from pectus excavatum. Saddle chest is a depression on both sides of the lower chest wall, which is significantly different from the single depression in the middle of pectus excavatum. The chest wall of a flat chicken chest is obviously convex and has a wide range, but there is a depression in the middle. The depression is small and limited to the sternum. This depression is obviously different from the independent depression of the funnel chest. Wenlin chest also has a depression, which is located in the middle and high. The upper edge is the convex sternal angle, the two sides are the drooping convex costal cartilage and ribs, the lower edge is open, the bottom of the depression is the sternum body and the lower end of the sternum, the sternum is thickened as a whole, and the side view is "S" shaped. The above three deformities are equivalent to actual compound deformities. Because of the obvious deformity characteristics and fixed structure, they are specially named. There are also a large number of compound deformities without fixed shapes in clinical practice, which also have depressions. These depressions also need to be distinguished from the funnel chest. The most obvious sign of these compound deformities is that they are all combined with convex deformity, while the chest wall of the funnel chest does not have any form of convexity.

When diagnosing pectus excavatum, it is important not only to perform standard differential diagnosis but also to exclude the possibility of associated pathological conditions. The most common comorbidities involve the lungs and the heart. These conditions can generally be identified with routine imaging examinations such as chest X-rays, CT scans, or echocardiography.

In addition to confirming the presence of pectus excavatum, assessing the severity of the deformity is also essential. Traditionally, the Haller Index has been used for this purpose. However, this method has several limitations and may not provide an accurate representation in all cases. As an alternative, the Wenlin Index offers a simpler and more practical approach. It allows for a more objective evaluation of the deformity's severity and is therefore considered a more ideal method in clinical practice [24].

6.Surgical Indications

The issue of surgical indications for pectus excavatum is one of the most frequently debated topics in clinical practice and also one of the most controversial. Some individuals summarize their so-called experiences and share them with others, while others go so far as to idolize these opinions, even incorporating them into so-called guidelines or consensus statements. However, this approach is not scientifically sound. Blindly following such content without critical evaluation can not only cause complications in clinical work, but more importantly, harm patients. Therefore, it is essential to approach published literature with rationality and caution, and not treat it as absolute truth.

In real-world clinical practice, two extreme situations are often encountered: one in which the deformity is very severe, but the patient firmly refuses surgery; and another in which the deformity is not severe, yet the patient strongly demands surgery. Both scenarios directly challenge the validity of so-called guidelines and consensus statements.

As physicians, we must recognize that we can neither force a patient to undergo surgery, nor refuse surgery outright to a willing patient without due reason. Rigidly adhering to externally created guidelines in such cases may result in significant complications in our professional responsibilities. Within the field of chest wall surgery, the involvement of cosmetic and reconstructive elements allows for a decision-making approach that differs from traditional medical paradigms. This means greater flexibility and personalization are not only possible but often necessary. Objectively speaking, for a benign condition like pectus excavatum, the decision to undergo surgery should not be made by the doctor, but rather by the patient and their family. The general principle is simple and practical: If the patient feels uncomfortable physically or is bothered by the appearance, then surgery is warranted. If the patient feels neither physical discomfort nor aesthetic concern, then surgery is not necessary [1]. This principle is both scientific and pragmatic, and avoids the vague and impractical nature of some so-called consensus statements or guidelines. Communicating with patients based on this principle can prevent unnecessary complications and is more conducive to the smooth progress of clinical work.

7. Surgical Treatment

The treatment history of pectus excavatum is long-standing. As early as 1911, a doctor named Meyer pioneered pectus excavatum surgery by directly removing costal cartilage [28]. Although the original intention of this approach is unclear, its significance is undeniable, as he initiated the surgical treatment of pectus excavatum. Subsequently, others performed more extensive costal cartilage resections with great success. Based on this, various surgical techniques have since emerged, allowing an increasing number of pectus excavatum patients to receive treatment.

Reviewing the history of surgical treatment for pectus excavatum, it can be roughly divided into two eras: the open surgery era and the minimally invasive surgery era. The representative open surgeries include two types: the Ravitch procedure and the sternal turnover surgery. The representative minimally invasive surgeries also include two types: the Nuss procedure and the Wang procedure. With technological advancements, these surgical techniques have been continuously improved, providing more treatment options for pectus excavatum.

(1) Ravitch Procedure

The Ravitch procedure, named after Dr. Ravitch, does not refer to a single fixed method but rather encompasses a broad category of traditional open techniques [29]. The procedure mainly consists of two key elements: (1) localized resection or excision of severely affected areas and (2) stabilization of the treated areas. Its defining feature is that the operation is performed under direct vision, allowing for thorough correction of deformity details. When performed by highly skilled surgeons, this procedure can achieve excellent correction of bony structures. However, it also has significant drawbacks: (1) substantial surgical trauma thoracic deformities often involve multiple regions, and direct correction requires wide exposure, resulting in major tissue damage; (2) long surgical scars because direct correction targets specific deformity details, extensive incisions are needed to expose these areas, leading to large scars that can compromise postoperative aesthetics; and (3) suboptimal corrective results while direct correction can, in theory, provide precise and satisfactory outcomes, it requires specialized concepts, techniques, and materials that were often unavailable in the early days of pectus excavatum surgery, leading to overall unsatisfactory results. Moreover, due to the disruption of chest wall integrity, postoperative healing and repair may also pose challenges, potentially affecting the final shaping outcome.

(2) Sternum Rotation Surgery

This surgery is also an open procedure. The specific method involves completely cutting and detaching the sunken anterior chest wall, then thoroughly rotating it before fixing it to the surrounding chest wall structures [30]. This approach can directly eliminate depression, providing a definite and thorough surgical effect. However, this surgery also has several drawbacks: ① Large trauma and many complications. During the procedure, a relatively long incision must first be made, then the sunken part of the chest wall is completely freed, followed by detachment, rotation, and fixation of the related ribs, costal cartilages, and sternum. Due to the extensive area of invasion, the trauma is significant, and multiple complications may occur. ② Unsatisfactory cosmetic effect. From the perspective of eliminating depression, this surgery is very thorough. However, it replaces the depression deformity with a protrusion deformity. In the early postoperative period, when the skin is not fully adhered to the bony structures, the appearance may seem better, but later, when the skin fully adheres to the bone, an irregular new deformity often forms, resulting in unsatisfactory long-term cosmetic results. ③ Long postoperative scar. This surgery requires a long incision, at least extending from below the xiphoid process to the level of the sternal angle. Because the incision is located in the midline and is quite long, the resulting scar significantly affects the aesthetic appearance.

(3) Nuss Surgery

The Nuss procedure was officially introduced in 1998 and immediately attracted worldwide attention due to its completely different surgical concept compared to traditional methods [31]. This surgery uses a specially designed steel bar to support and lift the sunken chest wall, thereby correcting the deformity (Figure 2-4-13). Since its introduction, the Nuss procedure has become popular globally and has undergone various modifications, leading to multiple improved versions. It remains the most widely influential surgical method for correcting pectus excavatum to date.

(1) Basic Principle

The Nuss procedure has been in use for many years, with surgeons worldwide performing this operation. However, the fundamental principles behind the surgery have never been clearly explained. When the underlying principle is unclear, the surgery becomes highly blind in nature, inevitably leading to failure. After extensive observation, we analyzed the procedure using principles of physics and ultimately discovered that the fundamental mechanism of the Nuss procedure is based on a simple lever principle [32]. This discovery provides direct theoretical guidance for surgical execution, effectively reducing the occurrence of surgical failures.

Essentially, the Nuss procedure is a typical example of mechanical force-based reshaping surgery. This type of surgery uses specially designed materials to indirectly correct the deformity. It is fundamentally different from destructive reshaping and template-guided reshaping. This distinction represents the core characteristic of the Nuss procedure.

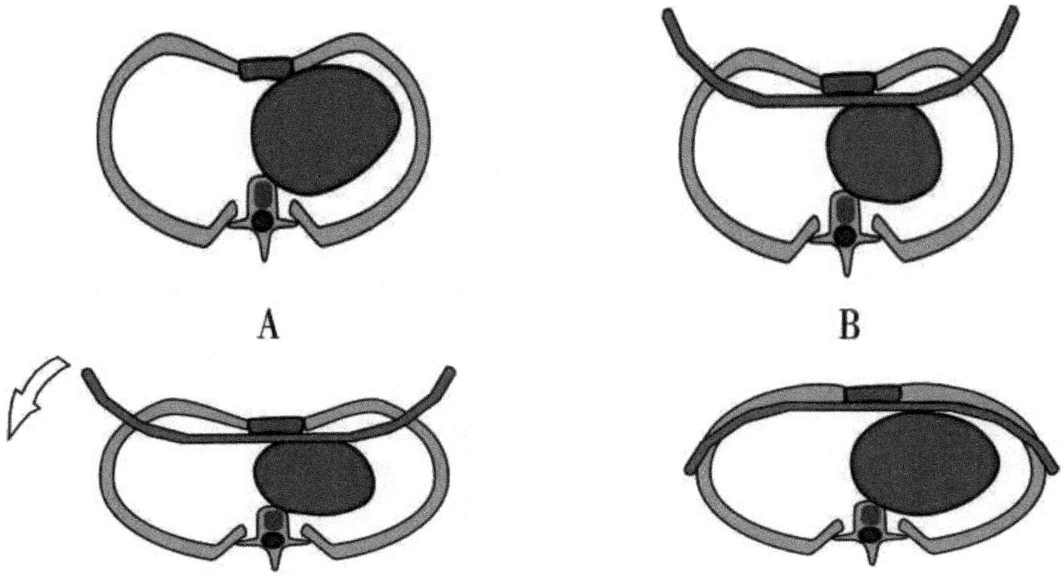

Figure 2-4-13 Diagram of the Nuss Procedure. (A. Cross-sectional view of pectus excavatum, showing the shape of the anterior chest wall and its relation to the heart; B. Placement of the curved steel bar at the bottom of the depression, with both ends of the bar exiting through incisions on either side of the chest wall; C. Rotation of the steel bar to lift the chest wall depression; D. After the anterior chest wall is lifted, fixation is performed at both ends of the steel bar.)

(2) Standard Nuss Procedure Operation

(1) Preoperative Preparation: Preoperative preparation mainly involves preparation of the steel bar and instruments. Preparation of the steel bar includes determining the number and length required. The number depends on the severity and extent of the deformity, and also on the surgeon's personal preference. The length of the bar depends on the width of the depression and likewise on the surgeon's preference.

(2) Intraoperative Preparation: Intraoperative preparation primarily involves shaping the steel bar. Since the bar is used to directly support and elevate the depressed chest wall, its shape must be determined by the characteristics of the

depression. During surgery, the bar should be molded according to the specific features of the depression to meet surgical requirements. Additionally, since most surgeons perform the procedure under Thoracoscopy, it is necessary to prepare the thoracoscopic equipment.

(3) Surgical Procedure: The standard Nuss procedure follows a relatively fixed sequence. First, incisions are made at appropriate positions on the lateral chest wall, followed by dissection of local soft tissue to expose the ribs. Then, entry into the thoracic cavity is made at a suitable site. Under thoracoscopic guidance, an introducer is inserted through one chest wall incision into the thoracic cavity, passed through the mediastinum, and exits through the contralateral chest wall incision. The introducer is connected to the steel bar, which is pulled into the thoracic cavity and across the mediastinum, exiting from the chest wall incision. A rotating wrench is used to rotate the bar, elevating the depressed anterior chest wall. Specially designed short stabilizers are placed at both ends of the bar to fix it firmly. The incisions are then closed, marking the end of the procedure (Figure 2-4-14). In this method, the introducer is directly connected to the steel bar and used to pull it into the thoracic cavity. Since the connection between the introducer and the bar is usually made with a strap, the joint may not be smooth, and resistance can be encountered while passing through the mediastinum. To overcome this issue, a guide tube can first be inserted through both chest wall incisions, and then the steel bar can be introduced. This allows for a smoother and safer placement of the bar (Figure 2-4-15).

(3) Advantages of the Nuss Procedure

After the Nuss procedure was introduced, it quickly garnered widespread attention, indicating that the surgery itself offered clear advantages. At the time, its benefits were especially evident when compared with open surgical techniques. The main advantages include: ① Simple Operation: The Nuss procedure corrects the depression using a specially designed steel bar without requiring direct manipulation of the depressed area. Essentially, it is an indirect reshaping method. Because it avoids the need for detailed structural dissection, the procedure is significantly simpler. With sufficient experience, surgeons can complete the operation in a very short time. ② Minimal Trauma: The Nuss procedure is performed through small incisions on the lateral chest wall, which are considerably smaller than those required in open surgery. Since most surgical trauma is confined to the areas around the incisions, overall trauma is much less than that of open procedures. ③ Small and Hidden Scars: The incisions made during the Nuss procedure are small and located on the side of the chest, making the resulting scars less noticeable. This leads to a better cosmetic outcome, which is often important for patients especially adolescents.

④ Satisfactory Results: The Nuss procedure has specific and well-defined indications. When patients are selected appropriately, the surgical outcomes are often very good. In such cases, the results can be clearly superior to those achieved through open surgery.

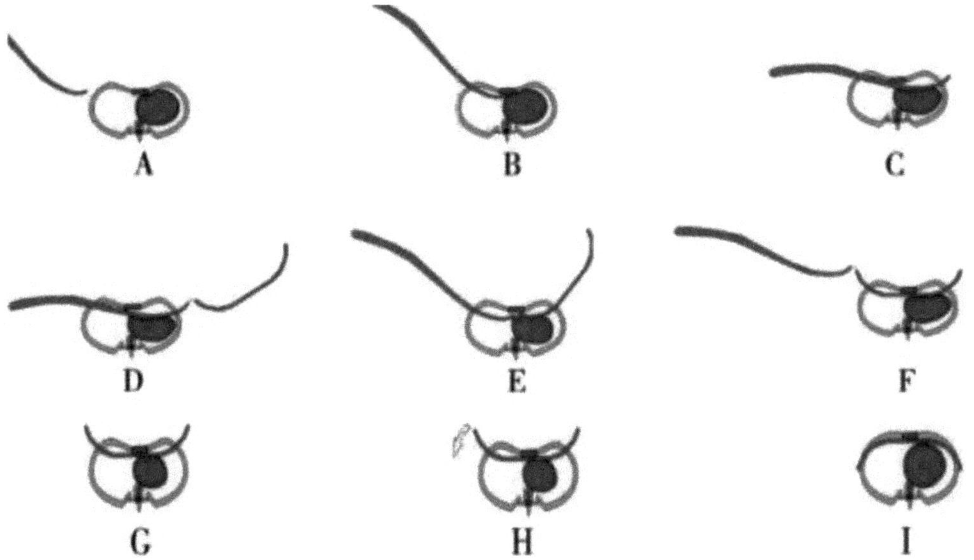

Figure 2–4–14: Schematic Illustration of Nuss Procedure (Introducing the bar directly into the thoracic cavity with the introducer) A. The introducer enters the thoracic cavity through an incision on one side of the chest wall. B. The tip of the introducer dissects the space between the heart and the anterior chest wall. C. The introducer passes through the space between the heart and chest wall and exits through the contralateral chest wall incision. D. The tip of the introducer is directly tied to the steel bar. E. The introducer is pulled back along the same route, dragging the steel bar across the mediastinum. F. The introducer brings the steel bar out through the incision on the surgeon's side of the chest wall. G. The steel bar is placed at the base of the depression, with both ends located inside the lateral chest wall incisions. H. The steel bar is flipped to lift the anterior chest wall. I. After the depression in the anterior chest wall is lifted, both ends of the steel bar are fixed in place.

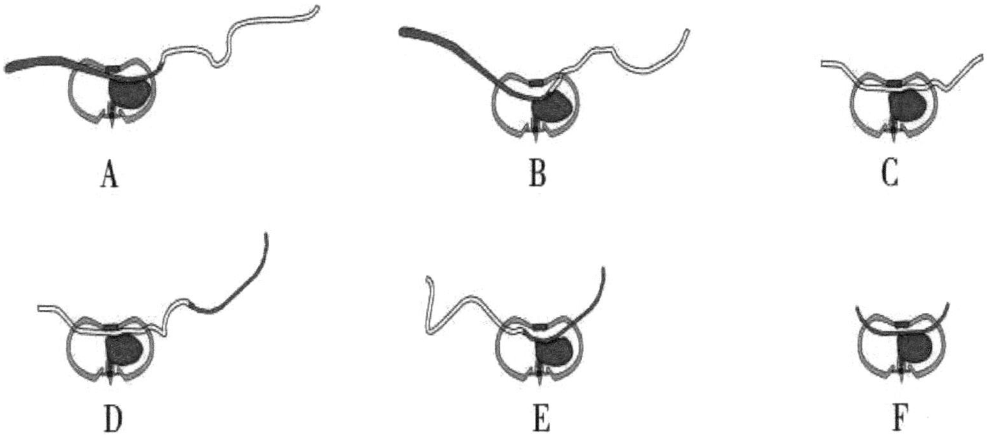

Figure 2–4–15: Schematic Illustration of Inserting the Steel Bar Using a Guiding Tube. A. After the introducer exits from the contralateral chest wall incision, it is not directly connected to the steel bar but instead linked to the guiding tube for the steel bar. B. The guiding tube is pulled into the thoracic cavity, passing through the mediastinum. C. The guiding tube is pulled out through the chest wall incision on the surgeon's side. D. One end of the guiding tube is connected to the steel bar. E. The guiding tube is used to pull the steel bar into the thoracic cavity and across the mediastinum. F. The steel bar is placed at the base of the depressed chest wall.

(4) Drawbacks of the Nuss Procedure

Although the Nuss procedure is an ingeniously designed operation with numerous clear advantages, like all other surgeries, it also has its own shortcomings. These are specifically reflected in the following aspects [33–38]:

(1) High surgical risk: Many people harbor mixed feelings about the Nuss procedure. On one hand, they perceive it as a very simple surgery, but on the other, they hesitate to attempt it due to its significant risks. In the actual execution of the Nuss procedure, the most critical step involves inserting the steel bar beneath the depressed area of the chest wall. This step must be performed in close proximity to the heart, often under conditions of poor visibility, which makes the operation highly blind and risky (Figure 2-4-16). If a mistake is made during this step, the introducer or steel bar could be accidentally inserted into the heart, potentially causing the patient's immediate death. This risk is not hypothetical such tragedies unfortunately occur every year. The accumulation of these incidents has instilled deep fear in many aspiring surgeons. As a result, even experienced thoracic surgeons may feel terrified at the thought of inserting the bar and dare not perform the procedure

at all.

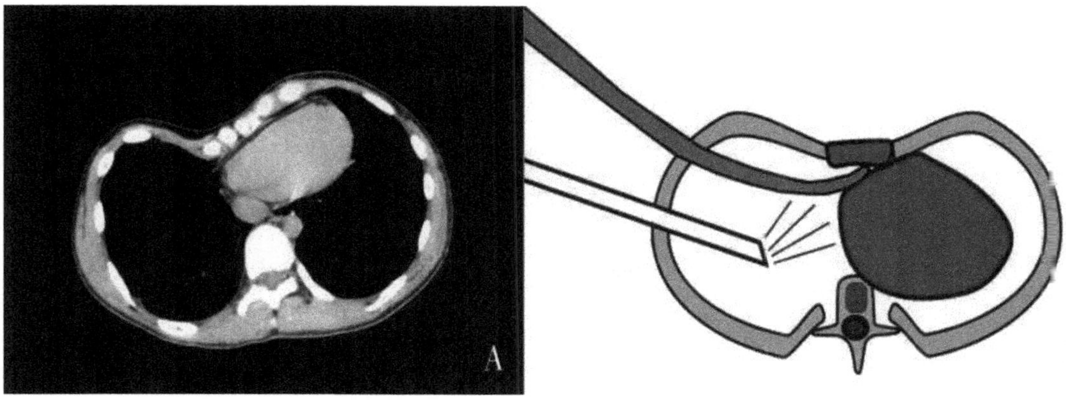

Figure 2-4-16 Risks of the Nuss Procedure (In patients with pectus excavatum, the heart lies very close to the anterior chest wall, and in severe cases, there is no gap between the two. Even with the aid of Thoracoscopy, it is difficult to visualize the entire operative process under such conditions. The passage of the steel bar through the bottom of the depression is the most dangerous part of the procedure, and this step makes it impossible to completely eliminate surgical risk.) A. The heart is tightly adhered to the anterior chest wall, and in severe cases, this area of contact may be extensive. When the steel bar passes through this region, if an appropriate method is not used, there is a high risk of injuring the heart. B. Thoracoscopy can only provide a view of one side of the mediastinum and does not reveal the trajectory of the bar within the narrow space. Even if thoracoscopes are used on both sides of the chest, the passage within this space remains invisible especially in cases of severe pectus excavatum. Clearly, Thoracoscopy often cannot visualize these critical areas, which represents a major limitation of thoracoscopic surgery and, even more so, a fundamental shortcoming of the Nuss procedure itself.

(2) Effectiveness of the Surgery: Compared to open surgery, the Nuss procedure can yield very good results when the indications are appropriately selected. However, such ideal scenarios are not commonly encountered. The most severe deformity in pectus excavatum is typically located at the deepest point of the depression. This region often protrudes toward the mediastinum, forming a distinct local deformity. To achieve a complete correction, this specific deformity must be addressed directly. Doing so not only ensures a more satisfactory aesthetic outcome but also helps prevent recurrence of the deformity. However, the Nuss procedure is a classic example of indirect reshaping; it relies on a steel bar to indirectly elevate the depression. This type

of operation does not focus on the detailed structure of the most deformed area. Consequently, in many cases, the Nuss procedure fails to correct the most crucial part of the deformity, resulting in suboptimal outcomes and an increased risk of postoperative relapse.

It primarily focuses on the overall appearance rather than the specific localized deformities. As a result, the most severely depressed part often remains uncorrected, which significantly compromises the surgical outcome. Such cases are frequently observed in clinical practice. This problem becomes even more pronounced when the steel bar is not positioned ideally, leading to unsatisfactory correction results (Figure 2-4-17).

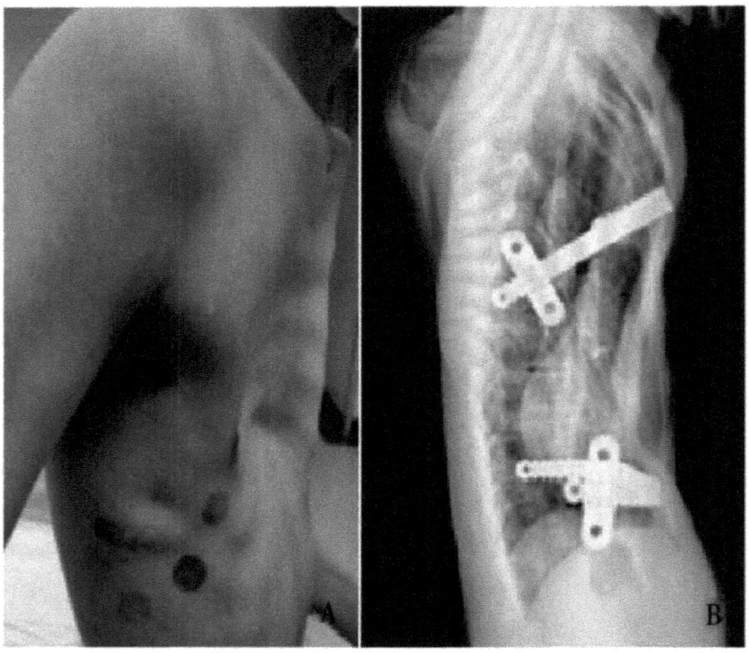

Figure 2-4-17 Failed Case of Nuss Procedure (According to the fundamental principle of the procedure, the steel bar must support the bottom of the depression to be effective. In this case, the bar clearly supports an incorrect position. This is the fundamental cause of surgical failure. A. External appearance of the chest wall: there is a distinct depression on the anterior chest wall, with old surgical scars visible on the lateral chest wall. B. Lateral X-ray shows the position of the bars. Both bars are placed away from the bottom of the depression and fail to perform corrective support, thus resulting in surgical failure.)

(3) formation of New Deformities: During the Nuss procedure, in order to elevate the depressed area, sufficient force must be applied via the steel bar to prop up the chest wall. However, this force requires a point of application or a fulcrum, which is typically located on the lateral chest wall. If this fulcrum is not strong enough, the pressure from the steel bar can cause a depression at the point of support. The appearance of such a depression indicates the formation

of a new deformity. The most common of these is the secondary saddle chest (Figure 2-4-18). If this occurs in conjunction with displacement of the steel bar, it may lead to a very severe deformity (Figure 2-4-19).

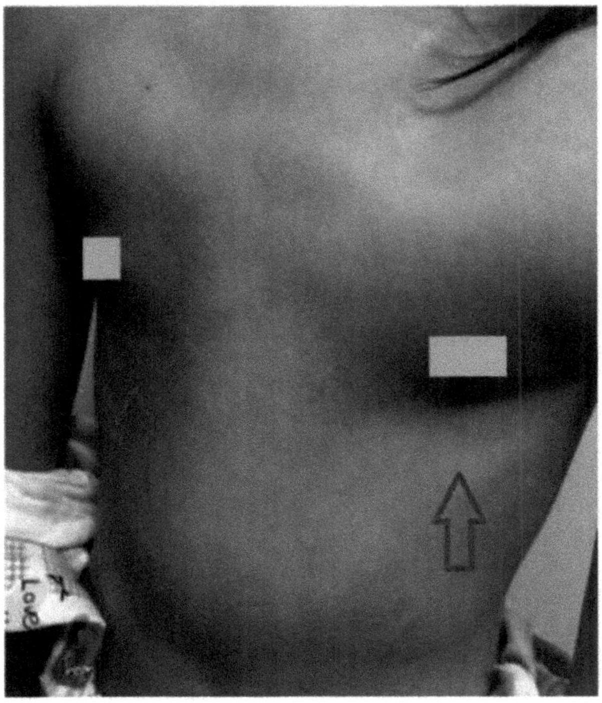

Figure 2-4-18: Secondary Saddle Chest after Nuss Procedure. The support points of the Nuss procedure's steel bar are located on the ribs of the lateral chest wall. If the ribs are not sufficiently rigid, they may be depressed by the pressure from the bar, resulting in a localized indentation. At this point, since the central depression has already been elevated, a new deformity emerges that is known as secondary saddle chest.

(4) Restriction on the Thoracic Cage: After the Nuss procedure, the ends of the steel bar exit through the intercostal spaces of the lateral chest wall and lie tightly along the outer sides of the ribs. This positioning creates a significant constraint on the thoracic cage. In younger children or prepubescent patients, due to the rapid growth of the chest, the implanted bar which neither adjusts its curvature nor increases in length over time imposes unavoidable restrictions. The most notable consequence is a pronounced depression in the thoracic wall beneath the bar, exacerbating the previously mentioned secondary saddle chest deformity.

(5) Age Limitation: The Nuss procedure requires a relatively rigid anchor point. If the patient is too young and the bones are too soft, the lateral thoracic structure cannot provide adequate support for the bar, making this procedure unsuitable for very young children. Additionally, since the skeletal growth rate in younger patients is high, an early Nuss procedure can severely constrain thoracic development. This is one of the main reasons why this procedure is not recommended for younger children. The general consensus is that the Nuss procedure should be used only in children older than 5 years. Some aggressive

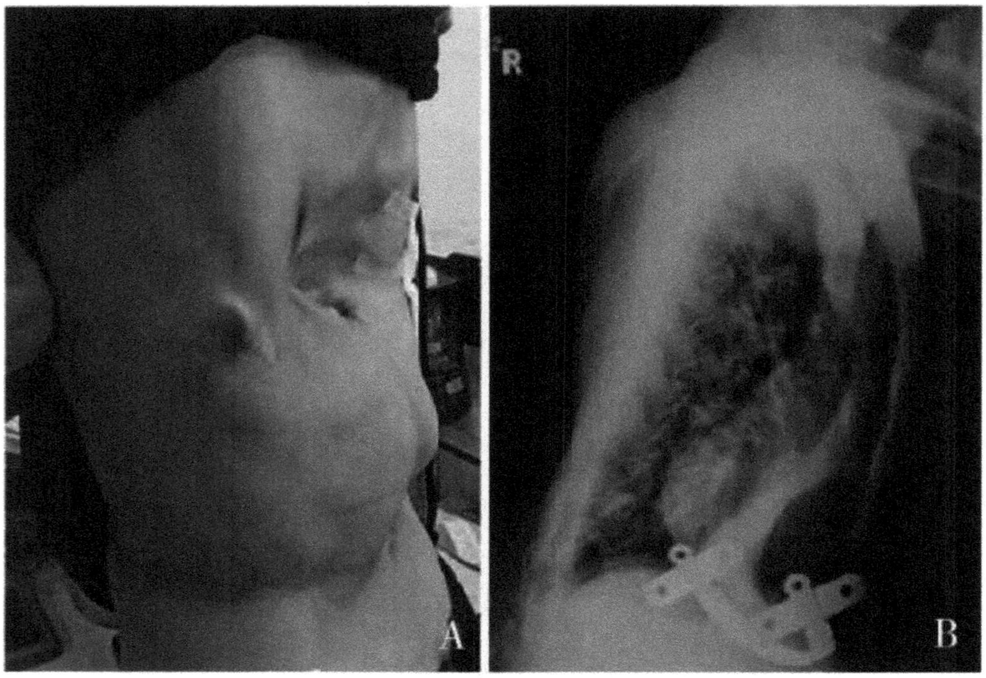

Figure 2-4-19: New Deformity After Failed Nuss Procedure. (A) Severe deformity of the anterior chest wall, with visible signs of the steel bar's end protruding. (B) Lateral X-ray image shows displacement of the steel bar, providing no support to the base of the depression.

authors lower the threshold to 3 years. However, the widely accepted view is that it should not be used in patients under 3. In principle, an ideal surgical technique should not be restricted by age. However, the age limitations of the Nuss procedure are so universally accepted that few dare to challenge them. Many infants are born with chest wall depressions, some of which are extremely severe and even life-threatening. Before the advent of the Nuss technique, such patients would undergo surgery early. But after the introduction of Nuss, the lack of alternatives and fear of revisiting open procedures have rendered some of these deformities "incurable." With no suitable options available, these infants are forced to suffer until they reach the age of 3 before undergoing Nuss surgery. This situation is highly abnormal. A more appropriate surgical method must be found to treat these patients in a timely manner.

(6) Limitations of Materials and Instruments: The original design of the Nuss procedure is based on a complete set of specially designed materials and instruments, which are essential for the surgery to be performed. Without these specific tools and implants, the procedure simply cannot be carried out.

Although the required materials and instruments have become more accessible over time, their specialized nature continues to restrict the widespread application of the surgery. In some lower-tier or rural medical facilities, the unavailability of these tools has made it impossible to perform the operation.

(7) Design Flaws in the Materials Themselves: The traditional Nuss bar features multiple notches at both ends and requires specially designed stabilizers for fixation. While this design may have some rationale, it is also one of the biggest shortcomings of the procedure. The presence of the notches significantly increases the risks associated with both the insertion and removal of the bar. The use of short stabilizers is particularly problematic; not only do they fail to enhance bar fixation effectively, but they also introduce unnecessary complications. Using stabilizers requires relatively long incisions, leading to more visible and aesthetically unappealing scars post-surgery. To properly embed the stabilizers, a significant amount of soft tissue is needed. Incomplete embedding can result in poor wound healing. Furthermore, in thin or underweight patients, the bar and stabilizers are positioned close to the skin surface, making them prone to injury if subjected to impact.

(5) Complications of the Nuss Procedure

The inherent shortcomings of the Nuss procedure not only limit its widespread application but also introduce numerous potential risks. If the procedure is not performed properly, it may lead to a variety of complications. The specific complications may include the following:

Cardiac rupture is the most serious complication of the Nuss procedure [39] It occurs when the introducer or the steel bar directly damages the heart during the operation.

The insertion of the steel bar into the heart is what causes cardiac rupture; this is the most severe complication of the Nuss procedure. Once it occurs, there is almost no time to rescue the patient; death can be immediate. The root cause of cardiac rupture lies in poor visibility; the most dangerous part of the procedure is performed without direct vision, which inherently carries enormous risk. To improve visibility, many surgeons use Thoracoscopy during the operation. While this method theoretically reduces risk, in practice it presents major issues. In cases of severe pectus excavatum, there is often no gap between the anterior chest wall and the heart, especially at the most sunken area. This severely limits the thoracoscopic view. Even if one side of the mediastinum is visible, the opposite side is often still obscured. As a result, the procedure remains largely blind. Ironically, nearly all reported cases of cardiac rupture so far have occurred during thoracoscopic-assisted Nuss procedures. This highlights the limited effectiveness of Thoracoscopy in preventing this

complication. To truly avoid such tragedies, improvements must be made from a technical standpoint, rather than relying solely on thoracoscopic visualization.
(2) Bleeding refers to hemorrhage originating from the chest wall and the surgical field. The injured vessels may include the intercostal arteries, and in severe cases, the internal thoracic (mammary) artery.
If active bleeding is identified during the surgery, immediate and effective hemostasis is required. If bleeding occurs postoperatively, the management should be based on the specific clinical situation.
(3) Rib Fracture: During the flipping of the steel bar in a Nuss procedure, if the depressed area creates significant resistance against the bar and the surgeon applies greater force to complete the maneuver, that resistance may be transferred through the bar to the supporting ribs. If the force is strong enough, it can cause a local rib fracture. In the Nuss surgery, ribs act as fulcrums. If the integrity of the rib is compromised, the fulcrum loses its function, and the surgery is bound to fail. Therefore, it's critical to protect the ribs during the bar-flipping process to prevent fractures. If a fracture occurs, remedial measures must be taken. The best option is to use another intact rib as a new support point; this is often the only feasible solution. However, if the issue of excessive resistance is not resolved, fractures may still occur in other ribs. Thus, the most fundamental solution is to effectively reduce the resistance. Through long-term clinical experience, we have developed a comprehensive method to eliminate resistance, collectively referred to as pre-shaping technology. With proper pre-shaping, local stress can be significantly reduced, minimizing resistance during bar flipping. This not only prevents rib fractures but also helps achieve a more satisfactory correction of the deformity.

(4) Abnormal positioning of the steel bar is a relatively common complication [40]. Since the position of the steel bar directly affects the contour of the chest wall, any deviation from the intended placement can significantly impact the surgical outcome (Figure 2-4-20) Abnormal positioning of the steel bar can be classified into two categories: displacement (Figure 2-4-21) and rotation (Figure 2-4-22). Displacement refers to the overall movement of the steel bar from its original position and can occur in three directions: Lateral (sideways), Vertical (up or down), Anteroposterior (front to back) Rotation, on the other hand, involves axial movement of the steel bar, leading to abnormal positioning without necessarily shifting the bar as a whole. The axis of rotation can be one of the standard three-dimensional axes or any arbitrary axis. In many cases, both displacement and rotation may occur simultaneously, resulting in a particularly complex positional change of the steel bar.

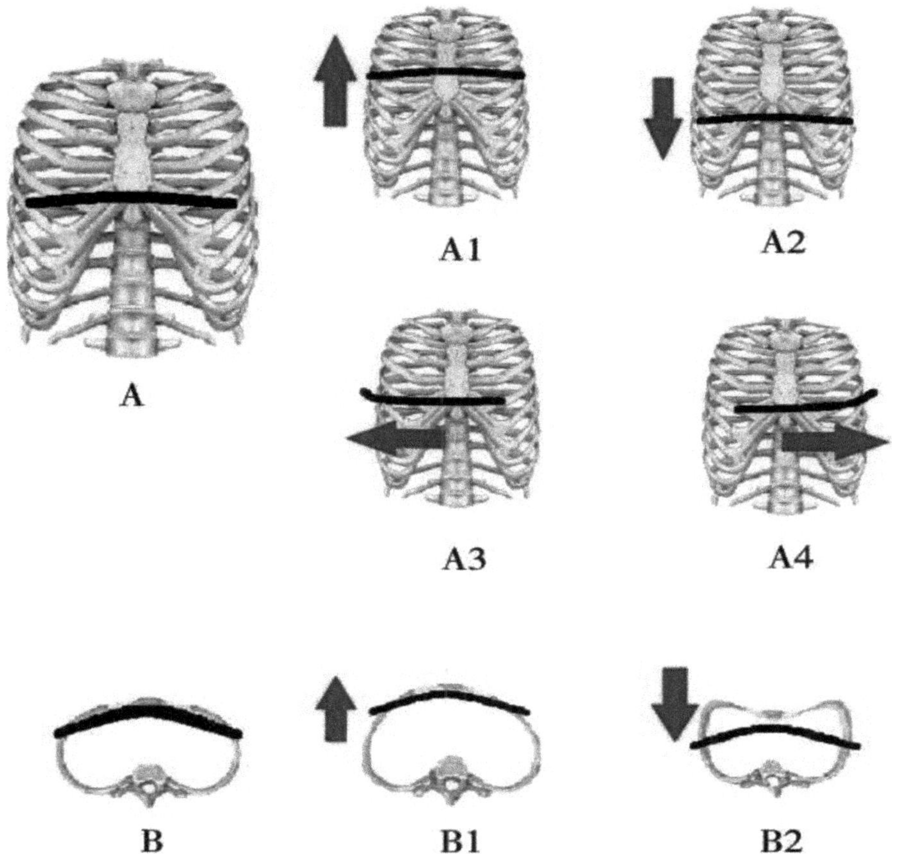

Figure 2-4-20 Cases of Various Steel Bar Displacements (When the steel bar shifts, its support function is lost, inevitably leading to surgical failure. Furthermore, the displaced bar may cause additional damage, resulting in various unforeseen consequences.) A. The steel bar is located beneath the depressed chest wall, offering no support function. B. One end of the bar slants downward, making it unable to support the depression. C. The steel bar shifts toward the right side, compromising its supporting effect. D. Neither of the two bars is positioned at the deepest part of the depression, thus failing to provide support. E. The bar is placed on the upper inner surface of the chest

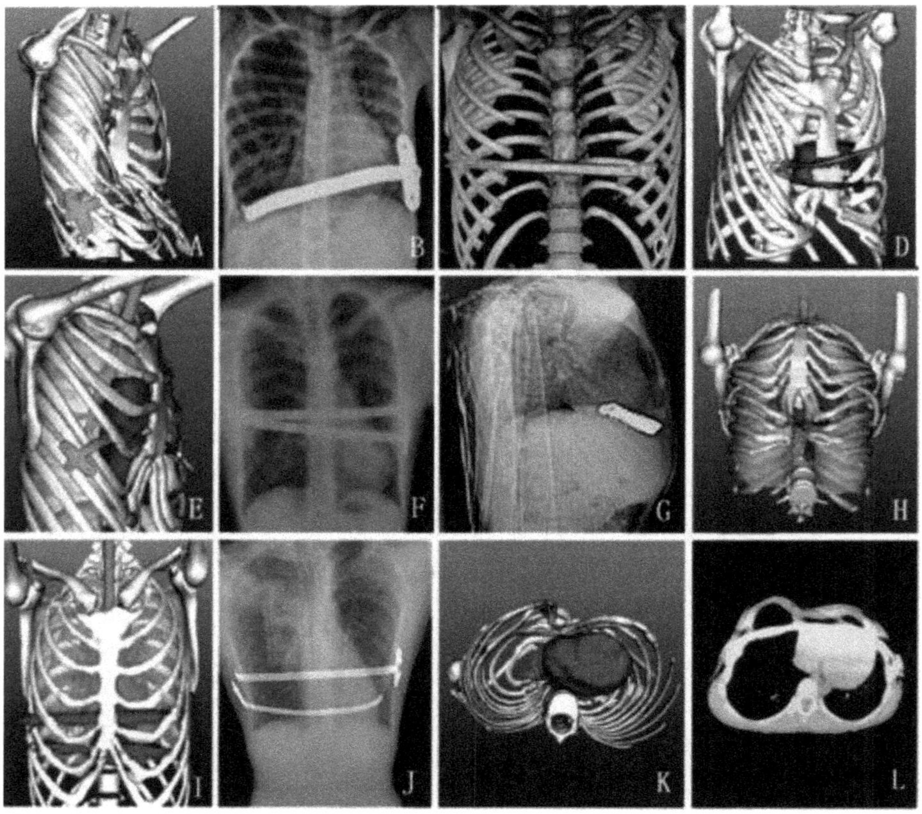

Figure 2-4-21: Displacement of the Steel Bar. A. Normal position of the steel bar in the coronal plane A1 & A2: Displacement in the vertical direction (upward and downward) A3 & A4: Displacement in the horizontal direction (left and right) B. Normal position of the steel bar in the cross-sectional (transverse) plane. B1 & B2: Displacement in the anteroposterior direction (forward and backward)wall, with no supporting function. F. The bar has slid to the right side, affecting its support capability. G. The central portion of the bar has rotated downward, preventing it from providing support. H. The bar has rotated upward, rendering it ineffective in supporting the chest wall. I. Both bars are not positioned at the deepest point of the depression; the upper bar is abnormally placed on the right side. J. The bar is not securely fixed; the fixation plate has detached from the main bar, resulting in displacement. K. The bar is abnormally positioned and unable to support the depressed area. L. The placement is suboptimal; the support point is too low to serve its function.

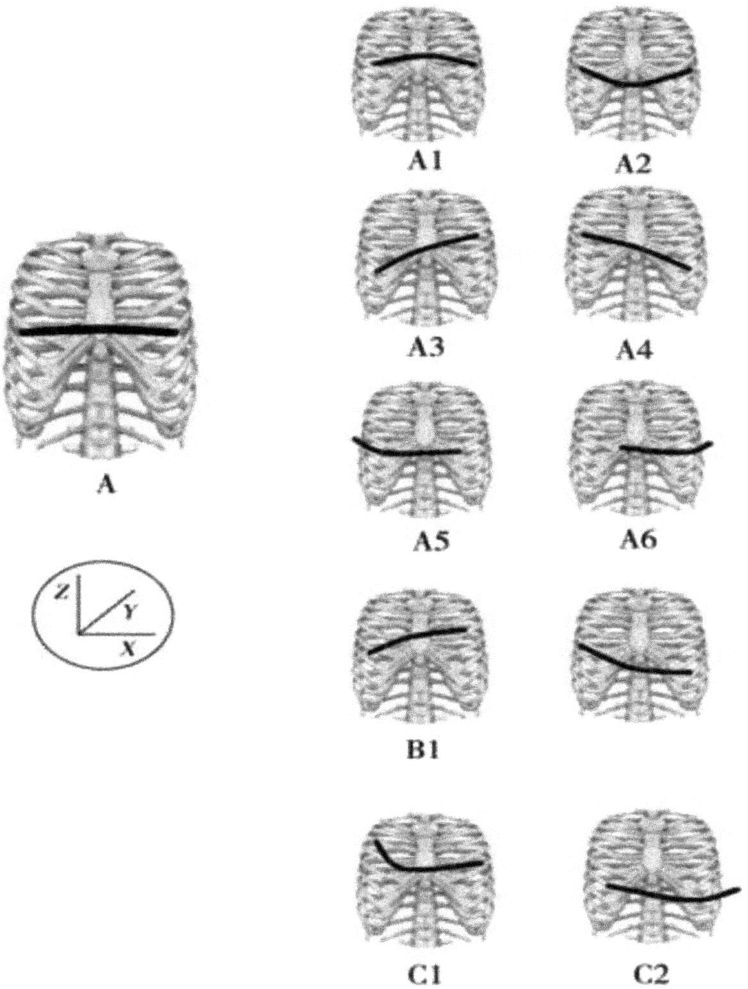

Figure 2-4-22: Rotation and Other Positional Abnormalities of the Steel Bar. A. Normal position of the steel bar A1 & A2: Rotation of the steel bar around the X-axis. A3 & A4: Rotation of the steel bar around the Y-axis. A5 & A6: Rotation of the steel bar around the Z-axis. B1 & B2: Rotation of the steel bar around non-standard axes (other axes of movement). C1 & C2: Combined rotation and displacement, resulting in complex positional abnormalities

Steel bar malposition is associated with various factors, among which the most common are: Surgeon-related factors: The primary cause of abnormal steel bar positioning is either insufficient fixation or incorrect placement during the procedure. Both issues arise directly from the surgeon's technique. If the surgeon ensures proper placement and secure fixation during surgery, postoperative displacement or malposition of the steel bar is almost impossible. Patient-related factors: In the early postoperative period, excessive physical activity by the patient can also lead to displacement of the steel bar. However, such occurrences often have an underlying technical flaw, typically inadequate fixation by the surgeon. If the steel bar is fixed firmly and properly, normal or even mildly intense patient movements should not cause any positional abnormalities. Abnormal positioning due to the movement of the subject. Thirdly, the issue of delayed shaping. Delayed molding is an inevitable change, and such a change can affect the position of the steel plate. One of the impacts is the change in the position of the steel plate. However, such displacement mostly occurs at a later stage, and if the steel plate is placed satisfactorily, it generally does not have a significant impact on the surgical outcome.

(5) Pneumothorax, pleural effusion. Nuss surgery requires entering the thoracic cavity, so all complications related to thoracotomy may occur. Pneumothorax and pleural effusion are relatively common complications. To prevent the harm it may cause, a prophylactic closed thoracic drainage device can be placed.

(6) Delayed incision healing. Delayed wound healing is a relatively common complication and is related to various factors, among which suturing technique is the most critical factor. Since there is a steel plate within the incision, it is necessary to use sufficient soft tissue to embed it during suturing. If such an operation is not performed, it may easily affect healing. Additionally, the issue of incision healing is also related to factors inherent to the patient. If the patient allows the incision to get wet prematurely or handles it improperly, it can also affect healing (Figure: 2-4-23).

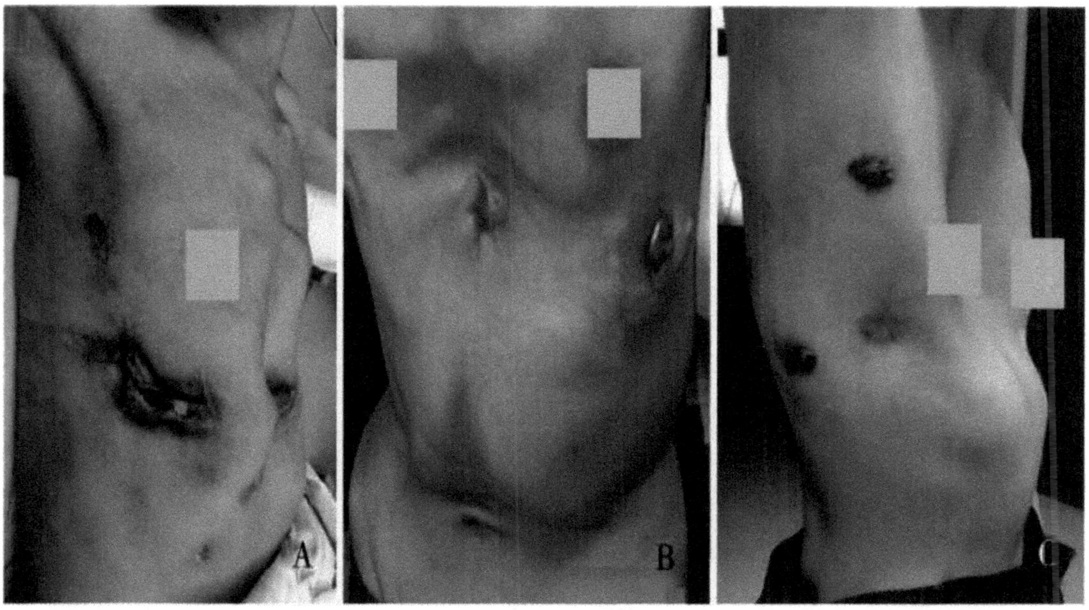

Figure 2-4-23 Poor postoperative incision healing (A. The patient has several steel plates placed inside, with multiple plates protruding through the skin, exposed externally; B. The fixed plate on the patient's left side is exposed on one end; C. Poor incision healing on the patient's right side)

(7) Scoliosis. Scoliosis may occur before surgery as a secondary condition, and it can also occur after surgery. Many patients may develop noticeable scoliosis postoperatively. There are two reasons for the occurrence of scoliosis: one is related to the surgery, and the other is related to the patient's own posture. The surgery for pectus excavatum involves the application of external force using a steel plate to forcibly alter the shape of the bones in the anterior chest wall. Since the thorax is a whole, when the shape of the chest wall skeleton is altered, every part of the thorax may be affected. The spine is a component of the thorax and will inevitably be affected during the orthopedics process. If the steel plate is not applied with appropriate force, it may lead to scoliosis (Fig. 2-4-24). This is a relatively common situation, often occurring in the early postoperative period, and is clearly causally related to the surgery. In addition to surgical reasons, scoliosis is also related to the patient's posture. After surgery, if the patient experiences asymmetrical pain in both sides of the chest wall, they may adopt a protective posture to alleviate the pain. This posture can cause the spine to bend to one side, resulting in uneven shoulders. If it persists for too long, it may lead to a permanent curvature.

This type of scoliosis is mainly caused by the patient themselves. To prevent it, the patient needs to actively adjust their posture. If the patient is a young child who cannot actively adjust their posture, external braces can be used for correction.

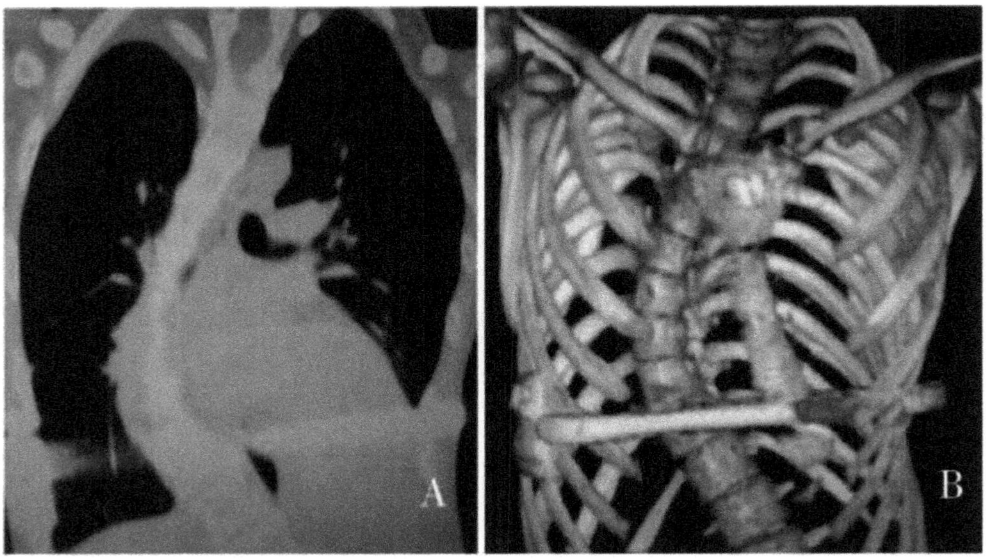

Figure 2-4-24 Scoliosis caused by surgery (The patient had no scoliosis before surgery, but showed significant scoliosis early after the surgery, clearly related to the surgery). A. CT images show significant spinal scoliosis.

(6) Improved Nuss surgery

The Nuss procedure quickly became popular after its inception due to its distinct advantages, with many doctors attempting to use it. However, this type of surgery has inherent design flaws, and it is difficult to achieve good results without making improvements. Precisely because of this understanding, doctors worldwide have been making various efforts over the years to improve it, aiming to reduce risks and achieve more satisfactory results. This is the so-called modified Nuss procedure. There are various improvements to the Nuss procedure, mainly in terms of materials, instruments, and techniques.

(1) Improvements in materials and instruments. Improvements in materials mainly involve redesigning the steel plate to eliminate the drawbacks of the classic Nuss surgical steel plate from various angles. The improvements in the instruments involve better design of special instruments necessary for surgery, making the surgical operations more convenient and safer.

(2) Improvements in operational methods. The improvement of the operation method mainly targets certain operational details, such as the method of passing steel plates, the method of fixing steel plates, and the positioning of the fixed steel plates. These improvements may have different effects.

(3) Improvement of auxiliary methods. In order to avoid the risks of surgery, some authors have designed various methods to enhance the safety of surgical procedures. For example, the process of penetrating the steel plate can be monitored using an electrocardiogram or transesophageal echocardiography. Some authors have designed a visual lens at the front end of the introducer to facilitate placement. These methods each have their own design rationale, but it must be pointed out that the operation involving the passage through the steel plate tests the doctor's skills. If the doctor does not possess such skills, or even lacks basic competence, no matter how advanced the auxiliary means are, it may lead to surgical failure. From this perspective, similar approaches are almost futile and may make doctors more fearful of the surgery.

(7). Wung Surgery

Among the various modified surgeries for Nuss procedure, it is necessary to mention a surgical method that is completely different from the classic procedure or all other authors' modified surgeries, namely the Wung procedure we designed [41]. The surgery is specifically named because it has distinct characteristics, which are introduced here in detail. (Figures 2-4-25 and 2-4-26)Wung, the basic surgical technique is: first, make an incision on the lateral chest wall at the plane of the deepest depression, which generally only needs to be 1~1.5cm. Whether placing one steel plate or two or even three steel plates, only such a length of incision is required. Incise the subcutaneous tissue and muscle tissue to directly expose the ribs beneath the incision, then dissect along the surface of the ribs to expose multiple surrounding ribs. Expose the intercostal space at the upper edge of the rib intended to serve as the pivot, and incise the intercostal muscle, approximately 2cm in size. Place a wire guide near the pivot point of the rib for standby. The procedures on the lateral chest wall incisions and their underlying areas are exactly the same. After completing these steps, insert the introducer through an incision on one side of the chest wall, enter the thoracic cavity through an intercostal incision, then pass through the mediastinum into the opposite thoracic cavity, and finally exit through an incision on the opposite chest wall. Connect the guiding tube of the steel plate to the end of the guide, and use the guide to introduce the guiding tube through the thoracic cavity and mediastinum from one incision to the other. Thread the steel plate into the guide tube, use the guide tube to pull the steel plate into the mediastinum and thoracic cavity, and pass it through the incision in the lateral chest wall, ensuring both ends of the steel plate are outside the incision, with the middle of the steel plate positioned at the base of the depression on the anterior chest wall. Use a turning wrench to maneuver the steel plate, positioning it correctly and lifting the depression. Then, guide the wire with a lead wire to wrap the wire around the ribs and the steel plate. Tighten the wire to securely fasten the metal plate. Close the incision, the surgery is complete.

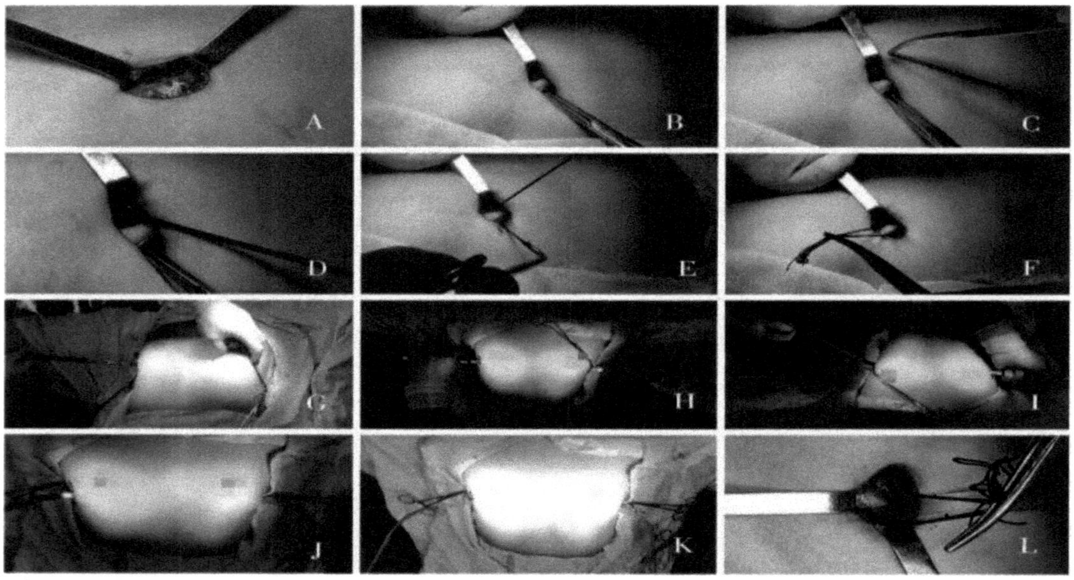

Figure 2-4-25 Wung Surgical Operation Diagram (1) (which includes the standard fixation plate technique of Wang [42]) (A. A small incision is made on the lateral chest wall, generally not exceeding 2cm. Cut the muscle tissue to expose the ribs. Further dissection along the rib to reveal the appropriate site for the plate's fulcrum. Use a right-angle clamp across the rib at the pivot point. Use a vascular clamp to hold the middle of the wire guide, and hand over the right-angle clamp. Clamp the middle of the guidewire using an angle clamp. Use an angle clamp to guide the steel wire lead out around the rib, with the position still located at the fulcrum of the steel plate. Reserve angle pliers for clamping the steel wire guide. Insert the introducer through an incision on one side of the chest wall and pass it through the mediastinum to exit from an incision on the opposite side of the chest wall, without using a thoracoscope. H. The introducer emerges from the contralateral chest wall incision. The introducer connects the steel plate guiding tube. J. The introducer guides the steel plate guide tube into the thoracic cavity, passing through the mediastinum. The steel plate guide tube is led out from the incision on the other side of the chest wall. Adjust the guidewire to ensure that it encircles both the rib and the steel plate simultaneously.

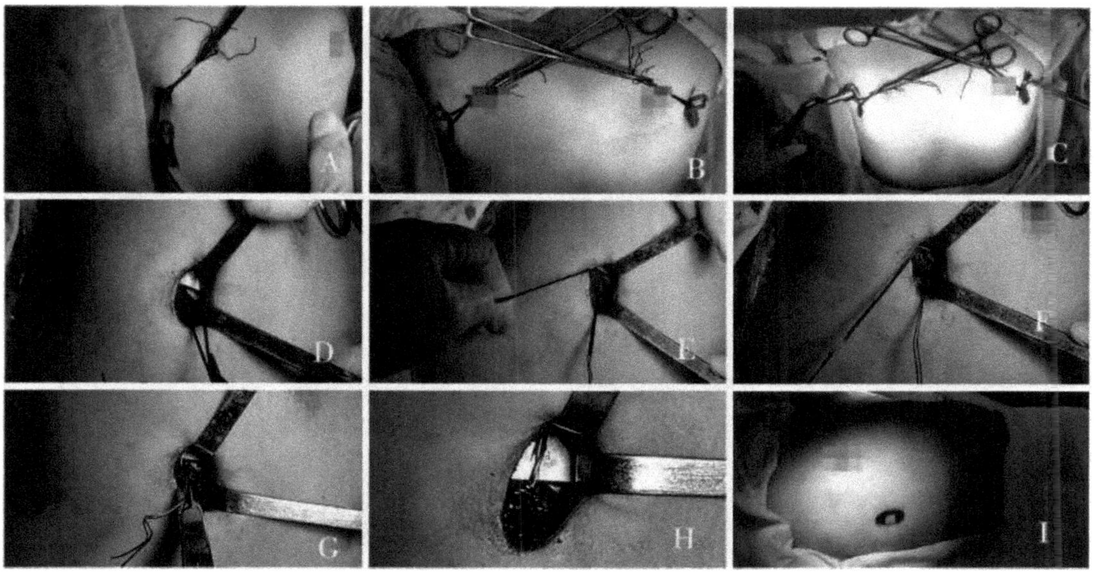

Figure 2-4-26: Wung Procedure Operation Diagram (2) (This includes the standard Wang technique for fixing the steel plate [42]) A. The guiding tube connects to the steel plate, dragging it into the thoracic cavity and exiting through the contralateral chest wall incision via the mediastinum. B. After removing the guiding tube, both ends of the plate are located within the bilateral chest wall incisions, with the main body of the plate positioned beneath the depression. C. Use a wrench to rotate the plate, lifting the depressed chest wall. D. At this point, the guiding wire encircles both the rib and the plate. E. Insert a folded steel wire into the guiding wire loop. F. Pull the guiding wire to wrap the steel wire around the rib, simultaneously encircling the rib and the plate. G. Tighten the wire to fix the plate and rib together. H. Cut the wire, placing the remaining end deep beneath the plate. I. Close the incision; the surgery is complete.

Compared to the classic Nuss procedure, the advantages of the Wung procedure are as follows [1]: ① Easier operation. During the surgery, we simplified many operational details, making the entire procedure extremely straightforward. First, we have completely abandoned thoracoscopy, all operations are performed without the use of an endoscope. This procedure greatly simplifies the surgery. Secondly, we have simplified the method of fixing the steel plate. Instead of using short fixation plates, the steel plate is now directly fixed to the ribs. Due to the use of a special Wung technique [42], the entire fixation process becomes extremely simple and easy. ② The operation is safer. Passing through the steel plate is the most dangerous process. We perform this operation without

the use of a thoracoscope, relying entirely on the sense of touch. This sensation is more precise and sensitive. As long as the technique is mastered, it is impossible to harm the heart, making it safer. Additionally, to ensure smoother placement of the steel plates, we use a special guiding tube for direction, thereby avoiding adverse factors during the placement process. ③The procedure is less invasive. By no longer using Thoracoscopy, the corresponding operational injuries are avoided. Additionally, the use of Wung technique for fixing steel plates significantly reduces the size of the surgical incision and also minimizes the corresponding damage [42]. The implementation of these techniques significantly reduces the overall damage of surgery, making it more minimally invasive. ④ the operation is more reasonable. The plate is directly fixed at the pivot point during surgery, ensuring the most reliable support and elevation effect. The technique of fixing the steel plate, Wang, is itself an ingenious design. This design facilitates other intraoperative procedures, making it very reasonable. ⑤ the scar is smaller. Since short fixed plates are no longer used for fixation, and especially with the application of the special Wung technique, all procedures can be performed within a very small incision, minimizing the incision to generally no more than 2cm, resulting in smaller postoperative scars.
After the introduction of the surgical procedure, we have fully adopted this technique in all pectus excavatum surgeries. By the end of 2021 in December(12), we completed over 3,500 cases of Wung surgeries, achieving satisfactory outcomes. Additionally, we have been invited to assist in performing this surgery in over 300 hospitals nationwide, which has significantly promoted the widespread adoption of this surgical method. It is particularly important to emphasize that the Wang technique for fixing steel plates that we designed has become the standard procedure in all thoracic deformity surgeries. It is not only applied to pectus excavatum but is also widely used in other deformity surgeries, and this technique has become recognized as a revolutionary technique[42].

(4) Wang surgery

Wang surgery is a special surgical method designed by us, officially announced in 2018. This surgery is completely different from the Nuss procedure and represents a new generation of pectus excavatum treatment technology [43]. The surgery was included in the "National Clinical Version of the Surgical Procedure Classification Codes" in 2019 as version 3.0, becoming another officially recognized surgery following the Nuss procedure.

Basic Principles

Nuss surgery fundamentally operates by using a steel bar to elevate the depression, while Wang surgery corrects the depression from a different angle. Some believe that the essence of this surgery is lifting or suspension, a view that essentially reflects the principle of the procedure. However, from the nature of the surgery, this type of surgery is a true template shaping, which is completely different from the mechanical force shaping of the Nuss procedure (Fig. 2-4-27)

The original intention of designing Wang's surgery is to treat young children with pectus excavatum. Since the Nuss procedure cannot be used for the treatment of younger patients with pectus excavatum, and many young patients have extremely severe chest wall depression, we have designed this procedure to treat this group of patients. In subsequent clinical practice, the indications for this surgery have been expanded, allowing consideration for use in some older pediatric patients.

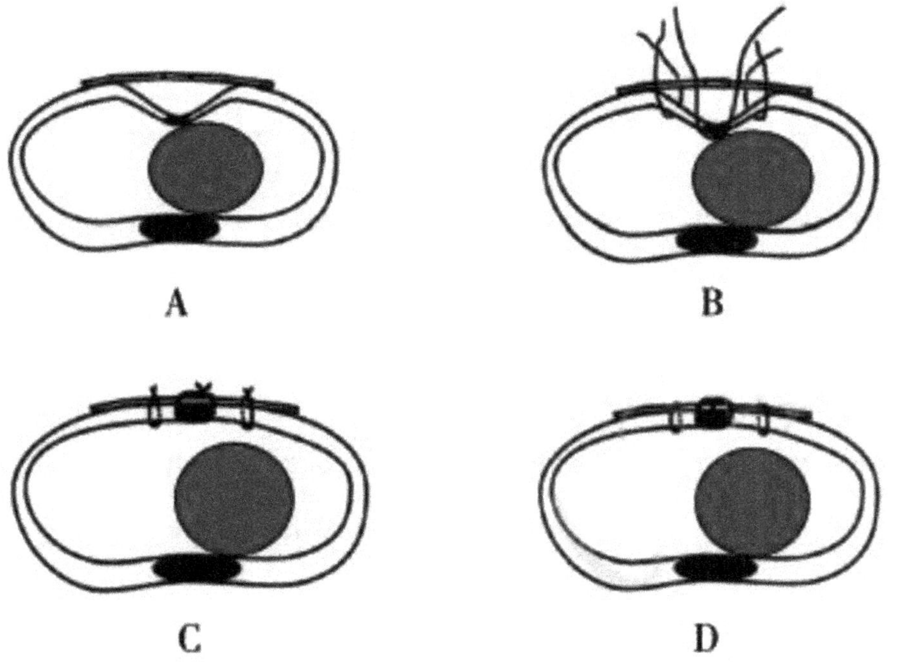

Figure 2-4-27 Wang Schematic diagram of the surgery (The basic principle is to use a steel plate to lift the depressed chest wall to eliminate the depression). The steel plate is placed on the surface of the bony structure of the concave surface.

(1) Indication

The original intention of designing Wang's surgery is to treat young children with pectus excavatum. Since the Nuss procedure cannot be used for the treatment of younger patients with pectus excavatum, and many young patients have extremely severe chest wall depression; we have designed this procedure to treat this group of patients. In subsequent clinical practice, the indications for this surgery have been expanded, allowing consideration for use in sone older pediatric patients.

(2) Surgical Method

Make a longitudinal incision below the xiphoid process and split it. First, perform dissection on the surface of the lower end of the sternum and surrounding bony structures to expose the relevant structures, then perform dissection behind the sternum. On the plane of the deepest depression, create a steel plate tunnel through the incision extending to both sides of the chest wall. Use a needle-equipped wire to suture the bilateral costal arch and the lower end of the sternum, placing the wire at the corresponding positions for later use. Place the specially made steel plates into both sides of the tunnel. After aligning the center of the steel plates, lift the sunken chest wall with the reserved steel wire so that the chest wall fits snugly against the steel plates. Then, tighten the wires to secure them, eliminating the sunken chest wall. Suture the incision, end of surgery (Fig. 2-4-28).

(3) Key Points of Operation

1. The position where the steel plate is placed. The steel plate should be placed in front of the deepest recessed plane. This is the best position for contouring. If deviated from this position, it will affect the surgical outcome.
2. The position of the wire suspension. The wire suspension is generally fixed at three points, which is the most ideal position and also the position where the force is optimal. If the suturing deviates from these areas due to technical issues, it may affect the surgical outcome.
3. The sequence of operations. Since all operations are performed within an extremely narrow incision, the order of operations is very important. If the order is improper, it can cause significant trouble for the surgery.

Figure 2-4-28 Wang's surgical procedure (A. Make a longitudinal incision at the bottom of the depression, with a length of 1 to 1.5 cm; B. Free the subcutaneous tissue on the surface of the bony structure to expose the bony structure; C. Use vascular forceps to bluntly separate the chest wall on both sides to make a tunnel for the steel plate; D. Use a steel wire with a needle to penetrate the chest wall structure at the bottom of the depression for suturing; E. Use the same method to place an appropriate number of steel wires; F. Unfold the steel wire to expose the surgical field; G. Place the steel plate in the tunnel; H. Pull up and tighten the steel wire to eliminate the depression; I. Cut off the steel wire, deal with the remaining end of the steel wire, suture the incision, and the operation is over)

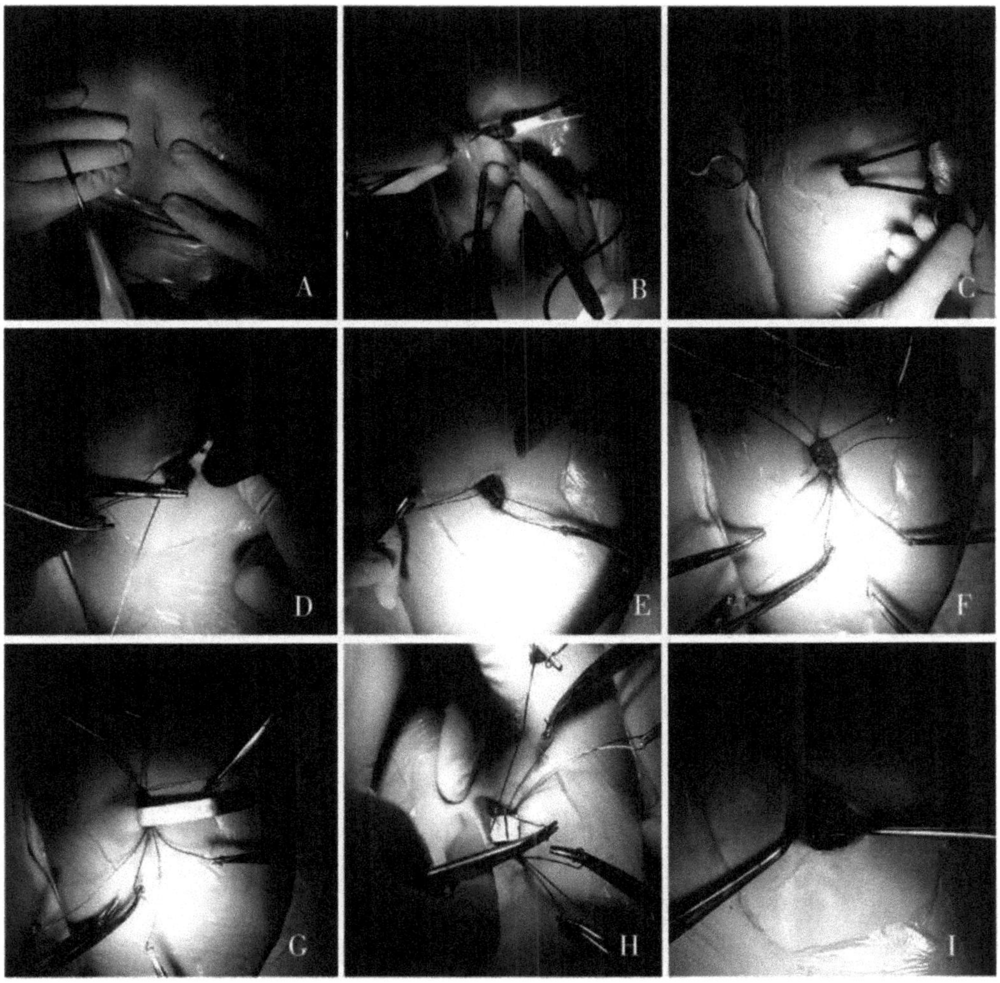

4. Understanding the shaping of the template. The essence of template shaping is to make the deformed chest wall structure fit closely to the steel plate. To achieve this objective, the chest wall structure must be firmly fixed to the steel plate, which is a fundamental requirement to ensure the surgical outcome.
5. Issues with incision suturing. Due to the presence of a steel plate within the incision, if the suturing is not ideal, it will affect the healing of the incision. The key point of suturing is to encapsulate with as much soft tissue as possible. In addition, proper hemostasis should be achieved to prevent local exudation, which is also a key point in avoiding poor wound healing.

(4) The advantages of surgery

The surgical operation details by Wang show that this kind of surgery has the following advantages [44]: ① Simple operation. All operations are performed under direct vision, requiring only the insertion of the steel plate into the chest wall and securing it by pulling the wire, making the procedure extremely simple and easy to implement. ② Operational Safety. The main operations are completed on the surface of the bony structure, eliminating the need to place a steel plate on the surface of the heart, thereby greatly reducing the risk. Additionally, since all operations are performed under direct vision, the risk of blind procedures is completely eliminated, significantly increasing the safety factor. ③ Precise operation. The operation is completed under direct vision, greatly improving the accuracy of the procedure; additionally, since the operation directly targets the most severe localized depression, it effectively eliminates the drawbacks associated with the Nuss procedure. Reduced scars. ④This surgery requires only a small incision to complete all operations, significantly reducing the number of incisions and consequently the number of postoperative scars. ⑤ The effect is better. This surgery directly targets the most severely affected area of the depressed lesion, ensuring the effectiveness of the treatment. Additionally, due to its fundamental nature as a molding template, this characteristic greatly enhances its molding effect. ⑥ Avoids a large number of complications. The plate in the Wang surgery is located on the surface of the bony structure. Since it "floats" on the bony structure rather than being "wedged" between the ribs like in the Nuss surgery, all related complications are absent. Additionally, since the plate in the Wang surgery is placed over multiple ribs, unlike the Nuss surgery which uses a single rib as a fulcrum, it effectively overcomes the issue of soft ribs in younger patients, making it suitable for use in younger children.

(5) Limitations of Surgery

(1) Age restrictions. Wang surgery is a procedure designed for younger children with pectus excavatum, and it is most suitable for use in this specific group of patients. For patients in other age groups, due to their bones being too hard, it is difficult to elevate these structures, which can affect the surgical outcome. Therefore, this procedure is not suitable for use in older patients. We advocate that children over 10 years old should avoid this surgery as much as possible [43]. of course, age is an uncertain factor, but the key is to look at the local pathological characteristics of pectus excavatum. If the child is relatively thin, with localized depressions that are not too hard, the age limit can be appropriately relaxed. The maximum age for performing the Wang surgery is 14 years, and the surgical outcome is satisfactory. On the contrary, in some cases, although the child is not over 10 years old, their bones are unusually dense, making them unsuitable for this surgery as well.

(2) Deformity limitation. The Wang surgery is designed for pectus excavatum, but it does not have good treatment effects for all types of pectus excavatum. Generally, the more localized and smaller the area of the deformity, the more satisfactory the surgical outcome. If the area is too large, it is difficult to perform extensive operations through smaller incisions, resulting in suboptimal outcomes.

(6) Complications

Any surgery may have complications, and Wang's surgery is no exception. The occurrence of complications is related to many factors, including Factors related to the surgery itself, as well as factors related to the operator's technique. No matter what factors are involved, they must be given attention.

(1) Bleeding. Wang the surgical field of Wang's operation does not involve the heart, and there is basically no possibility of massive bleeding. However, during the process of stitching with wire, it is sometimes possible to puncture the blood vessels of the chest wall. The blood vessels that are more prone to injury are the intercostal vessels. This type of blood vessel is relatively fine, with a small amount of bleeding, and cauterization with an electrosurgical knife can easily stop the bleeding. The vessel with less damage is the internal thoracic artery. If this blood vessel is damaged, it may lead to significant bleeding. At this point, an electric cautery can also be directly used for hemostasis. If the effect is not satisfactory, you can slightly extend the incision and suture it with silk thread, which generally can easily stop the bleeding.

(2) Wire breakage. The suspended steel wires and plates may repeatedly rub against each other due to the child's movements, which could lead to the wires breaking. Early wire breakage may affect shaping, while later wire breakage

will not have a significant impact. To avoid this complication, it is necessary to choose wires of appropriate thickness, which not only need to have sufficient strength but also be present in adequate quantity.

(3) Delayed incision healing. The steel plate is located within the incision. If suturing is not ideal, it may lead to the exposure of the steel plate, affecting the healing of the incision (Fig. 2-4-29)

.

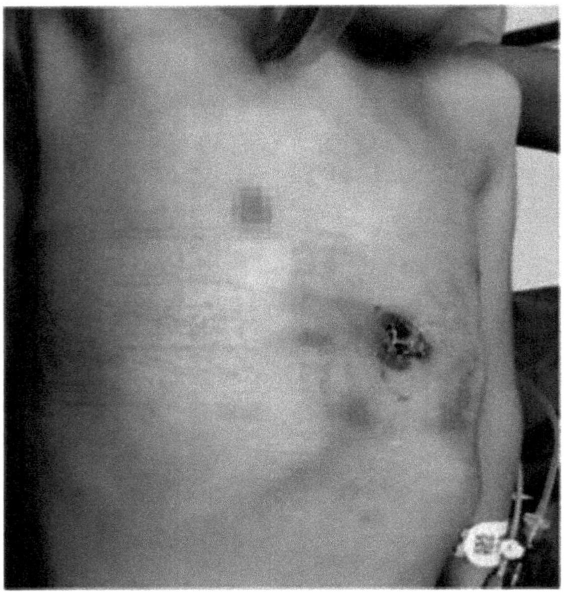

Figure 2-4-29 Wang Surgery- The incision healed poorly after surgery. Due to the small amount of local soft tissue, if not handled properly, it is easy to cause the steel plate to be exposed

8 Time to remove steel plate

Initially, we believed that the steel plate could be removed 1 year after surgery, but some children experienced a recurrence of depression after the removal of the steel plate. Research has found that 1 year is not sufficient for the complete disappearance of chest wall deformities in children. In order to consolidate the therapeutic effect, we will ultimately

The time for removing the metal plate is extended to 2 years post-surgery. After this extension, relapses almost never occurred again.

9. Surgical Outcome

In past clinical work, we have used the Wang surgery to treat a large number of children with pectus excavatum, achieving very satisfactory results (Fig. 2-4-30).

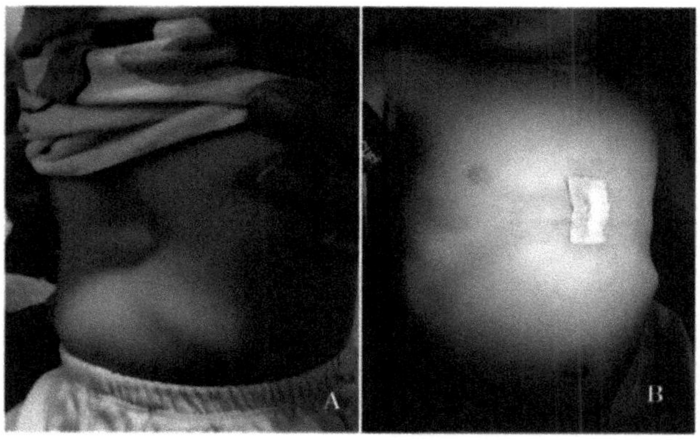

Figure 2-4-30 Results of Wang's procedure (Since the template molding principle was adopted, the appearance is almost entirely normal. A. Pectus excavatum deformity of the anterior chest wall; B. Postoperative chest wall appearance)

(5) Complex Pectus Excavatum Surgery

In clinical practice, aside from typical or simple pectus excavatum, there are also complex cases such as high-position pectus excavatum, large-area pectus excavatum, asymmetric pectus excavatum, pectus excavatum with rib arch protrusion, and extremely deep pectus excavatum. These special types require special techniques for correction. To achieve satisfactory results, the following principles must be adhered to during the procedure[1]:

(1) Flexibly choose surgical procedures. So far, there are various surgical methods available for clinical use. Each surgical method has its own advantages, and it is necessary to flexibly choose the surgical method according to the characteristics of the deformity. This approach can fully utilize the advantages of the surgery to achieve the most ideal results.

(2) Combination of different surgical techniques. For some patients, the surgery is too complex, and a single approach is insufficient to meet orthopedics needs. At this time, different surgical methods can be combined for correction, fully utilizing the advantages of each type of surgery in service of orthopedics to ensure a successful operation.

(3) Use other materials. The materials currently used in pectus excavatum surgery have essentially been standardized. For most deformity surgeries, these materials are already sufficient. However, for some special deformities, if other materials are involved in the correction, it might achieve unexpected results.
Not restricted to minimally invasive surgery. When faced with particularly complex cases, if minimally invasive surgery cannot achieve correction or poses significant risks, it is necessary to adopt open surgical procedures for treatment.

(5) Cannot do without Thoracoscopy. Thoracoscopy is a device used for operations within the thoracic cavity and offers certain assistance when passing through the mediastinum. However, this device is not necessary. If you can master other methods proficiently, you can completely do without such a device.

10. Steel Plate Removal Surgery

The steel plates implanted during pectus excavatum repair generally requires removal. The timing depends on the surgical method and individual recovery. Typically, plates from the Nuss procedure are removed after 3 years, while those from the Wang procedure are extracted at 2 years. Special circumstances may warrant earlier or delayed removal.

(1). Plate Removal in Nuss Procedure

The patient is placed in a supine position. Incisions are made along the old surgical scars on both sides of the chest wall to expose the plate. After removing the stabilizer bars and fixation wires, the plate is maneuvered out of the incision. A wrench is used to straighten the plate as much as possible before extracting it through one side.

While plate removal is usually straightforward, challenges may arise in the following scenarios:
① Prolonged implantation with callus formation. If the plate remains for over 3 years, callus may encase it, making extraction difficult.
② Plate notches lodged in the mediastinum or chest wall. If the plate's serrated edges embed in bony structures, bone rongeurs may be needed to clear the callus. If stuck in the mediastinum, forceful extraction must be avoided gentle repositioning is required.
③ Plate migration into the thoracic cavity. Poor initial fixation may cause the plate to slip between ribs into the chest. Prolonged placement can also lead to rib erosion, allowing the plate to penetrate the lung, causing atelectasis, inflammation, or functional loss. Removal in such cases may require partial rib resection and subsequent lung repair to prevent bleeding or air leaks.
The removal of the steel plate is relatively straightforward but can still lead to complications. The most serious complication is cardiac injury. Some plates have serrated ends that may cut into the heart, resulting in cardiac damage. There have been reports of patient deaths caused by heart injuries during plate removal, which represent extreme complications [45]. In addition to cardiac injury, massive bleeding can occasionally occur, primarily due to damage to chest wall or intrapulmonary blood vessels. Furthermore, removal of the plate

may injure lung tissue, leading to air leakage and bleeding.

Plate removal in Nuss surgery is often viewed as minor, but it can be highly complex in certain cases, with life-threatening risks. Thus, the procedure must never be underestimated.

(2) Wang Surgical Removal of Steel Plate

Wang, the surgery can be performed using two different types of plates, and the procedures for plate removal also differ. If a standard Wang surgical plate is used, the surgery can be completed with just a small incision at the site of the original surgical scar. The specific operation involves loosening the screw in the middle after exposing the steel plate, and then removing the two halves of the steel plate to complete the procedure. If the Nuss surgical plate is used, it is best to make a new incision on one side of the chest wall. First, loosen the central wire, and then remove the steel plate from the incision on the lateral chest wall. Relatively speaking, the procedure to remove the steel plate from Wang is easier, and complications are rare.

11. The prognosis of funnel chest surgery

(1). Criteria for evaluating effectiveness

The evaluation of the effectiveness of pectus excavatum surgery is a very subjective process, influenced by many factors. A more objective evaluation requires considering the opinions of multiple parties, rather than relying solely on the opinions of doctors or patients themselves. We once designed an evaluation system that fully considers the opinions of doctors, patients, and their families. The system scores according to different weights and ultimately evaluates the results based on the scores. This is a relatively satisfactory evaluation system.

(2) Surgical Outcome

The outcome of surgery can be one of four basic results: first, satisfactory; second, improvement; third, no change; and fourth, deterioration. For pectus excavatum, a type of depression deformity, a satisfactory result is achieved if the depression can be completely eliminated, bringing the appearance of the thorax to the level of a normal person. If the desired result is not achieved and the depth of the depression is only reduced, such a result can only be considered an improvement. If there is no change in the appearance of the thorax before and after the surgery, it is equivalent to no change. In some patients, the deformity becomes more severe after undergoing surgery, which is a very regrettable outcome, as it essentially leads to the worsening of the deformity.

For most people, whether doctors or patients, there are only two outcomes for surgery: either a successful surgery or a failed one. It's a binary choice with no middle ground [1]. Therefore, even if there is some improvement, many people still regard it as a failed surgery, which is an outcome that many patients and their families find unacceptable. This characteristic of evaluating surgical outcomes is unique to thoracic deformities, which places extremely high demands on the doctor's skills.

(3) Recurrence issue

Recurrence refers to the situation where the depression of the patient's anterior chest wall reappears after a successful surgery. Recurrence can occur before the removal of the plate, or it can occur after the removal of the plate. The recurrence time varies, and the reasons also differ.

Recurrence before removing the steel plate is often related to the displacement of the steel plate. Plate displacement is primarily related to surgical procedures and secondarily to individual patient factors. If the fixation is not secure or the method is problematic, the metal plate may undergo significant displacement. Once displacement occurs, the function of the steel plate to support the depression will be lost, and the depression will inevitably recur. The factors related to the patient are mainly associated with improper exercise or posture. If the patient engages in intense physical activity in the early postoperative period, it may cause the displacement of the plate, leading to a recurrence of the depression. Similarly, incorrect posture can also lead to recurrence. For example, adopting a lateral position too early may affect the position of the plate and, in severe cases, may lead to recurrence. It must be pointed out that although patient factors may cause a recurrence, such factors are secondary. If the fixation procedure during surgery is flawless, no matter how the patient moves or what posture they adopt, it will not affect the position of the plate, making recurrence impossible.

The recurrence after plate removal is also influenced by many factors: ① Issues related to surgical design. Some surgical designs are not very reasonable, which may leave hidden risks for recurrence. For example, during the Nuss procedure, the deepest part of the depression is not addressed, which is the area with the most severe deformity. This deformity persisted throughout the years of corrective post-operative care and remained even after the removal of the steel plate. This sets the stage for the recurrence of the depression. In contrast, the surgical operation performed by Wang was precisely located at the deepest point of the depression, which is the most severely deformed area. The likelihood of recurrence of the depression is significantly reduced by directly disrupting this area and providing thorough contouring. ② Doctor operation issue. The level of skill with which the doctor operates is directly related to the effectiveness of deformity correction. If there is a problem with the operation itself, it may cause a relapse. Some occurrences of pectus excavatum are related to the pulling of the underlying fibers. The safest method for such deformities is to eliminate local traction. If the doctor does not address the local traction during the procedure, once the plate is removed and the force supporting the depression is eliminated, the fibers may pull on the anterior chest wall and cause the depression to reappear. Such recurrences are clearly related to the physician's operational techniques. There are many other procedures in clinical practice that also affect the recurrence of deformities, such as the critical pre-shaping. If the doctor does not understand this procedure, postoperative complications may also lead to deformity recurrence. Issue of timing for removing the steel plate. No matter what type of surgery it is, postoperative healing is a long process that requires sufficient time. If the steel plate is removed too early, the likelihood of recurrence will increase.

Recurrence is a very troublesome outcome, signifying a complete failure of the surgery for the patient, who will suffer greatly as a result. For this reason, it is essential to take every patient seriously and strive to prevent recurrence.

12. Postoperative Rehabilitation Issues for Pectus Excavatum

After being discharged, patients with pectus excavatum face rehabilitation issues. The quality of recovery has a significant impact on the quality of surgery; therefore, doctors must provide professional guidance to patients during their recovery. Postoperative rehabilitation is generally divided into three stages [46]. The main purposes of hospitalization after surgery are to alleviate pain, promote incision healing, and prevent complications. During this time, some simple activities can be performed. The main goal from discharge to within three months after surgery is to eliminate the impact of surgical trauma, quickly regain physical strength, and resume normal daily activities. During this time, you can gradually increase your activity level and nutrition to allow the body to recover quickly. Three months after the surgery, the bone repair is basically complete, and the position of the steel plate is relatively fixed. At this time, patients can engage in general exercises and physical labor, but bodybuilding exercises are not recommended. Bodybuilding increases the volume of pectoral muscles, and if the muscles are too bulky, it can complicate the procedure of removing the steel plate. Therefore, it should be avoided as much as possible. Many patients are relatively thin and weak. To enhance the aesthetic appearance of the chest wall post-surgery, engaging in bodybuilding exercises after removing the steel plate can be beneficial. This will further help in altering the overall appearance of the chest wall, achieving a more perfect result.

REFERENCES

[1] Wang, W. L. 2021a. "Clarifications on Several Issues Regarding Pectus Excavatum." *Thoracic Deformity Surgery Expert*, November 6.

[2] Nuss, D., R. E. Kelly, D. P. Croitoru, et al. 1998. "A 10-Year Review of a Minimally Invasive Technique for the Correction of Pectus Excavatum." *Journal of Pediatric Surgery* 33: 545–552.

[3] Wang, W. L. 2016a. "Two Opposing Mechanisms in Pectus Excavatum Formation." *Thoracic Deformity Surgery Expert*, June 20.

[4] Wang, W. L. 2014. "Genetic Factors in Pectus Excavatum." *Thoracic Deformity Surgery Expert*, August 29.

[5] Wang, W. L. 2015. "Pathogenesis of Pectus Excavatum in Twins." *Thoracic Deformity Surgery Expert*, November 3.

[6] Wang, W. L. 2020a. "Direct Evidence of Genetic Factors in Pectus Excavatum: Wang Procedure Performed on Identical Twin Brothers." *Thoracic Deformity Surgery Expert*, November 9.

[7] Wang, W. L. 2020b. "Pectus Excavatum Following Pulmonary Cystadenoma Surgery." *Thoracic Deformity Surgery Expert*, October 24.

[8] Wang, W. L. 2020c. "Mechanism of Pectus Excavatum Formation after Congenital Diaphragmatic Hernia Repair." *Thoracic Deformity Surgery Expert*, November 24.

[9] Wang, W. L. 2013. "Thoracic Deformities Following Congenital Heart Surgery." *Thoracic Deformity Surgery Expert*, September 28.

[10] Wang, W. L. 2020d. "Secondary Pectus Excavatum." *Thoracic Deformity Surgery Expert*, April 6.

[11] Wang, W. L. 2021b. "MatrixRIB Chest Wall Reconstruction for Secondary Unilateral Thoracic Collapse." *Thoracic Deformity Surgery Expert*, July 7.

[12] Wang, W. L., C. M. Chen, W. G. Long, et al. 2015a. "Preliminary Study on the 'Thoracic Defect Hypothesis' in Pectus Excavatum Pathogenesis." *Journal of Practical Medicine* 31 (Suppl): 200–201.

[13] Wang, W. L. 2021c. "The Most Distinctive Characteristics of Pectus Excavatum." *Thoracic Deformity Surgery Expert*, July 7.

[14] Wang, W. L. 2021d. "Generalized Asymmetric Pectus Excavatum." *Thoracic Deformity Surgery Expert*, September 15.

[15] Wang, W. L. 2019. "Modified Wang Procedure for Extensive Pectus Excavatum." *Thoracic Deformity Surgery Expert*, May 31.

[16] Wang, W. L. 2021e. "Wing Procedure for High-Position Pectus Excavatum." *Thoracic Deformity Surgery Expert*, January 30.

[17] Wang, W. L. 2018a. "Off-the-Charts Haller Index: Minimally Invasive Surgery for Severe Grand Canyon-Type Pectus Excavatum." *Thoracic Deformity Surgery Expert*, November 21.

[18] Wang, W. L. 2021f. "Surgical Considerations for Acute Angle Deformities." *Thoracic Deformity Surgery Expert*, September 8.

[19] Wang, W. L., C. M. Chen, X. J. Li, et al. 2018. "Comprehensive Classification System for Thoracic Deformities." *Chinese Journal of Clinical Thoracic and Cardiovascular Surgery* 25 (11): 981–985.

[20] Wang, W. L. 2021g. "Acute Angle Deformities." *Thoracic Deformity Surgery Expert*, August 18.

[21] Sesia, S. B., M. Heitzelmann, S. Schaedelin, et al. 2019. "Standardized Haller and Asymmetry Index Combined for More Accurate Assessment of Pectus Excavatum." *Annals of Thoracic Surgery*

107 (1): 271–276.
[22] Wang, W. L. 2016b. "'Off-the-Charts' Haller Index: Successful Surgery for Extremely Severe Pectus Excavatum." *Thoracic Deformity Surgery Expert*, October 25.
[23] Wang, W. L. 2020e. "Negative Haller Index: Wang Procedure + Wenlin Procedure after Failed NUSS Surgery for Severe Pectus Excavatum." *Thoracic Deformity Surgery Expert*, November 17.
[24] Wang, W., W. Long, Y. Liu, et al. 2022a. "Wenlin Index of Pectus Excavatum." *International Journal of Surgery Science* 6 (3): 84–87.
[25] Wang, W. L. 2021h. "Another Serious Complication of Pectus Excavatum: Scoliosis." *Thoracic Deformity Surgery Expert*, May 12.
[26] Wang, W. L. 2021i. "Malignant Thoracic Deformity." *Thoracic Deformity Surgery Expert*, March 18.
[27] Wang, W., W. Long, Y. Liu, et al. 2022b. "Wenlin Triad of Pectus Excavatum." *International Journal of Case Reports in Surgery* 4 (1): 16–18.
[28] Brochhausen, C., S. Turial, F. K. P. Müller, et al. 2012. "Pectus Excavatum: History, Hypotheses and Treatment Options." *Interactive Cardiovascular and Thoracic Surgery* 14 (6): 801–806.
[29] Kanagaratnam, A., S. Phan, V. Tchantchaleishvili, et al. 2016. "Ravitch versus Nuss Procedure for Pectus Excavatum: Systematic Review and Meta-Analysis." *Annals of Cardiothoracic Surgery* 5 (5): 409–421.
[30] Liu, T., H. Liu, and Y. Li. 2014. "Comparison of the Nuss and Sternal Turnover Procedures for Primary Repair of Pectus Excavatum." *Asian Journal of Surgery* 37 (1): 30–34.
[31] Notrica, D. M. 2018. "Modifications to the Nuss Procedure for Pectus Excavatum Repair: A 20-Year Review." *Seminars in Pediatric Surgery* 27 (3): 133–150.
[32] Wang, W. L. 2017. "Structural Basis of NUSS Procedure." *Thoracic Deformity Surgery Expert*, September 24.
[33] Wang, W. L. 2018b. "Critique of Nuss Procedure Part 1: Trauma Issues." *Thoracic Deformity Surgery Expert*, February 26.
[34] Wang, W. L. 2018c. "Critique of Nuss Procedure Part 2: Age Limitations." *Thoracic Deformity Surgery Expert*, February 27.
[35] Wang, W. L. 2018d. "Critique of Nuss Procedure Part 3: Problems with Steel Plates." *Thoracic Deformity Surgery Expert*, February 28.
[36] Wang, W. L. 2018e. "Critique of Nuss Procedure Part 4: Recurrence Issues." *Thoracic Deformity Surgery Expert*, March 1.
[37] Wang, W. L. 2018f. "Critique of Nuss Procedure Part 5: Global Remodeling vs Micro-Remodeling." *Thoracic Deformity Surgery Expert*, March 2.
[38] Wang, W. L. 2018g. "Critique of Nuss Procedure Part 6: The Impact of Blind Worship on Treatment (Final Chapter)." *Thoracic Deformity Surgery Expert*, March 5.
[39] Wang, W. L. 2019b. "Fatal Complications of NUSS Procedure." *Thoracic Deformity Surgery Expert*, December 4.
[40] Wang, W. L. 2019c. "Plate-Related Complications after NUSS Procedure." *Thoracic Deformity Surgery Expert*, May 21.
[41] Wang, W. L. 2021j. "Wang Procedure vs Wang Procedure." *Thoracic Deformity Surgery Expert*, March 29.
[42] Wang, W., W. Long, Y. Liu, et al. 2022c. "Wang Technique: A Simple and Practical Steel Bar Fixation Technique in Thoracic Deformity Surgery." *International Journal of Surgery Science* 6 (3): 78–83.
[43] Wang, W. L., W. G. Long, and C. M. Chen. 2019. "Application of Wang Procedure in Pediatric Pectus Excavatum Treatment." *Journal of Southern Medical University* 39 (2): 249–252.
[44] Wang, W. L. 2019d. "Wang Procedure vs NUSS Procedure." *Thoracic Deformity Surgery Expert*, June 21.

[45] Wang, W. L. 2017b. "Fatal Complications during Plate Removal Surgery." *Thoracic Deformity Surgery Expert*, July 17.
[46] Wang, W. L. 2021k. "Rehabilitation Considerations after Thoracic Wall Surgery." *Jinri Toutiao*, November 2.

Pectus carinatum is the most common form of protrusive chest wall deformity and is considered by many to be the second most frequent chest wall deformity after pectus excavatum (Fig.2-5-1). However, this viewpoint is not supported by specific statistical data, and from the general public's perception, pectus carinatum seems to be more common than pectus excavatum. On one hand, this is related to the fact that pectus carinatum is more easily noticeable; on the other hand, it may also be related to its actual incidence. To thoroughly investigate the specific incidence rate, extensive survey data is required for support. Unfortunately, such data is currently lacking.

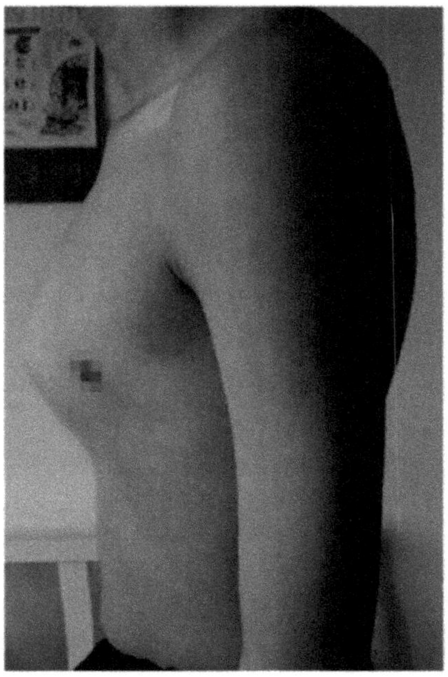

Figure 2-5-1 Appearance of Pectus Carinatum. The anterior chest wall exhibits significant protrusion, severely compromising aesthetic appearance.

1. Pathogenesis

There are many theories about the pathogenesis of chicken breast, the most common being that it is related to calcium deficiency and is a manifestation of rickets. Such a possibility exists, and it can be theoretically explained clearly [1,2]. However, in some identical twins, almost identical cases of pectus carinatum can be found, indicating that in addition to calcium deficiency, there are other causes that can lead to pectus carinatum [3]. Chicken breast can also occur after a median sternotomy, in which case it is referred to as secondary pectus carinatum, whereas those with unknown causes are referred to as primary pectus carinatum.

Secondary pectus carinatum is more common after cardiac surgery in young children (Fig. 2-5-2). Due to the sternum being split, the integrity of the thoracic cage is affected. At this time, the bone of the child patient is relatively soft, making it impossible to securely fix with wire. The deep surface of the incision is the heart, which is a structure filled with positive pressure fluid. Such a structure will continuously impact the anterior chest wall. Under the impact of this force, the damaged chest wall of the structure may gradually protrude forward, eventually forming a condition known as pigeon chest. This is a good explanation for the frequent occurrence of pectus carinatum after congenital heart disease surgery [4].

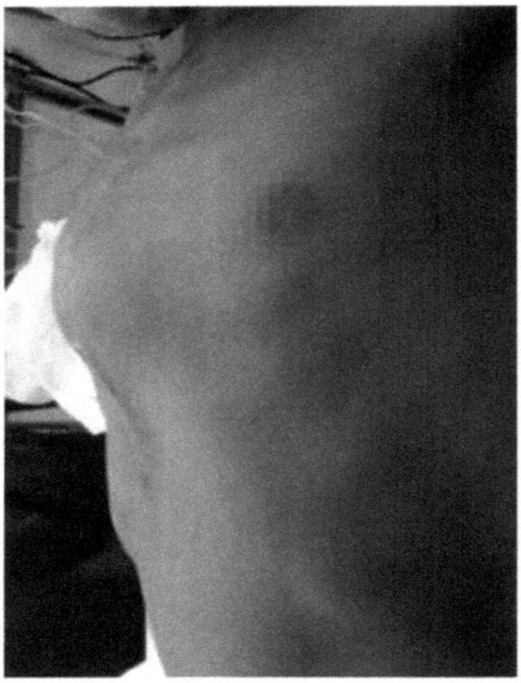

Figure 2 -5 -2 Secondary pectus carinatum post-cardiac surgery. This type of deformity is the most common thoracic deformity after cardiac surgery.

The mechanism by which rickets leads to pigeon chest is similar. Rickets is a manifestation of a systemic calcium deficiency, where the calcification of all bones is problematic, and the hardness of the bones is significantly insufficient. Since many muscles attach to the bones, in order to maintain human posture or perform certain movements, the muscles will exhibit continuous or intermittent tension. The location of muscle action is generally on the skeleton. When bone hardness is normal, its shape will not change. If there is an issue with hardness, the shape of the bones will change under the continuous tension of the muscles. For this reason, the bones that change shape in patients with rickets are typically those most affected by external forces, such as the bones of the lower limbs, which are the most commonly impacted areas. The mechanism of anterior chest wall protrusion deformity is similar. The reduction in the hardness of the bony structure of the chest wall, coupled with the heart continuously exerting positive pressure against the anterior chest wall, can similarly cause the chest wall to protrude forward and form a deformity (Figure 2-5-3)[1].

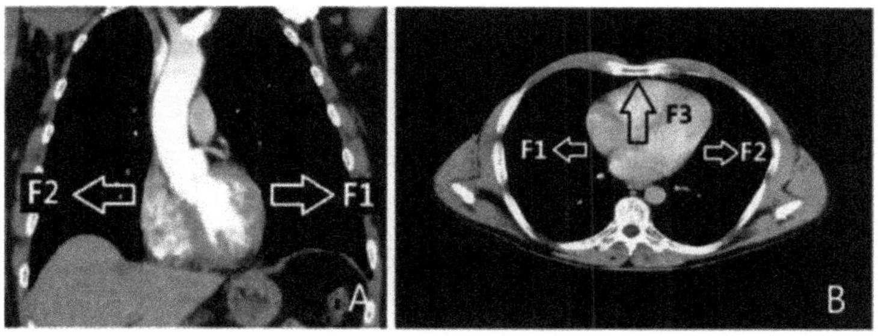

Figure 2-5-3 Mechanism of Chicken Breast Occurrence (A. The heart is a structure filled with high-pressure fluid, and its pressure varies with the heartbeat, resulting in intermittent impact force. This force can be released in all directions, including towards both sides of the chest cavity and the anterior chest wall. Releasing into both sides of the thoracic cavity has no substantial meaning. When the impact force of the heart is released to the anterior chest wall, if the anterior chest wall is relatively weak, it may protrude, eventually forming a pectus carinatum.

2. Pathological Characteristics

Pectus carinatum is a forward protrusion deformity of the anterior chest wall, where the local structure is significantly pushed forward, rising above the surrounding structures. This type of deformity generally involves the sternum. Deformities that involve only the ribs or costal cartilage with anterior protrusion are extremely rare and are mostly localized protrusion deformities. After the bony structure of the chest wall protrudes beyond the surface of the chest wall, it indicates that the local pathological structure is relatively longer than the normal structure, which is an objective fact. This matter provides a theoretical basis for the surgical removal of certain structures. However, clinical experience shows that such an operation is not necessary. Even without excision, a good corrective effect can still be achieved.

The chest wall deformity can be a symmetrical protrusion, or asymmetrical; the position can be high or low, and the extent can vary from large to small. Absolute or relative depressions beneath the protrusion can be consolidated. Absolute depression is an objectively existing visible depression. At this time, the deformity is a compound deformity, and related content will be discussed in other chapters. Relative depressions are actually just areas on the raised slope. Theoretically, there are no obvious depressions, but they are related to the outcome of the surgery. At this time, the deformity is still a simple pectus carinatum, and additional treatment is needed for the relative depression during surgery.

Pathological changes in the chicken breast have distinct age-related characteristics. Pathological changes in younger children are often not severe. With age, the anterior protrusion will gradually worsen. Particularly after reaching puberty, most children with anterior protrusion deformity experience a sudden worsening, not only in severity but also in the extent of the condition. Many children and their parents only become alert at this time and seek medical attention.

3. Clinical Manifestations

The sternum is located on the anterior chest wall. As with all thoracic deformities, if symptoms are present, they are certainly related to the organs within the thoracic cavity. Pectus carinatum, or pigeon chest, is a forward protrusion deformity that does not affect the organs within the thoracic cavity, and therefore, symptoms related to the respiratory or circulatory systems are rarely observed. However, his deformity can have a noticeable impact on appearance. Abnormalities in appearance can affect the patient's psyche, leading to various psychological issues [5]. Psychological issues can, in turn, affect the patient's physical health, leading to various related symptoms such as chest tightness and chest pain. It must be made clear that the appearance of these symptoms is not related to pressure on the lungs and heart or their functional abnormalities, but rather is an indirect effect caused by psychological issues.

The signs of pectus carinatum are very distinct, primarily manifested by the protrusion of the bony structure on the anterior chest wall. Generally, it is clearly visible to the naked eye, and apart from that, there are no other specific signs.

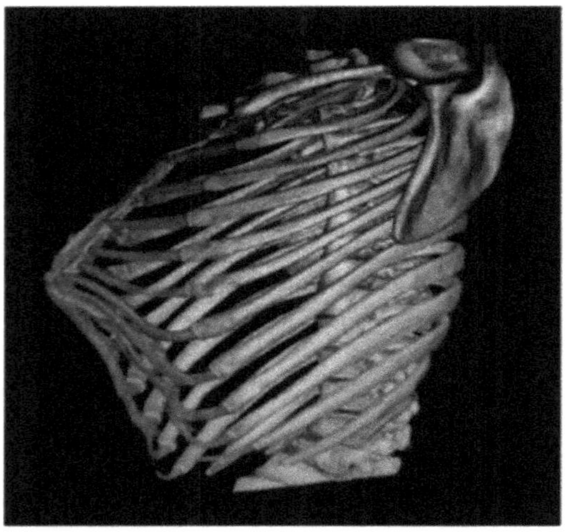

Figure 2-5-4
3-D reconstruction of pectus carinatum, demonstrating comprehensive visualization of the thoracic cage and the deformed region.

4. Examination

As with all other thoracic deformities, the examination of pectus carinatum begins with a basic physical examination, which generally provides the main information about pectus carinatum. Imaging examinations can clarify the specific shape of bones and provide information about the condition of thoracic organs. Three-dimensional reconstruction examination can clarify the overall structure of the thorax, which is very helpful for a comprehensive understanding of the characteristics of pectus carinatum (Figure 2-5-4). However, these checks are not necessary. Generally speaking, preoperative procedures only require an electrocardiogram and chest X-ray examination (Figure 2-5-5). Further examination is only necessary when there is suspicion of other combined lesions, and a CT scan may be considered (Figure 2-5-6).

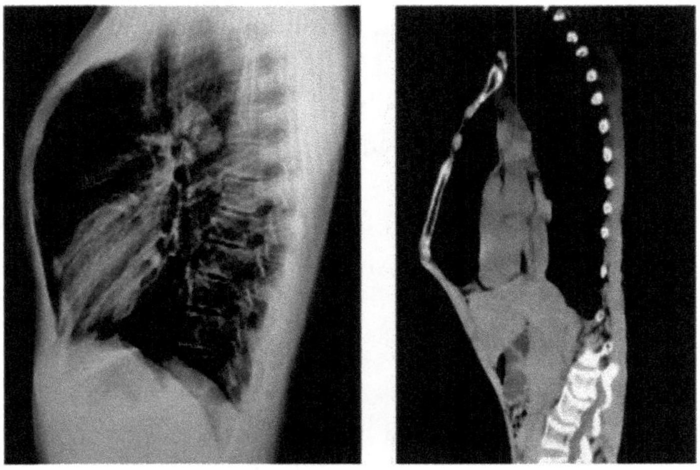

Figure 2-5-5 Radiographic findings of pectus carinatum. The lateral view demonstrates a 3 cm anterior chest wall protrusion

5. Diagnosis and Differential Diagnosis

The diagnosis of pectus carinatum is relatively straightforward, with the only diagnostic criterion being the protrusion of the bony structure of the anterior chest wall. Differential diagnosis needs to differentiate from Wenlin chest, localized protrusion deformity, Poland syndrome, combined deformity, saddle chest, and asphyxiating thoracic dystrophy (Jeune syndrome). Wenlin chest was previously mistaken for a type of pectus carinatum, but it is completely different from typical pectus carinatum, and the surgical concepts and methods are also entirely different, making it necessary to distinguish between them [6]. Wenlin. The chest protrusion is located at the level of the sternal angle. In addition to the sternal angle, the costal cartilage and ribs connected on both sides may also present an anterior protrusion. This type of anterior protrusion is relatively broad but is limited to the sternal angle and its sides, with a noticeable depression directly below it. The base of the depression is the sternum, which is thickened overall and appears as an "S" shape from the side. Localized protruding deformity is a local protrusion occurring in the ribs or costal cartilage. This deformity does not involve the sternum and is not a true pectus carinatum. Poland syndrome is characterized by underdevelopment of one side of the chest wall, making the unaffected side appear significantly higher than the affected side, which resembles an asymmetrical form of pectus carinatum. For female patients, due to the complete lack of development on one side of the chest wall, it is more likely to be considered as asymmetric pectus carinatum. This understanding is actually a form of bias. The so-called protrusion on the healthy side is only a relative protrusion, not an actual protrusion, and therefore cannot be diagnosed as pectus carinatum. Compound deformities have a noticeable protrusion of the chest wall, but because there is also a definite depression present, it cannot be considered a simple pectus carinatum. Saddle chest is a relatively rare deformity [8], characterized typically by depressions on both sides of the chest wall. Due to a significant difference in height, it appears as a protruding deformity, also known as pigeon chest. In fact, this protrusion does not actually exist; it is a relative protrusion caused by depressions on both sides. Such a deformity is not pectus carinatum. Patients with asphyxiating thoracic dystrophy often exhibit a protrusion deformity. This protrusion is actually a relative protrusion caused by the depression of the lateral chest walls and is therefore not a true pectus carinatum [9].

6. Indications for Surgery

The primary concern with pectus excavatum for patients is the appearance of the chest wall, and since most patients do not experience physiological harm, deciding on surgery is often a rather difficult decision. If surgical indications are deliberately set for such patients, it will instead bring a lot of trouble. To this end, our consistent practice is to leave the decision of whether to undergo surgery to the patient and their family. If the patient feels that it looks unattractive or is uncomfortable, surgery is necessary. If the patient neither feels uncomfortable nor finds it unsightly, surgery is not necessary. This principle is actually exactly the same as the principles of all other thoracic deformity surgeries.

7. Timing of Surgery

Chicken breast can occur at almost any age. Considering the natural development of the thorax and the progression of chicken breast itself, surgery is not suitable for every age. For younger children, due to the chest's strong self-repair capability, early surgical intervention for pectus carinatum is not recommended. However, if the deformity is too severe, the age restriction may not be considered. The most common patients in clinical practice are adolescents. This is mainly related to the characteristics of chest development. Such patients must undergo surgery as early as possible, otherwise, it will become increasingly severe. For pectus carinatum following heart surgery, since the cause is clear, the condition is almost impossible to resolve on its own. Therefore, once detected, surgery should be performed as soon as possible, regardless of the patient's age.

8. Surgical Treatment

Chicken breast is a very ancient disease, and its treatment also has a long history. The early surgical method was open surgery. In recent years, some minimally invasive surgical methods have gradually been used in clinical practice, leading to significant improvements in the treatment of pectus carinatum.

(1) Open Surgery

Open surgery primarily involves performing corrective procedures on deformities through a relatively long incision [10]. There are various specific methods, and one of the more commonly used methods is the sternal retraction technique. The basic theoretical basis of this method comes from a certain understanding of the onset of chicken breast. The theory suggests that pectus carinatum is caused by the overgrowth of ribs or costal cartilage. Since there is overgrowth, it should be excised. The specific method is to first expose all the costal cartilage, then remove all the costal cartilage, and finally fix the ribs to the sternum. Through such treatment, the protrusion deformity may be eliminated.

Open surgery is performed entirely under direct vision, making the operation relatively straightforward. However, there are many drawbacks to this type of surgery. First, the trauma is significant and the damage is apparent. This surgery requires the removal of all costal cartilage and entry into both pleural cavities. The extensive surgical field makes its damage particularly noticeable. The result is often unsatisfactory and cannot completely eliminate the anterior convexity, especially when there is a significant localized deformity of the sternum, and the result is difficult to guarantee. Fourth, it may lead to secondary thoracic dysplasia. After the rib cartilage is removed, the thorax itself becomes narrower. If the patient is an adolescent or young child, the removal of the costal cartilage will stunt the development of the thorax, resulting in secondary thoracic hypoplasia. When this occurs, another, more severe deformity develops.

(2) Minimally invasive surgery

(1) Abramson surgery
In 2005, Abramson reported a specific surgical approach [11]. In this method, a special Nuss surgical plate is used to compress the chest wall bulge, and then the plate is fixed to the ribs on both sides of the chest wall to correct the chicken breast. The Abramson procedure is performed by making an incision on both sides of the chest wall, parallel to the plane of the bulge at its highest level. The ribs inside the incision are freed, and a short fixation plate is fixed on top of the ribs, then a tunnel is made on the surface of the ribs towards the highest part of the projection in the centre, a steel plate is put into the tunnel, and a steel plate is pressed against the projections on the chest wall, and then both ends of the steel plate are inserted into the grooves in the middle of the plate to fix it, and then the incision is closed, and the operation is finished.
This method is generally the opposite of the Nuss procedure in principle, and has been called the “anti-Nuss procedure”. As a term of endearment, there is nothing wrong with describing the procedure in this way. However, if the details of the operation are carefully analysed, the two surgeries are not completely opposite, and therefore this name is inappropriate.
Naming a procedure after a familiar name is an ordinary thing to do. However, it reflects the fact that there is an unrealistic worship of a certain type of surgery. If one surgical concept is used to dictate the treatment of other deformities, it tends to have a direct influence on the design of the surgical procedure. This influence can lead the surgeon to incorporate other surgical concepts and materials into the new procedure, which is not only detrimental to the surgical process, but can also be very problematic.

The biggest disadvantage of the Abramson procedure is that it is heavily influenced by the Nuss procedure. This influence is manifested in two aspects: one is the surgical material, and the other is the surgical method. In terms of surgical materials, the use of the Nuss procedure's special steel plates was not inappropriate, but the use of fixation plates for immobilization was clearly an unwise choice. In terms of surgical method, the main issue is the fixation method of the plate. This is in fact a reference to the Nuss fixation method. In the Abramson procedure, the plate is first fixed to the rib, and then the main plate is inserted into the groove of the plate for fixation. This method may be easier to perform in a completely disembodied state, but in the actual operation of chicken breast surgery, it is extremely difficult to fix the plate with sufficient pressure. In addition, indirect fixation is generally unsatisfactory, which inevitably affects the final result of contouring. The Abramson procedure is a great success because of its borrowing from the Nuss procedure, but the Abramson procedure is a major drawback because of the problems associated with over-borrowing from the Nuss procedure (Figs. 2 - 5 - 7). In any case, the Abramson procedure was a revolution in the treatment of chicken breast and laid the foundation for the emergence of other excellent surgeries.

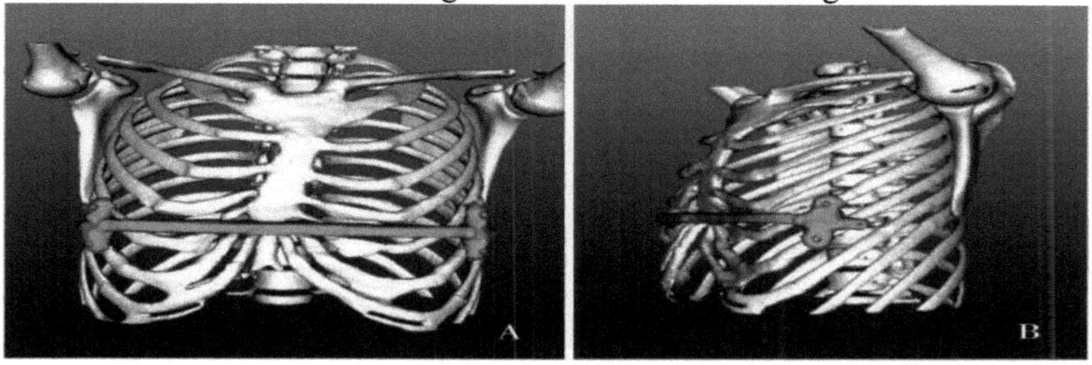

Figure 2-5-7 Position and fixation of the Abramson surgical plate (A. Both sides are fixed with short fixation plates; B. First, the short fixation plates are fixed to the ribs, and then the main plate is fixed, with the main plate indirectly fixed to the ribs)

(2) Wenlin Surgery

For a long time, we have been treating chicken breast deformity. Initially, we performed open surgery, but the results were unsatisfactory. Later, we began performing minimally invasive surgery, and the method we focus on is fundamentally different from the Abramson procedure. To distinguish it from this procedure, we named it the Wenlin procedure [12].

(i) Method of operation.

A longitudinal skin incision is made in the lateral chest wall parallel to the highest plane of the bulge, and the subcutaneous and muscular tissues are freed to reveal the ribs within the incision. Wire guides are placed around the ribs at the proposed fixation points. Tunnels are made deep into the chest wall muscle along the rib surfaces. After the chest wall tunnels on both sides have been passed through in the center, the introducer is placed into the tunnel, first guiding the plate guide tube, and then using the guide tube to guide the plate into the tunnel. The steel plate is placed into the tunnel. The steel wire is guided through the tunnel with a steel wire guide so that the steel wire encircles the rib and the steel plate at the same time. The steel wire is tightened sequentially to flatten the raised chest wall, and the two ends of the steel plate are securely fastened to the ribs on the lateral chest wall. The incision is closed and the procedure is completed (Figures 2-5-8 through 2-5-11).

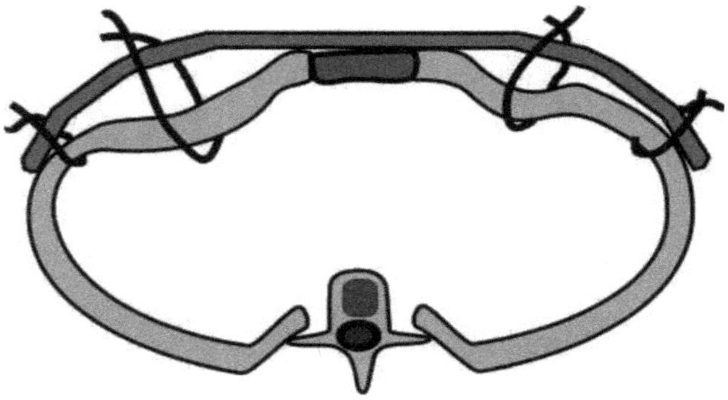

Figure 2-5-8 Schematic diagram of the Wenlin procedure. The procedure is a classic template Plasty, in which a steel plate is used as a template to Mold the chest wall structure to the shape of the plate.

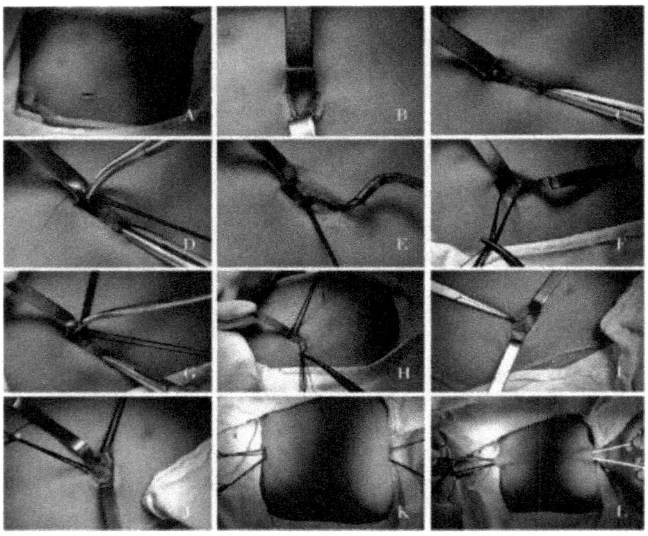

Figure 2-5-9 Wenlin procedure (1) (A. Make an incision in the lateral chest wall, the length of the incision is 1-2 cm; B. Expose the ribs; C. Place the wire guide across the ribs with a right-angle forceps, which is the position for fixation of the plate; D. Clamp the middle part of the wire guide with vascular pliers, and intersect it with the right-angle forceps; E. The right-angle forceps pulls the wire guide around the ribs; F. The vascular pliers clamp the wire guide in a standby; G. A second wire guide is placed in the same manner; H. Both wires are placed; I. An incision is made in the contralateral chest wall to expose the rib; J. Two wires are placed in the same manner on the contralateral side; K. Two wires are placed on each side; and L. Two vascular forceps are used to make a plate tunnel through the incision from both sides toward the center of the plate, with the tunnel located on the surface of the bony structure. The Wang technique for fixation of plates is routinely used in this procedure)

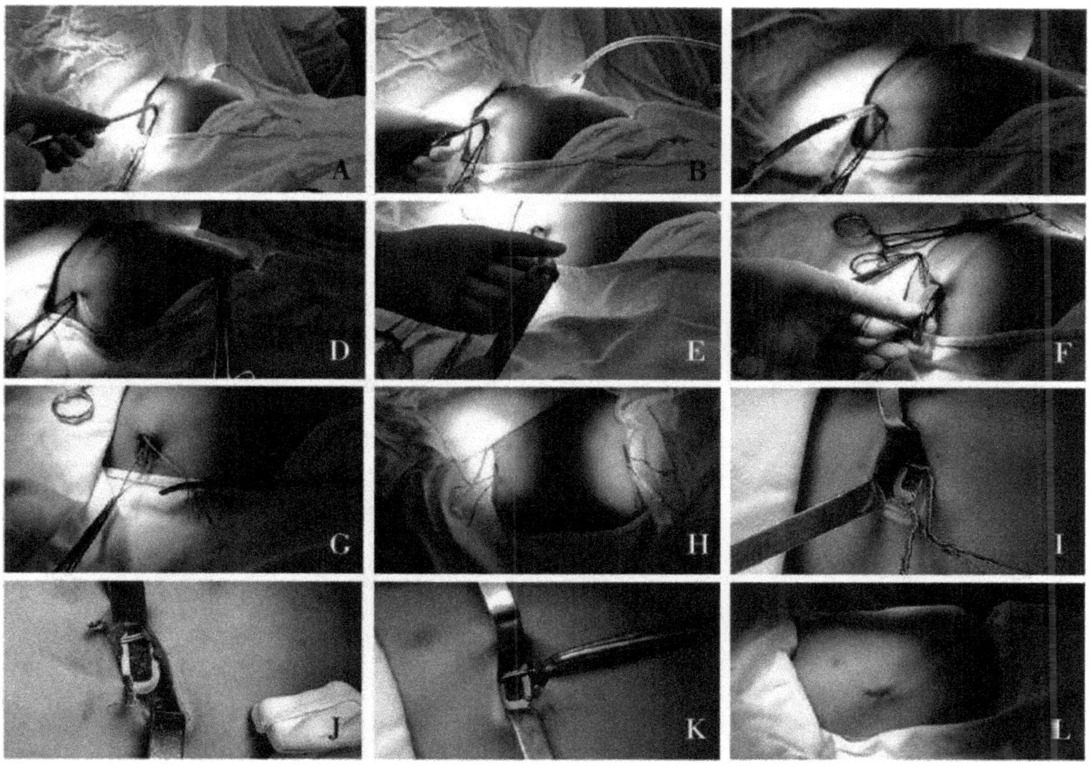

Figure 2-5-10 Wenlin Surgical Procedure Method (2): (A. The introducer is passed through the tunnel, entering through an incision on one side of the chest wall and exiting from the incision on the opposite side. B. The introducer is connected to the steel plate guide tube; C. The introducer pulls the steel plate guide tube into the tunnel, entering from one side and exiting from the other side; D. The steel plate guide tube is positioned within the tunnel, with both ends extending outside the chest wall incisions on both sides; E. The steel plate guide tube is connected to the steel plate; F. The steel plate is pulled into the tunnel, with both ends of the plate located outside the chest wall incisions on both sides; G. The steel wire guide line guides the steel wire, which just wraps around the ribs and the steel plate; H. Four steel wires on both sides are tightened simultaneously to fix the steel plate onto the ribs; I. Local view of the steel wire fixation; J. Cut the steel wires; K. Embed the cut ends of the steel wires; L. Close the incision to complete the surgery. In this procedure, the Wang technique for fixing the steel plate is routinely used.

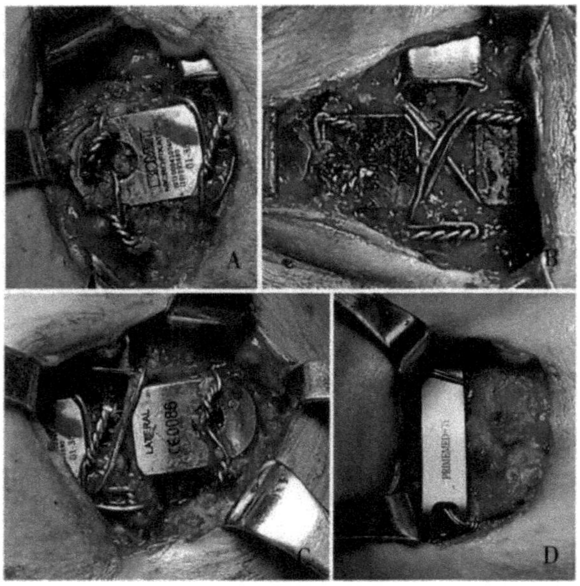

Figure 2 - 5 - 11 Differences between the Wenlin procedure and the Abramson procedure for fixation of the ends (A, B, C. The Abramson procedure has a standard indirect fixation of the main plate over the rib by means of a short fixation plate. This method is highly injurious, takes up a lot of space, and is complicated to perform. D. The Wenlin procedure, in which the plates are fixed directly to the ribs, is simple to perform and takes up very little space.)

(ii) Operative points.

The Wenlin procedure is a safe and simple operation, but to obtain good results, it is necessary to master the basic operating principles. These include, first, choosing the right length of plate. The length of the plate is essential to the completion of the contouring process, and should be neither too long nor too short. Generally, the length of the plate should be determined in relation to the site of fixation, and this should be done during the preoperative preparation. Secondly, the curvature of the plate should be reasonably shaped. If the curvature of the plate is too large, it will not be possible to produce enough compression and will not be able to shape the plate; if the curvature of the plate is too small, it will be counterproductive and will not give a good result. The setting of the curvature of the plate can be done at the surgical site. Adjustments are made while compression is being applied, so that the optimal curvature can be obtained. Third, the right number of plates should be prepared. for chicken breast with limited bulge, one steel plate may obtain good results. However, if the bulge is more severe, or if the bulge is more extensive, two or even more plates are needed to fulfill the needs of the surgery. The number of plates needs to be decided before surgery. Fourth, the appropriate fixation position should be chosen. There are two factors to consider, one is the need for contouring and the other is the need for stress distribution. The need for contouring is mainly due to the need for template shaping, and fixation should be done in every relatively concave area. The need for stress dispersion, on the other hand, requires fixing in different areas. The fixing should not only take into account the part of the rib, but also the part of the steel plate. This is the basic requirement for stress dispersion. Its Fifth, to master the appropriate fixation strength. The fixation of chicken breast is fundamentally different from the fixation of funnel chest. The fixation of the funnel chest is for simple fixation, but the essence of chicken chest fixation is for pulling, so we can't screw all the wires extra tightly. Too tight wire may not only lead to overkill, but also cause fracture, leading to surgical failure, so the fixation of the wire must have an appropriate degree, and moderation is the basic principle. Sixth, the principle of gradual progress should be followed. In the process of fixation, because it is impossible to start fixation after all plates have been placed, there must be a sequence. After placing the first steel plate, not all the wires can be tightened. If this is done too tightly, extreme stresses will be generated, which can lead directly to breakage of the wires or ribs, and should therefore be avoided as much as possible. A reasonable operation should be to apply force in several places at the same time and to fixate evenly, and only in this way can complications be avoided. Seventh, the order of operations should be clarified. Since all operations are completed in a very small operating space, if the order of operation is too arbitrary, it will make the whole operation confused and seriously affect the operation process. Eighth, to deal with relative depression. Many chicken breasts will have relative depression. In order to avoid the appearance of depression deformity, I need to be orthopedics. The specific method is to correct the depression by placing a wire in the depression. This serves two purposes: one is to lift the depression directly and the other is for plate fixation. Both of these roles are in fact the basic requirements of moldboard shaping.

(iii) Main advantages

The Wenlin procedure also uses a steel plate to directly compress the anterior chest wall bulge, but the specific method is significantly different from that of the Abramson procedure. This difference is mainly reflected in the most crucial fixation method: first, the concept of fixation is different; the concept of fixation in the Abramson operation is only to provide sufficient force for the compression of the plate, and this concept is the basis for the completion of the operation. However, this concept ignored the mechanical properties of the fixation site and did not even carefully consider the characteristics of the fixation device, which ultimately made the fixation an indirect fixation, i.e., indirectly fixing to the ribs by means of a short fixation plate. This type of fixation is not only weak, but also extremely difficult to manipulate. In contrast, the concept of Wenlin's surgical fixation is to contour, and to do so in the most direct way possible with a template. The ultimate goal of this molding is not to compress the chest wall, but rather to bring the various parts of the chest wall in close proximity to the chest wall. This philosophy is clearly different from that of the Abramson procedure. In order to achieve a tight fit to the chest wall, the Wenlin procedure directly fixes the plate to the ribs, which not only simplifies the procedure, but also provides a more accurate result (Figures 2-5-8 through 2-5-12). Secondly, the method of fixation is different. Almost all of the details of fixation in the Wenlin procedure are different from those in the Abramson procedure, which utilizes the revolutionary Wang technique of plate fixation, whereas the Abramson procedure is very outdated, and the Wenlin procedure is extremely simple, whereas the latter's fixation is quite complex and difficult. Thirdly, the fixation sites are different, Wenlin surgery has fully considered the limit of the ribs to withstand the tension of fixation, in order to avoid the fracture of the ribs under the strong external force, it is common to use two or even three ribs for fixation, so that the stress of the plate can be effectively dispersed. In addition, since the fixation area is located either on the inside or near the end of the plate, it is possible to realize the molding function of the template, which results in a better molding effect (Fig. 2-5-13). This feature is particularly important in the case of particularly severe types of localization, which is an advantage that the Abramson procedure cannot match. Fourth, the number of fixations is different. In order to adequately distribute the stresses, the number of fixations is randomized and flexible. The number of fixation sites is mainly related to two factors: one is the site of fixation, and the other is the number of plates to be fixed. The number of fixing points can be two or three, depending on the requirements. The number of fixation plates can be one, two or even three plates as required. This is the basic requirement for Wenlin surgical fixation. Through the reasonable allocation of the number of plates, the stress can be fully dispersed, and therefore the fixation effect can be minimized. In contrast, the Abramson procedure has only one fixation site. In contrast, the Abramson procedure has only one fixation site, which is obviously not conducive to the distribution of stress, and therefore the results are not satisfactory. If two or more plates are used in the Abramson procedure, the fixation area will be extremely constricted and crowded due to the presence of the fixation plates, which not only affects the fixation effect, but also necessitates a large incision, which is a disadvantage of the surgical design.

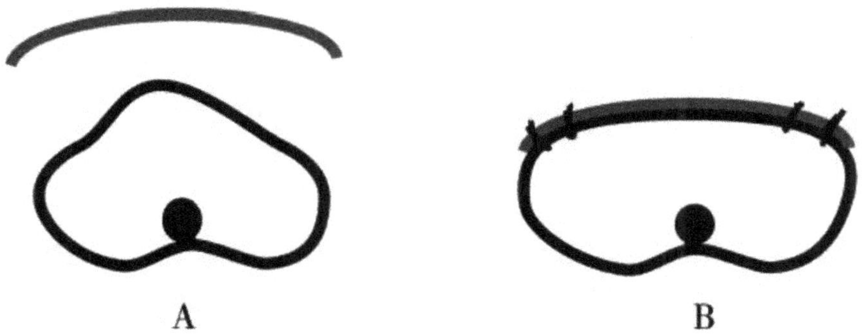

Figure 2 - 5 - 12 Principles of template shaping for the Wenlin procedure (two key elements: first, the template must be close to the shape of the normal target thorax; second, it must be securely fastened. A. Shape of the template in relation to the anterior thoracic wall; B. Shape of the template after shaping)

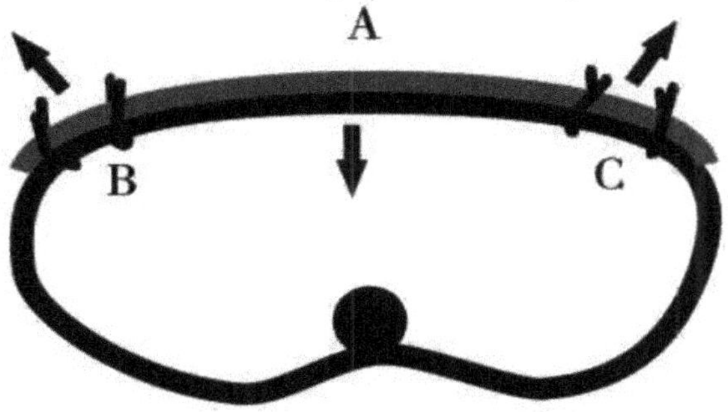

Figure 2 - 5 - 13 force analysis of the Wenlin procedure. Pressure is exerted on the anteriorly convex chest wall in the center of the plate, and external forces are exerted on both sides of the plate, first by the operator and then, through fixation, on the ribs on both sides of the chest wall, resulting in an equilibrium of forces, and the resultant contouring.

In addition to the advantages of fixation, the Wenlin procedure has the following advantages: First, it is minimally invasive. The procedure requires only a small operation on the lateral chest wall to complete the contouring, so the trauma is minimal and it is truly minimally invasive. Secondly, the postoperative scars are small and hidden: Wenlin incisions are small, usually less than 1.5cm in length, and are located on the lateral chest wall, which makes the postoperative scars more aesthetically pleasing. Thirdly, the surgery is safe and reliable. All operations are performed on the surface of the bony structures. Since it does not enter the chest cavity, it will not cause damage to important

organs, so it is very safe and generally will not lead to serious complications. Fourthly, the effect of molding is ideal. Through standardized operation, perfect results can generally be obtained. This fully reflects
the. superiority of template shaping

(iv) Major flaws.
No surgery can be perfect, and the Wenlin procedure, too, has its own drawbacks. for one thing, the shallow location of the plate has a negative effect on the soft tissues of the body surface. If the patient is thin and weak, localized soft tissue necrosis in the vicinity of the plate may occur, resulting in related complications. Second, in some patients, obvious traces of the plate can be seen on the body surface, which may affect the appearance of the thorax before the plate is removed. Thirdly, the stress is concentrated on the ribs of the lateral chest wall, if the ribs themselves are thin and cannot provide enough counter force, the surgical effect will be affected.
Minimally invasive surgery for chicken breast is a more popular surgical procedure nowadays, and the Abramson procedure is mainly performed abroad, but it is not widely carried out, and a few hospitals in China are also using the Abramson procedure. In recent years, we have assisted a large number of hospitals in China to carry out Wenlin surgery. Due to the obvious advantages of this surgery, it was quickly popularized in a large area, and now it has become the mainstream technique of chicken breast correction.

(3) Surgical complications
Whether it is Abramson surgery or Wenlin surgery, complications may occur during the operation, these complications include the following:

(1) Wire breakage. Since the plate is secured to the rib by means of a wire, the wire will ultimately bear the force, whether the fixation is indirect or direct. If the force is too great and the steel wire is not hard enough, it may result in the wire breaking. When the wire breaks, the forces loaded on the plate will be released, causing the end of the plate to buckle, which may puncture the incision and protrude out of the body, resulting in failure of the surgery. Wire breakage is a purely technical problem that needs to be prevented from a technical point of view.

(2) Rib fracture. Rib fracture is similar to, but different from, wire fracture. Rib fracture indicates an over-concentration of localized stress, and to prevent this complication, measures must be taken to disperse the stress.

(3)Delayed healing of the incision. Due to the presence of a steel plate in the incision, delayed healing of the incision may occur if there is little local soft tissue or if there is poor circulation. If not handled properly, the plate may have to be removed, which will result in surgical failure.

(4)Secondary concave deformity. Many anterior convex deformities that are flattened develop structural changes in the opposite direction and may be localized as depressions. This deformity becomes more pronounced over time. Depression of the deformity occurs in association with relatively long ribs or rib cartilage at the site of the convexity, which is a relatively common complication. There are three basic measures that can be taken to avoid the development of a depression: firstly, compression should be moderate and not excessive; secondly, the plate should be removed early; and thirdly, an additional plate can be used to support the base of the depression. With these three measures, the development of depressed deformity can usually be avoided.

(5)Impairment of lung function. In some patients, respiratory compromise occurs after resolution of the anterior convexity deformity. This is related on the one hand to the decrease in thoracic volume and on the other hand to the compression of the lungs. However, this impairment is usually relative or temporary, and the symptoms will disappear with time.

9. Plate removal surgery

In all minimally invasive surgeries for chicken breast, a special plate is used for correction. The plate is a foreign body and cannot be retained for life, but must be removed after a certain period of time. Generally, the plates can be removed within 1 - 2 years after surgery, depending on the recovery. If there are complications, the plate may need to be removed earlier. If the chest looks good after surgery, it can be left in place for a longer period of time.

Chicken breast surgery is very safe as the plate is completely on the surface of the bony structure and does not involve any organs in the chest cavity. The plate can be removed by completely loosening the wire. Since most of the plates are straight, there is no need to straighten them and they are easy to remove.

10. Prognosis

The vast majority of patients with chicken breast can achieve satisfactory results after surgery. In the case of pre-pubertal patients, no recurrence can be ensured in adulthood. The results are equally satisfactory in adult patients with chicken breasts (Figures 2-5-14 and 2-5-15). Of course, a successful prognosis is based on successful surgery. If the surgery itself is unsuccessful, or if there are complications associated with it, the outcome can be seriously compromised.

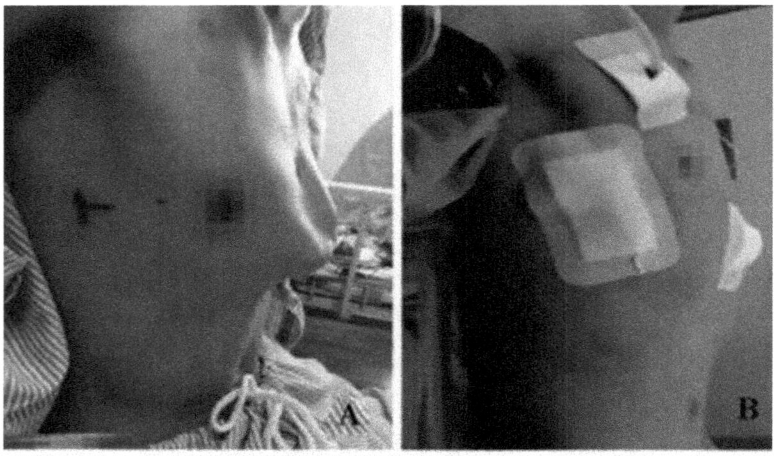

Figure 2 - 5 - 14 Wenlin procedure for chicken breast (A. Preoperative chest wall appearance of an extremely severe chicken breast; B. Results after Wenlin procedure)

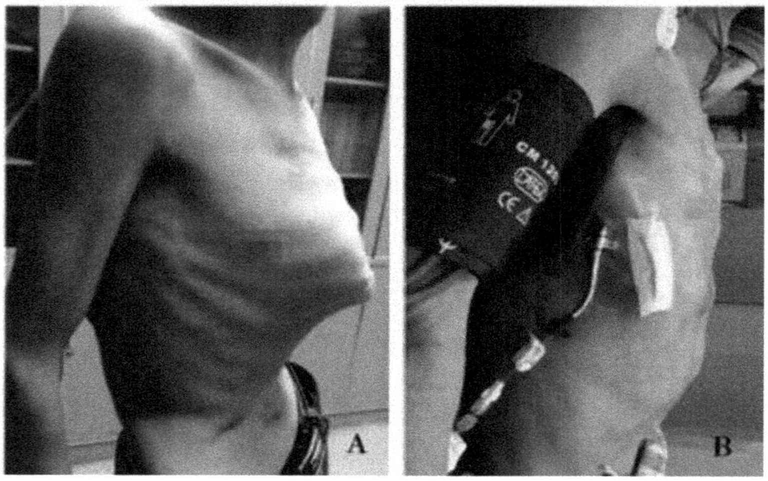

Figure. 2 - 5 - 15 Wenlin operation for severe chicken breast (A. Severe anterior chest wall anterior convexity, large and extensive, with invagination of the costal arches; B. Wenlin operation with three plates, with satisfactory results)

REFERENCES

[1] Wang, W. L. 2017a. "Why Do Patients with Rickets Tend to Form Chicken Chest Rather than Funnel Chest?" *Thoracic Deformity Surgery Specialist*, February 19.
[2] Wang, W. L. 2021a. "Not All Protuberance Development Is Associated with Rickets." *Thoracic Deformity Surgery Specialist*, September 10.
[3] Wang, W. L. 2017b. "Evidence for the Inheritance of Chicken Chest: The Li Sheng Brothers and Their Family." *Thoracic Deformity Surgery Specialist*, February 20.
[4] Wang, W. L. 2020a. "Nanning Surgery Today: The Wenlin Procedure for Severe Chicken Chest after Cardiac Surgery." *Thoracic Deformity Surgery Specialist*, May 16.
[5] Wang, W. L. 2021b. "Heart Disease and Mental Illness in Patients with Chicken Breast." *Thoracic Deformity Surgery Specialist*, April 28.

[6] Wang, W. L. 2021c. "Wenlin Chest: Not Chicken Chest + Funnel Chest." *Thoracic Deformity Surgery Specialist*, October 24.
[7] Xu, B., T. Liu, and C. J. Liu. 2020. "Breast Reconstruction with Perforator Flaps in Poland Syndrome: Report of a Two-Stage Strategy and Literature Review." *Breast Care (Basel)* 15 (4): 421–427.
[8] Wang, W. L. 2017c. "Nomenclature and Morphological Features of Saddle Chest." *Journal of Practical Medicine* 33 (Suppl): 380–381.
[9] Wang, W. 2022. "Surgical Treatment of a 36-Year-Old Patient with Asphyxiating Thoracic Dysplasia." *Interactive Cardiovascular and Thoracic Surgery* 34 (1): 153–155.
[10] Scarci, M., L. Bertolaccini, N. Panagiotopoulos, et al. 2016. "Open Repair of Pectus Carinatum." *Journal of Visualized Surgery* 2: 50.
[11] Abramson, H., X. Aragone, J. B. Blanco, et al. 2016. "Minimally Invasive Repair of Pectus Carinatum and How to Deal with Complications." *Journal of Visualized Surgery* 2: 64.
[12] Wang, W. L. 2019. "Wenlin Procedure for Severe Chicken Breast in Women." *Thoracic Deformity Surgery Specialist*, March 26.

Section 6

Flat Chest

Flat chest is one of the four most traditional types of thoracic deformities. There are no precise data on its incidence, but it is generally believed to be lower than that of pectus excavatum and pectus carinatum. However, this perception is actually inaccurate, and the underlying reason is closely related to the level of attention it receives. Pectus excavatum and pectus carinatum are widely recognized as diseases that attract significant attention from both clinicians and patients. Once a condition is acknowledged as a disease, the number of patients seeking medical attention naturally increases. Typically, incidence rates are calculated based on hospital statistics: the more patients who seek treatment, the higher the recorded incidence. This is the fundamental reason why the reported incidence of pectus excavatum and pectus carinatum appears relatively high. In contrast, a flat chest receives far less attention. Patients and their families often do not regard it as a disease, and even many healthcare professionals do not recognize it as such. When a deformity is widely overlooked as a disease, its true incidence inevitably appears low. From a clinical perspective, however, flat chest is a very real thoracic deformity. It is classified as such in various medical textbooks precisely because it possesses the essential characteristics of a deformity—therefore, it must be regarded as a disease, and an important one at that.

As one of the common thoracic deformities, flat chest has distinct structural characteristics: the anteroposterior diameter of the thorax is significantly shortened, the normal curvature of the anterior chest wall is lost, and the chest appears flat in outward appearance. This deformity is named precisely for the flat appearance of the chest wall.

1.Incidence

Flat Chest is a deformity closely related to age.

Before puberty, children rarely have a flat chest. Clinically, patients with flat chest are generally seen during or after puberty. This characteristic is associated with the natural development of the thorax. At birth, the anteroposterior diameter of the thorax is relatively large, and the chest typically appears barrel-shaped. With increasing age, the anteroposterior diameter gradually shortens, forming a slightly flattened shape. However, the physiological flattening is not the same as pathological flat chest. Pathological flat chest usually begins during puberty and represents a more pronounced flattening (Figure 2-6-1).

The pathogenesis of the flat chest remains unclear. Due to its morphological similarity to large-area pectus excavatum, the two conditions may share a similar mechanism of development. However, since the pathogenesis of pectus excavatum itself has not been definitively explained, the mechanism underlying flat chest also remains uncertain. The underlying mechanisms still require further investigation.

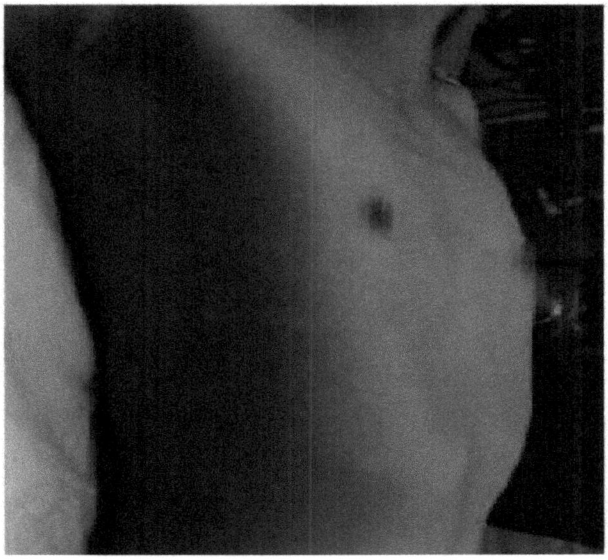

Figure 2-6-1 Appearance of thin gauze. The chest wall does not have a normal curvature, and the large thin gauze

2. Hazards

As with all other thoracic deformities, pectus planum (flat chest) poses two main types of harm: physiological and psychological. The physiological harm is primarily related to compression by the anterior chest wall. Because both the lungs and the heart may be compressed, patients can develop corresponding functional problems. Many patients with pectus planum are markedly thin, which may be associated with impaired digestive function. The digestive issues may result either from direct compression of the stomach by the lower anterior chest wall or indirectly from the effects of respiratory and circulatory compromise on the digestive system. The psychological harm stems from the impact on physical appearance. Many patients experience feelings of inferiority due to the shape of the chest, which can lead to a range of psychological issues.

3. Clinical Manifestations

Flat chest is commonly seen in tall, slender young individuals. Due to excessive thinness, in many cases the condition is not recognized as a thoracic deformity but is instead regarded simply as leanness. Because patients may be asymptomatic, it is often difficult to consider this a disease.

Flat chest is prone to be associated with spontaneous pneumothorax. In many cases, the flat chest is first identified when the patient seeks treatment for spontaneous pneumothorax [1]. This is a distinguishing feature of this deformity. The mechanism by which flat chest predisposes to spontaneous pneumothorax is complex, and although many have attempted to elucidate the connection, the results remain inconclusive.

Most patients with a flat chest have no symptoms. In severe cases, patients may experience mild exertional dyspnea, but symptoms are generally not significant. Some patients are dissatisfied with the appearance of the chest wall, and in severe cases, psychological problems may arise.

The physical signs of flat chest are fairly typical: physical examination reveals a flat anterior chest wall, and signs of cardiac compression may be present. If spontaneous pneumothorax is present, related signs may be observed. On lateral chest X-ray, the anterior chest wall appears flattened, with evidence of cardiac compression; the frontal view generally shows no positive findings. CT scans may demonstrate loss of the normal anterior chest wall curvature, cardiac compression with slight leftward displacement, and occasionally apical pulmonary bullae (Figure 2–6–2).

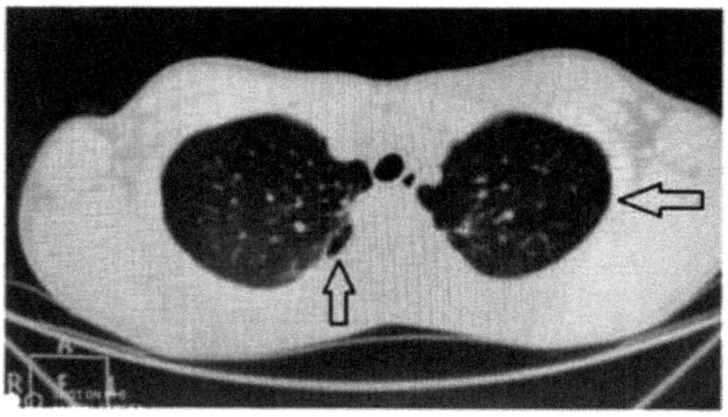

Figure 2–6–2. Patients with flat chest often have concomitant pulmonary bullae, which may rupture and cause spontaneous pneumothorax. Such patients frequently present for medical attention due to spontaneous pneumothorax.

4. Diagnosis and Differential Diagnosis

The diagnosis of flat chest (pectus planus) is relatively straightforward and can be confirmed through a simple physical examination. Imaging studies can help assess whether there is cardiac compression or the presence of pulmonary bullae, which is useful for surgical planning. Flat chest needs to be differentiated from extensive pectus excavatum [2]. Pectus excavatum is a type of depression deformity, in which depression is the sole pathological feature In a flat chest, there is no actual depression in the anterior chest wall, so the distinction is clear. However, a flat chest can sometimes be combined with pectus excavatum. In this combined deformity, the entire anterior chest wall is generally flattened, with a local depression in the center, forming a composite deformity of flat chest with pectus excavatum. The treatment for such a composite deformity is different from that for simple flat chest or isolated pectus excavatum, and requires a specialized approach for correction.

When making a differential diagnosis of flat chest, another condition to consider is straight back syndrome [3]. Also known as "pseudo-heart disease," the primary pathology of straight back syndrome is in the spine rather than the heart. The loss of the normal physiological curvature of the thoracic spine reduces the distance between the spine and the anterior chest wall, causing compression of the heart and other vital organs, which leads to a series of clinical symptoms. Patients with straight back syndrome often also have flat chests. The presence of a flat chest may further aggravate cardiac compression, significantly worsening the symptoms. In such cases, surgical correction of the flat chest is almost the only way to relieve symptoms.

In addition to the above conditions, it is also important in clinical practice to distinguish flat chest from a generally slender body habitus. Patients with a true flat chest have obvious chest wall features: the entire chest is flat, and the anterior chest wall lacks the normal curvature. By contrast, a slender physique mainly shows reduced soft tissue coverage, but the anteroposterior diameter is not shortened, and the anterior chest wall maintains a normal curvature, resulting in a normal-appearing chest with no deformity. Such a chest should not undergo surgery.

5. Surgical Treatment

Once the diagnosis of flat chest is confirmed, the next issue to consider is surgery, which is a major concern for both patients and doctors. Unlike pectus excavatum and pectus carinatum, opinions on surgery for flat chest vary greatly. One relatively conservative view does not regard this deformity as a disease and strongly rejects surgical treatment—especially when the patient has no symptoms. The second view is more proactive and supports undergoing surgery. Regarding the need for surgery, doctors must adhere to a basic principle: the decision should ultimately rest with the patient and their family. If the patient feels that the appearance is unsightly or experiences discomfort, then it amounts to both a physical and psychological condition. Since it is a disease, it should be treated, and if conservative methods cannot resolve it, surgery must be performed. Conversely, if the patient does not feel self-conscious or uncomfortable, then the deformity is essentially not seen as a disease. In that case, there is no need for treatment, and certainly no need for surgery.

(1) Surgery for isolated flat chest

From the overall classification of chest wall deformities, flat chest belongs to Type I deformities, specifically the I-g subtype [4]. The most distinctive feature of this type of deformity is depression. Flat chest is regarded as an overall depression of the anterior chest wall. This understanding is significant for treating flat chest, because for depression-type deformities, two relatively mature surgical methods currently exist: one is the Nuss procedure, and the other is the Wang procedure. Viewing flat chest as a depression-type deformity is essentially to better apply these existing techniques for its treatment.

However, it must be acknowledged that this so-called depression is not a true depression in the strict sense — its essence is still flatness. Therefore, when using surgical methods specifically designed for true depression deformities, adjustments must be made based on the actual situation. The Nuss procedure is designed for classic pectus excavatum. It relies on two structural elements: a central depression and relatively elevated surrounding edges. These two elements provide the basic conditions needed for the Nuss procedure to work. As previously discussed, the fundamental principle of the Nuss method is the lever principle, which involves lifting the depression by using the raised surrounding structures as a fulcrum. Pectus excavatum naturally has this structural basis, so the Nuss procedure can be effective. However, the flat chest does not have this structural foundation; in other words, the flat chest lacks sufficiently high fulcrums. Without high enough fulcrums, the lever cannot function properly, and the procedure is unlikely to succeed. Clinically, there are often cases where the Nuss procedure has failed for flat chest patients. The root cause is clear: the structural characteristics of a flat chest make it unsuitable for this procedure. Such failed cases seem to contradict the logic of classifying flat chest as a depression-type deformity since flat chest is treated as a type of depression and the Nuss procedure is specifically for treating depressions, it should theoretically be effective. Yet, in reality, it often fails. From this analysis, it becomes clear that the cause of failure is obvious: it is the problem of the fulcrum. The "depression" in flat chest is visually obvious, but what is conspicuously missing is the fulcrum. If the issue of the fulcrum can be resolved, then the surgical challenge is no longer an issue.

According to the basic principles of the lever mechanism, a fulcrum should have three essential properties: 1. sufficient height; 2. sufficient rigidity; 3. satisfactory stability. Based on these three requirements, a fulcrum with adequate height must be positioned close to the plane of the anterior chest wall. Such a location is generally much higher than the fulcrum position used in a standard Nuss procedure for pectus excavatum — meaning it is closer to the midline. Selecting this type of fulcrum can satisfy the requirement for height. The anterior chest wall bones of patients with flat chest deformity are generally quite rigid, so the requirement for rigidity can also be met. If height and rigidity are relatively easy to secure, the critical issue then becomes the third factor — stability. In practice, the stability of the fulcrum is the decisive factor that determines whether the surgery will succeed. Considering the direction of the ribs and the position of the implanted steel bar, the most stable fulcrum position should ideally be on a rib surface that is perpendicular to the direction of the bar. However, this is practically impossible, because almost no ribs on the lateral chest wall can be perfectly perpendicular to the bar. Since perfect perpendicularity is not feasible, the rib that forms the largest angle with the bar should be selected — this rib will most likely provide maximum stability. Once the issue of stability is resolved, a successful Nuss procedure becomes possible. of course, the choice of fulcrum is only one key factor for surgical success; achieving the final desired result still requires careful planning of all operative details — only with this level of precision can an optimal corrective outcome be achieved.

Just like the Nuss procedure, the Wang procedure is also designed for correcting depression-type deformities. Flat chest does not present an actual depression, so using a standard Wang procedure might seem impossible to succeed. However, one must not overlook another fundamental aspect of the Wang procedure — its core principle of template shaping. Once this core feature is fully understood, it becomes clear that even without an actual depression, a flat chest can still potentially be corrected using the Wang technique.

(2) Surgery for Flat Chest Combined with Pectus Excavatum

Surgery for flat chest combined with pectus excavatum can be approached from two perspectives. From the perspective of pectus excavatum, this type belongs to a relatively complex category. Its complexity stems from the fact that the area of the depression is large and the surrounding support points are low, making both the Nuss procedure and the Wang procedure technically demanding. However, when this condition is approached from the perspective of flat chest surgery, the surgical difficulty seems somewhat reduced. The main

reason is the presence of the central depression. This depression creates a relative height difference compared to the surrounding flat area. This position conveniently provides a higher support point for the surgery, making the operation easier to complete.
Although the deformity is the same, looking at it from different perspectives reveals two entirely different impressions — illustrating a simple truth: flat chest surgery is clearly more challenging than funnel chest (pectus excavatum) surgery. Surgeons who have never performed flat chest procedures often cannot appreciate this fact, and some may even underestimate the difficulty of flat chest operations — a mindset that is entirely mistaken. Approaching flat chest surgery with such an attitude is highly likely to lead to surgical failure.

(3) Simultaneous Surgery for Flat Chest Combined with Pulmonary Bullae (Spontaneous Pneumothorax)

Flat chest is often discovered when a patient seeks treatment for spontaneous pneumothorax. The correct approach is to surgically treat both conditions at the same time [1]. However, for various reasons, many
patients undergo surgery only for pneumothorax and are unable to receive surgery for flat chest. These reasons include: 1. Failure to recognize the necessity of flat chest surgery. Many doctors do not view flat chest as an actual medical condition, and patients themselves are even less likely to see it as a disease. If neither the doctor nor the patient considers it a disease, surgery naturally will not be considered. 2. Spontaneous pneumothorax requires emergency surgery, while flat chest surgery is an elective procedure that demands special materials and instruments. Because of this, some doctors have no choice but to perform only the pneumothorax surgery and abandon the flat chest procedure. 3. The surgeon does not know how to perform flat chest surgery. Flat chest correction is technically demanding, and many doctors do not have the necessary skills. Since spontaneous pneumothorax requires urgent care and patients cannot be transferred long distances, only the pneumothorax surgery is performed. 4. Other personal factors. Flat chest surgery requires specialized materials and instruments, which can be expensive. Some patients cannot afford these costs and therefore cannot undergo the procedure. Performing flat chest and pneumothorax surgery simultaneously is the most reasonable option. To properly address both conditions, detailed surgical planning is essential.

First, there is the issue of using Thoracoscopy. To achieve a truly minimally invasive effect, using Thoracoscopy is the best approach. of course, it is also possible to perform the procedure through small incisions directly without using Thoracoscopy, and this approach is not particularly difficult. Second, there is the issue of incision selection. Considering the cosmetic outcome after surgery, the incisions must be used to their fullest advantage. Generally speaking, flat chest surgery only requires one incision on each side of the chest wall. As long as the incisions are properly positioned, both procedures can be completed through them.

(4) Flat Chest Surgery After Spontaneous Pneumothorax Surgery

As described above, many flat chest patients do not receive simultaneous correction surgery when they develop spontaneous pneumothorax. If these patients later undergo corrective surgery, it becomes a true second surgery in practice. Like all other second surgeries, the risks and technical difficulty will be higher. The main challenge lies in managing intrathoracic adhesions. If a patient previously underwent spontaneous pneumothorax surgery on one side, the adhesions will be limited to that side; if pneumothorax surgery was performed on both sides, then adhesions will exist in both pleural cavities. If the Nuss procedure is chosen for treatment, it requires placing the steel bar through the thoracic cavity, which poses significant risks. The most critical step at this point is to separate the adhesions. Since the adhesions are confined to the thoracic cavity, the mediastinum is usually. When there are no adhesions, the surgical risk can be significantly reduced as long as pleural adhesions are properly separated (see Figure 2-6-3). If separating the intrathoracic adhesions proves difficult, then using the Nuss procedure for correction is no longer the ideal choice. In such cases, the possibility of performing a Wang procedure should be considered instead. The Wang procedure is performed along the surface of the bony structures and does not require separation of intrathoracic adhesions, effectively avoiding this risk and greatly increasing the safety of the operation. Additionally, since the Wang procedure eliminates the need to separate intrathoracic adhesions, the overall surgical difficulty is significantly reduced.

Performing flat chest surgery after surgery for spontaneous pneumothorax not only increases the difficulty and risk of the operation but also adds to the patient's pain and burden. This is clearly an unfortunate outcome. To avoid this situation, the ideal approach is to address the pneumothorax and the flat chest in the same operation whenever possible. If there is not enough time to perform flat chest surgery immediately, conservative treatment for the pneumothorax can be carried out first, while making thorough preparations for the flat chest surgery. This approach generally does not pose significant problems. Of course, this approach is based on the premise that the surgeon has the capability to perform flat chest surgery. If the surgeon is not able to carry out this procedure, then the pneumothorax surgery must be done first.

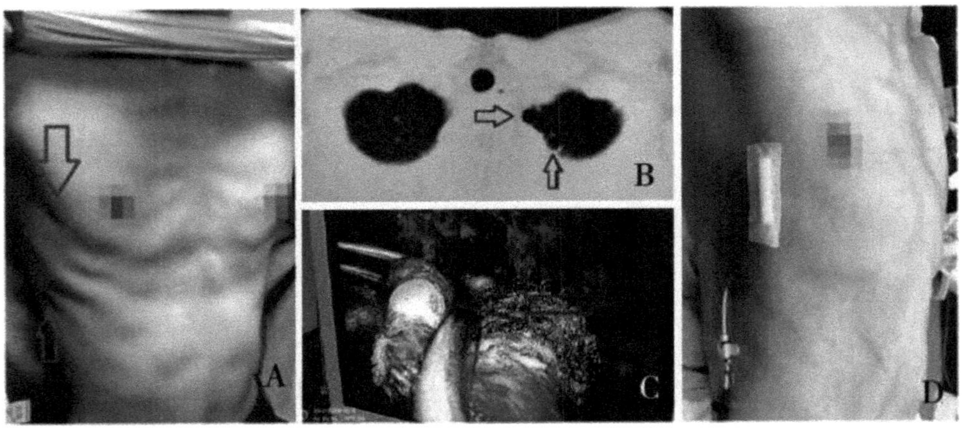

Figure 2-6-3 Flat Chest Surgery Combined with Pulmonary Bulla Ligation After Spontaneous Pneumothorax Surgery (A) The patient had previously undergone surgery for spontaneous pneumothorax, but the result was incomplete and pulmonary bullae remained. (B) Preoperative CT shows apical pulmonary bullae. (C) The pulmonary bullae were ligated and resected under Thoracoscopy. (D) Because Thoracoscopy allowed for effective dissection of intrathoracic adhesions, the Wong procedure could be performed without needing an additional incision for the Wang procedure. After the Wang procedure, the outcome was satisfactory and the chest wall appearance was completely normal

(5) Surgery for Spontaneous Pneumothorax After Flat Chest Procedures

After chest wall surgery became an independent specialty, operations inside the thoracic cavity were no longer categorized as part of chest wall surgery. Strictly speaking, then, surgery for spontaneous pneumothorax does not fall under the scope of chest wall surgery and should instead be classified as thoracic surgery. Since it belongs to thoracic surgery, chest wall surgeons theoretically should not perform such procedures. However, it must be clearly stated that even though intrathoracic disease surgery is not officially classified under chest wall surgery, chest wall surgeons have always performed such operations especially when chest wall diseases are complicated by intrathoracic conditions. It is not feasible for a surgeon to call in a thoracic surgeon intraoperatively to handle these conditions on the spot. Therefore, for certain common thoracic diseases, treatment by a chest wall surgeon does not constitute overstepping professional boundaries especially when a chest wall disease already exists and addressing an intrathoracic condition concurrently is entirely reasonable. A typical example is the occurrence of spontaneous pneumothorax after flat chest surgery. Because this relates to the initial flat chest operation, the chest wall surgeon has every justification to manage it. In such cases, the surgeon may encounter three scenarios: 1. The flat chest surgery was performed recently, and the steel plate cannot yet be removed; 2. A considerable time has passed since the flat chest surgery, so steel plate removal should be considered at the same time; 3. The flat chest surgery is complete and the steel plate has already been removed. Spontaneous pneumothorax can occur in all three situations, but the specifics differ entirely. However, they all involve one critical issue: intrathoracic adhesions. Adhesions can be severe or mild, and careful dissection of these adhesions is key to the success of the surgery. In the first scenario, if the steel plate cannot yet be removed, only surgery for the spontaneous pneumothorax is needed. In the second scenario, the steel plate must be removed at the same time. The third scenario means the patient has already undergone two surgeries, so intrathoracic adhesions may be more severe. Therefore, careful management of the adhesions is even more important to ensure the surgery proceeds smoothly.

(6) Revision Surgery After Failed Flat Chest Procedures

Compared to more common deformities, surgery for flat chest is generally more technically demanding and greater difficulty naturally increases the likelihood of surgical failure. Patients with flat chest have noticeably different attitudes toward surgery: some are eager to undergo surgery, while others refuse it altogether. However, for patients who have already undergone an unsuccessful procedure, most tend to want a revision surgery. This reflects a strong psychological factor at play. When a second surgery is performed to correct a failed procedure, the level of difficulty inevitably increases significantly. If the Nuss procedure is attempted again, the risks may be even higher, making revision surgery a major challenge. The challenge lies not only in the increased technical demands and risks but also in the uncertainty of the postoperative outcome. To achieve good results, careful surgical planning is essential not only must the appropriate surgical method be chosen, but meticulous attention must be paid to technical details. Only in this way can a successful operation be ensured (see Figure 2–6–4).

6. Surgical complications

Although the shape of the flat chest is different from that of the funnel chest, the surgery used is basically the same, which makes the complications basically the same. In summary, these complications include the following: (1) complications related to the position of the plate, such as displacement and transposition of the plate, which may directly affect the contouring; (2) complications related to the operation into the chest cavity, such as pneumothorax, lung injury, etc., which may affect postoperative recovery; (3) complications related to the local operation of the incision, such as fracture of the ribs, broken wires, etc., which directly affects the operation; (4) complications related to the healing of the incision, such as cracking of the incision, infection, etc., which directly leads to the incision Complications related to incision healing, such as incision cracking, infection, etc., which will directly lead to delayed healing or non-healing of the incision; (5) Complications related to contouring, including overkill, ineffective, or the emergence of new deformities, which will ultimately lead to surgical failure. Flat chest surgery is significantly more difficult than funnel chest surgery. More difficulty means more challenges, and without a convincing technique, complications are bound to be higher. This is one of the key features that distinguishes flat chest surgery from funnel chest surgery.

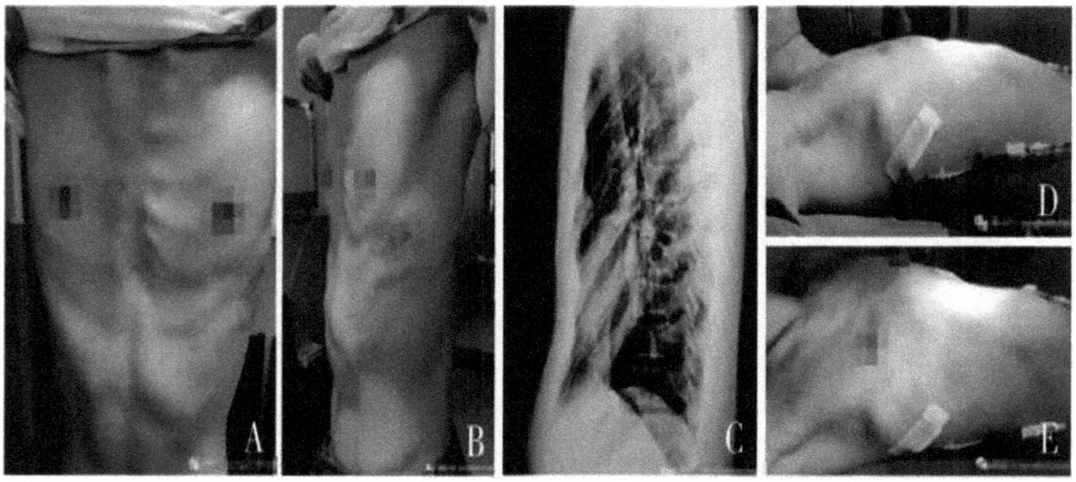

Figure 2-6-4 Revision Surgery After Failed Flat Chest Operation (A) The flat chest patient incorrectly underwent a standard Nuss procedure, resulting in surgical failure; frontal view shows the anterior chest wall remains flat. (B) Lateral view shows the anterior chest wall is still flat, with no correction achieved. (C) Lateral X-ray image indicates a flat anterior chest wall. (D) A revision surgery using the Wung procedure was performed for correction, with incisions made on both sides of the chest wall to complete the correction. (E) Postoperative chest wall shows an essentially normal contour

7. Surgical effects

Flat chest is not a particularly complex deformity. However, because there is still no specifically designed, targeted surgical procedure for it, achieving good treatment outcomes has always been a significant challenge. In particular, when many surgeons mistakenly assume that the Nuss procedure will produce satisfactory results, the outcome is often disappointing. It is no exaggeration to say that the failure rate of flat chest surgeries in clinical practice is much higher than that of other deformity surgeries. The reasons for this are mainly twofold: first, insufficient attention and understanding of the condition; second, inadequate surgical technique. It is clear that to achieve good results, both awareness and technical proficiency must be improved — otherwise, effective treatment for this deformity will not be possible.

REFERENCES

[1] Wang, W. L. 2020. "One-Stage Surgery for Flat Chest Combined with Pulmonary Bullae." *Thoracic Deformity Surgery Expert*, June 29.

[2] Wang, W. L. 2018. "Flat Chest and Depression-Type Deformities." *Thoracic Deformity Surgery Expert*, December 24.

[3] Lou, Y., W. Wang, W. Long, et al. 2021. "Chest Wall Reconstruction with Digitally Designed Materials for Straight Back Syndrome with Tracheal Stenosis: A Case Report." *Annals of Translational Medicine* 9 (16): 1357.

[4] Wang, W. L., C. M. Chen, X. J. Li, et al. 2018. "A Comprehensive Classification System for Thoracic Deformities." *Chinese Journal of Clinical Thoracic and Cardiovascular Surgery* 25 (11): 981–985.

Section 7

BARREL CHEST

Barrel chest is a relatively common thoracic deformity and is one of the most basic thoracic deformities. However, the perception of this deformity is quite different from that of other deformities. Whereas other deformities are generally recognized as congenital or primary, barrel chest is almost exclusively recognized as a secondary thoracic deformity from chronic respiratory disease. Medical students are taught that barrel chest occurs almost exclusively in the setting of chronic respiratory disease [1], and as a result, the deformity becomes a standard feature of the disease or an accessory to the disease, while its own problems are ignored, and the possibility of a primary barrel chest is not even considered. However, barrel chest is not uncommon in the clinical work of chest wall surgery, and almost all of them are primary malformations (Fig. 2 - 7 - 1)[2]. The prevalence of this deformity has not been standardized but in our experience the actual number of cases is not insignificant. These patients are often very distressed and eager for help, which makes it necessary to study this malformation in detail.

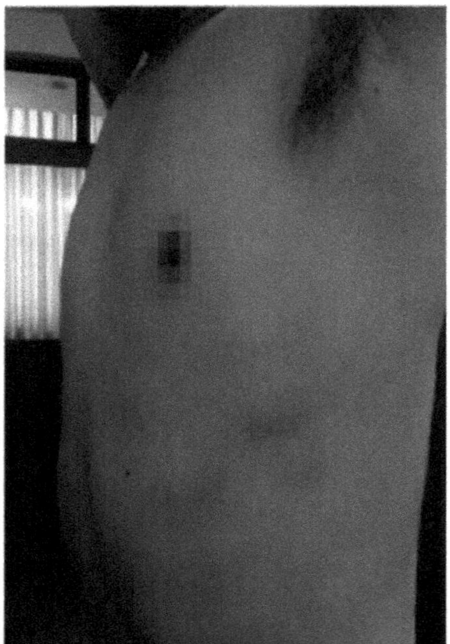

Figure 2-7-1 Barrel-shaped chest wall appearance

1. Pathogenesis

In infancy and childhood, the normal human thorax is usually barrel-shaped. This shape is inherited from the shape of the thorax during fetal life and is the original shape of the thorax. After the birth of the fetus, the negative pressure in the thoracic cavity increases as a result of respiratory movements. Negative pressure acts evenly around the chest wall, but the anterior chest wall is relatively weak. Under the influence of negative pressure, the anterior chest wall gradually sinks, gradually shortening the anterior and posterior diameters and creating a slightly flattened shape [3]. During this process, the respiratory muscles are also involved in the movement of the anterior chest wall, which together contribute to the

development of the thorax. The developing thorax is no longer barrel-shaped and is completely different from the shape at the beginning of life.
The change in the shape of the thorax is gradual and is usually completed by the age of 8 years. If the chest remains barrel-shaped thereafter, it becomes pathologically barrel-shaped, or primary barrel chest. The pathogenesis of primary barrel chest is unknown, but it is present from childhood. This means that the shape of the chest is not altered by respiratory movements. Mechanically
In these patients, the thoracic structure seems to be more rigid, especially in the anterior and posterior diameters, and is not easily altered by external forces; the reason for this characteristic is not known. Secondary barrel chest occurs in patients with chronic respiratory disease. The mechanism may be related to compensatory muscle work. In the presence of lung disease, respiratory function is impaired. In order to get more oxygen, the patient has to make an active effort to breathe. Such work is mainly caused by active contraction of the respiratory muscles of the chest. After prolonged active contraction, the muscles pull on the thorax, expanding the volume and causing irreversible compensatory changes in the skeleton, resulting in a barrel-shaped chest. This can also occur in people living in the highlands in an oxygen-deprived environment. The lack of oxygen makes it necessary to breathe hard in order to meet the demands of life activities, and the result is an alteration of the thorax similar to that seen in patients with chronic lung disease.

2. Pathological features
The barrel chest is so named because of the barrel-shaped appearance of the thorax. The patient's ribs and costal cartilages are long, and the overall anterior-posterior diameter of the thorax is increased without significant shortening of the right and left diameters, and the cross-section is essentially round. In order to establish a link with other types of thoracic deformities, the barrel-shaped thorax is viewed in the systematic classification system as a generalized anterior convexity of the anterior thorax. This understanding helps in the treatment of this deformity. In addition to the thoracic changes, patients with barrel chest may have lung disease. Primary barrel chest may be absent, but secondary patients may have changes such as emphysema.

3. Hazards
Barrel chest is a specific thoracic deformity in which the patient is usually not physiologically at risk due to the absence of localized or global depression of the anterior chest wall. In the secondary barrel chest, the alterations in the thorax are compensatory lesions, again posing no harm in themselves.

However, the markedly abnormal appearance often results in definite psychological harm to the patient. Barrel chest patients have a thorax that is difficult to conceal with clothing, and therefore the degree of psychological harm is often greater than with other deformities.

4. Clinical manifestations

Primary barrel chest is usually asymptomatic and the most common complaint is dissatisfaction with the appearance of the chest wall. The most common complaint is dissatisfaction with the appearance of the chest wall. The patient may suffer from low self-esteem because of its appearance, which can lead to a range of psychological problems. Secondary barrel chest is usually symptomatic and is characterized by respiratory symptoms. These symptoms predate the development of barrel chest and are exacerbated by the presence of barrel chest. This exacerbation is not caused by the barrel chest, but is the result of an exacerbation of the lung disease.

Barrel chest patients typically have a barrel-shaped chest wall with an overall anterior chest wall convexity and enlarged intercostal spaces. In the presence of chronic lung disease, the "triple concave sign" can be seen.

5. Inspection

Like other types of thoracic deformities, the examination of barrel chest relies heavily on physical examination. A definitive diagnosis can usually be made by examining the external appearance: X-ray is the most basic examination (Fig. 2-7-2), CT shows an almost circular skeletal section of the chest wall (Fig. 2-7-3), and three-dimensional reconstruction shows the overall shape of the thorax (Fig. 2-7-4). These examinations are helpful, but are not essential, and are only necessary if there is a suspicion of pulmonary co-morbidity. Imaging

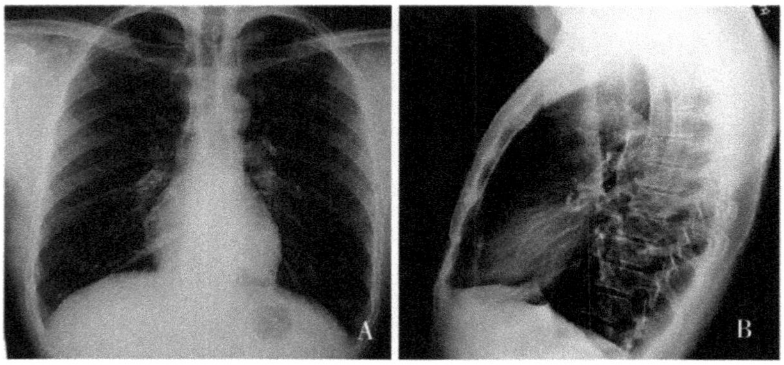

Figure 2-7-2 X-ray signs of barrel chest (A. Frontal view is nonspecific; B. Lateral view shows a markedly enlarged anteroposterior diameter of the chest)

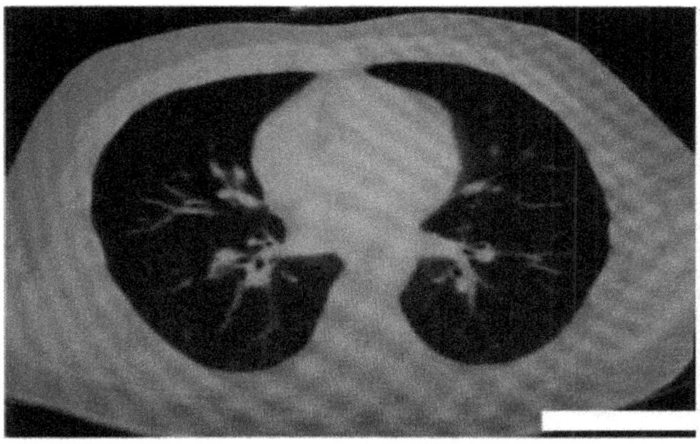

Figure. 2-7-3 CT sign of barrel chest with significantly enlarged anterior and posterior diameters and nearly circular cross-section

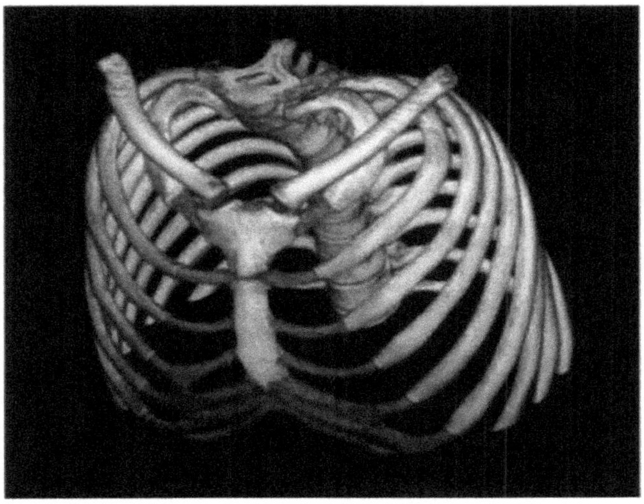

Figure 2-7-4 Three-dimensional reconstruction of the barrel chest sign.

6. Diagnosis and Differential Diagnosis

In most cases, the diagnosis of barrel chest is not difficult and can be clarified by appearance and imaging. The differential diagnosis needs to focus on two issues: first, the difference between primary and secondary barrel chest. One of the main criteria for differentiating between the two is age, and the other depends on the medical history and the environment in which the child was raised. Primary barrel chest is most common in young adults, but chronic lung disease must be excluded. Secondary patients are more common in the elderly and tend to have a long history of lung disease. Second, the difference between true barrel chest and pseudo barrel chest. Pseudo-barrel chest is firstly a sign of obesity, due to the patient's obesity, the normal shape of bony structure is covered by the fat tissue on the surface of the body and disappears, showing the appearance of a barrel, which constitutes a pseudo-barrel chest. Pseudo-barrel-shaped chest can also be seen in some special healthy women, due to the crossing of breast tissues in the midline, resulting in the illusion of protruding anterior chest wall, which can also constitute pseudo-barrel-shaped chest. Pseudo-barrel chest has a completely normal thorax, and the identification method is very simple, and the diagnosis can be clearly made through imaging examination.

In addition to the above two problems, there are other thoracic deformities that need to be differentiated from each other in clinical practice: (1) massive chicken chest. When there is a large anterior convexity of the anterior chest wall, it is easy to be confused with barrel chest. The main method of differentiation is to look at the extent of the convexity. If the bulge is localized and does not involve the entire anterior chest wall, then it is a chicken chest; if the whole anterior chest wall is anteriorly convex and has the appearance of a barrel, then it is a typical barrel chest. (2) If the whole anterior chest wall is anteriorly convex and has a barrel-shaped appearance, it is a typical barrel chest. The anterior sternal angle is not a deformity in itself, but the presence of the mammary glands may cause the anterior chest wall to be elevated in the center, giving the whole appearance of a barrel shape. This shape is cosmetically displeasing and can be a source of concern for many people. This is completely different from barrel chest and can be differentiated by physical examination and imaging. (3) Complex thoracic deformities. This type of deformity is often associated with severe spinal deformity. The spinal deformity is so severe that the overall shape of the thorax is altered. The front and side of the thorax appear to be barrel-shaped, but in fact they are complex irregular deformities. This deformity is distinctly different from barrel chest, and the difference can be easily detected on imaging.

7. Indications for surgery

Barrel chest secondary to chronic lung disease is a compensatory pathologic change. This change cannot be treated surgically and is a contraindication to surgery. Patients living in a chronic hypoxic environment who are dissatisfied with the appearance of their chest may be considered for treatment. However, it is advisable to change the living environment after surgery and not to continue to live in an anoxic environment. The main problem with primary barrel chest is cosmetic abnormality, and there is usually no physiologic harm. If the patient has no cosmetic needs, surgery may not be considered. Surgery may be considered if the patient or family wishes to improve the appearance of the chest. Since no physical harm is involved, the decision to operate should not be left to the surgeon, but to the patient and family!

8. Surgical treatment

Barrel chest is a very old thoracic deformity that has been recognized for many years. However, the treatment of this deformity has not been satisfactory. The earliest treatment came from Naef, who reported surgery for the treatment of barrel chest in 1953, but the exact method was unknown [4].In 1976, another author, Witz, reported surgery for barrel chest, and the method of treatment was also unclear [5]. For a long time since then, no one has treated this deformity. In recent years, we have been the first to perform surgery for this deformity using minimally invasive techniques with satisfactory results [6]. The method we used was the Wenlin procedure for proptosis. This procedure is practically the same as the Wenlin procedure for chicken breast. However, the details of the procedure differ due to the extent of the proptosis deformity

(1) Pre-operative preparation

Barrel chest is an overall proptosis of the anterior chest wall. Of all the anterior chest wall deformities, barrel chest is probably the most severe due to the large size and extent of the anterior chest wall. Surgery for this deformity requires adequate preoperative preparation. First, the patient must be prepared psychologically. Because of the severity of the deformity, the surgery, although minimally invasive, can be quite traumatic. Patients may experience significant discomfort or pain after surgery. It is necessary to give patients a good explanation before the operation, on the one hand, to make them psychologically prepared, and on the other hand, to eliminate their fear. Secondly, it is necessary to prepare the materials. The barrel-shaped chest has a wide range and large area, and the operation requires more materials, which is the basic guarantee for the completion of the operation. For this reason, it is necessary to prepare the specification and quantity of the materials before the operation to lay the foundation for the success of the operation. Thirdly, the preparation of instruments should be done well. The preparation of instruments mainly involves the conventional instruments for thoracic deformity correction surgery, in addition to some special instruments. It is necessary to prepare the instruments well before the operation to ensure the successful completion of the operation. Fourth, technical preparation. Technical preparation mainly refers to the preparation of surgical strategies and methods. Although the method of barrel chest surgery is relatively mature, there are some special cases, such as the combination of rib arch proptosis or intraoperative complications, which need to be well prepared before surgery to avoid trouble during surgery.

(2) Surgical methods

The standard Wenlin procedure is used. A longitudinal incision is made in the lateral chest wall, usually 2-3 cm in length. The skin and subcutaneous tissues are incised, and the musculature is incised longitudinally to expose the ribs and the ribs are freed along the rib surfaces to expose the ribs in and around the incision. The fixation position is selected in the plane of the proposed plate, and the fixation is performed using the Wang technique, in which a wire guide is placed around the rib in the fixation position. A tunnel is made on the bony surface of the anterior chest wall where the plate is to be placed. The tunnel converges from the lateral chest wall to the center, connecting the left and right sides, and a guide is placed into the tunnel, which pulls the plate guide tube into the tunnel, and then the plate guide tube pulls the plate into the tunnel on the chest wall. The steel wires are introduced through the wire guides at each fixation site, wrapped around the ribs and the plate, and tightened sequentially to secure the plate to the ribs. After fixation, the incision is closed and the procedure is completed.

(3) Surgical points

The basic principles of surgery must be understood. The principles of the Wenlin procedure can be understood in two ways. The first is a visual understanding, i.e., compression of the raised chest wall with a steel plate; the other is template shaping, i.e., using a steel plate as a template to directly shape the deformed chest wall. This understanding is more abstract, but not difficult, and the only requirement is that the structures of the chest wall be placed against the plate to achieve the shape. The two understandings are quite different but directly related. Compression requires firm fixation, and the result of this fixation is a tight fit of the chest wall against the plate, which is exactly what is required for template contouring. This is exactly what is required for template molding. It can be seen that the two understandings are just different angles, and the actual results are exactly the same.

Every detail of the operation must be emphasized. Wenlin surgery for barrel chest is a huge systematic project, which involves a large number of operational details, each of which has a bearing on the success or failure of the operation, and therefore extra attention must be paid.

Key techniques must be mastered. Objectively speaking, every detail of Wenlin surgery is critical and requires careful attention. The key techniques here are those that are not so easy to handle. The first critical technique is the specific operation technique, which is related to the handling of the plate, and mainly includes plate selection, handling, and fixation, etc. The selection of the plate is mainly about the handling of the plate, and the fixation of the plate. The selection of a steel plate is mainly the selection of its specification and quantity; the treatment is the intraoperative shaping of the steel plate; and the fixation includes the location, site, and method of fixation, etc. These contents are directly related to the placement of steel plates. These elements are directly related to the placement and fixation of the steel plate, which is a key technology. The second critical technique is more abstract and refers to the overall operating procedure, which is set up to accomplish the surgery in a more organized manner. In order to obtain the best operating procedure, it is necessary to optimize and simplify the whole process, and to develop the simplest and most reasonable operating procedure; once such a procedure is completed, it cannot be changed arbitrarily during the operation, or it will bring unexpected trouble.

There must be a sense of the big picture. Although there are similarities between Wenlin surgery for barrel chest and Wenlin surgery for chicken breast in general, there are too many differences, and the main difference lies in the content of the operation. In the specific operation process, due to the small incision, the limited field of operation, and the various tubes, sutures and other contents, if there is no sense of the big picture, it will be difficult to deal with the various contents clearly, which will seriously affect the process of the operation.

Good knowledge of mechanics is necessary. The reason for considering barrel chest as a convex type of deformity is to make it easier to perform surgery, especially Its a targeted approach to performing surgery for bulge type deformities. This view itself is the most basic perception of the mechanics of surgical correction. The large number of mechanical issues involved in the process, such as the problem of stress dispersion and the mechanical strength of wires and ribs, are critical mechanical issues that are crucial to the success or failure of the surgery, and may lead to failure of the surgery if they are not adequately understood.

Must be well organized. One of the important features of Wenlin's surgery is that it is minimally invasive, and the distinguishing feature is the miniscule size of the incision. A large number of operations are performed through such a small incision, and a large number of retractor wires, wires, retractor catheters, plates, etc., are placed successively, which will make the whole operation a mess if there is no good organization. Therefore, during the operation, you must always know the progress of the operation and the order of the operation, and only when each step is carried out in an orderly manner according to a fixed order can you ensure that the operation is completed smoothly. Once any program or step goes wrong, it will bring great trouble to the operation.
It is necessary to proceed step by step. In completing the orthopedics process, one of the important operative elements is to tighten the wires so that the steel plate will be tightened against the ribs and pressure will be exerted on the

anterior chest wall. This is a process that involves a large change in stress, and if the distribution of stress is not taken into account, the wires may be tightened as soon as the compression of the first plate is completed. Such a maneuver would result in the ribs being severed by the wire due to the concentration of stress, or the wire itself being pulled apart. Such an accident, should it occur, would have an extremely unfavorable effect on the operation. To avoid such accidents, the principle of gradualness must always be observed. When fixing the steel plate, the steel wire should not be tightened all at once, but should be tightened gradually between each fixation point, alternately, so that the stress of each fixation site is maximally dispersed, to ensure that both the completion of the shaping operation and not to the occurrence of accidents.

Must be appropriate. This is actually a question of degree. In the process of orthodontic treatment, the tighter the wire is fixed, the better the result. If the wires are not completely tightened, and if they still serve to apply stress, the fixation is just right. One of the most important concepts that must always be kept in mind when performing the Wenlin procedure is that the wires are pulling, not fixing. This role is completely different from that of the Nuss procedure for funnel chest. It is only by understanding this difference that the essence of the Wenlin procedure can be truly understood.

(4) Complications

Although minimally invasive, the Wenlin procedure for barrel chest is a huge systematic project due to the wide range of deformities. During the specific operation, each link is related to the success or failure of the surgery, and requires the operator to be very careful in the operation. However, because of the magnitude of the project, even with the best of care at every stage, certain problems may still occur. This leads to various complications.

Broken ribs. The root cause of rib fracture is excessive localized stress. Once the fracture has occurred, the area is no longer suitable for immobilization. If a suitable replacement cannot be found in the surrounding area, the orthopedics result will be adversely affected. If a rib fracture occurs postoperatively, the fixation of the plate disappears and the end of the plate will push up against the skin, and in severe cases, it may protrude from the incision or even break through the skin. Problems with the plate itself will cause severe discomfort to the patient and, in more serious cases, lead to surgical failure. When this happens, a second surgery is required. During the operation, the exposed plate has to be sterilized and a suitable site has to be found to re-fix it. If there is no suitable local fixation site and the plate is heavily contaminated, the plate should be removed.

Wire breakage: Wire breakage is also due to excessive localized stress. After the breakage, new steel wire can be used to replace the broken wire.

Replacement. However, placing the wire will be very difficult due to the presence of the plate already in place. Wire breakage, if it occurs after surgery, has exactly the same consequences as a broken rib. The same treatment is required in order to eliminate the danger.
Hemothorax. Placement of the wire involves right-angle forceps, wire guides, and wire threading around the ribs, all of which are performed between the ribs. Since multiple parts of the bilateral chest wall are involved in multiple intercostal spaces, there may be intercostal vascular injuries, and gas may enter the thoracic cavity, resulting in hemopneumothorax. This is usually not serious and can be effectively eliminated by routine placement of a closed chest drain after surgery.
Localized depression of the anterior chest wall. In the process of compression of the anterior chest wall, if the appropriate degree is not grasped, overkill may occur, resulting in a concave deformity of the anterior chest wall. Such a deformity may be transient or permanent. The degree of compression must always be observed in order to avoid the appearance of depression. As long as the compression is not overdone, it does not usually result in a depressed deformity. When depressions do occur, if they are more severe, the plate needs to be removed earlier. If the depression is not severe, it can be observed and usually improves or disappears with the removal of the plate.
Relative Anterior Convexity of the Rib Arches. The aim of barrel chest surgery is to lower the whole anterior chest wall and restore the normal height and curvature. However, the extent of the anterior chest wall is often extremely large. Multiple plates are required to lower such a large area of the chest wall. In general, 3 plates are used to perform the operation. However, if the area is too large, there will not be enough plates, and if there are not enough plates to orthopedically lower the anterior chest wall, the rib arch will not be able to descend, resulting in a relatively convex deformity. This deformity will have an impact on the overall contouring result. If spare plates are available, they must be contoured. Shaping is simple and can still be corrected using the Wenlin procedure.

Delayed healing of the incision. Barrel chests use a lot of plates and wires, which are located inside the incision and need to be embedded with sufficient soft tissue during suturing. If the embedding is not adequate, healing may be compromised. In addition to embedding, other factors may affect healing and must be carefully managed during and after surgery.

9. Plate removal surgery
The time for removal of the plates for barrel chest Wenlin surgery is

approximately the same as that for chicken breast Wenlin surgery, and they are usually removed 1 - 2 years after surgery. The specific method is to make an incision at the scar of the first surgery to reveal the plate, cut the wire and remove it, and then pull the plate out of the body separately. The removal of the plates is a very safe and simple procedure, and there are usually no complications.

10. Prognosis

Barrel chest surgery is equivalent to severe chicken breast surgery, which is difficult and high-risk, and it is difficult to obtain good results if the technique is not excellent. In the past, we have optimized our technique and completed nearly 100-barrel chest surgeries, which has made this technique mature. Our experience has shown that, as long as the technique is strictly adhered to, the results are basically good and acceptable to the patient (Figures 2-7-5 and 2-7-6). However, it has to be noted that there are many problems caused by surgery that are complex and challenging, and if you do not master this technique perfectly, you may experience more serious consequences after the surgery. This is what must be reminded

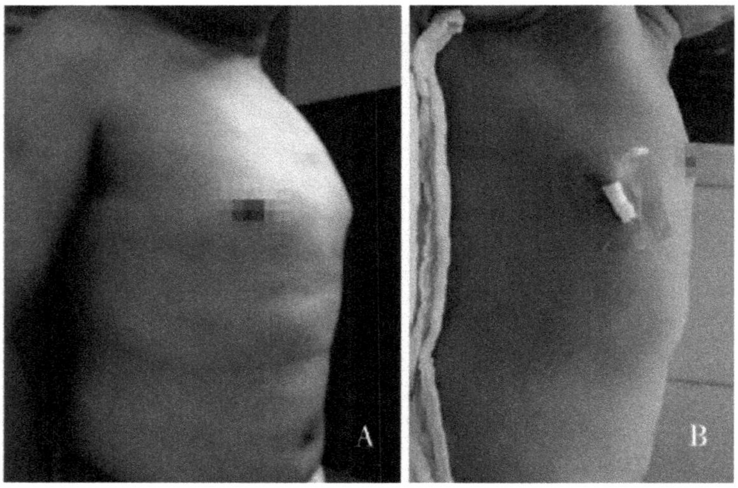

Figure 2 - 7 - 5 Wenlin procedure for barrel chest
(A. Preoperative chest wall appearance; B.Postoperative chest wall appearance)

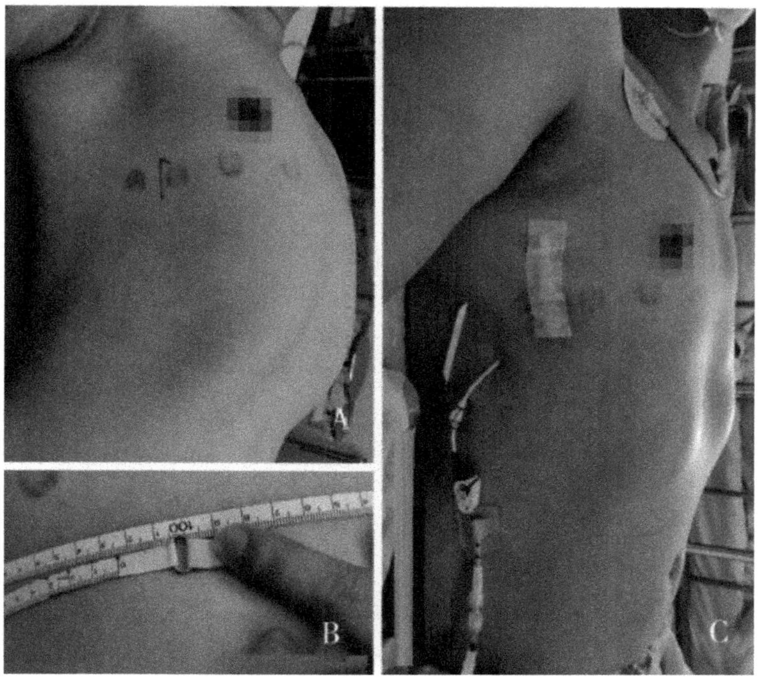

Figure 2 -7 -6 Wenlin procedure for severe barrel chest (A. Appearance of severe barrel chest; B. Chest circumference of 102.5 cm; C. Postoperative thoracic appearance)

REFERENCES

[1] Pierce, J. A., and R. V. Ebert. 1958. "The Barrel Deformity of the Chest, the Senile Lung and Obstructive Pulmonary Emphysema." *American Journal of Medicine* 25 (1): 13–22.

[2] Wang, W. L. 2021. "The Particularity of Barrel Chest." *Thoracic Deformity Surgery Specialist*, May 10.

[3] Wang, W. L. 2018a. "Congenital 'Barrel Chest' and Minimally Invasive Surgery in Young Children." *Thoracic Deformity Surgery Specialist*, February 23.

[4] Naef, A. P. 1953. "The Surgical Treatment of Barrel-Shaped Thorax." *Praxis* 42 (5): 73–77.

[5] Witz, J. P., G. Morand, and J. M. Wihlm. 1976. "Funnel Chest and Barrel Chest: Treatment by Stern Chondroplasty with Reference to 43 Operations." *Annales de Chirurgie Thoracique et Cardiovasculaire* 15 (2): 157–160.

[6] Wang, W. L. 2018b. "Minimally Invasive Surgical Technique for Barrel Chest." *Surgical Case Reports* 1 (2): 1–2.

For a long time, all depression-type deformities of the anterior chest wall were referred to as pectus excavatum. Although the appearance of these depressions rarely truly resembled a funnel shape, no one questioned this terminology. The fundamental reason for this concept lay in the surgical approach. In the early days, nearly all anterior chest wall depression deformities were treated with open surgery. Open surgery involved large incisions to expose the bony structures of the deformity, which were then deliberately disrupted and reshaped using special materials and techniques to achieve a relatively satisfactory appearance. This type of surgery was essentially destructive, comparable to a major overhaul of a car no matter how complex the deformity, it could be corrected. Because the surgical methods for all depression-type deformities were basically the same even down to the surgical details — it seemed unnecessary to distinguish these deformities in detail. So, classifying all such deformities simply as pectus excavatum was reasonable. Against this background, more detailed classification seemed redundant. However, with advances in surgical techniques, minimally invasive surgery has gradually become the mainstream in all surgical fields, and chest wall deformity surgery has entered the minimally invasive era. When the Nuss procedure became the representative minimally invasive surgery for pectus excavatum, new questions about the naming of these deformities arose [1–3]. The Nuss procedure was specifically designed for standard pectus excavatum, which represents only one type of anterior chest wall depression. Besides this, there are other depression deformities with different characteristics. Because the Nuss procedure places specific demands on the subtle structural features of the deformity, if the structural features differ from those of standard pectus excavatum, the Nuss procedure is no longer suitable for correction. In early practice, few people recognized the impact of structural differences on surgical outcomes, and the Nuss procedure was applied to all depression-type deformities. As a result, some surgeries ultimately failed. The reason for these failures was precisely the failure to recognize the structural differences. When these differences became apparent, the need for new distinctions and terminology became real [4]. "Groove chest" was named in this context.

The term pectus excavatum has a long history. In theory, this name should not change just because surgical methods have changed — especially not for a new procedure that has been around for only about 20 years. However, the fact that the naming issue for pectus excavatum has truly emerged shows, on one hand, that the original naming itself had shortcomings and, on the other hand, that this reflects practical clinical needs. When the Nuss procedure came to be widely regarded as the only option for treating pectus excavatum, deformities that did not fit the criteria for the Nuss procedure naturally came under scrutiny and were ultimately excluded from the category of pectus excavatum and recognized as new deformities [1-5]

From an etiological perspective, a furrowed chest can be considered a variant of pectus excavatum. However, when the definition of pectus excavatum is strictly defined, a furrowed chest becomes a distinct deformity separate from pectus excavatum. This deformity features a depression located on the anterior chest wall, appearing as a furrow that runs horizontally across the lower portion of the anterior chest wall. In pectus excavatum, the depression is pit-like, with a midpoint indent and raised edges surrounding it. In contrast, the depression in the furrowed chest is a distinct groove, with the upper part elevated, extending laterally to the side chest wall without elevated edges. The lower sides are elevated rib arches, with the central part located near the xiphoid process, without elevation, extending downward to the abdominal wall (Figure 2-8-1) [1-3,5].From a surgical treatment perspective, the Nuss procedure is not suitable for this model, so it is necessary to separate the grooved chest as an independent model from the funnel chest.It is located near the xiphoid process, without any protrusion, and extends downward to the abdominal wall (Figure 2-8-1) [1-3,5].From a surgical treatment perspective, the Nuss procedure is not suitable for this model, so it is necessary to separate the grooved chest as an independent model from the funnel chest.

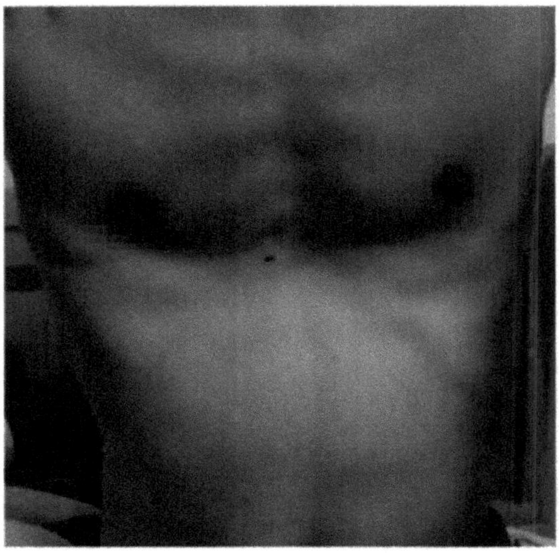

Figure 2-8-1 External appearance of groove-shaped chest

1. Etiology and Pathophysiology

Groove chest is a type of anterior chest wall depression deformity. According to the general pathogenesis of deformities, the formation of this depression may be related to two factors: one is weakness of the chest wall, and the other is the effect of external forces. In newborns or young children, the Harrison groove (also called the coastal diaphragmatic groove) is often seen. This groove is formed by the inward traction of the ribs at the diaphragm attachment, creating a horizontal groove [6,7]. This groove is considered to be related to calcium deficiency. Calcium deficiency softens the bony structures, and under the traction of the diaphragm, the local bone changes shape and forms a depression; this is the mechanism of Harrison groove formation. The Harrison groove affects the appearance of the thorax and can be regarded as an early manifestation of groove chest. If this change persists, it will result in an actual groove chest. This should be the mechanism behind the formation of groove chest. The pathogenesis of pectus excavatum is complex and is generally believed to be unrelated to calcium deficiency. However, the above analysis shows that groove chest is closely related to calcium deficiency, which is a clear difference between the two deformities.The above is one explanation for the pathogenesis of groove chest, but it does not seem to fully explain all cases. One phenomenon worth noting is that groove chest in adults differs significantly in shape from Harrison grooves seen in young children. Although it cannot be ruled out that a Harrison groove may develop into a groove chest, it is undeniable that other possibilities exist, since their appearances do indeed differ.Referring to the pathogenesis of pectus excavatum, it is also possible that other forces are involved in the formation of the groove chest. The specific mechanism requires further research.

Groove chest is located in the lower part of the anterior chest wall. In addition to the heart and lungs, the deep surface of the depression also involves upper abdominal organs. The presence of the depression exerts pressure on all these organs, ultimately leading to related symptoms that constitute its physiological harm. In addition to these effects, depression severely impacts the appearance of the thorax, causing a significant chest wall deformity, which can also have psychological effects on the patient.

2. Clinical Manifestations

The clinical manifestations of groove chest are similar to those of pectus excavatum, which is one reason this deformity has long been mistaken for pectus excavatum. The main clinical symptoms are related to compression caused by depression. Mild depressions have no obvious symptoms, while severe depressions can cause clear compression-related symptoms. These symptoms may originate from the cardiovascular system or the respiratory system. Some patients may also experience digestive system symptoms or even systemic symptoms. Symptoms generally worsen progressively and become more pronounced with age. In addition, symptoms tend to worsen during intense physical activity. The physical signs of groove chest are quite characteristic: the lower anterior chest wall shows a transverse, groove-like depression. The depression can be located above the level of the xiphoid process or may extend across it. Cardiac pulsation can often be seen on the left side of the depression, and in severe cases, a heart murmur may be heard. This murmur is mostly functional and differs from structural murmurs caused by cardiac structural abnormalities. In addition, depression can also shift the heart to the left and change the stress distribution on both sides of the spine, which may lead to scoliosis and result in a more severe deformity.

3. Examination

A general physical examination can clearly establish the diagnosis. If it is necessary to understand the relationship between the depression and the heart and lungs, or to assess possible intrathoracic complications, imaging studies can be performed. A lateral X-ray will show the characteristic depression in the lower anterior chest wall with obvious cardiac compression; a frontal X-ray may show an enlarged cardiac silhouette, leftward displacement, and possible scoliosis. A CT scan will show a normal cross-section of the upper chest wall, while the lower chest wall will display signs of a flattened chest with cardiac compression. A 3D reconstruction can display the complete outline of the thoracic cage, clearly showing the groove-like depression.

4. Diagnosis and Differential Diagnosis

Groove chest has a typical shape, making diagnosis relatively easy, physical examination alone is generally sufficient for diagnosis, while imaging studies can assist in confirming the diagnosis and help rule out intrathoracic diseases. The differential diagnosis mainly includes distinguishing groove chest from pectus excavatum, saddle chest, and flat chest. Groove chest and typical pectus excavatum are clearly different, but when pectus excavatum is extensive and located low on the chest, it can sometimes be confused with groove chest. The key point of distinction lies in the difference between a “groove” and a “pit”: the depression in pectus excavatum is surrounded by a raised edge, whereas groove chest only has raised edges at the upper and lower borders, with no elevation on either side, resulting in an open boundary. This is the fundamental difference between the two. The location of the saddle chest is similar to that of the groove chest, and it also presents with depression.

However, in the saddle chest, the depressions are located on both sides of the chest wall and are not connected in the center. In groove chest, the depression is a continuous groove extending from left to right without any separation in the middle. Flat chest presents as a generally flattened anterior chest wall without a distinct depression, so it is also relatively easy to differentiate it from groove chest.

5. Surgical Indications

In the past, patients with a groove chest were always treated as having pectus excavatum, so the surgical indications were basically the same as those for pectus excavatum. Various criteria for surgical indications of pectus excavatum in the literature have also been applied to groove chest, but these clearly have many issues. Like all other thoracic deformities, the fundamental principle for surgical indications is that the decision should not be made by the doctor alone, but rather by the patient and their family. If the patient and family feel that the deformity is unsightly or causes discomfort, surgery should be performed; if they do not feel it is unsightly or uncomfortable, surgery can be avoided.

When deciding on surgery, special attention must be paid to young children. Since the deformity in these patients may develop normally or lessen as they grow, early surgery is not recommended. However, if the deformity appears as a distinct transverse groove that is clearly different from the shape of a Harrison groove, it may indicate a more severe groove chest, and early surgery may be considered.

6. Surgical Treatment

As mentioned above, groove chest is named separately because the Nuss procedure is not suitable for its treatment. According to the basic principle of the Nuss procedure, it works based on the lever principle [8,9]. Since it relies on a lever, there are special requirements for the related structures, and the key to the success of the procedure is the fulcrum. The fulcrum must have sufficient height, adequate rigidity, and enough stability. For standard pectus excavatum, the edges of the depression on the lateral chest wall can meet all three requirements for a fulcrum, making it easy to perform the Nuss procedure. However, the biggest issue with groove chest is the height of the fulcrum. Because the sides of the groove are open and lack raised edges, using this area as the fulcrum for the steel bar makes it almost impossible to achieve the leverage needed for support. This is the fundamental reason why previous attempts to treat groove chest with the Nuss procedure have failed. Therefore, to ensure surgical success, the related details must be redesigned.

(1) Transverse Procedure

The direction of the depression in the groove chest is transverse. Before groove chest was given its own name, this type of deformity was always treated with the Nuss procedure. The direction of the Nuss procedure is parallel to the groove, that is, it is a transverse operation or transverse procedure. The Wang procedure, which is also designed for treating depressed deformities, is likewise a transverse operation. Groove chest is a type of depressed deformity, so theoretically, using either the Nuss procedure or the Wang procedure is reasonable. However, the standard procedures clearly cannot achieve satisfactory correction; modifications or adjustments to the details are necessary to meet the requirements of proper deformity correction.

(1) Modified Nuss Procedure

The standard Nuss procedure cannot achieve satisfactory correction of groove chest, and its biggest problem is the lack of an ideal fulcrum. So, in order to successfully perform surgery for a groove chest, it is necessary. To achieve correction using the Nuss procedure, a suitable fulcrum must be found. However, the structural feature of groove chest is that both ends are open with no raised edges, making it impossible to find a natural fulcrum. In this situation, the only feasible approach is to artificially create a fulcrum. There are many ways to achieve these special materials that can be used, or a suitable fulcrum can be created by carefully selecting its position and applying special techniques.

In this process, relying solely on the original concept of the Nuss procedure will not yield good results; it is essential to fully incorporate the principle of template shaping this is the only way to achieve an ideal outcome.In essence, the Nuss procedure is a mechanical reshaping using external force, while template shaping is fundamentally a different approach. Combining these two different techniques into a modified Nuss procedure may seem impossible. However, it must be clearly understood that the purpose of the modified Nuss procedure is precisely to make what is impossible with the standard Nuss procedure possible. As long as the surgical details are carefully designed, both techniques can be integrated into a single operation and function together effectively [10].

(2) Modified Wang Procedure

Unlike the Nuss procedure, the Wang procedure also requires a fulcrum, but the fulcrum can be positioned lower even below the level of the depression. As long as the end of the steel bar has a fixed position with sufficient rigidity, the Wang

procedure can be successfully completed. Although the lateral chest wall in groove chest is relatively low, it is sufficient to provide a fulcrum for the steel bar. This feature lays the foundation for performing the Wang procedure.
In the specific operation, incisions are first made on both sides of the chest wall. The ends of the steel bar are firmly fixed to the fulcrum on the lateral chest wall, causing the steel bar to arch in the middle. Then, the depressed central structures are lifted and fixed onto the steel bar, completing the reshaping [11].

(3) Key Technical Points

Both the modified Nuss procedure and the modified Wang procedure have their own specific technical points, which are critical to the success of the surgery. In addition to these individual points, there are some common technical aspects that require special attention: First, Pre-Shaping. Generally speaking, whether it is the modified Nuss procedure or the modified Wang procedure, an important operative mechanism involved is template shaping. Template shaping requires thorough pre-shaping of the chest wall structures. Especially for groove chest, which has a lower fulcrum with potentially insufficient rigidity, effective pre-shaping will significantly improve the success rate of the operation. Therefore, it is essential to ensure that pre-shaping is properly carried out. Second, the implementation of template shaping. Template shaping requires the chest wall structures to fit tightly against the steel bar — the closer the fit, the better the result. In the process of performing the modified Nuss procedure and the modified Wang procedure, the tight fit between the steel bar and the chest wall is particularly important and is a key factor for the success of the surgery.

(4) Combined Procedure Considerations

Groove chest is a special type of deformity although it appears as a form of depression, it is still different from a typical depression. If you look only at the base of the depression, this type of depression is more similar to flat chest, so certain surgical principles used for flat chest are worth referencing. In addition, when dealing with this unique deformity, it is helpful to broaden the perspective rather than stick to a single surgical method. The Nuss procedure, Wang procedure, or even the Wenlin procedure can be combined. When different procedures are reasonably combined, the function of each can be effectively utilized, ultimately achieving an ideal result [12,13].

(1) Longitudinal Procedure

The Nuss procedure and the Wang procedure are both corrective procedures performed along the direction of the depression, which are essentially transverse procedures. Considering, the raised upper and lower edges of the depression can be used to reshape the depression, which leads to another surgical design: the longitudinal procedure. The specific operation of the longitudinal procedure uses a specially designed steel plate to correct the deformity in a direction perpendicular to the groove-shaped depression. There are two ways to perform it: one is to prop up the bottom of the depression, and the other is to lift the surface of the depression (Figure 2-8-2). The propping method is similar to the Nuss procedure. Since all operations are done on one side of the chest wall without passing through the mediastinum, the procedure is simple, feasible, and risk-free in theory, making it easier to achieve good results. However, this procedure also has some problems: (1) The lower edge of the depression is near the costal arch. Although this structure may be relatively high, its hardness may not be sufficient. When used as a support point for propping up the bony structure, insufficient hardness may directly affect the outcome. (2) Corrective surgery must consider postoperative physiological function. All previous procedures have used a transverse approach because such operations do not affect the anteroposterior movement of the chest wall after surgery. If a longitudinal procedure is used, the presence of the steel plate may restrict forward bending, not only limiting movement but also causing discomfort. (3) Since the depression is broad, supporting the entire depression completely may not be achievable with just one steel plate on each side of the chest wall. If two plates are used, multiple incisions will be needed, which will affect the appearance of the chest wall after surgery. Using a steel plate to lift the surface of the depression is also an option. Since the steel plate "floats" on the chest wall surface, the actual operation is similar to the Wang procedure. However, this approach also faces a series of problems in practice. Thus, in theory, the longitudinal procedure seems feasible, but in actual implementation, many challenges must be addressed through careful design to achieve a good outcome.

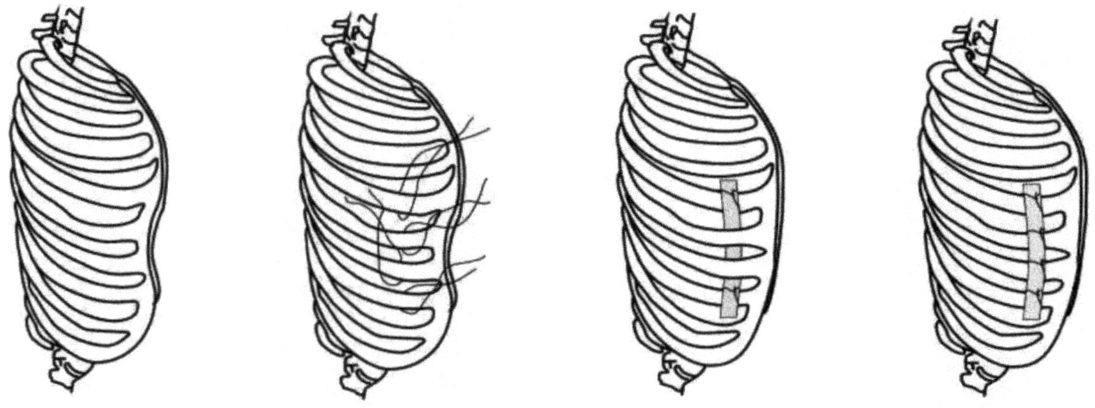

A B C D

Figure 2-8-2 Schematic diagram of the longitudinal procedure (A. Structural diagram of the groove-shaped chest; B. Placement of wires at different positions of the groove-shaped chest as needed; C. The steel plate is placed on the deep side of the depressed ribs to prop up the depression; D. The steel plate is placed on the surface of the depressed ribs to lift the depression.)

(2) Semi-open procedure

The surgical techniques discussed above are all minimally invasive procedures. In actual practice, sometimes minimally invasive surgery cannot achieve good results. In such cases, another option must be considered: the semi-open procedure. Considering that the depression usually involves only one or two ribs, a MatrixRIB plate can be used to directly reshape the ribs, restoring their physiological curvature to achieve the purpose of correction, the surgical objective is clear, and the results are more satisfactory. The plate can remain permanently in the body without the need for a second surgery for removal. However, this procedure is more invasive, with a longer incision, so if there are better options available, it is generally not considered.

(3) Open Surgery

In certain special cases, minimally invasive and semi-open surgeries cannot achieve the treatment goal. For example, in some adult patients with a gutter chest, the bone is abnormally hard, making minimally invasive or semi-open procedures difficult. In such cases, open surgery can be considered. The specific procedure involves performing a wedge-shaped osteotomy on the upper edge of the sternum at the depression, lifting the central depressed area, then reshaping and fixing the depressions on both sides to complete the surgery. This operation directly targets the key part of the deformity for reshaping, providing more precise correction and satisfactory results. However, the concept of open surgery completely contradicts the modern trend of minimally invasive techniques, and some patients may not accept this approach. Therefore, unless absolutely necessary, this technique is not recommended.

(4) Surgical Complications

As mentioned above, there are multiple treatment methods for gutter chest, and each method has different procedural details and possible complications. Considering that the types of surgeries are not significantly different from general chest wall deformity surgeries, the complications are also generally similar. A unique complication occurs in vertical surgeries since the ends of the plates are near the body surface and the ribs used for fixation may shift with changes in body position, this can lead to related complications. To avoid such complications, necessary measures must be taken during the operation. Semi-open and open surgeries are techniques now rarely used in modern chest wall surgery. These techniques also carry risks of complications, so extra caution is required during their execution. Among all complications, the most common and serious is surgical failure. Surgical failure can result from many factors, but the most fundamental reason is surgical technique. If the special characteristics of the deformity are not fully understood and the Nuss procedure is hastily applied, success is almost impossible. Using other methods can also lead to failure. This shows that surgical techniques still need improvement.

7. Secondary Surgery for Gutter Chest

In the past, many patients with gutter chest were mistakenly treated as having pectus excavatum and underwent the Nuss procedure. Due to misunderstandings of key technical points, these surgeries almost universally failed. After such failed surgeries, the deformity often still appears as a gutter chest, or even transforms into a more complex deformity. Faced with this outcome, patients often strongly desire a revision surgery.

When performing secondary surgery for gutter chest, the difficulty is undoubtedly much greater (Figure 2-8-3). To ensure surgical success, efforts must be made on multiple fronts: First, regarding the choice of surgical method the best option at this point is the modified Wang procedure. Since this operation is carried out entirely on the surface of the bony structures, it can effectively reduce surgical risks and difficulty. Of course, a semi-open or open surgery can also be directly considered. These approaches provide good exposure and direct manipulation, which not only effectively lowers the difficulty but also reduces surgical risks, and they are reasonable choices for secondary operations.

Second, there is the issue of adhesion management. In general revision surgeries, special measures for adhesion handling may not be required, but for failed gutter chest operations, this must be carefully addressed.

Adhesions mean there is severe traction on the anterior chest wall. To ensure a better surgical outcome, it is necessary to separate these adhesions. Even when performing the Wang procedure, adhesiolysis is needed, as it helps achieve good surgical results. When performing semi-open or open surgery, separating adhesions is relatively simple and can be done during the procedure, but given the nature of these surgeries, the significance of adhesiolysis is limited and therefore often unnecessary.

Besides failed gutter chest cases, there are also gutter chest deformities secondary to other surgeries (Figures 2-8-4 and 2-8-5). The surgical approach for these deformities is similar to that for secondary gutter chest correction and requires the same effort in the aspects mentioned above.

During secondary surgery, if a minimally invasive approach is used, the risk and difficulty are high, making it a true test of the surgeon's skill. Only by paying close attention to surgical details and performing all steps carefully can good results be achieved. Otherwise, the surgery may fail again, causing the patient even greater suffering [14].

8. Prognosis

The overall outcome of the various thoracic deformities is generally low in terms of the success rate of sulcus thoracic surgery, with a variety of postoperative problems. This is mainly due to the lack of understanding of the nature of the deformity. If it is treated as a common funnel chest, it will definitely lead to surgical failure. Therefore, it is necessary to recognise the special characteristics of this deformity from the ideological perspective, and on this basis, adopt appropriate methods and special techniques to ensure the success of the surgery.

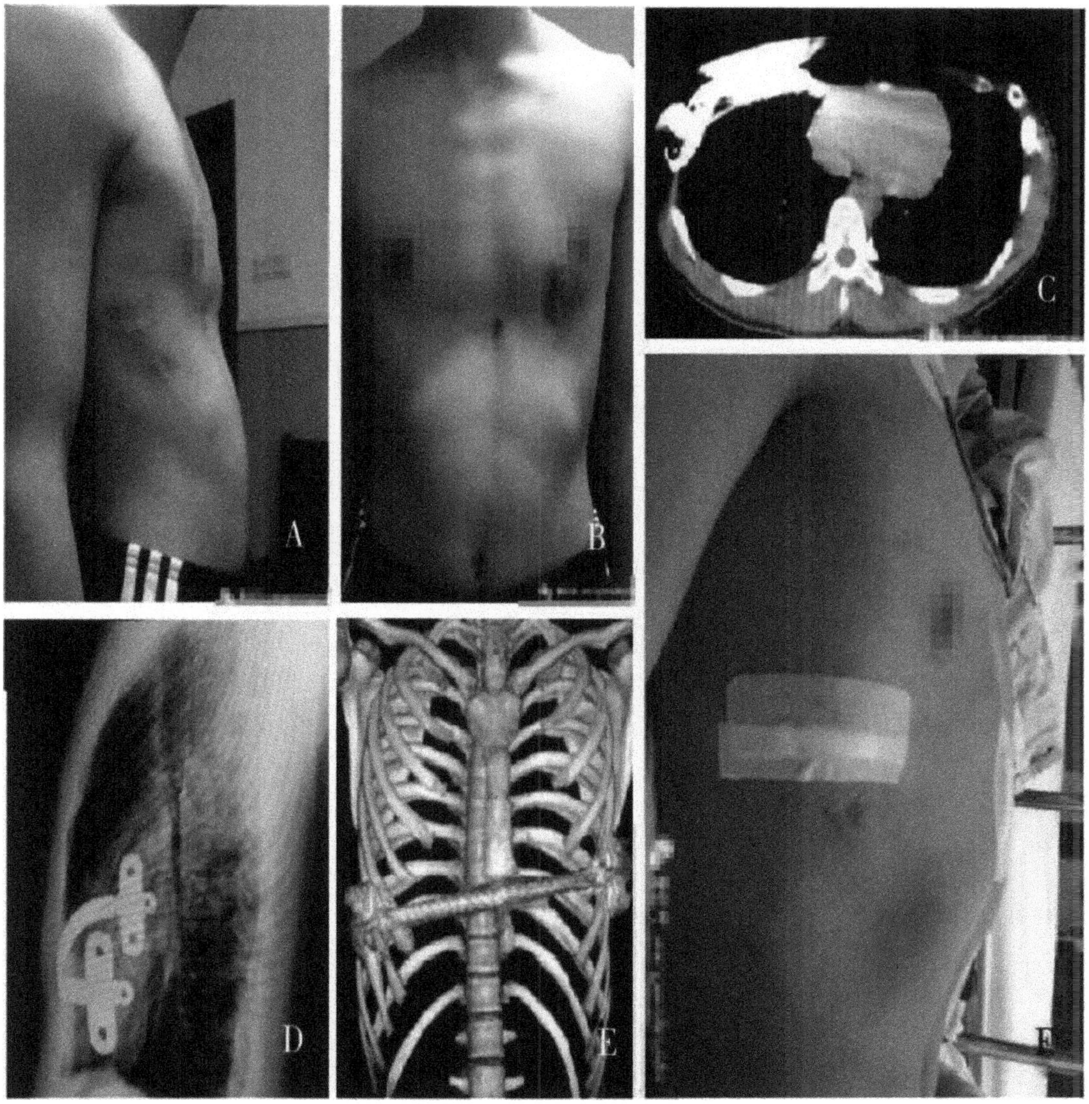

Figure 2-8-3 Secondary surgery after failed gutter chest Nuss procedure (A, B. External appearance of the thorax, showing a distinct gutter-like depression on the anterior chest wall with visible old surgical scars; C. CT cross-sectional image indicating severe adhesions around the plate; D. In the first surgery, the plate was positioned on the deep surface of the chest wall above the depression, providing no supporting effect; E. 3D reconstruction showing the position of the plate; F. Post-secondary surgery appearance of the chest wall, with the deformity completely corrected.)

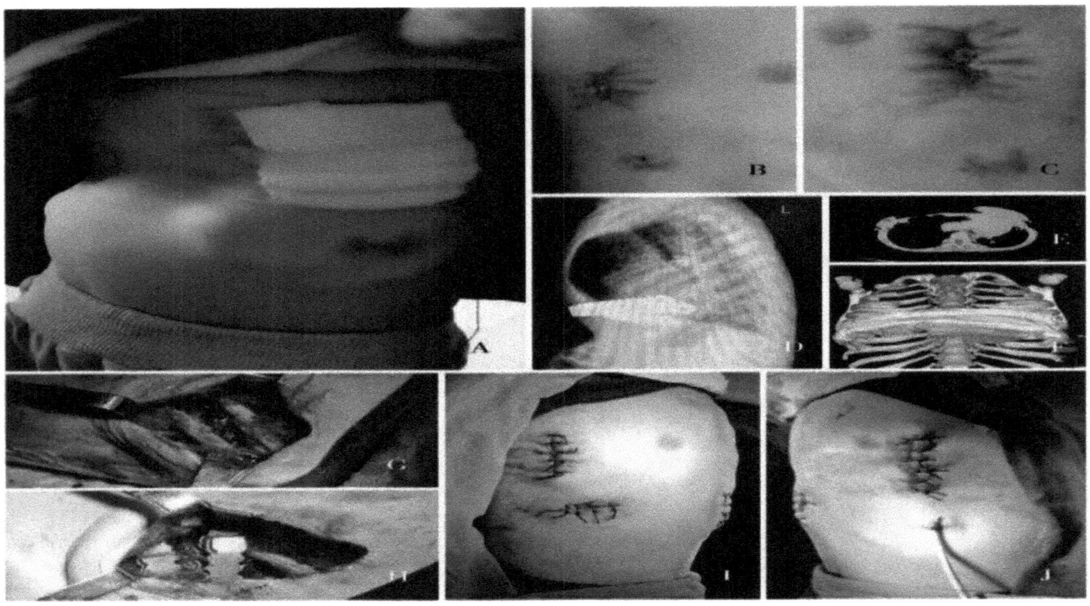

Figure 2-8-4 Secondary gutter chest after pectus carinatum surgery corrected by Wenlin procedure + Wung procedure(A. The child underwent surgery for pectus carinatum at a local hospital, where two plates were used: one plate to press down the protrusion and another plate to support the depression, but a significant gutter-like depression deformity developed postoperatively; B. Surgical scar on the right side; C. Poor healing of the left-side incision with the plate exposed outside the body; D. Lateral X-ray showing abnormal positions of both plates; E. CT cross-sectional image showing adhesions around the plates; F. 3D reconstruction showing plate positions; G. During the secondary surgery, the original plates were removed, exposing the ribs used for fixation;H. Correction was performed with two plates: the upper plate for the Wenlin procedure and the lower plate for the Wung procedure;I, J. Postoperative appearance of the chest wall with the deformity completely corrected.)

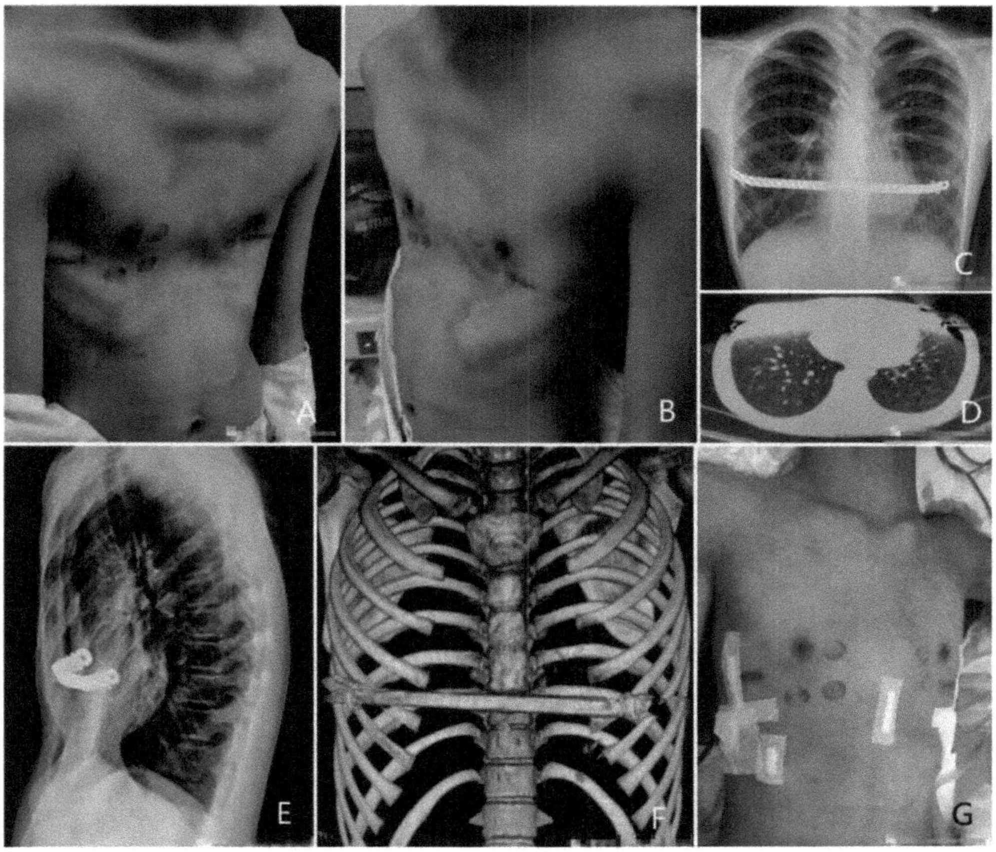

Figure 2-8-5 Gutter chest surgery after failed funnel chest Nuss procedure(A. The anterior chest wall shows a clear gutter-like depression; B. Old surgical scar visible on the chest wall;C. Frontal X-ray showing the plate shifted to one side; D. CT cross-sectional image showing obvious adhesions around the plate; E. Lateral X-ray showing the plate located deep on the upper chest wall above the depression, providing no supporting effect for the depression; F. 3D reconstruction showing a single plate deviated to the right side; G. Chest wall appearance after the revision surgery.)

REFERENCES

[1] Wang, W. L. 2018a. "The Difference between Groove Chest and Funnel Chest." *Thoracic Deformity Surgery Specialist*, March 14.

[2] Wang, W. L. 2018b. "Groove Chest: This Groove Is Not That Groove." *Thoracic Deformity Surgery Specialist*, March 12.

[3] Wang, W. L. 2021a. "Not All Depressions Are Funnel Chests." *Thoracic Deformity Surgery Specialist*, July 1.

[4] Wang, W. L. 2021b. "The Particularity of Surgery Determines the Naming of the Deformity." *Thoracic Deformity Surgery Specialist*, June 11.

[5] Wang, W. L. 2016. "Naming and Morphological Characteristics of Groove Chest." *Journal of Practical Medicine* 32 (2): 335–336.

[6] Wang, W. L. 2017a. "Does Harrison's Groove Affect Breathing?" *Thoracic Deformity Surgery Specialist*, March 11.

[7] Herlitz, G. 1945. "What Is the Cause of Harrison's Groove in Rickety Infants." *Acta Paediatrica* 32 (3–4): 439–444.

[8] Wang, W. L. 2017b. "Basic Principles of the Nuss Procedure (1)." *Thoracic Deformity Surgery Specialist*, December 1.

[9] Wang, W. L. 2017c. "Basic Principles of the Nuss Procedure (2)." *Thoracic Deformity Surgery Specialist*, December 2.

[10] Wang, W. L. 2021c. "The Wang Procedure for Groove Chest." *Thoracic Deformity Surgery Specialist*, April 4.

[11] Wang, W. L. 2019. "Today's Modified Wang Procedure for Groove Chest." *Thoracic Deformity Surgery Specialist*, April 17.

[12] Wang, W. L. 2020. "Today's Surgery: Minimally Invasive Surgery for Groove Chest." *Thoracic Deformity Surgery Specialist*, January 9.

[13] Wang, W. L. 2021d. "Today's Groove Chest Surgery." *Thoracic Deformity Surgery Specialist*, March 21.

[14] Wang, W. L. 2012. "Analysis of Reasons for Surgical Failure of Groove Chest." *Thoracic Deformity Surgery Specialist*, December 18.

LATERAL CHEST WALL DEPRESSION DEFORMITY

Depression-type deformities are the most common thoracic deformities. The depression may be located in the midline of the anterior chest wall, off the midline of the anterior chest wall, or on the lateral chest wall. In the past, all chest wall depressions were referred to as pectus excavatum. If treatment specifically, the choice of surgical method is not considered, this naming is not a major issue. However, after the advent of the Nuss procedure, which has been recognized as the standard surgical method for pectus excavatum, some authors indiscriminately applied it to all types of chest wall depressions. The misuse of surgery inevitably extended beyond the applicable scope of the Nuss procedure, resulting in many failed deformity surgeries. This serves as a warning that not all depression-type deformities should be treated as pectus excavatum. Only depressions located on the anterior chest wall are true pectus excavatum; depressions in other areas should not be regarded as pectus excavatum. To better understand and treat various depression deformities, we have successively named different related deformities. Depressions located on the lateral chest wall are named lateral chest wall depression deformity to emphasize their particularity (Figure 2-9-1) [1]. Lateral chest wall depression deformity is a relatively rare thoracic deformity. Since no other authors have focused on this type of deformity, there is no reported incidence rate.

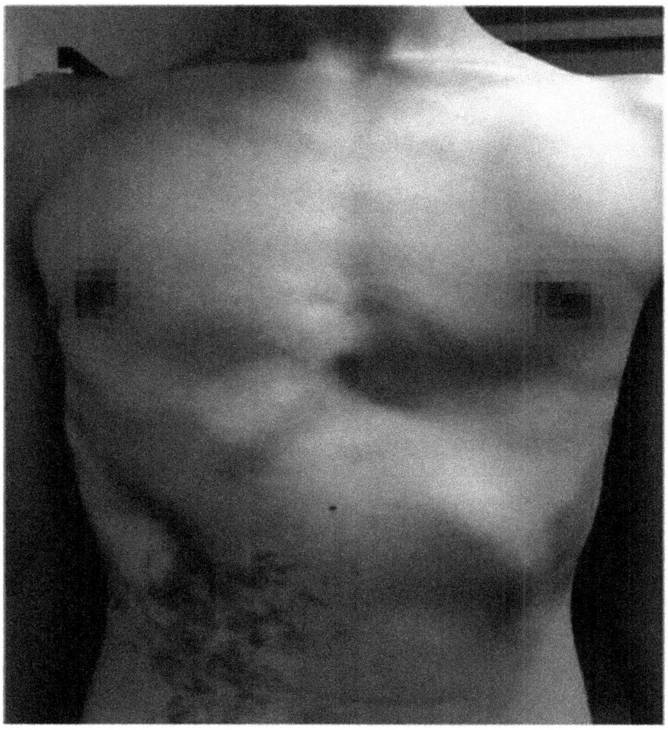

Figure 2-9-1 Chest wall appearance of lateral chest wall depression deformity. Depression on the left lateral chest wall, with the corresponding area on the right side essentially normal.

In our clinical practice, we often encounter this deformity, but its incidence is significantly lower compared to depressions located on the anterior chest wall (i.e., pectus excavatum).This deformity has its own unique characteristics, and although its incidence is not high, it requires special treatment methods. Therefore, it is necessary to regard it as an independent deformity.

1. Causes and Pathogenesis
According to the different causes, lateral chest wall depression deformity can be divided into primary and secondary types. Primary lateral chest wall depression deformity. The cause of primary lateral chest wall depression deformity is unclear. Generally speaking, the development of depression-type deformities is related to two factors: one is changes in the chest wall's own structure, and the other is the action of external forces. The lateral chest wall depression deformity is located on the lateral chest wall, with the bottom of the depression facing the thoracic cavity and having no direct contact with any structures, so traction from the bottom is unlikely. However, there is negative pressure inside the thoracic cavity, which also acts as an external force on the chest wall. If this negative pressure continuously increases due to certain factors, it may cause the chest wall to depress. In addition to forces from beneath the depression, external forces can also come from outside the chest wall. External compression or other forms of external force may also cause lateral chest wall depression.

Secondary depression deformity has a clear cause. Clinically, the most common cause is chest wall depression resulting from empyema, which originates from the traction of the inner fibrous structures of the chest wall due to pleural thickening. This is a relatively specific deformity that often occurs in remote areas and is rarely seen in regions with good hygiene conditions. Besides empyema, secondary lateral chest wall depression deformity can also occur after chest wall trauma. If there is extensive damage to bony structures and no timely fixation is performed after surgery; a depression deformity may develop. There are many differences between secondary and primary depression deformities, which will be described in other chapters.

2. Pathological Characteristics
Lateral chest wall depression deformity is a depression located on the lateral chest wall, with a clear base and raised edges, similar to the "pit" seen in pectus excavatum. However, this deformity does not involve the sternum; the shape and height of the sternum remain normal, without any protrusion or depression.

The degree of depression in this type of deformity is generally not severe, meaning the depression is neither very deep nor extensive. When the deformity occurs on the right side, the chest wall depression may compress the right lung. When it occurs on the left side, the depression may compress both the left lung and the heart, and in such cases, the clinical symptoms may be more severe. In addition, the lateral chest wall depression can cause uneven stress on both sides of the spine, and some patients may develop significant scoliosis.

3.Clinical Manifestations

When the degree of lateral chest wall depression deformity is mild, there may be no clinical symptoms. If the depression is more severe—especially when the lesion is located on the left lateral chest wall more obvious compression symptoms may appear, manifesting as discomfort in the respiratory and circulatory systems. Physical examination may reveal a clear abnormal chest shape, asymmetry between the left and right sides, and occasional scoliosis.

Since the depression is located on the lateral chest wall and relatively hidden, its impact on appearance is less pronounced than a midline depression, so patients generally have fewer aesthetic complaints. However, if there is a large-area depression on one side of the chest wall, especially when the spine is involved, the overall body shape may be affected. If the patient is very concerned about their appearance, psychological issues may arise, along with related symptoms.

4. Examination

Physical examination can confirm the diagnosis, while imaging studies help to clarify the characteristics of the depression itself and its relationship with the intrathoracic structures relationship. Three-dimensional reconstruction can show the overall contour of the thorax and is very helpful for understanding the characteristics of the deformity.

5. Diagnosis and Differential Diagnosis

The diagnosis of lateral chest wall depression deformity is relatively straightforward. The key points for diagnosis are: (1) The presence of depression in the chest wall. Depression is the most basic feature of this deformity. It is relatively localized, mostly involving the ribs, sometimes the costal cartilage, but not the sternum. The depression is typically a “pit” ; the centre is the lowest point, surrounded by a raised edge that does not exceed the normal chest wall height. (2) The depression is located on the lateral chest wall. The main part of the depression is entirely on the lateral chest wall and may partly involve the anterior chest wall, but it can never be completely on the anterior chest wall. (3) The sternum is normal. The structure, shape, and height of the sternum are completely normal and unrelated to the deformity.

The main differential diagnosis is with pectus excavatum, saddle chest [2], Poland syndrome [3], and thoracic dysplasia syndrome [4]. The difference from pectus excavatum is mainly in the location and structures involved. Standard symmetrical pectus excavatum is located on the anterior chest wall and involves the sternum, while lateral chest wall depression deformity is located on the lateral chest wall and does not involve the sternum. The difference is clear and easy to distinguish. Asymmetrical pectus excavatum may have its deepest point on the lateral chest wall, which can be confused with lateral chest wall depression deformity. The key point for differentiation is the shape and height of the sternum, that is, whether the sternum is affected. If the sternum is involved and also shows some degree of depression, it is asymmetrical pectus excavatum. If the sternum is completely normal, it is lateral chest wall depression deformity. Saddle chest is a depression on both sides of the chest wall, with a low position, and the midline separated by a normal-height sternum or lower structures. Lateral chest wall depression deformity only affects one side and does not involve both sides of the chest wall,

so, it is relatively easy to distinguish.

Poland syndrome involves abnormal development of the bony structures and soft tissues of the chest wall, which can appear as a depression of the unilateral upper chest wall. This depression may seem similar to a high-position lateral chest wall depression deformity, but they differ essentially. The distinguishing points are: (1) Poland syndrome often involves absence or fusion of ribs or costal cartilage, whereas lateral chest wall depression deformity does not have such local abnormalities. (2) Poland syndrome involves hypoplasia or absence of soft tissue, which is also not present in lateral chest wall depression deformity. Thoracic dysplasia syndrome should also be differentiated. (3) This deformity mainly involves abnormal thoracic structures and scoliosis. Local ribs may be absent or fused, but the location is posterior, mainly near the spine. The chest wall may show localized collapse, but the depression is usually not pronounced. In contrast, lateral chest wall depression deformity is located more anteriorly, is localized, and does not have structural absence or fusion at the base of the depression. The difference between the two is clear.

In diagnosis, in addition to differentiating from the above deformities, it is also necessary to distinguish whether the lateral chest wall depression deformity is primary or secondary. Primary deformity has no obvious cause, is smaller in scope, and milder in severity. Secondary deformity has a clear cause with a definite causal relationship, tends to be larger in scope, and more severe. Treatment of secondary deformity is relatively complex and involves treating the primary condition. Therefore, it is important not only to differentiate it from primary deformity but also to identify the underlying disease as accurately as possible. This is key to successful correction.

6. Indications for Surgery

If lateral chest wall depression deformity does not cause obvious symptoms and the patient is not concerned about the deformity, surgery may not be necessary. Conversely, if there are symptoms or if the patient is dissatisfied with the appearance of the deformity, surgery should be performed. In general, as with all other deformity surgeries, the decision for surgery should ultimately rest with the patient and their family.

7. Surgical Treatment

Surgery for thoracic deformities is highly variable and requires flexible selection of surgical techniques based on the characteristics of the deformity. Although lateral chest wall depression deformity has clear features, there are many individual variations among patients, which places high demands on the choice of surgical method. In general, lateral chest wall depression deformity is not very severe especially for primary cases, where the depression is relatively mild and commonly used minimally invasive procedures can achieve good results. However, in certain special cases, minimally invasive surgery may not fully correct the deformity, and in such cases, an open surgery must be performed as an unavoidable option.

(1) Minimally Invasive Surgery

From an overall classification perspective, lateral chest wall depression deformity belongs to a Class I deformity [5], and in principle, this type of deformity can be treated with the Nuss procedure [6] or the Wang procedure [7]. However, in actual clinical practice, if the special characteristics of this deformity are not fully understood, these two procedures are highly likely to fail. On the surface, this may seem to contradict the general treatment principles, but there are underlying reasons for this. Take the Nuss procedure as an example. Its failure may be related to the following factors: (1) Treating lateral chest wall depression deformity as a typical pectus excavatum without making any special modifications to the surgical details, and directly applying the standard Nuss procedure, which leads to surgical failure. This is actually a very basic mistake. When the standard symmetrical Nuss procedure for typical pectus excavatum is used without careful consideration, the incisions and supports are placed on both lateral chest walls, and the metal bar is shaped symmetrically. The healthy side can have a suitable support point selected according to the standard Nuss procedure, but the support point on the affected side even if positioned at the outer edge of the depression will not have a height suitable for the Nuss technique. Such a structural setup cannot meet the basic requirements of the Nuss procedure, resulting in inevitable failure. (2) Treating lateral chest wall depression deformity as an asymmetrical pectus excavatum and making some technical adjustments, but the modifications are inappropriate, resulting in surgical failure.

Compared with the first situation, this approach is a step forward but still has clear flaws. When lateral chest wall depression deformity is mistaken for asymmetrical pectus excavatum, surgeons often use an asymmetrical metal bar to achieve a good outcome, but all other steps are still performed according to the standard Nuss procedure meaning the incision and support points are still chosen on the lateral chest wall, and the bar still passes behind the sternum. This approach should theoretically yield relatively good results, but since the chest wall structure still cannot meet the basic requirements of the procedure, it will ultimately fail as well. From the reasons for the Nuss procedure's failure, it is clear that mechanically applying the Nuss technique without understanding its core principle is the root cause of failure. Essentially, the Nuss procedure is effective for all depression-type deformities. Its working principle is to use a symmetrical bar to support and lift the centre of the depression. This is the most fundamental part of its mechanism. To achieve this, the support points for the Nuss procedure must always be located at the highest edges of the depression. This is the key to success for the Nuss procedure. For symmetrical pectus excavatum, the support points happen to be located symmetrically on both sides of the chest wall, which makes incision placement selection much easier in most surgeries, the incisions are placed symmetrically on both sides of the chest wall. For asymmetrical pectus excavatum, if only the need to correct the depression is considered, the support points should still be chosen at the highest edges of the depression. In this case, the ideal incision position should also be near the support points. However, such an incision obviously deviates from the basic principle of incision placement, because its location may affect the cosmetic result. Therefore, in clinical practice, surgeons still choose to make the incision on the lateral chest wall. Since this incision is far from the ideal support point, to perform the surgery, the support point has to be selected near the incision instead. Such a support point is clearly no longer ideal. To compensate for this inadequate support point position, surgeons have to use other methods namely, changing the shape of the metal bar and using an asymmetrically shaped bar during the procedure. Although this approach may be effective, it is not the best solution.

In lateral chest wall depression deformity, the deformity is located on the lateral chest wall. According to the basic requirements of the Nuss procedure, the ideal support point should be at the edge of the depression. Using this area as the support point provides the structural foundation needed for the Nuss procedure to work properly, making surgical failure unlikely. Similarly, the Wang procedure has a similar issue using the sides of the depression as support points instead of the lateral chest wall. Once this principle is understood, the Wang procedure can also be easily performed and can achieve very good surgical results.
From the above analysis, it can be seen that when using the Nuss procedure or the Wang procedure, it is essential to understand the surgery with a broad perspective not narrowly focus only on the standard approach used for pectus excavatum. These two surgical methods are intended for all depression-type deformities, not just for pectus excavatum. When they are applied to other depression deformities, it is critical to fully understand the principles behind the procedures and go beyond or even forget the standard pectus excavatum technique. Only in this way can the surgery fully achieve its intended effect and produce good outcomes.

(A) Modified Nuss Procedure

To distinguish the Nuss procedure used for lateral chest wall depression deformity from the standard Nuss procedure, it is referred to here as the modified Nuss procedure. There are three specific operative approaches: First, the Nuss procedure specifically for lateral chest wall depression deformity; Second, a method similar to the Nuss procedure used for asymmetrical pectus excavatum; Third, a further improved version of the Nuss procedure.

(i) The Nuss procedure specifically for lateral chest wall depression deformity

When the Nuss procedure directly targets the depression of the lateral chest wall, the incision can be made right at the edge of the depression without considering the usual incision restrictions. The rib structure at the elevated edge is exposed, and a symmetrical bar is placed under the depression to lift it. After fixing the bar, the surgery is completed. If only the correction effect of the depression itself is considered, this approach is undoubtedly the ideal method. However, the resulting scar from the incision may cause cosmetic concerns; this is the biggest drawback of this technique. If the patient can accept the cosmetic cost, then this approach is reasonable. Unfortunately, some patients cannot accept this trade-off, which greatly limits the feasibility of this method.

(ii) The Nuss procedure similar to that used for asymmetrical pectus excavatum

The biggest problem with the above approach is the placement of the incision. To avoid the drawback of having an anterior chest wall incision, the incision has to be made on the lateral chest wall, making the surgery similar to the Nuss procedure used for asymmetrical pectus excavatum. The shortcomings of this approach have already been mentioned previously. To minimize these drawbacks, the specific surgical details must be carefully optimized and designed during the operation only then can good results be achieved

(iii) Further Improved Nuss Procedure

Both of the above methods have their own advantages: the first directly targets the depression, while the second offers a more satisfactory incision location. When used independently, each has clear drawbacks. However, combining the two can produce an excellent surgical approach. After extensive observation and study, we designed a modified Nuss procedure specifically for lateral chest wall depression deformity. The specific method is as follows: incisions are made on both sides of the chest wall, in the same positions as a standard Nuss procedure. A tunnel for the bar is created with the following route: it enters the edge of the depression on the affected side, passes through the bottom of the depression, exits from the other edge of the depression, continues to the opposite side, passes in front of the sternum, and follows the healthy side's rib surface to the opposite incision. From this route, it can be seen that although the incisions are still on the lateral chest wall, the support points are at the edges of the depression, thus combining the advantages of both previous methods into a more ideal procedure (Figure 2-9-2).

This further improved Nuss procedure is completely different in technique from other types of Nuss procedures. However, since it still directly targets the depression and lifts it from the bottom, it remains within the scope of the Nuss procedure. When performing this specific operation, several key points require special attention: First, the working principle of the bar must be fully understood only then can the key points of the operation be mastered to ensure a smooth procedure. Second, the fixation point for the bar on the affected side must be carefully planned to ensure it is in the correct position. Third, the shape of the bar must be properly designed to ensure it not only lifts the depression but also does not affect the appearance of the healthy side of the chest wall. Fourth, the technical details of placing the bar must be well designed to avoid damage to thoracic organs and ensure smooth completion of the surgery. Fifth, the incision must follow the basic requirements: it should be as hidden as possible while still allowing smooth operation.

The further improved Nuss procedure is a completely new technique designed specifically for lateral chest wall depression deformity and may be challenging for inexperienced surgeons. However, as long as the principles of the procedure are fully understood and the details are carefully handled, it is not difficult to perform. On the contrary, since the bar does not need to pass through the mediastinum, the surgical risk is greatly reduced, making it easier to master

Figure 2-9-2 Further Improved Nuss Procedure (A. Lateral chest wall

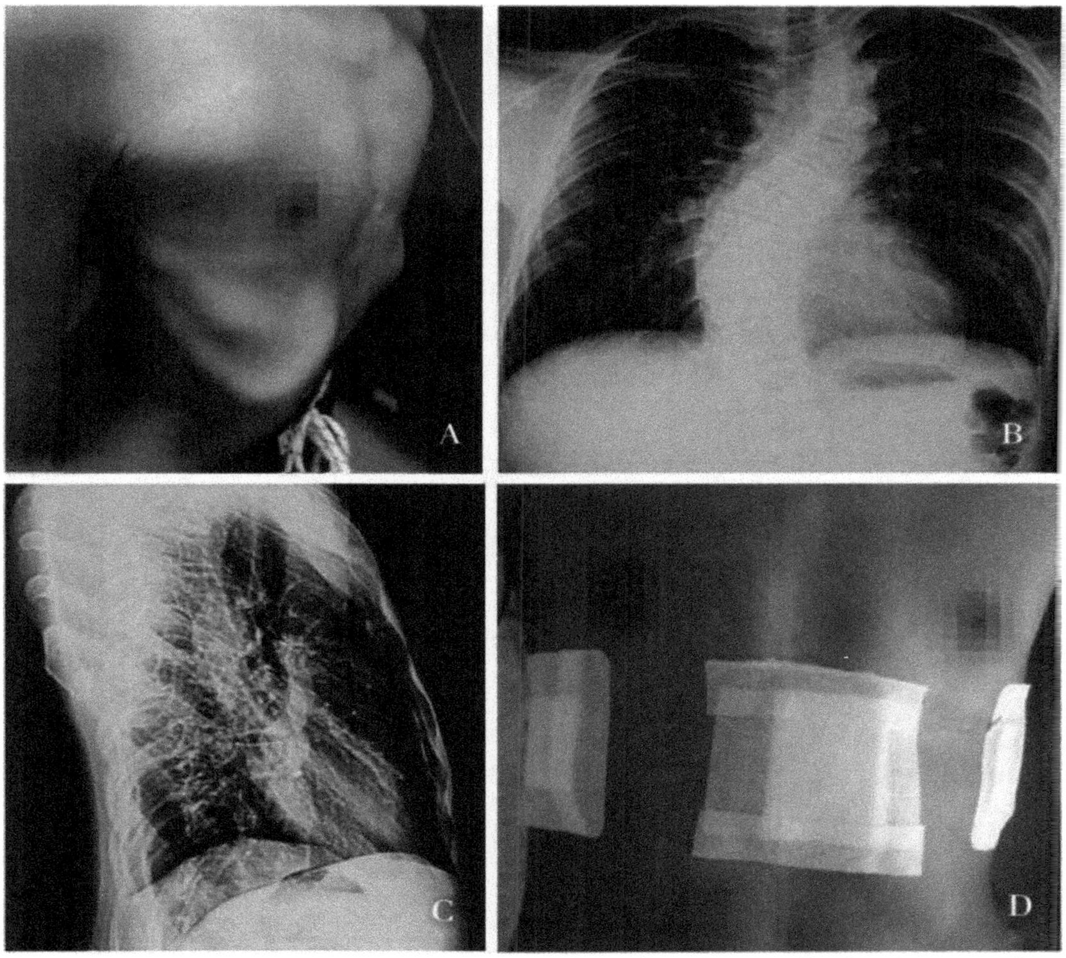

depression deformity; B. X-ray frontal view showing scoliosis; C. X-ray lateral view showing no obvious abnormal signs; D. Postoperative chest wall appearance, basically restored to normal shape)

(B) Modified Wang Procedure

The standard Wang procedure is used for correcting midline pectus excavatum, but this does not mean the Wang procedure can only be used for pectus excavatum. Like the Nuss procedure, the Wang procedure can also be applied to all depression-type deformities, including lateral chest wall depression deformity. In actual practice, since there are differences from the Wang procedure for pectus excavatum, it is referred to here as the modified Wang procedure. In this case, the metal bar can also be placed over the top of the depression. During the operation, as long as the bar extends beyond the edges of the depression, the surgical requirements are met. Once the bar is placed, the bony structure at the bottom of the depression is lifted and securely fixed, and the deformity can then be completely corrected (Figure 2-9-3).

From the above operative details, performing a modified Wang procedure for lateral chest wall depression deformity is also an extremely simple operation. As long as the operative concept of the Wang procedure is applied to the lateral chest wall depression, the surgery is almost effortless. Considering that there are no special structures deep within the depression, the Wang procedure in this case is not only safer but also easier to perform.

(C) Longitudinal Surgery

The Nuss procedure and Wang procedure are both performed in the transverse direction. Since they usually require the ribs as support points, and considering the orientation of the ribs, this support is not always ideal.

(2) Open Surgery

A lateral chest wall depression deformity is located on the lateral chest wall, which is relatively concealed, so making a larger local incision generally does not cause significant aesthetic issues. This feature makes open surgery feasible. The basic principle of open surgery is destructive reshaping: a wedge resection or transection of the depressed ribs or costal cartilage is performed first, then special materials are used for fixation and reshaping. This is the essence of open surgery. For this specific type of deformity, the actual trauma of open surgery may not be significant, and the incision can be designed to be small, so the real damage may be much less than that of traditional open surgery. During the operation, MatrixRIB material can be used for reshaping, which can achieve very good results. In addition, since this material does not need to be removed, the pain of a second surgery can be avoided.

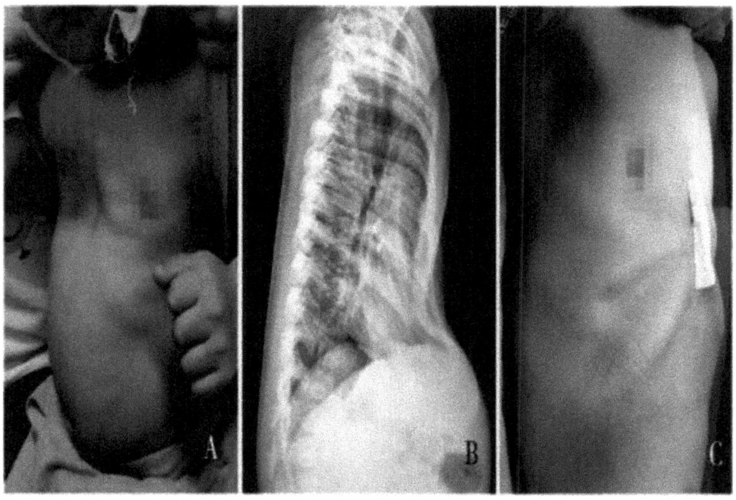

Figure 2-9-3 Modified Wang Procedure (A. Lateral chest wall depression deformity obvious depression of the right chest wall, no abnormality on the left side; B. X-ray lateral view showing clear chest wall depression; C. Deformity completely corrected postoperatively using the Wang procedure)

However, if the operation is performed from a different direction — that is, in the longitudinal direction — the implant (steel bar) will be oriented perpendicular to the ribs, making the ribs more suitable as support points. Given that a lateral chest wall depression is essentially a "pit" with an intact edge, performing the correction longitudinally is also reasonable and entirely feasible. In practice, either the Nuss procedure or the Wang procedure can be adapted for this approach. With proper design, good results can be achieved. However, this type of surgery has certain drawbacks, and if the transverse procedure can yield satisfactory outcomes, the longitudinal approach should be avoided whenever possible.

8. Surgical Complications

As a type of thoracic deformity, the basic nature of surgery for a lateral chest wall depression deformity is essentially the same as that for other deformities, so the surgery involves roughly the same complications. Since complications are closely related to the choice of surgical method, the occurrence of complications varies with different approaches. However, this does not mean that open surgery necessarily has more complications than minimally invasive surgery. In many cases, minimally invasive surgery may actually have more complications. Therefore, in practice, the more minimally invasive the procedure, the more carefully and cautiously it should be performed to minimize the risk of complications. From the above operative details, performing a modified Wang procedure for lateral chest wall depression deformity is also an extremely simple operation. As long as the operative concept of the Wang procedure is applied to the lateral chest wall depression, the surgery is almost effortless. Considering that there are no special structures deep within the depression, the Wang procedure in this case is not only safer but also easier to perform.

9. Reoperation After Failed Lateral Chest Wall Depression Surgery

Although a lateral chest wall depression deformity is technically just a simple depression deformity, its unique location makes the surgery significantly more challenging than a typical pectus excavatum procedure, and therefore it is not easy to achieve a successful outcome. In particular, when most surgeons regard it simply as a type of pectus excavatum and readily choose the Nuss procedure, the likelihood of success becomes even lower. In our clinical practice, we have encountered many such cases. We have encountered many cases of surgical failure, and most of these patients require revision surgery.

Most cases of failed lateral chest wall depression surgery still present as lateral chest wall depression, while a few patients develop a new deformity. If the deformity remains a lateral chest wall depression, the difficulty of revision surgery will be significantly increased due to the previous failed operation, and an appropriate surgical method must be selected according to the specific situation. If a new deformity is present, the situation may be more complex and requires intraoperative adjustments and appropriate techniques based on the characteristics of the deformity. In the most complicated cases, if a standard minimally invasive procedure cannot achieve correction, an open procedure should be considered, which would be the final and most reasonable option.

10. Prognosis

A lateral chest wall depression deformity is usually relatively localized and mild, so the treatment outcome should generally be favourable. However, because few people recognize its unique characteristics, surgical failure often occurs. In fact, achieving a good result is not complicated — as long as the nature of the depression is correctly understood and the proper method is applied, the surgery can certainly be successful.

REFERENCES

[1] Wang Wenlin. Naming of Localized Lateral Chest Wall Depression. Practical Journal of Medicine, 2015, 31 (Supplement): 196.
[2] Wang Wenlin. Lateral Chest Wall Depression Deformity and Saddle Chest. Thoracic Deformity Surgery Expert, 18-09-2021
[3] Wang Wenlin. Correction of Poland Syndrome Using MatrixRIB. Thoracic Deformity Surgery Expert, 23-10-2021
[4] Wang Wenlin. On Thoracic Dysplasia Syndrome. Thoracic Deformity Surgery Expert, 19-09-2021
[5] Wang Wenlin, Chen Chunmei, Li Xuejun, et al. Overall Classification System for Thoracic Deformities. Chinese Journal of Clinical Thoracic and Cardiovascular Surgery, 2018, 25 (11): 981–985.
[6] Wang Wenlin. Surgical Issues of Lateral Chest Wall Depression Deformity. Thoracic Deformity Surgery Expert, 16-09-2021.
[7] Wang Wenlin. Wang Procedure for Lateral Chest Wall Depression Deformity. Thoracic Deformity Surgery Expert, 25-10-2021

Section 10

SADDLE CHEST

Saddle chest is a special type of deformity that we have identified and named in recent years, so named because its appearance resembles a saddle [1]. This deformity is a relatively rare thoracic deformity, and due to limited research, its exact incidence is unknown. It has distinct characteristics and requires specific surgical techniques for correction, so it is necessary to describe it as a separate type of deformity.

1. Basic Concept

Saddle chest is a special deformity of the lower chest wall, characterized mainly by symmetrical depressions on both sides of the chest wall. The central area between the depressions remains at a normal height, with no significant protrusion or depression. The bilateral depressions are separated by the central chest wall, giving the deformity a saddle-like appearance (Figure 2-10-1) [1]. Essentially, saddle chest is a compound deformity, equivalent to a combination of two lateral chest wall depressions [2]. Because the positions of the two depressions are unique and form a fixed pattern, it is necessary to name it separately. This combination is similar to other special compound deformities, such as flat pectus carinatum [3] and Wenlin chest [4], but it differs from common compound deformities.

A compound deformity has a common feature: the deformity is not singular, and such patients generally have both protrusions and depressions at the same time. When the protrusion and depression occur in random positions without fixed characteristics, it is considered a general compound deformity. If the protrusion and depression have fixed positions and shapes, it is no longer a general compound deformity but a special compound deformity. Saddle chest falls within the category of compound deformities but differs from flat pectus carinatum and Wenlin chest. The saddle chest does not have a protrusion; it is simply a combination of two depressions. Because the depressions are not in the same location, it differs from all single depression deformities and is therefore classified as a type of compound deformity. Strictly speaking, the depressions of the saddle chest are not located entirely on the lateral chest wall but rather at the junction between the anterior chest wall and the lateral chest wall.

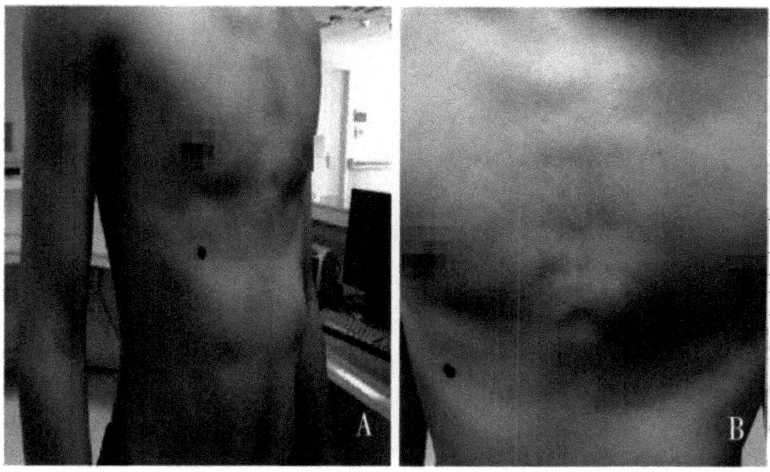

Figure 2-10-1 Appearance of Saddle Chest (A. Lateral view: depressions on both sides of the chest wall, with normal height in the midline; B. Frontal view: obvious depressions on both sides of the chest wall)

This special location makes it difficult to form a “pit” type depression like pectus excavatum; more often, it appears as a gentle slope. The central area is generally near the xiphoid process, consisting of the bony structures near the costal arch and the upper portion of the abdominal muscles, forming a direct extension of the midline anterior chest wall. Saddle chest can be classified into primary and secondary types. The cause of primary saddle chest is unknown; it can occur in childhood or during adolescence. Secondary saddle chest specifically refers to deformities that develop after a Nuss procedure and is a complication unique to this surgery [5] (Figure 2-10-2).

2. Pathogenesis

The pathogenesis of the primary saddle chest is unclear. Based on the general pathogenesis of thoracic deformities, there are two possible mechanisms: one is weakness of the chest wall, and the other is the effect of external forces. Since the location of the depression roughly corresponds to the Harrison groove, it may be related to the formation of this groove [6]. The Harrison groove is caused by the diaphragm pulling on the chest wall structures, and this mechanism may play a role in the development of the saddle chest. When the chest wall undergoes internal structural changes for various reasons, its rigidity will significantly decrease. If the pulling force of the diaphragm continues to increase at this point, it may cause a local depression of the chest wall. Such situations can occur in cases of calcium deficiency and prolonged respiratory distress or asthma. In the chapter on groove chest, we mentioned the relationship between the Harrison groove and the formation of groove chest, and the mechanism of saddle chest formation may be similar to that of groove chest.

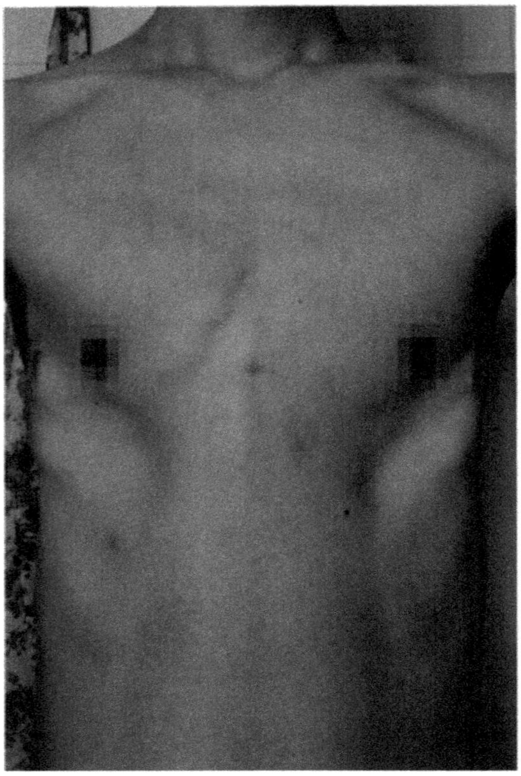

Figure 2-10-2 Saddle Chest Secondary to the Nuss Procedure. When the steel bar lifts the central depression, all the stress is borne by the bar itself. The support points of the bar are located on the lateral chest wall. If the stress becomes too great and the ribs of the lateral chest wall are relatively soft, a local depression may occur. However, since the central depression has already been lifted, this results in the appearance of a saddle chest.

Secondary saddle chest is commonly seen after the Nuss procedure for pectus excavatum. When a steel bar is used to support the depression in the midline of the anterior chest wall

When the steel bar lifts the midline depression, its support points are located on the lateral chest wall, which must bear the significant stress generated during elevation. If the support area is sufficiently strong, its shape and height will remain unchanged. If the support is relatively weak, it may collapse under the stress. Because the collapse occurs symmetrically on both sides of the chest wall while the central depression has already been lifted, this can result in a typical saddle chest. This is a common complication of the Nuss procedure. The occurrence of this complication is unrelated to the surgeon's technique and is instead an inherent flaw in the design of the procedure [5].

3. Risks

The risks of saddle chest also come from two aspects: one is the physiological harm caused by structural abnormalities, and the other is the psychological harm caused by the abnormal appearance. The physiological harm is mainly due to depression, which can compress the heart and lungs, leading to functional abnormalities. The psychological harm mainly stems from the abnormal appearance, which can cause various psychological issues.

4. Clinical Manifestations

The pathological changes of the saddle chest are mainly located on the lower parts of both sides of the chest wall. The deep area of the right-side depression involves lung tissue and the right diaphragm, while the left-side depression may compress the heart. Patients may feel breathing discomfort due to the compression and sometimes experience palpitations or chest pain; in severe cases, they may have dyspnea. These are the clinical manifestations of physiological harm. Since many patients are dissatisfied with the appearance of the chest wall, they may develop psychological problems of varying forms and degrees. Psychological problems can inturn affect the patient's physiological functions, leading to various complex clinical symptoms.

In terms of physical signs, the saddle chest has distinct features marked by two main characteristics: first, the characteristic depressions on both sides of the chest wall; second, the normal-height midline separation, which can be seen as a relative elevation rather than an actual protrusion.

From the perspective of the thoracic deformity classification system, since saddle chest only involves depressions and no protrusions, it is classified as a Type I deformity, specifically Type I-e [7]. This deformity can be regarded as a combination of two lateral chest wall depressions, but they are located on both sides of the chest wall rather than two depressions on the same side. This is what distinguishes it from a simple lateral chest wall depression deformity.

5. Examination

Saddle chest should first be assessed through a physical examination, with visual inspection being the most important component. By observing the appearance, the main features of the deformity can be identified. X-ray examination can reveal the depression of the anterior chest wall and its compression of the heart, and can also show the condition of the spine. CT scanning can provide detailed images of the depressions on both sides and their relationship to the heart, and can also give information about the internal condition of the thoracic cavity. If a heart murmur is present, an echocardiogram should be performed. Three-dimensional reconstruction can display the entire contour of the thorax and the structures of the intrathoracic organs; it is the most advanced examination method but is usually unnecessary.

6. Diagnosis and Differential Diagnosis

The diagnosis of saddle chest is generally confirmed through visual observation of the appearance, while imaging examinations can rule out any associated intrathoracic lesions and provide additional information about the condition.

The differential diagnosis mainly includes three other deformities: the first is pectus carinatum, the second is compound deformity, and the third is asphyxiating thoracic dystrophy (Jeune syndrome). When the depressions in a saddle chest are deep, the midline separation can appear as a relative protrusion. From a local external view, this can closely resemble typical pectus carinatum, which makes misdiagnosis possible. The key point for differentiation is its relationship with the upper chest wall: if the protrusion rises above the plane of the upper chest wall, it is pectus carinatum; otherwise, it is a saddling chest. A compound deformity is mainly a combination of a protrusion and a depression. In such cases, the arrangement of the depression and protrusion is random and does not precisely occur symmetrically on both sides of the chest wall. The saddle chest, however, consists of only two depressions with no actual protrusion, and the midline separation does not rise above the normal chest wall plane, so it is only a relative protrusion. This clearly distinguishes it from a typical compound deformity. Asphyxiating thoracic dystrophy (Jeune syndrome) is a rare thoracic deformity characterized by abnormal growth directions of the ribs and costal cartilages [8,9]. This deformity can also present with depressions on both sides of the chest wall. When these depressions are located lower, the appearance may resemble the saddle chest. However, the two conditions differ significantly in essence. The depressions in asphyxiating thoracic dystrophy are broader in scope, the base of the depression is severely affected and may sharply protrude inward into the thoracic cavity, and there is usually a large, midline anterior protrusion as well. These features are markedly different from the saddle chest. On CT imaging, the characteristic "凸" (convex) shape of asphyxiating thoracic dystrophy can appear across multiple scan layers, whereas in saddle chest it is seen mainly in the lower layers.

7. Surgical Indications

From a physiological perspective, if a patient with saddle chest develops obvious symptoms due to the depression compressing intrathoracic organs, this indicates pathological harm and surgery should be considered. From a psychological perspective, the same principle applies: psychological distress is also a form of illness and should likewise be treated. Therefore, as with other deformities, whether to undergo surgery should ultimately be decided by the patient and their family. If the patient and family feel that the appearance is unacceptable or that there is significant discomfort, then surgery is necessary;

if they feel neither concern about the appearance nor discomfort, then surgery is not necessary.
Contraindications for surgery mainly come from two aspects: psychological condition and physiological condition. Since patients with deformities often have psychological issues, if these problems are too severe, surgery should not be performed. The physiological condition mainly refers to the patient's overall health status. If the patient cannot tolerate surgery, then surgery should likewise not be performed.

8. Preoperative Preparation

Preoperative preparation can be carried out according to the standard protocol for general anesthesia surgery. Since a minimally invasive procedure is used during the operation, with a short operating time and limited steps, overly complex preparation is unnecessary; preparation should follow the principle of simplicity.

9. Surgical Treatment

(1) Basic Principles

Saddle chest involves two depressions at the same time, and the basic surgical principle is to treat it as a depression-type deformity. There are generally only two surgical options for treating depression deformities: the Nuss procedure and the Wang procedure. In principle, either procedure can be used to treat the saddle chest. However, since both sides must be corrected simultaneously, the use of materials and the efficiency of the operation must be carefully considered. When examining the entire procedure from a broader perspective, there may be different understandings of the surgical approach, and the Wenlin procedure may be used. In this context, the Wenlin procedure does not address an actual protrusion but instead targets the bilateral depressions. From another perspective, it is equivalent to a combination of two Wang procedures [10]. Therefore, the Wenlin procedure in this situation is actually a special operation under a special surgical perspective and is completely different from the typical Wenlin procedure for protrusion deformities. In any case, the name of the procedure is just a label — what matters is the fundamental surgical principle. Only by truly understanding the essence of the procedure can the deformity be effectively corrected.

(2) Surgical Methods

(i) Nuss Procedure

The saddle chest has two depressions, and each depression can be treated using the Nuss procedure. Theoretically, the saddle chest can be corrected with two completely independent Nuss procedures. In other words, two steel bars can be used to correct the depressions on both sides of the chest wall separately. However, putting this theoretical possibility into practice requires careful consideration of its feasibility. The Nuss procedure relies on the principle of leverage, with its most critical structural basis being the support points. The lateral support point of the depression is the rib, which, if sufficiently strong, can meet the surgical requirements. However, the central support point is the midline separation. Although its height may be adequate for the procedure, its rigidity is often insufficient, making it difficult to perform two independent Nuss procedures successfully. Objectively analyzing this approach, even if technically feasible, it is entirely unnecessary for several reasons: (1) Operations on both sides may interfere with each other in the middle; (2) Even if the midline operation is feasible, it would lead to redundant steps; (3) The position of the midline steel bar would be too superficial, negatively affecting both aesthetics and incision healing. Because of these issues, using two separate Nuss procedures to treat saddle chest is impractical. To eliminate these drawbacks, both sides can be treated with a single, combined Nuss procedure, that is, using one steel bar to correct both sides simultaneously. In this method, the path of the steel bar is as follows: it first enters the thoracic cavity through an incision on one side, passes beneath the base of the depression, then exits the same side's thoracic cavity and travels over the surface of the midline separation, enters the contralateral thoracic cavity, passes beneath the depression on the opposite side, and finally exits through an incision on the opposite chest wall. From the path of the steel bar, this method is equivalent to overlapping two Nuss procedures. Although the midline area still acts as a support point, since the steel bar is unified, all the stress is ultimately borne by its two ends. Therefore, as long as the support points at both ends are strong enough, the procedure can be successfully completed. However, this approach is not easy to implement, with the main challenge being the placement of the steel bar. To overcome this difficulty, the procedure can be further simplified by placing the midline portion of the steel bar beneath the surface of the midline separation rather than on its surface. In this way, for each side's depression deformity. In this sense, it is essentially a single Nuss procedure. The steel bar still has two support points: one is the outer edge of the depression on the same side of the chest wall, and the other is the outer edge of the depression on the opposite side. If the contralateral depression is not considered, this approach is clearly a standard Nuss procedure. When both depressions are included, the overall operation becomes an overlap of two Nuss procedures, ultimately forming a single Nuss procedure. This cycle shows that although the two depressions of the saddle chest are fundamentally different from pectus excavatum, another name has to be used to describe it. However, when the two depressions are corrected separately using the Nuss procedure, it ultimately returns to being a single Nuss procedure. This cycle is not a coincidence but rather a deeper understanding of the principle behind the Nuss procedure. This understanding shows that the Nuss procedure can be applied to depression deformities of various forms, whether it is a single depression or a double depression like saddle chest. As long as the basic requirements for the Nuss procedure are met, surgical success can be achieved.

Key points of the procedure: (1) Support points: Regardless of the form of the Nuss procedure, it is based on the principle of leverage and thus always involves the fundamental issue of support points. for the saddle chest, the support points on both sides are located more posteriorly; their relative height is not a problem, but their rigidity often is. Therefore, appropriate measures must be taken during the operation, and this is the key to success. (2) Curvature: The curvature of the steel bar is always one of the basic conditions for successfully completing the procedure. When both depressions need to be lifted, each side of the steel bar must have a proper curvature; only then can good correction results be achieved. To meet this requirement, the overall shape of the steel bar can be designed in a butterfly shape, with both sides shaped to effectively lift the depressions. (3) Technical skill: If the steel bar needs to pass in front of the midline separation, the operation becomes very challenging and requires special techniques. If the bar passes through the mediastinum, although this is similar to an ordinary Nuss procedure, it must pass near or even through the diaphragm's attachment or the diaphragm itself. In this case, more tissue is traversed, increasing the difficulty, so the procedure must be performed with great care.

(ii) Wang Procedure

Since saddle chest involves depressions, it is possible to use the Wang procedure [10]. Similar to the Nuss procedure, the Wang procedure can be performed by addressing the depressions on both sides separately. The specific method involves placing two steel bars over the surfaces of the depressions and then lifting the base of each depression. However, performing two separate Wang procedures is also impractical, so it is likewise necessary to combine both sides into one operation, using a single steel bar to correct both depressions simultaneously. From a broader perspective, this essentially becomes a Wenlin procedure in practice. The Wenlin procedure was originally designed to treat protrusion deformities. Although the saddle chest has no actual protrusion, it does have a relative protrusion, which forms the working basis for the Wenlin procedure. This shows that in certain special situations, different procedures can be converted into one another — the foundation for this conversion is the unique structure of the chest wall. Wherever there is a depression, there will always be a protrusion; this protrusion can be absolute or relative. Regardless of its nature, as long as there is a relative height difference, it can lead to a change in the surgical approach.

Key points of the procedure: (1) Support Points: Although support points are not as critical in the Wang procedure, they gain special importance when the midline separation is not sufficiently rigid, so appropriate measures must be taken to handle this properly. (2) Lifting points: The key to the Wang procedure's success is the lifting mechanism. To completely eliminate depression, it is essential to lift the most important structures. In the saddle chest, the only suitable structures for lifting are the ribs. However, since the intercostal spaces in this area may be wide, lifting only one rib would affect the surgical outcome; therefore, it is necessary to lift all relevant areas as needed. (3) Incision Placement: The Wang procedure requires the incision to be located at the deepest part of the depression. Considering aesthetic concerns, the incision can be made slightly more lateral.

If this is regarded as a Wenlin procedure, then an incision only needs to be made on the lateral chest wall. In this case, the incision position is basically the same as that described for the Wang procedure above. However, when performing the Wenlin procedure, it is essential to remember that the inner wires are not solely for fixation; their more important function is lifting. Guided by this concept, it becomes easy to unify the Wang procedure and the Wenlin procedure. This approach is more beneficial for correcting the deformity.

(iii) Longitudinal Procedure

This procedure is similar to the longitudinal procedure used for groove-shaped chest deformities. It makes use of the higher edges above and below the depression to design the operation. In this procedure, a specially designed steel plate can be placed longitudinally on the surface or deep inside the depression, and the deformity is corrected by lifting or supporting the depressed area. Although this method is theoretically feasible, achieving good results requires careful and detailed planning; otherwise, not only will it fail to produce good outcomes, but it may also lead to surgical failure.

(iv) Open Procedure

The depressions on both sides of the chest wall in saddle chest can be regarded as being caused by localized insufficiency in the length of the ribs or costal cartilage. for this reason, open surgery can be used to reshape the local bony structures. During the procedure, MatrixRIB can be used to lengthen and reshape the bony structures. Considering the issue of surgical trauma, the operation can be performed through the smallest possible incision, which can effectively eliminate the drawbacks of open surgery.

10. Surgical Complications

There are various specific surgical methods for treating saddle chest, and different procedures may have different complications, so the range of possible complications is relatively complex. However, overall, this type of surgery is not fundamentally different from other thoracic deformity surgeries, so the complications are generally similar. The most common complications include Hemothorax or pneumothorax, displacement of the steel plate, wire breakage, rib fracture, and delayed wound healing. In addition, since the operation site is relatively low, the diaphragm may also be injured — this is another possible complication.

Once a complication occurs, it can cause varying degrees of harm and requires appropriate management. Among these, one of the more troublesome outcomes is surgical failure. There can be many causes for surgical failure, but regardless of the cause, a repeat surgery is necessary if failure occurs. A second surgery involves many specific challenges — such as dealing with adhesions, managing the steel plate from the first surgery, and selecting the appropriate surgical method — all of which are difficult issues that require careful consideration by the surgeon to make good decisions. Otherwise, it will be very difficult to successfully complete the second operation.

11. Surgery for Saddle Chest After Nuss Procedure

Apart from primary saddle chest, the most commonly seen form in clinical practice is saddle chest that occurs after a Nuss procedure. The incidence of this form is even higher than that of primary saddle chest. Considering the inherent design flaws of the Nuss procedure, many people take a lenient attitude toward this complication and do not regard it as a complication or defect. However, some patients may feel anxious about it and wish to have it thoroughly corrected. This creates a demand for further surgical treatment.

Surgery for secondary saddle chest can be divided into two situations: one is surgery performed before removal of the Nuss procedure steel bar, and the other is surgery performed after its removal. When the Nuss steel bar is still in place, the midline separation can provide a very firm support point, which is beneficial for treating the bilateral depressions. However, since the depressions are mainly caused by the pressure from the Nuss steel bar, if the bar has not been removed, it will obstruct the treatment of the depressions, making any corrective method quite challenging. To make the best surgical decision, it is necessary to first check how long the bar has been in place. If it is possible to remove the bar earlier than planned, the surgery becomes easier to perform. The bar can be removed first, and then a Wenlin procedure can be used for correction, which can yield satisfactory results. If it is not yet time for bar removal, another approach should be designed. In this case, the Wenlin procedure can still be used, but due to the presence of the steel bar, the operation may be more difficult and the results may not be ideal. Because of these drawbacks, the best option is to wait until the bar has been removed before performing the corrective procedure.The second situation is surgery performed after the Nuss steel bar has been removed. Besides the Wenlin procedure, another Nuss procedure can also be considered for correction. In this case, the Nuss procedure is clearly different from the first one; the focus is on the design of the bar's curvature and the choice of the supporting position, which need to be handled according to the specific intraoperative conditions.

12. Prognosis

Saddle chest is a very unique type of thoracic deformity. Although it involves depressions, they are different from the typical "pit"-shaped depressions. Considering that most current techniques are designed for typical "pit"-shaped depressions, none of these techniques are an ideal choice for saddle chest. Therefore, surgery for the saddle chest is a serious test of a surgeon's technical skills. If the surgeon does not understand and master the essence of these techniques, it is very difficult to achieve a good result. On the other hand, as long as the surgeon carefully analyzes the structural characteristics of the saddle chest and fully utilizes the special features of different procedures, good results can definitely be achieved, ensuring the surgery is successfully completed (see Figure 2-10-3).

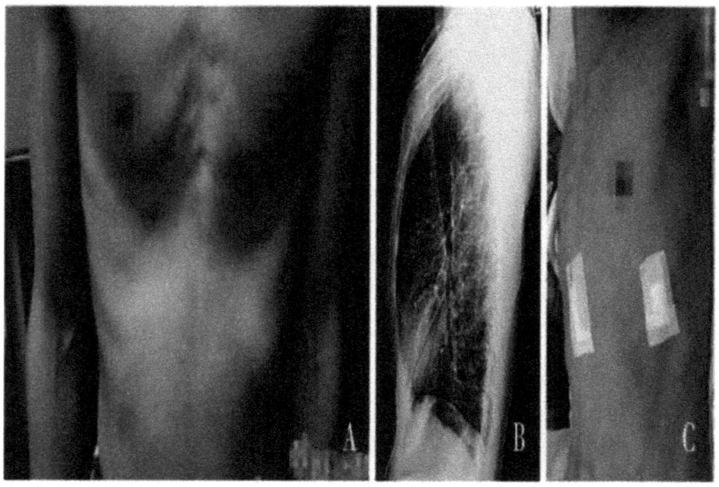

Figure 2-10-3 Surgical outcome for saddle chest (A) Appearance of saddle chest; (B) X-ray lateral view findings; (C) Postoperative appearance of the chest wall showing complete correction of the deformity.

REFERENCES

[1] Wang, W. L. 2017. "The Naming and Morphological Characteristics of Saddle Chest." *Journal of Practical Medicine* 33 (Suppl): 380–381.

[2] Wang, W. L. 2021a. "Lateral Chest Wall Depression Deformity and Saddle Chest." *Expert in Thoracic Deformity Surgery*, September 19.

[3] Wang, W. L. 2019. "The Naming of Flat Pectus Carinatum: A Special Thoracic Deformity." *Expert in Thoracic Deformity Surgery*, May 23.

[4] Wang, W. L. 2021b. "The Particularity of Wenlin Chest." *Expert in Thoracic Deformity Surgery*, June 10.

[5] Wang, W. L. 2021c. "Common Complication of the Nuss Procedure: Secondary Saddle Chest." *Expert in Thoracic Deformity Surgery*, May 17.

[6] Naish, J., and H. R. E. Wallis. 1948. "Significance of Harrison's Grooves." *British Medical Journal* 1 (4550): 541–544.

[7] Wang, W. L., C. M. Chen, X. J. Li, et al. 2018. "Overall Classification Method for Thoracic Deformities." *Chinese Journal of Clinical Thoracic and Cardiovascular Surgery* 25 (11): 981–985.

[8] Wang, W. L., W. G. Long, C. M. Chen, et al. 2021. "Surgical Treatment of Asphyxiating Thoracic Dystrophy." *Chinese Journal of Clinical Thoracic and Cardiovascular Surgery* 28 (8): 984–989.

[9] Wang, W. 2022. "Surgical Treatment of a 36-Year-Old Patient with Asphyxiating Thoracic Dysplasia." *Interactive Cardiovascular and Thoracic Surgery* 34 (1): 153–155.

[10] Wang, W. L., C. M. Chen, W. G. Long, et al. 2018. "Wang Procedure: Novel Minimally Invasive Procedure for Pectus Excavatum Children with Low Age." *Case Reports and Images in Surgery* 1 (1): 1–2.

Section 11

FLAT PIGEON CHEST

Flat Pectus Carinatum is a special type of thoracic deformity that we have named. Its appearance is similar to pectus carinatum (pigeon chest) but also has features that differ from typical pectus carinatum — there is a localized depression in the center, and the anterior chest wall appears flat when viewed from the side. Therefore, we call it flat pectus carinatum [1]. This deformity has distinct characteristics and a fixed structural pattern, and it differs significantly from classic pectus carinatum; therefore, it cannot be treated using the same surgical methods as pectus carinatum. For this reason, it is necessary to study it as an independent deformity. Flat pectus carinatum is relatively rare. Because no one else has paid much attention to this deformity, its exact incidence is unknown. It is more commonly seen in people after puberty (Figure 2-11-1), but it is not impossible for it to occur in younger children — some young children can also present with the typical appearance of this deformity (Figure 2-11-2).

This essentially, flat pectus carinatum is a type of compound deformity — it involves both a protrusion of the anterior chest wall and a depression. However, this combination of protrusion and depression is different from more common

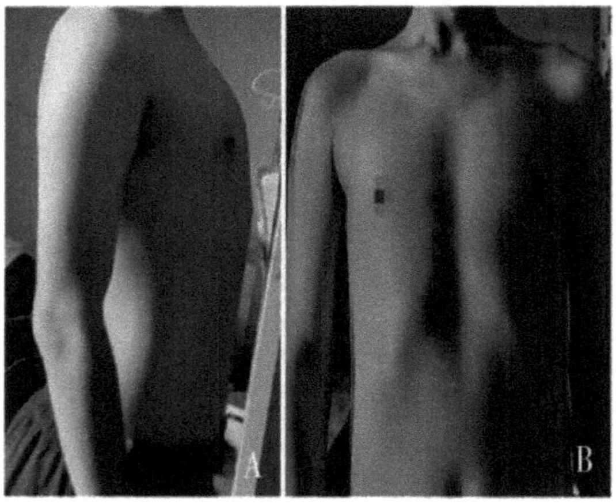

Figure 2-11-1 Post pubertal patient with a flat chicken chest (A. Lateral view of the thorax suggests an overall anterior chest wall convexity; B. median limited depression of the anterior chest wall).

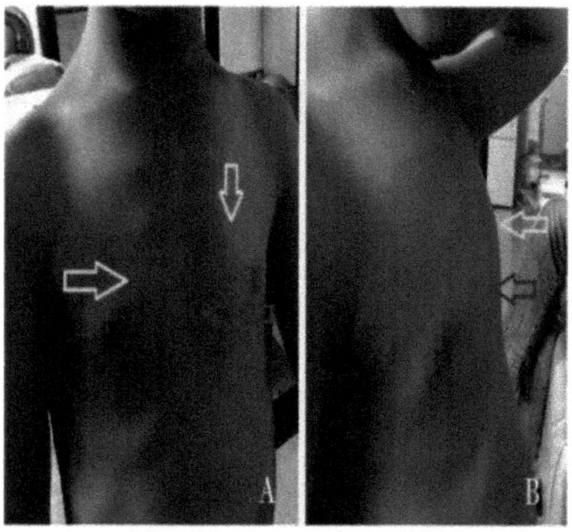

Figure 2-11-2 Flat pectus carinatum in a young child (A) Central depression in the anterior chest wall with protrusion on both sides; (B) Lateral view showing anterior protrusion of the chest wall.

combinations, which may be arranged vertically or horizontally. In flat pectus carinatum, the combination is an inclusive pattern: the entire anterior chest wall protrudes forward, while a localized depression exists in the center of the anterior chest wall — precisely at the point where pectus carinatum typically protrudes the most. This depression is localized and groove-like, running vertically, and is different from the typical depression seen in pectus excavatum. The presence of this depression causes the highest point of the anterior chest wall's protrusion to collapse slightly, giving the side profile of the anterior chest wall a flat appearance that forms the most distinct difference from classic pectus carinatum (Figure 2-11-3).

2. Pathological Features

Structurally, flat pectus carinatum is a special type of compound deformity. The entire anterior chest wall is protruded forward, forming the main structure of the deformity. However, a depression appears in the center, specifically at the location of the sternum. This depression generally involves only the sternum and costal cartilage. The costal cartilage forms an angle at its junction with the ribs, and the sternum forms the bottom of the depression. Because the depressed area is small and localized, it has very poor plasticity and is difficult to reshape through general external force. This presents challenges for surgical correction.

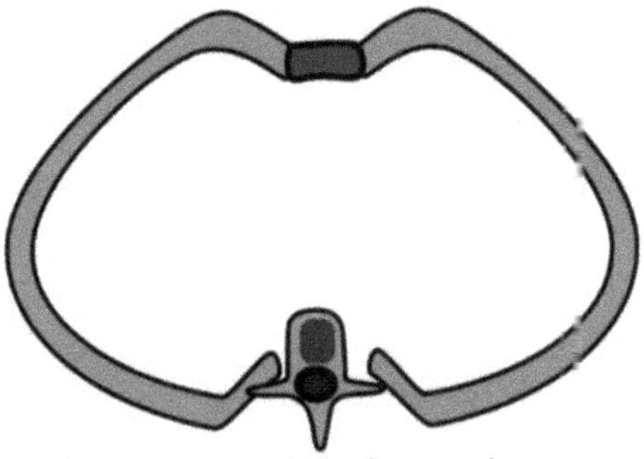

Figure 2-11-3 Schematic diagram of flat pectus carinatum

The protrusion in flat pectus carinatum is not typical of classic pectus carinatum, and the depression is not typical of pectus excavatum. The depression in the flat pectus carinatum does not have closed edges but is a longitudinal groove running in the same direction as the sternum. Furthermore, due to its narrow range, the depth is limited and generally does not form a very deep depression.

3. Clinical Manifestations

Although flat pectus carinatum involves a depression, the depression is localized and generally does not cause significant compression; therefore, obvious symptoms are usually absent. In terms of appearance, the main feature is anterior protrusion, similar to classic pectus carinatum or barrel chest. Patients are often distressed by their appearance, which can lead to a variety of psychological issues. On physical examination, the primary finding is an abnormal chest wall appearance. This distinctive external feature is markedly different from all other types of deformities, making it easy to recognize.

4. Inspection

A physical examination is generally sufficient to establish a definitive diagnosis. A standard posteroanterior chest X-ray typically shows no significant abnormalities, while a lateral view may reveal a double shadow on the anterior chest wall, and the heart may appear compressed. CT scans can show characteristic changes in cross-sectional images, presenting a 'concave' shape; however, the extent and degree of the depression are relatively mild and differ from the more pronounced deformity seen in pectus excavatum. Three-dimensional reconstruction can provide a complete and detailed image of the thoracic structure, but such imaging is generally not necessary in routine clinical practice

5. Diagnosis and Differential Diagnosis

The features of flat pectus carinatum (flattened pigeon chest) are quite distinct, and diagnosis mainly relies on its external appearance. X-ray and CT imaging can serve as auxiliary diagnostic tools. Overall, diagnosing flat pectus carinatum is relatively straightforward. However, due to the rarity and limited awareness of this deformity, it is often misdiagnosed as other thoracic deformities. The main conditions to be differentiated from it are three: barrel chest, large-area pectus carinatum, and pectus excavatum.

The barrel chest is characterized by a generalized anterior protrusion of the chest wall, giving it a barrel-like appearance, and its cross-section on CT imaging is typically round. The midline of the anterior chest wall may be slightly protruding or relatively flat but shows no depression. The main differences between flat pectus carinatum and barrel chest are twofold: first,

flat pectus carinatum has a central depression, whereas barrel chest has a slight anterior bulge; second, the lateral chest wall in flat pectus carinatum is relatively flat with minimal curvature, while in barrel chest, the lateral chest wall is more curved, forming a round or elliptical shape.
Large-area pectus carinatum also presents as a broad anterior protrusion of the chest wall, with the most anterior point of the midline projecting forward in a sharp angular deformity or a relatively flat structure, but a depression is never present. Although flat pectus carinatum shows some anterior protrusion, there is a distinct central depression. This is the most obvious difference between the two.
Pectus excavatum is a typical depression-type deformity, characterized by a large area of anterior chest wall depression. The surrounding area may appear elevated, but this is only a relative protrusion — its height remains within the normal range of the chest wall and never actually projects beyond the body surface. In flat pectus carinatum, the depression is localized and shallow with an incomplete edge, which makes it clearly different from pectus excavatum

6. Indications for Surgery
Flat pectus carinatum generally does not cause clinical symptoms; its main issue is cosmetic appearance. Therefore, the decision to undergo surgery primarily depends on the patient's own perception and preference. If the patient has a strong desire for corrective treatment, surgery may be considered."

7. Surgical Treatment
Flat pectus carinatum is a complex deformity involving two different types of structural abnormalities that must be corrected simultaneously. According to the general principles of deformity correction, two surgical approaches can be considered. The first method is open surgery. Flat pectus carinatum is a complex deformity that involves two different structural abnormalities, both of which must be corrected simultaneously. According to general principles of deformity correction, two surgical approaches can be used. The first method is open surgery, and the second is minimally invasive surgery. In open surgery, a midline incision is made. The deformed costal cartilages and ribs at the site of the depression are cut or resected, and then the entire anterior chest wall structure is reshaped as needed. Finally, fixation is achieved using shaping materials. Open surgery does not place excessive constraints on the size of the incision or the degree of tissue disruption, so various techniques can be employed. However, it is clear that this is not the ideal option; the preferred approach should be minimally invasive surgery.
Based on the characteristics of this deformity, we have designed a composite

minimally invasive procedure. Specifically, small incisions about 2 cm in length are made on both sides of the chest wall, positioned in the plane of the central depression. The subcutaneous tissue and muscle are dissected to expose the ribs of the lateral chest wall. Guidewires are placed on two ribs and tunneled along the bony structures toward the midline, passing deep to the chest wall muscles to meet in front of the sternum.

A vertical incision, 1–2 cm long, is made anterior to the xiphoid process, which is then split longitudinally. The sternum and structures behind both costal arches are freed, and the soft tissues of the anterior chest wall are dissected along the sternum up to the plane of the tunnel. Guidewires are passed across both coastal arches. A guiding device is inserted into the tunnel to introduce the steel plate. The guidewires are used to draw the relevant wires into the incision, encircling and fixing them around the bony structures and the steel plate. The wires in the midline incision are tightened first, followed by the wires in the lateral chest wall incisions, securely fixing the steel plate to the bony structures of the chest wall. The incisions are then closed, completing the procedure. A review of the entire surgical procedure shows that it also consists of two fundamental steps: one addressing the protrusion and the other addressing the depression. The former is the Wenlin procedure [2], and the latter is the Wang procedure (Figure 2-11-4) [3]. This combined approach has the following advantages: 1) High efficiency: Both steps are accomplished using the same steel plate, achieving dual correction in one operation. This not only saves material but also eliminates a large amount of redundant work. 2) Minimal trauma: Each of these procedures is minimally invasive on its own, and performing them together does not significantly increase tissue trauma, so the overall procedure remains a typical minimally invasive surgery.3) Minimal postoperative scarring: The entire surgery requires only three small incisions, each generally no longer than 2 cm. Such small incisions typically do not result in significant scarring.4) Satisfactory results: Both procedures are specifically designed for distinct aspects of the deformity. The Wenlin procedure directly corrects the anterior protrusion, while the Wang procedure addresses the depression, allowing for highly satisfactory outcomes. This procedure successfully combines the Wenlin procedure and the Wang procedure, allowing for simultaneous correction of the two deformities present in flat pectus carinatum [1]. However, this combination is entirely different from the usual combination of surgeries for other composite deformities. In typical composite deformities, the two procedures are performed independently and have little to do with each other. In flat pectus carinatum, however, the two procedures are integrated into a single operation, which places specific technical demands on the surgeon. To perform this procedure successfully, the following technical points must be noted: 1) Number of steel plates: The standard surgical approach is designed to use a single steel plate, which is sufficient for younger patients or those with less rigid bony structures. However, when the area of deformity is large, especially when the depression spans a wide region — more than one plate may be required. Additionally, when the anterior protrusion is broad and extensive, a single plate may not be enough for correction, and two or even three plates may be needed. In this case, the functions of each plate must be managed flexibly. If two plates are required, the Wang procedure can be performed with one plate and a separate Wenlin procedure with the other. This approach satisfies the corrective requirements without increasing surgical complexity. 2) Curvature of the steel plate: The steel plate must serve both procedures simultaneously. Since the curvature requirements for the two procedures do not conflict, priority can be given to the Wenlin procedure. Generally, to flatten the anterior protrusion, the plate's curvature should not be excessive — a relatively straight plate is preferable. Such curvature is also suitable for depression correction. A plate with excessive curvature is strongly discouraged, as it may aid the depression correction but will fail to adequately flatten the protrusion. 3) Incision placement: The exposure provided by the lateral chest wall incisions can be freely adjusted and generally does not pose a problem during the procedure. The midline incision is positioned lower on the chest; if the lifting effect is poor, the surgical outcome may be affected. To improve the lifting effect, the incision can be moved to the center of the depression, where the wires can cross the costal cartilage or sternum. This placement facilitates depression correction but may result in more visible scarring due to its higher position on the chest, making it less ideal. The optimal choice remains an incision near the xiphoid process. To achieve better lifting, the span of wire placement can be extended, crossing more ribs or other structures above the incision to facilitate the procedure. 4) Number of wires: Fixation at both ends of the steel plate primarily serves to apply pressure to flatten the protrusion. Double-point fixation is generally required to effectively distribute stress. The midline wires are for lifting; because the resistance here is greater, special attention must be paid to the number of wires and the exact lifting position. Only when the stress is well-distributed can the operation proceed smoothly. 5) force applied to the lifting wires: Since the steel plate is positioned higher and the lifting point is lower, the force may not be applied evenly. It is crucial to control both the direction and the amount of force to prevent the plate from being pulled off-axis, which would compromise the shaping effect. 6) Pre-shaping: As described above, the central depression is generally localized and rigid, making the operation technically demanding. Appropriate pre-shaping is therefore necessary. There are various methods for pre-shaping, which can be selected according to the specific situation. This greatly facilitates the procedure.

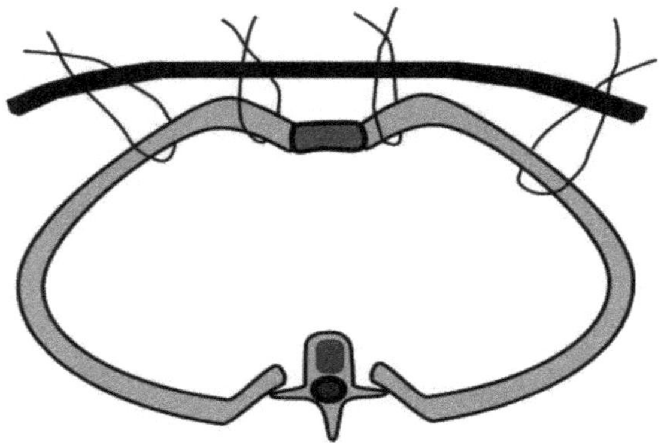

Figure 2-11-4 Minimally invasive surgery for flat pectus carinatum. This procedure is essentially a combination of the Wenlin procedure and the Wang process.

Flat pectus carinatum is, in essence, a composite deformity. The surgical plan described above fully takes into account its unique features and is therefore a rational approach. However, in clinical practice, a lack of awareness of this deformity's special characteristics can lead to various problems: 1. Treating the deformity as ordinary pectus carinatum. Due to the obvious anterior protrusion, it is often misdiagnosed as typical pectus carinatum. In such cases, only the protrusion is compressed, without addressing the central depression, which can actually worsen the depression (Figure 2-11-5). 2. Treating the deformity as pectus excavatum. Some physicians see only the central depression and overlook the protrusion. In such cases, the Nuss procedure may be used. The mechanism of the Nuss procedure is based on the principle of a lever, which requires an optimal fulcrum located at the edge of the depression. This is the most fundamental requirement of the Nuss procedure. However, in flat pectus carinatum, the depression is too localized, so the fulcrum of the steel bar actually ends up being on the lateral chest wall rather than at the edge of the depression. This fulcrum is not ideal. Using it to push up the depression is almost impossible, as the depression cannot be adequately elevated. If one tries to establish a fulcrum at the edge of the depression, it would require making an incision near the midline, which would disrupt the entire surgical plan and is not acceptable in practice (Figure 2-11-6) [4]. 3. Using the sandwich procedure: In general, the sandwich procedure can be used for most similar composite deformities. However, flat pectus carinatum is an exception, mainly due to the localized nature of the depression. As mentioned above, because the depression is not suitable for the Nuss procedure, the sandwich technique can only correct the protrusion but cannot address the depression. Therefore, this approach cannot be used for this deformity.

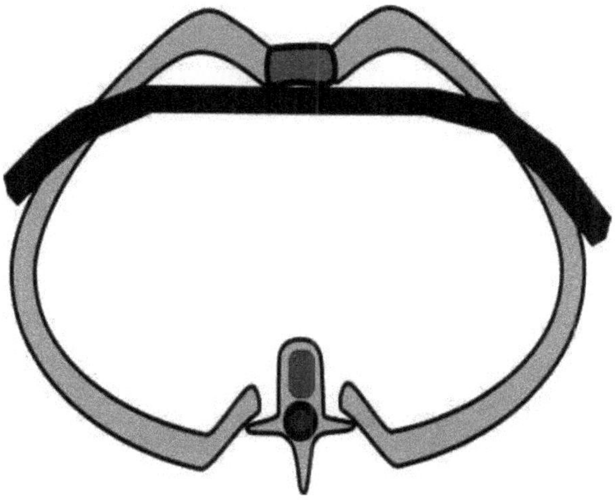

Figure 2-11-5 Treating flat pectus carinatum as ordinary pectus carinatum — the central depression remains uncorrected

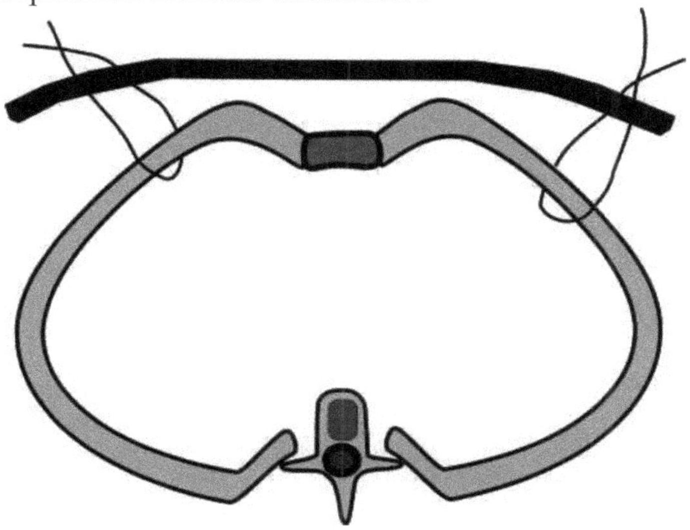

Figure 2-11-6 Treating flat pectus carinatum as pectus excavatum — the fulcrum is too low, making it impossible to correct the depression

8. Complications

Although surgery for flat chicken chest is relatively complex, it remains a deformity correction procedure performed on the chest wall, so its complications are generally similar to those of other chest wall deformity surgeries. These may include complications related to the Wenlin procedure as well as those associated with the Wang procedure. These aspects are described in detail in the relevant sections and will not be repeated here.

9. Revision Surgery After Failed Procedures

The three most common failure scenarios for flat chicken chest are: first, failure caused by treating it as pectus excavatum; second, failure caused by treating it as pectus carinatum; and third, failure caused by treating it as flat chicken chest itself. Each of these failed procedures is different, leading to different outcomes, and the principles and approaches for revision surgery also differ.

First scenario: If the condition was mistakenly treated as pectus excavatum and the surgery failed, the initial procedure is usually the Nuss procedure (Figure 2-11-7) [4]. Due to the small area of depression and local rigidity, the Nuss procedure is unlikely to be effective, and the operation often has little to no impact on the deformity. When performing revision surgery, the deformity remains flat chicken chest. However, the situation is clearly more complex than during the first operation, mainly due to intrathoracic adhesions, which increase the risks and difficulties of a second surgery. The first operation typically involves manipulation near the lateral chest wall incision, which may lead to local structural changes. These changes usually have minimal impact on the revision procedure. The main challenge lies in adhesions inside the thoracic cavity, especially behind the mediastinum. When dissecting structures behind the sternum, extreme care must be taken to avoid unnecessary injury.

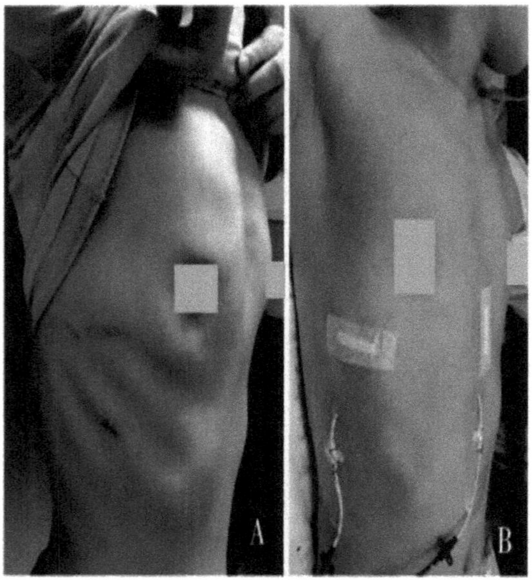

Figure 2-11-7 Failed Nuss Procedure for Flat Chicken Chest Corrected with Secondary Surgery Using the Wenlin Procedure + Wang Procedure, Achieving a Satisfactory Outcome. (A. Preoperative appearance of the thoracic cage showing residual surgical scars from the previous operation; B. Postoperative appearance of the thoracic cage, with the deformity completely corrected)

Scenario 2: If treatment as a chicken breast fails, the first procedure used may be a general bulge compression procedure. This procedure can be very effective. In other words, it will flatten the convex chest wall. However, a significant depression may form in its center. This depression resembles a small funnel chest. In this case, if reoperation is to be performed, the choice of procedure will depend on the circumstances. It may be a Wenlin procedure combined with a Wang procedure or a Wang procedure alone, but the Nuss procedure is preferable for the reasons described above, mainly the inability to identify a satisfactory fulcrum. The pivot point cannot be determined, and the Nuss operation is difficult to accomplish. In this case, the first operation is performed entirely outside the thoracic cavity, and no adhesions are created in the thoracic cavity, so there is no need to worry about intrathoracic operations. However, since the surface of the chest wall has already been completed once, if a tunnel needs to be constructed, there may be trouble with the operation, so the details of the operation need to be carefully designed to ensure its success. The third case: Failure of treatment as a flat chicken breast. In this case, the surgery used must be a combination of the Wenlin procedure and the Wang procedure described above. This surgery is based on a correct understanding of the deformity, so that even if it fails, it will not lead to a new deformity, but at most to an unsatisfactory result. If a second operation is required, it is necessary to work on the details of the operation. After continuous optimization of the technical details, a successful reoperation can usually be achieved.

10. Prognosis

Flat chicken chest surgery is a complicated surgery, which requires the surgeon to master not only the treatment techniques of funnel chest and chicken chest, but also the operation essentials of Wenlin surgery and Wang surgery. However, at present, there are not many doctors who can skillfully master the Nuss operation for funnel chest, let alone the Wenlin operation and Wang operation. Without proper techniques, it is difficult to complete the deformity surgery, therefore, most of the flat chicken chest surgeries in the clinic will end in failure. In addition, the recognition of the deformity directly determines the prognosis of the surgery. Flat chicken breast is a very specific deformity that has not been recognized as such in the past. Without understanding the characteristics of the deformity, it is impossible to use the appropriate method of orthopaedics, which has become the fundamental reason for the failure of the surgery. It can be seen that in order to change this situation completely, we should firstly recognize this deformity from the essence, and on this basis, we should carefully study the details of surgical operation, and only in this way can we avoid surgical failure and get good results.

REFERENCES

[1] Wang Wenlin. Naming of Flat Chicken Chest: A Special Type of Thoracic Deformity. Thoracic Deformity Surgery Expert, 2019-05-23.

[2] Wang W L. Minimally Invasive Surgical Technique for Barrel Chest. Surgical Case Re- Ports, 2018, 1 (2): 1-2.

[3] Wang WL, Chen CM, Long WG, Et Al. Wang Procedure: A Novel Minimally Invasive Procedure for Pectus Excavatum Children With Low Age. Case Reports and Images In Surgery. 2018;1(1):1–2.

[4] Wang Wenlin. A Painful Lesson: The Consequences of A Failed Nuss Procedure. Toutiao, 22-10-2021.

Section 12

WENLIN CHEST

Wenlin's chest is a very rare malformation with a very low incidence, with no more than 100 cases reported worldwide. In the early years of thoracic surgery, this deformity was not named independently, but was treated as a type of chicken breast and occasionally referred to as pigeon breast. However, due to the inherent confusion between the concepts of chicken breast and pigeon breast, little attention has been paid to this malformation [1,2]. Occasionally, the term "pigeon breast" has been used in China, but the combined funnel chest has also been described, which is tantamount to treating a complete deformity as if it were two separate deformities that are completely unrelated. This designation is neither scientific nor reasonable, as it severs the integrity of the deformity [3]. If such a concept is used to guide surgery, it is difficult to achieve good results. Overseas designations are even more varied, including Peutus Arcuatum, Currarino Silverman Syndrome, Pouter Pigeon Chest, Condromanurial Deformity and Type -2 Pectus Carinatum. The wide variety of names is a tribute to the rarity of the malformation, which is recognized by experts from all over the world. My department specializes in chest wall surgery and is the largest center for chest wall deformity correction in the country. We see many patients with this deformity in our clinic, and with a combined total of more than 100 surgeries, we have performed more surgeries than all other authors in the world combined, so we are more than qualified to give this deformity a name. In order to standardize the name of this deformity and to help in diagnosis and treatment, we finally came up with our own name, Wenlin's chest [4,5], which is unique because it is a complex deformity that is different from all others in that it is a special combination of a convexity and a depression [6]. Because it is different from the usual composite deformity, it places special demands on the treatment. In order to treat this deformity satisfactorily, the characteristics of the deformity need to be studied in depth.

1. Basic concepts

Morphologically, Wenlin's chest is a complex deformity with both a convexity and a depression. The combination of the bulges and depressions is not random, but has a clear pattern. The bulge is most pronounced at the level of the sternal angle, which is locally thickened, and the rib cartilage and ribs on both sides are concomitantly augmented by the connection to the sternal angle, resulting in a large transverse anterior convexity deformity (Figure 2-12-1) [7,8]. The bulge appears as a steep slope downward in the middle of the bulge and then continues as a depression, with the sternal body and infrasternal segment at the base of the steep slope and depression, and an overall thickening of the sternum. The lower edges of both sides of the bulge are curved downward, and the inner lower edges of the bulge form the lateral edges of the depression. The depression is mostly relative and not deep in actuality, with the lower margins open to the vicinity of the xiphoid process. In general, Wenlin's chest is a fixed combination of a bulge and a depression, but unlike a simple chicken chest combined with a funnel chest [6], the bulge is a characteristic bulge, unlike chicken chest. Unlike chicken breast, the projection of chicken breast is more limited and mostly longitudinal, with no obvious peripheral depression. In Wenlin's chest, the projection is located on the upper chest wall, is large and extensive, is transverse, and has a characteristic depression below it, this is completely different from chicken breast. The depression in Wenlin's chest is also different from the usual funnel chest. The depression in the funnel chest is a restricted pit, low in the center, at the base of which may be the sternal body, but the sternal body is not markedly thickened, and it is surrounded by a bulge with a complete rim. The depression of Wenlin's chest is a relative depression, generally not deep in extent, but falling away from the bulge above it; moreover, its periphery is incomplete, with only the upper and lateral margins, and it is open below, without margins.The bottom of Wenlin's chest is the body of the sternum, which is markedly thickened, and which is a marked departure from that of funnel chest depressions.

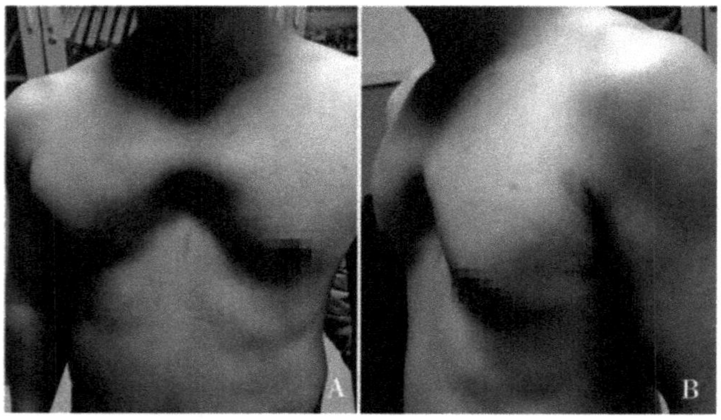

Figure 2-12-1 Appearance of Wenlin's Chest A. Frontal View, Typical Bulge and Depression Visible; B. Lateral View

2. Pathogenesis

Wenlin chest lesions are distinct and structurally fixed, and there must be a specific pathogenesis and mechanism when analyzed from an etiological point of view. However, the specific pathogenesis of this deformity is not clear because not many people have paid much attention to it in the past.

In our clinic, we found that although this deformity has two obvious lesions, i.e., convexity and depression, the fundamental lesion comes from the sternum, which consists of two main elements: the thickening of the sternum as a whole, and the change of its shape, i.e., a roughly "S"-shaped alteration (Fig. 2-12-2) [7]. The rib cartilage and ribs are also altered, but the basic shape does not change much, and since the rib cartilage is directly connected to the sternum, it can be considered as a secondary lesion. When analyzing the pathogenesis of Wenlin's Chest, it is possible that the following process occurs: the sternum itself undergoes a pathological change due to some specific factors, which then leads to a shift in the position of the associated costal cartilages and ribs, resulting in the formation of a specific convexity and depression. This is the possible pathogenesis of the deformity. of course, this is only speculation, and further research is needed to find a truly convincing mechanism.

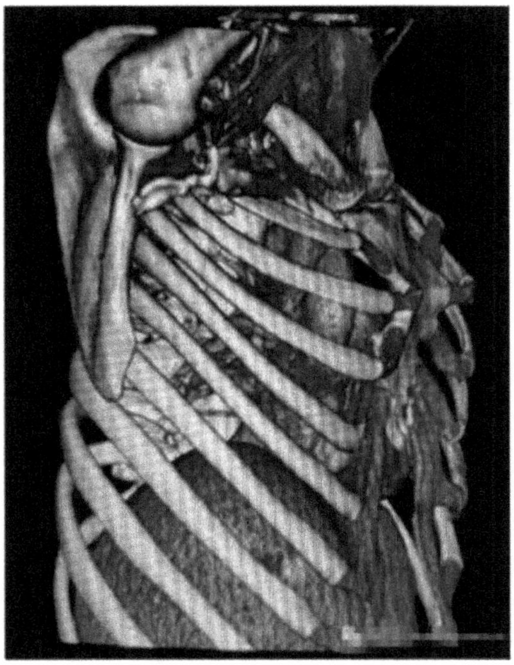

Figure 2-12-2 Three-dimensional reconstruction of Wenlin's chest, showing the shape of the bones

3. Clinical manifestations

The depression in the Wenlin chest is generally shallow and, although located in the precordial area, does not constitute a serious compression, so that symptoms of compression are not obvious. The patient's dissatisfaction with appearance is the biggest concern. Visually, the chest of a patient with Wenlin Chest can be mistaken for a sign of robustness, but in reality, it is a deformity. In severe cases, patients will feel uncomfortable when wearing clothes and certainly feel unsightly. Because of the obviousness of the bumps, it is almost impossible to hide the deformity, and most patients desire surgery. The bumps and depressions in the anterior chest wall of Wenlin's chest are unlike those found in any other deformity, and this constitutes the characteristic physical sign of the deformity. This is an important basis for the diagnosis of this deformity.

4. Inspection

The primary method for examining Wenlin chest deformity is physical examination, which can typically lead to a clear diagnosis. However, in clinical practice, imaging tests are often performed, mainly to observe the structure of the sternum. On lateral X-ray images, the sternum can be seen to have an approximately "S"-shaped change, and both the sternal angle and body appear significantly thickened (Figure 2-12-3). A CT scan can reveal a combination of protrusion and depression of the anterior chest wall (Figure 2-12-4).
3D reconstruction imaging can display the overall shape of the thorax at the affected site, which is helpful in surgical planning (Figure 2-12-5).

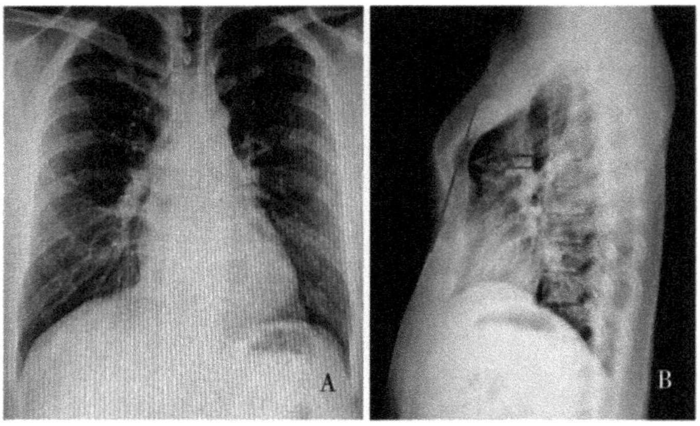

Figure 2-12-3 Radiograph of Wenlin's chest (A. Frontal view lacks specific signs; B. Lateral view suggests convexity of the sternal angle and relative depression of the body of the sternum below)

5. Diagnosis and Differential Diagnosis

Wenlin chest is well characterized and relatively simple to diagnose. The differential diagnosis mainly includes funnel chest, chicken chest and compound malformation [4]. Funnel chest is usually an isolated depression without a marginal bulge, so it is not difficult to differentiate. However, Wenlin's chest can develop at a young age, when the projection is present but

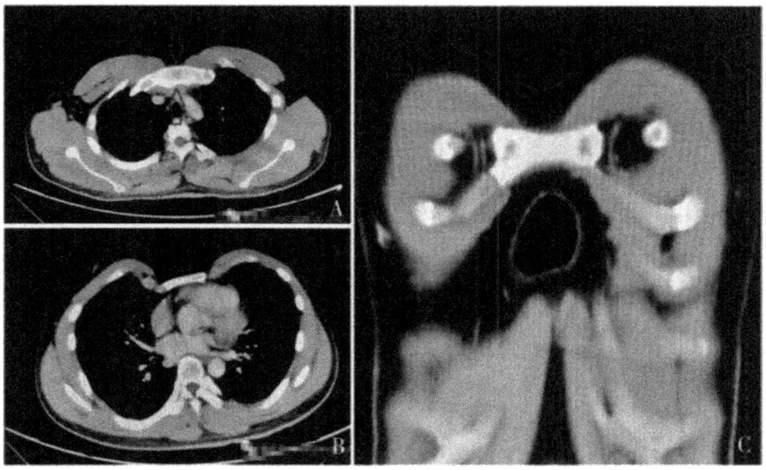

Figure 2-12-4 CT examination of Wenlin's chest (A. High CT cross-sectional view showing marked thickening of the sternal angle; B. Low CT cross-sectional view showing median depression of the anterior chest wall with convexity on both sides; C. CT coronal view showing convexity of the sternal angle with depression just below

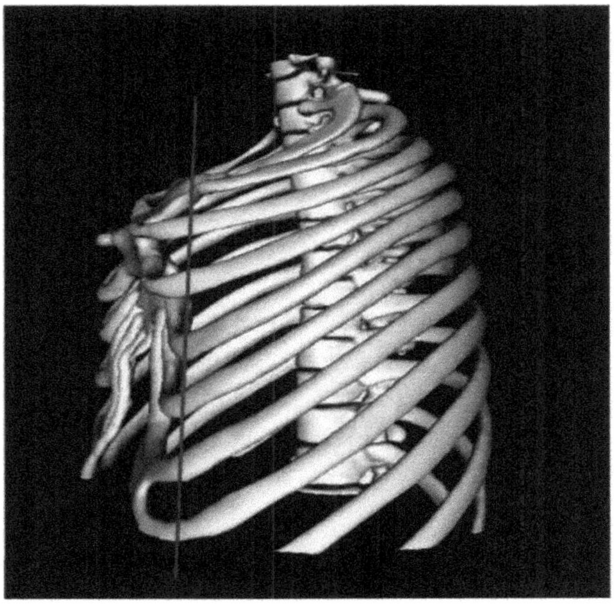

Figure 2-12-5 Three-dimensional reconstruction of Wenlin's chest.

not obvious, and can be easily recognized as a simple funnel chest if not observed carefully. It is important to distinguish between a normal sternal angle and a raised sternal angle. If there is a bulge, then it is a Wenlin chest, and the difference between a Wenlin chest and a chicken chest is not difficult to distinguish clinically. The distinction between Wenlin chest and chicken breast is more obvious and less difficult to make clinically. The usual complex deformity may have both a convexity and a depression, but the combination of the two is random, with no characteristic convexity or depression, and is therefore easier to distinguish from Wenlin chest[5-8].

6. Surgical treatment

In earlier years, Wenlin chest was mistaken for pectus carinatum (pigeon chest), and the unique nature of the deformity was not recognized. As a result, correction was attempted using treatment methods intended for pectus carinatum. The earliest surgeries were primarily open surgeries. The procedure involved making a midline incision to expose all the bony structures of the anterior chest wall affected by the deformity. Then, a thorough reshaping of these structures was performed. However, this method involved significant trauma and resulted in large scars.

The key to minimally invasive treatment of Wenlin's chest is to recognize the pathology of the deformity, which is essentially a composite deformity, a combination of bumps and depressions, and definitely not a single bump or depression. It is usually assumed that this deformity can be corrected by sandwich surgery. However, there is a problem with this procedure, and the source of this problem is the abnormally hard sternum. The hard sternum makes the convexity and concavity one and the same. It is difficult to correct both deformities at the same time when the operation is performed with a normal plate, and therefore the sandwich operation alone cannot be used for the treatment of Wenlin's chest. When this most basic method cannot be used for the treatment of the deformity, it is necessary to design other methods [9-12].

(1) Minimally invasive + semi-open surgery

This approach was the one we used in the early days, and the basic operation was equivalent to Wenlin's operation + Wang's operation. The combination of this procedure is similar to the sandwich procedure, but the key to the operation is the treatment of the hard sternum, that is, pre contouring, which is the most important part of the operation [9-12]. The specific method of pre contouring is as follows: a longitudinal incision is made near the sternal angle, the sternum is exposed, and the superficial layer of the raised sternum, including the anterior cortex and the medulla, is bitten off with bone-biting forceps; the rib cartilage attached to the sternum is cut off, and the sternum is transected at the slope where the sternal angle is attached to the sternal body. By doing this, the sternal structures at the level of the sternal angle are softened and the convexity is separated from the concavity, thus providing the basis for the correction of the two deformities separately. After pre contouring, an incision is made in the chest wall on both sides, a fixed wire retractor is placed, and tunnels are made to the middle of the chest in different planes for the Wenlin procedure and the Wang procedure; for the Wenlin procedure, the tunnels are located at the level of the sternal angle, and can be performed with a single plate, or with two plates if the area is larger; for the Wang procedure, the intermediate operation is performed through the median incision. Traction wires are placed across both rib arches, and then the corresponding plates are placed into the tunnels, tightened, and secured to correct the deformity. In practice, the Nuss procedure can be used instead of the Wang procedure. The operation can be performed as needed, but the pre contouring remains the same.

Both of these basic procedures fall into the category of minimally invasive surgery. However, there is a drawback in that the pre-contouring has to be done through a median incision, which is often more invasive. Although the median incision is not very long and the damage is not as great as in conventional open surgery, it cannot be considered a truly minimally invasive procedure because of the objective damage (Figure 2-12-6) [13,14].

In our early surgical practice, we used this method for Wenlin chest patients because we could not find a better surgical method to perform the operation. The results of the postoperative correction of the deformity were quite satisfactory, but the trauma and postoperative scarring were the major drawbacks of this method

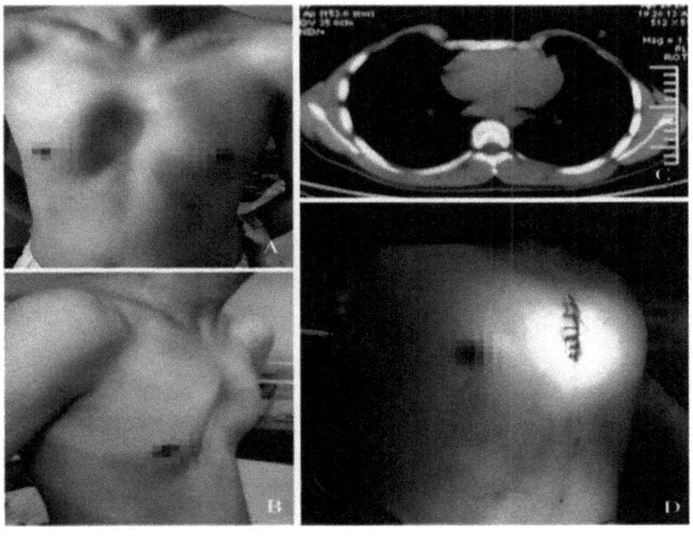

Figure 2-12-6 Minimally invasive + semi-open surgical treatment of Wenlin's chest (A, B. Appearance of the chest wall; C. CT cross-section showing the median depression; D. Postoperative thoracic appearance, with the deformity essentially disappearing)

(2) Attempted minimally invasive surgery

This is an experimental procedure because we have not used this technique on a large scale. It is performed by making a small incision in the center of the chest and using a bone biting forceps to remove the superficial cortex and medulla at the level of the sternal angle, cutting off the associated costal cartilage, and suturing the distal part of the costal cartilage to the edge of the sternum. These maneuvers result in a significant lowering of the chest wall in the vicinity of the sternal angle, eliminating the bulge. After completion of the operation, the ossified sternal bone structure is filled in the surface of the depression, and the incision is closed with a thorough soft-tissue encasement to complete the operation[13,14] .

This approach is an extremely simple and more minimally invasive procedure. It is based on: (1) the abnormal thickening of the sternal structures at the sternal angle, if all the bony structures before the posterior cortex are occluded, the sternum still has good stiffness and integrity; (2) the bulge on both sides of the sternal angle is an adjustable bulge, which can be effectively eliminated by partially resecting the rib cartilage, and then fixing the distal end of the rib cartilage to the edge of the sternum with a suture. (iii) The concavity of the anterior chest wall is not serious and can be treated with plastic surgery. Direct filling can be performed without the need to completely reshape the depressed chest wall. (4) The resected sternal bone can be used as filler material to eliminate the depression.

We have used this method in the surgery of one patient, and the outcome was relatively satisfactory. However, we have not applied this technique extensively, mainly due to certain concerns. The first concern relates to the management of the depression: since this procedure does not fundamentally eliminate the depression, there is a risk that using bone material as filler may actually increase the pressure on the depressed area. The second concern involves the healing of the free bone structure. Once the resected bone is placed in the depression, its viability cannot be guaranteed, which may lead to poor local healing. If poor healing occurs, the surgery may fail. For these reasons, we believe this technique requires further observation and refinement.

(3) Modified Sandwich Procedure

In the first surgical approach, open pre-shaping was performed to ensure the smooth execution of the Wenlin procedure and the Wang procedure, ultimately allowing the surgery to be completed. In this operation, if the Wang procedure is replaced by the Nuss procedure, it becomes an actual sandwich procedure. However, this type of operation is not a typical sandwich procedure, as a true sandwich procedure should not involve any open surgical steps. To eliminate

the drawbacks of open surgery, we developed a minimally invasive pre-shaping technique through repeated design and refinement. Based on this, performing the sandwich procedure again results in a completely new version, which we refer to as the modified sandwich procedure. The key technical point of the modified sandwich procedure is the midline pre-shaping. First, a small incision is made on the surface of the upper slope of the depression to expose the sternal body. Using a bone-biting forceps, the sternal body is resected, and then an elevator is used for traction and reshaping.
With this technique, the protrusion and the depression are completely separated and can be treated independently with minimally invasive surgical steps, making the sandwich procedure feasible (Figure 2-12-7).

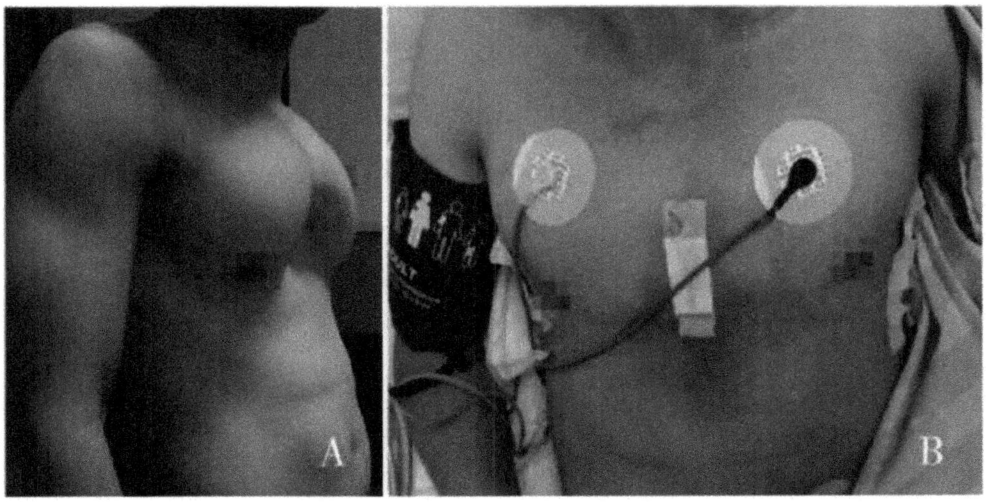

Figure 2-12-7 Modified sandwich procedure for Wenlin's chest (A. Preoperative appearance of the chest wall; B. Postoperative appearance of the chest wall, with the deformity essentially gone)

In performing this procedure, the concavity procedure is not so difficult; it is the maneuvering performed on the convexity that is more difficult. At this stage, using a single steel bar is often insufficient to achieve proper correction; typically, two steel bars are required — this is the basic surgical requirement. If performing the procedure directly with two steel bars is still challenging, further pre-shaping is needed. Of course, this pre-shaping must not be an open surgery, it must also be minimally invasive.
The modified sandwich procedure makes minimally invasive surgery for Wenlin chest possible. In this process, if the midline incision is positioned lower, the Wang procedure can be used instead of the Nuss procedure, thereby

providing more surgical options. However, in terms of its nature, this approach is no longer considered a true sandwich procedure.

(4) True Minimally Invasive Surgery: The Sandwich Procedure

The fundamental reason why Wenlin chest cannot be treated directly with minimally invasive surgery lies in the rigid structure of the sternum. This characteristic is the greatest obstacle during treatment of this deformity. In all the procedures described above, the core surgical techniques essentially revolve around overcoming this obstacle. However, there is one situation where this obstacle can be naturally resolved: performing surgery at a young age. This is the most suitable period for minimally invasive surgery.

In most cases, patients with Wenlin chest present at an older age, with many seeking treatments after puberty. By this time, the sternum is fully developed, thick, and rigid, making it extremely difficult to perform minimally invasive surgery directly. In contrast, in young children, the sternum can be directly reshaped, making minimally invasive surgery feasible [15–19]. At this stage, Wenlin chest can be treated as a typical complex deformity and corrected directly using the sandwich technique.

However, it must be emphasized that although Wenlin chest is a complex deformity, the depression it involves is still different from that of a typical pectus excavatum. When performing a Nuss procedure, strong pre-shaping is still necessary; otherwise, satisfactory results cannot be achieved. It is difficult to perform effective pre-shaping from a lateral chest wall incision during a standard Nuss procedure. The best approach is to perform pre-shaping through a midline incision, which is key to a successful operation. At this point, there is another more rational option: the Wang procedure. The Wang procedure requires a midline incision, and pre-shaping is also done through this approach, which makes it more reasonable for this condition (Figure 2-12-8).

7. Complications

The techniques used in Wenlin breast surgery are essentially the same as those used for other thoracic deformities, and therefore the complications are generally the same. The main focus here is on a more problematic complication, namely surgical failure. This can occur after different surgeries: (1) surgery for funnel chest, (2) surgery for chicken breast, (3) surgery for complex deformity, and (4) surgery for Wenlin chest.

When Wenlin's chest is treated as a funnel chest, the Nuss operation can only raise the bottom part of the depression, but it is impossible to eliminate the depression due to the extreme hardness of the sternum. This procedure is usually ineffective and is a common surgical failure (Figure 2-12-9) [10].

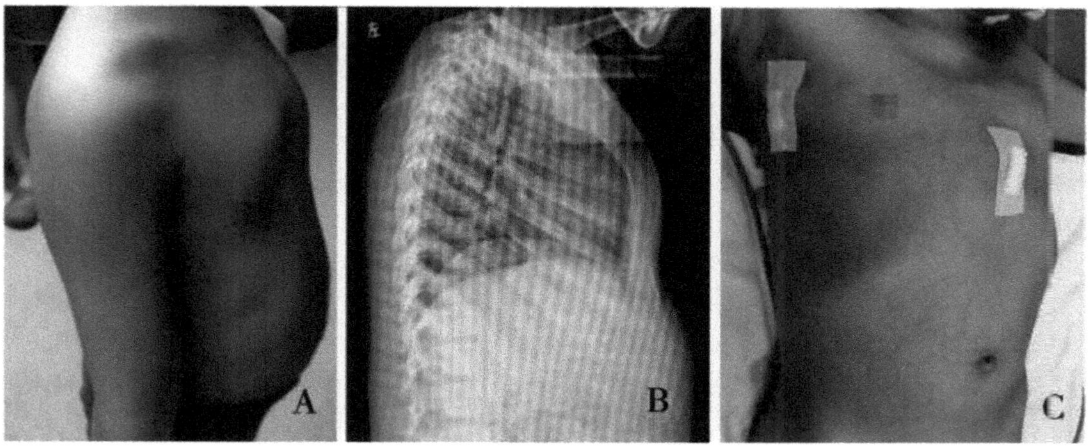

Figure 2-12-8 Minimally Invasive Surgery for Wenlin Chest (A. Preoperative appearance of the chest wall; B. Lateral X-ray showing anterior protrusion of the sternal angle with depression below; C. Postoperative appearance of the chest wall, with the deformity largely corrected)

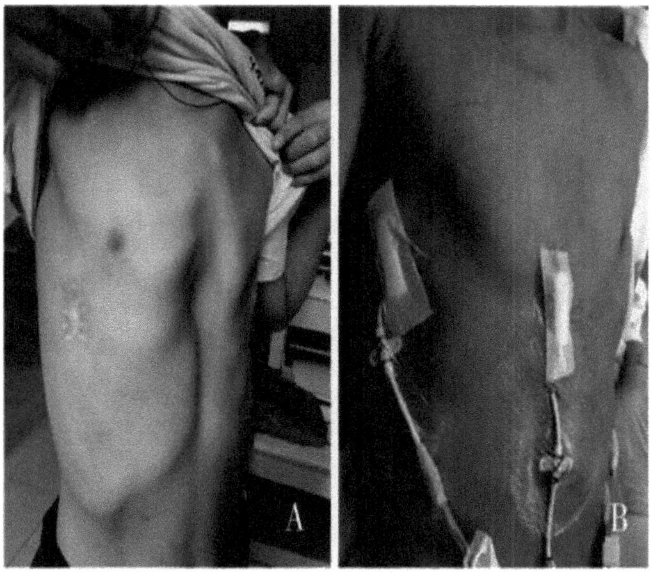

Figure 2-12-9 Secondary surgery after failed Nuss procedure for Wenlin's chest (A. Typical Wenlin's chest wall changes in the anterior chest wall with old surgical scars on the lateral chest wall; B. Minimally invasive secondary surgery, with complete disappearance of the deformity and essentially normal appearance of the thorax after surgery).

When Wenlin Chest is treated as a chicken breast, most of the time the surgery will not produce any results due to the fact that the sternal angle and surrounding structures are extremely hard and it is very difficult to flatten the bulge by normal means. Even if there is some success, the depression becomes deeper when the bulge is lowered, which is also a sign of surgical failure.

It is not a good idea to think of Wenlin's chest as a funnel chest or a chicken chest, but rather as a complex deformity, which may be corrected by a combination of surgeries that target both the convexity and the depression. However, the success of such a procedure is based on good technique, and failure is equally likely. The shape of a failed surgery can be complex, but the most likely result is that the shape remains unchanged, mainly due to the hard sternal angle and the sternal body.

When the basic structure of the Wenlin chest is recognized and corrected in an appropriate way, the results may be greatly improved, but there is also the possibility of complications and failure. Failure is mainly due to the degree of correction of the deformity. In most cases, the deformity may be improved, but not completely corrected.

8. Secondary surgery for Wenlin's chest

The biggest problem of Wenlin chest is the sternal angle and the hardness of the sternum itself. Since it is difficult to change its shape, it is very difficult to get good results according to the normal surgical methods, therefore, after the first failed surgery, the shape of the patient's chest is not likely to change too much, and only in a few cases will a new shape appear. The risks and difficulties of reoperation will not be the same depending on the method used for the first surgery. The key to the success of the reoperation is that it must be performed according to the characteristics of the first operation and the deformity

If the first operation is a simple Nuss procedure, the main postoperative problem will be intrathoracic adhesions. In addition, there may be scarring or fibroplasia near the incision in the lateral chest wall, with some local structural changes. All of these conditions can have an impact on the secondary surgery[10]. In this case, correction with the Wenlin procedure in combination with the Wang procedure can be effective (Fig. 2-12-10). Direct correction of the anterior chest wall structures with MatrixRIB material is also possible, depending on the characteristics of the deformity (Fig. 2-12-11).

If the first operation is a simple chicken breast operation, the main postoperative problem will be confined to the bony structures of the chest wall and there will not be much change in the thoracic cavity. The reoperation can be corrected with the Wenlin procedure combined with the Wang procedure or with the Wenlin procedure combined with the Nuss procedure.

If the first operation is a general complex deformity operation, i.e. a sandwich operation, the situation is often more complex and the choice of reoperation is based on the structural characteristics of the deformity and the details of the first operation.

If the specificity of the Wenlin breast is recognized and the procedure is

performed before the first operation, the deformity is usually significantly improved and the reoperation can be performed with good results if the technical aspects are adjusted.
Successful surgeries have the same outcome for all deformities, while failed surgeries are not uniform and can present a wide variety of shapes. Although in most cases the shape of the thorax does not change much after a failed Wenlin breast surgery, there are cases where the change is very significant, which means that a new deformity will develop. The new deformity will be more complex and varied, and its successful correction will require a more in-depth study of the characteristics of the deformity and an appropriate method of correction if the reoperation is to be successful.

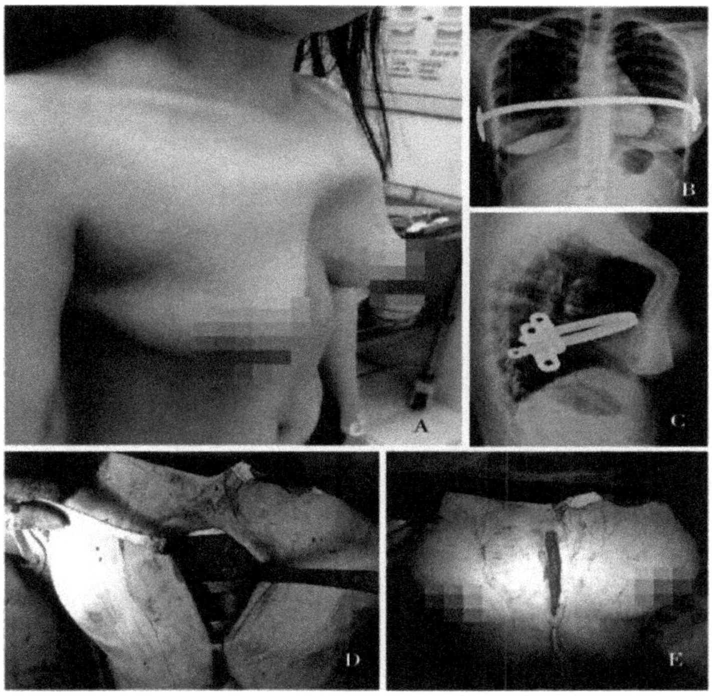

Figure 2-12-10 Secondary Surgery after Failed Nuss Surgery for Wenlin Chest (A. Preoperative chest wall appearance with typical Wenlin chest changes B, C. X-rays show the position of the plate inside the body, which is not able to play an orthopedics role; D. Correction was performed with Wenlin Surgery Wang Surgery; E. The deformity was completely eliminated after the surgery)

9. Prognosis
Wenlin's chest is extremely rare and has rarely been treated, so surgical experience is limited, and some authors' approaches have been extremely haphazard and unsatisfactory. We have seen a number of failed operations in patients who have undergone a variety of procedures. It is easy to see from these failed surgeries that the nature of the deformity is rarely investigated, and this is the root cause of the failure. The structural characteristics and surgical approaches to this deformity have been extensively studied, and a number of specific surgical procedures have been devised [20-27]. Each of these procedures

has its own characteristics and can correct the deformity from different perspectives. However, due to the special characteristics of the sternal structure, it is a great challenge to minimize the trauma and obtain better results while accomplishing the deformity. It is reasonable to believe that with the continuous progress of science and technology, the treatment of Wenlin's chest will be gradually improved, and ultimately achieve a perfect result.

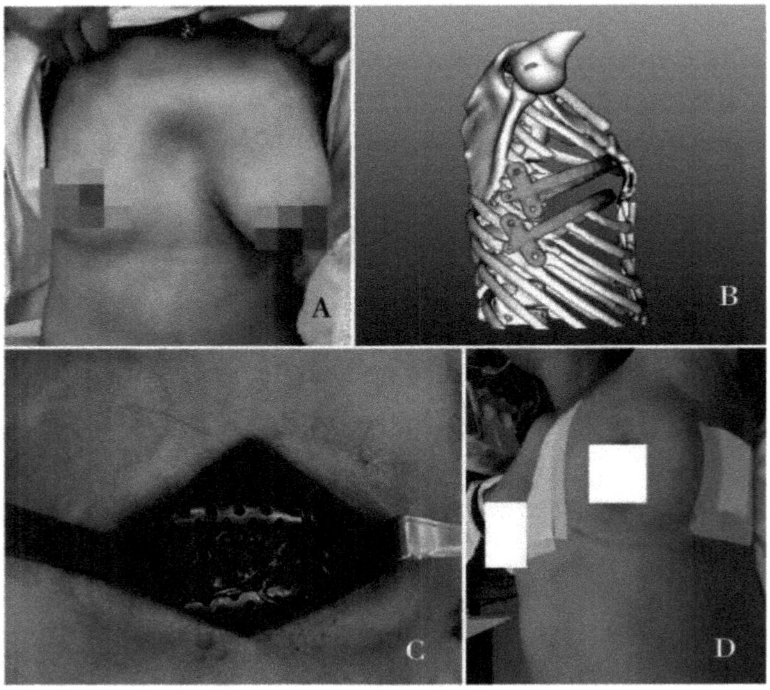

Figure 2-12-11 Wenlin's chest combined with Poland's syndrome in a patient who underwent a second surgery after a failed Nuss procedure (A. Right breast and soft tissue hypoplasia, thin bony structures, anteriorly projecting sternal angle, and anteriorly depressed sternal angle); B. Three-dimensional reconstruction showing two plates in the body, which have no orthopedics effect; C. Removal of the plates and complete localized orthopedics correction with MatrixRIB; C. Removal of the plates and complete localization with MatrixRIB; D. Complete disappearance of the deformity)

REFERENCES

[1] Lester, C. W. 1953. "Pigeon Breast (Pectus Carinatum) and Other Protrusion Deformities of the Chest of Developmental Origin." *Annals of Surgery* 137 (4): 482–489.
[2] Lester, C. W. 1954. "Pigeon Breast, Funnel Chest, and Other Congenital Deformities of the Chest." *Journal of the American Medical Association* 156 (11): 1063–1067.
[3] Shang, Z. Y., X. L. Duan, P. Zhang, et al. 2012. "Surgical Treatment of Pediatric Funnel Chest

Combined with Spherical Pigeon Chest." *Chinese Journal of Pediatric Surgery* 33 (2): 148–149.
[4] Wang, W. L. 2018a. "Wenlin Chest (Pigeon Chest), Chicken Chest and Funnel Chest." *Thoracic Deformity Surgery Specialist*, December 16.
[5] Wang, W. L. 2021a. "Wenlin Chest and Wenlin Surgery." *Thoracic Deformity Surgery Specialist*, June 22.
[6] Wang, W. L. 2021b. "Wenlin Chest: Not Chicken Chest + Funnel Chest." *Thoracic Deformity Surgery Specialist*, October 24.
[7] Wang, W. L. 2021c. "Minimally Invasive Options for Wenlin Chest (Pigeon Chest) Surgery." *Thoracic Deformity Surgery Specialist*, November 18.
[8] Wang, W. L. 2021d. "Specificity of Wenlin Chest." *Thoracic Surgery Specialist*, June 10.
[9] Wang, W. L. 2019a. "Difficulties in Wenlin Chest Surgery." *Thoracic Surgery Specialist*, September 29.
[10] Wang, W. L. 2019b. "Successful Wenlin Chest (Pigeon Chest) Surgery." *Thoracic Surgery Specialist*, March 4.
[11] Wang, W. L. 2019c. "Radical Surgery for Wenlin Chest after Spinal Surgery." *Thoracic Deformity Surgery Specialist*, March 3.
[12] Wang, W. L. 2021e. "Matrix Rib Plasty: Reoperation for Wenlin Chest with Poland Syndrome." *Thoracic Deformity Surgery Expert*, September 28.
[13] Wang, W. L. 2021f. "Changes in Wenlin Chest Surgery: From Open to Minimally Invasive to Absolutely Minimally Invasive." *Thoracic Deformity Surgery Specialist*, May 3.
[14] Wang, W. L. 2020a. "Minimally Invasive Solutions for Wenlin Chest: The Wenlin Procedure and the Wung Procedure." *Thoracic Deformity Surgery Expert*, December 24.
[15] Wang, W. L. 2019d. "Minimally Invasive Surgery for 4-Year-Old Wenlin Chest." *Thoracic Deformity Surgery Specialist*, June 5.
[16] Wang, W. L. 2021g. "Minimally Invasive Surgery of 5-Year-Old Wenlin Chest." *Thoracic Deformity Surgery Specialist*, July 9.
[17] Wang, W. L. 2019e. "Minimally Invasive Surgery of Wenlin Chest." *Thoracic Deformity Surgery Specialist*, September 9.
[18] Wang, W. L. 2019f. "Minimally Invasive Surgery of Wenlin Chest at Age 13." *Thoracic Deformity Surgery Specialist*, November 9.
[19] Wang, W. L. 2019g. "Minimally Invasive Wenlin Chest Surgery in a Young Child." *Thoracic Deformity Surgery Specialist*, September 6.
[20] Wang, W., W. Long, Y. Liu, et al. 2022a. "Minimally Invasive Operation der Wenlin-Brust." *International Journal of Case Reports in Surgery* 4 (2): 59–61.
[21] Wang, W., W. Long, Y. Liu, et al. 2022b. "Surgical Treatment of Wenlin Chest." *International Journal of Case Reports in Surgery* 4 (2): 62–64.
[22] Wang, W., W. Long, Y. Liu, et al. 2022c. "Surgical Treatment of Wenlin Chest after Spinal Orthopedics." *International Journal of Case Reports in Surgery* 4 (2): 65–67.
[23] Wang, W., W. Long, Y. Liu, et al. 2022d. "Operation of Wenlin Chest." *International Journal of Case Reports in Surgery* 4 (2): 68–71.
[24] Wang, W., W. Long, Y. Liu, et al. 2022e. "Wenlin Chest: An Independent Thoracic Deformity." *International Journal of Case Reports in Surgery* 4: 13–15.
[25] Wang, W., W. Long, Y. Liu, et al. 2022f. "Morphological Characteristics of Wenlin Chest." *International Journal of Case Reports in Surgery* 4: 22–24.
[26] Wang, W., W. Long, Y. Liu, et al. 2022g. "Reoperation after Failure of Nuss Procedure on Severe Wenlin Chest." *International Journal of Surgery Science* 6 (4): 14–17.
[27] Wang, W. 2022h. "Minimally Invasive Surgical Treatment for Severe Wenlin Chest." *International Journal of Case Reports in Surgery* 4 (2): 129–132.

Section 13

RIB ARCH DEFORMITY

A lesser-recognized deformity, the rib arch deformity is a separate deformity that can manifest itself in a variety of specific shapes. However, clinical references to this deformity refer to a specific deformity, namely the anterior convexity of the costal arch, which is commonly known as ectropion of the costal arch, which is in fact a less precise term [1]. Rib arch deformities can exist independently or in combination with other deformities, most commonly with funnel chest (Fig. 2-13-1), either before or after funnel chest surgery. In addition to the funnel chest, the arch deformity may be associated with other deformities. Due to the lack of awareness of this deformity in the past, little work has been done specifically on this deformity. In the past, we have done a lot of work not only on the anterior rib arch deformity, but also on other deformities of the rib arch. This work has led to a more comprehensive understanding of this deformity, which lays the foundation for its diagnosis and treatment [2].

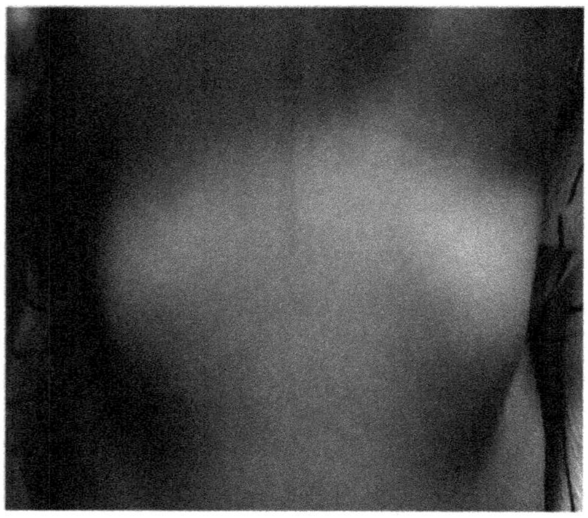

Figure 2-13-1 Rib Arch Deformity

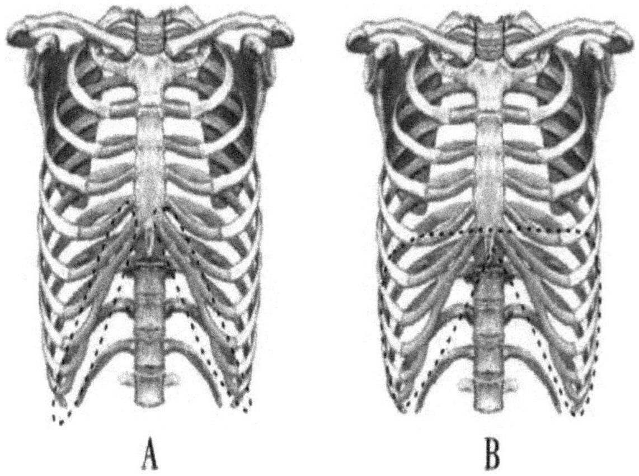

Figure 2-13-2 Definition of the Rib Arch (A. Conventional descriptive area of the rib arch; B. Actual rib arch area)

1. Pathologic typing

A rib arch deformity is a structural abnormality that occurs in the rib arch. In order to understand this deformity, it is important to know the exact definition of the coastal arch. While the concept of the arch is apparently anatomically clear, the definition is not. The term “costal arch” is used idiomatically to refer to the most marginal part of the lower edge of the anterior chest wall, which is imprecise because the area extending from the edge to the lateral chest wall can also be called a costal arch. for the purposes of this study, we have defined the arch as the area from the inner lower edge of the thorax to the lateral chest wall (Fig. 2-13-2). Under normal conditions, the rib arch is a continuous extension of the thorax from top to bottom, lying in the same plane as the entire thoracic cage. It is neither elevated nor depressed, and no localized deformities are present. If there is an abnormality in the shape of this region, it constitutes a rib arch deformity。

Rib arch deformities can present with various morphological characteristics. for research purposes, we classify them into three basic types (Figure 2-13-3) [3]: Type I: Global anterior protrusion deformity, characterized by a large area of the rib arch protruding anteriorly with raised edges. The entire region extends outward in a sloping manner, without any localized depressions. Type II: Localized anterior protrusion deformity, where the edge of the rib arch shows a confined anterior protrusion while other areas remain in normal position. The protrusion forms a distinct angle with the surrounding structures and is not accompanied by any localized depressions. Type III: Complex deformity, with marked anterior protrusion of the rib arch combined with localized depressions of the lateral chest wall. The area of depression is limited, and the rib arch shape is distorted.

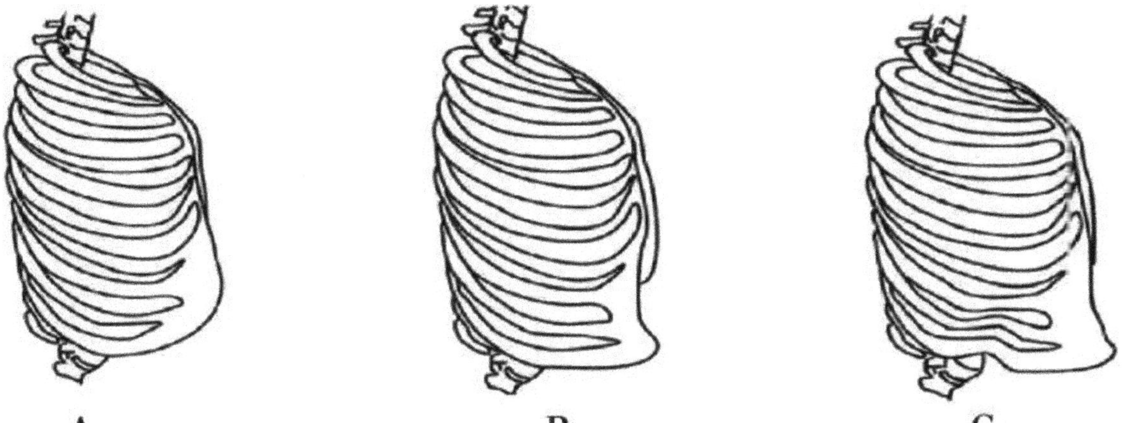

A B C

Figure 2-13-3 Classification of Rib Arch Deformities (A. Type I, generalized rib arch proptosis; B. Type II [limited rib arch marginal proptosis; C. Type III, rib arch proptosis combined with depressed deformity)

2. Etiology and pathogenesis

Rib arch deformities are complex, with multiple presentations and different pathogenesis for different types of deformities. Three types of costal arch All deformities have varying degrees of proptosis. Rib arch deformities can be categorized as primary or secondary proptosis depending on the cause. The cause of primary proptosis is unknown, whereas secondary proptosis has a clear cause. Common causes include: (1) relative proptosis due to superior concavity. This is quite common, as the actual height of the rib arch is not very high, but there is a significant depression above it. The difference in height creates a relative proptosis of the rib arch. (ii) Anterior convexity after surgery for funnel chest. During surgery for the funnel chest, the entire depressed chest wall is raised, and the rib arch attached to it is sometimes raised at the same time. Since the rib arch is higher than the normal plane of the chest wall, a secondary proptosis develops. The rib arch is higher than the normal plane of the chest wall, and a secondary proptosis is formed. The abdominal wall structure is weak in young children, due to the continuous positive pressure in the abdominal cavity, under the action of pressure, the abdomen will easily bulge, and in severe cases, the child may even show a "frog-like abdomen". As the upper end of the abdominal wall is mainly attached to the edge of the rib arch, when the abdominal wall is obviously bulging, the abdominal wall structure pulls the rib arch anteriorly, resulting in anterior projection of the rib arch, which ultimately leads to the formation of proptosis [4].

In addition to the proptosis, type III costal arch deformity is also characterized by depression, which is formed by a complex mechanism with no clear explanation. There are two possible reasons: (1) abnormal development of the rib arch, which eventually leads to localized depression due to its own structural mutation; and (2) due to the attachment of the diaphragm in the deep part of the rib arch, which may lead to localized depression when the diaphragmatic pull is too severe.

In rib arch deformities, bulging is the more common pathologic change, and depressions are less common. Once depression occurs, the deformity is generally more complex and troublesome to treat, requiring special skills to accomplish the procedure [5].

3. Clinical manifestations

The main pathologic feature of type I and type II costal arch deformities is the anterior convexity, which is usually asymptomatic because there is no compression and the patient's complaints are mostly cosmetic. Type III patients have a combination of depressed deformities, which may cause compression of the deeper structures, but because the depression is limited and is not deep, it is usually asymptomatic.

Relative proptosis is the more common deformity. This deformity is often associated with funnel chest deformity, but can also be seen as a sulcus or saddle chest deformity. When a depressed anterior chest wall deformity is corrected, there are two possible outcomes of anterior rib arch convexity: the first is seen in younger children with funnel chest [4]. In such children, the chest wall is weak, and when the depressed chest wall is corrected, the bracing forces are localized to the chest wall and do not reach the costal arch, and therefore do not result in continued anterior convexity of the wall at the costal arch. Since the rib arch was originally relatively anteriorly convex, its actual height is not very high, when the depression is eliminated, the height difference between the two disappears, and the relative anterior convexity will be significantly reduced or even completely disappeared at this time. This is the most satisfactory result. The second result is seen in older or adult patients with funnel chest [6]. In these patients, the chest wall is structurally rigid, and the depressed chest wall forms a rigid hole with the rib arch. If support is applied to the depression, the force of the support is transmitted to the coastal arch and the height of the arch is increased. This is tantamount to increasing the height of the rib arch, and it is impossible to eliminate the rib arch deformity. This result can be seen in many surgical procedures. It is clear that surgery of the upper chest wall depression does not change the shape of the rib arch deformity. It is clear that if only the depression above the relative proptosis is treated, the proptosis will have a different outcome depending on the age of the patient.

The relative deformity described above is a common secondary deformity that occurs as a result of an overlying concavity deformity. This deformity can be clinically significant in its own right, especially if the depression is severe. Other Secondary Anterior Convexity Deformities. There may also be specific causes, such as "froggy belly", surgery for depressed deformities, etc., which have their own specific clinical manifestations that can help in the diagnosis of costal arch deformities.

4. Inspection

Rib arch deformity is mainly based on physical examination, and observation of the appearance is important evidence for the diagnosis of the deformity. Imaging examination can clarify the general structure of the bony structures, but since the rib arch is mostly a cartilaginous structure, some imaging examinations cannot visualize it accurately. Three-dimensional reconstruction can clarify the overall structure and provide reference for surgery.

5. Diagnosis and Differential Diagnosis

The diagnosis of arch deformities is based on visualization and consists of two basic types of deformities, one anteriorly convex and the other concave. The distribution of the deformities is further characterized by three specific types. Differential diagnosis requires, firstly, a distinction between arch deformity and relative arch deformity, which is associated with a depressed deformity of the upper chest wall, while the position of the rib arches themselves is essentially normal, and, secondly, a distinction between primary deformity and secondary deformity. Secondly, it is necessary to distinguish between primary deformities and secondary deformities. Primary deformities do not have a clear cause, whereas secondary deformities have a clear cause, which can usually be found if the cause is carefully analyzed.

6. Indications for surgery

In the case of independent costal arch deformities, the basic pathologic change is the anterior convexity of the costal arch, and in a small percentage of patients there is a concave deformity. The anterior convexity is located directly in front of the trunk, and the most important hazard is its cosmetic impact. Even if a small percentage. If patients have a concavity present, it is rarely associated with serious symptoms, so most patients will seek medical attention because of its appearance. If the appearance of the deformity is unacceptable, treatment is definitely necessary; if one does not care about the appearance and at the same time does not have significant symptoms, treatment can be left untreated [7].

When a rib arch deformity exists in combination with other deformities, it is ideal to perform surgery for the other deformities at the same time as the rib arch deformity. This can lead to a more perfect surgical result. However, in practice there are many practical limitations, such as technical limitations, material limitations, and ability to pay, etc., and arch deformities are often untreatable because of these limitations. When surgeons and patients generally do not consider a combined rib arch deformity as a necessary surgical component, the chances of this deformity being treated are very low.

7. Surgical Treatment

Rib arch deformities can exist independently or in combination with other deformities. When discussing the surgical aspects of costal arch deformity, it is important to address each of the two specific situations

(1) Stand-alone surgery for costal arch deformity

The arch of the rib cage is a very specific deformity. Since the arch of the rib cage is part of the overall thorax, its characteristics are similar to those of the overall thoracic deformity, and it can basically be considered as a predominantly bulging deformity. In the orthopedics process, the surgery can be performed with the usual techniques for thoracic deformities. However, there is a definite difference between this area and the upper thoracic structures. The absence of bony structures in the middle of the rib arches on both sides, which are medial to the upper part of the abdominal wall, results in a relatively high degree of mobility of the rib arches, a characteristic that is completely different from that of the upper part of the thorax. Because of this characteristic, there are other options for the correction of the deformity, which can be completely different from the traditional concept of thoracic deformity surgery [7-10].

(1) Wenlin surgery

The basic lesion of the rib arch deformity is a proptosis, which is present in each of the three specific types, and can therefore be corrected using the Wenlin procedure, drawing on the general approach to proptosis in thoracic deformities (Fig. 2-13-4).

i. Wenlin procedure for type I rib arch deformity: this deformity is characterized by a large anterior convexity of the rib arch, which is similar to that of a large chicken breast and can be treated with the standard Wenlin procedure. The specific method is as follows: make incisions on both sides of the chest wall to reveal the ribs where the plates are fixed, place wire guides, make tunnels along the surface of the ribs in a median direction, and the tunnels are connected with the incisions on the opposite side of the chest wall; put the guides into the tunnels, introduce the guide tubes of the steel plates, connect the steel plates to the guide tubes, and pull the steel plates into the tunnels, and then introduce the wires with wire guides, encircle the ribs and the steel plates, tighten the wires to fix the steel plates to the ribs, and close the incisions, and the operation is finished. The incision is closed and the operation is finished. The main points to be noted during the operation are as follows: First, the plate must have the appropriate length and curvature. The length should be beyond the anterior axillary line, not too long or too short. The curvature should be that of normal chest wall appearance. Second, the location of steel plate placement. The steel plate should be placed in the most obvious part of the anterior convexity. Before the operation, the plate can be placed on the body surface for compression test, and the part with the best compression effect is the most appropriate. Third, the position of plate fixation.

Each end of the plate can be fixed in two places, on the one hand, to ensure that the plate is firmly fixed, and on the other hand, to spread the stress as much as possible. In specific operation, generally a single steel plate can obtain satisfactory results. If the area is wide and large, two plates can be used for shaping. The specific methods are basically the same.

ii. Wenlin's procedure for type II rib arch deformity: Since the anterior convexity is confined to the edge of the rib arch, there is a clear turn between the bulge and the surrounding structures, which corresponds to a relative depression. When the bulge is depressed, the neighboring areas are also depressed, and a relative depression deformity must exist. If this deformity is not dealt with, it will be detrimental to the overall shaping. In order to eliminate this disadvantage, when using the Wenlin procedure, it is important to make sure that the medial fixation is located on the medial side of the proptosis deformity, i.e., in the area of the relative depression. Fixation in this area is equivalent to a lifting action, which in essence is equivalent to the Wang procedure. In this way, the total operation can also be described as a combination of Wenlin surgery and Wang surgery. After the two operations, not only the bulge is corrected, but also the relative depression is eliminated, so the overall treatment result will be very satisfactory. This procedure usually requires only one plate to achieve satisfactory results. If the result is not satisfactory, two plates may be considered.

iii. Wenlin's procedure for type III rib arch deformity: The depression of type II deformity is a relative depression, and after depressing the bulge, the relative depression is removed. It will be clearly visible. In type III rib arch deformity, the depression is an objective deformity, an absolute depression. The deformity in this case is equivalent to a composite of two deformities at the same time. Since this is a composite deformity, it is objectively necessary to use both procedures to complete the treatment. In the case of a convex anterior deformity, the Wenlin procedure is generally used, whereas in the case of a depressed deformity, the Nuss procedure or the Wang procedure may be considered. Because of the small size of the rib arch and the fact that the convexity and depression lie in approximately the same plane, it is possible to perform both procedures with the same plate, the simplest being the combination of the Wenlin and Wang procedures.

The simplest operation is the combination of the Wenlin and Wang procedures. The median portion of the plate is used to compress the convexity of the arch, and then the depressed portion is lifted. This combination of two procedures is essentially the same as the Wenlin procedure alone, since the depressed lifting part can also be considered as a simple fixation of the plate. From this point of view, this procedure is no different from the Wenlin procedure in type II and type I surgery (Figures 2-13-4 and 2-13-5).

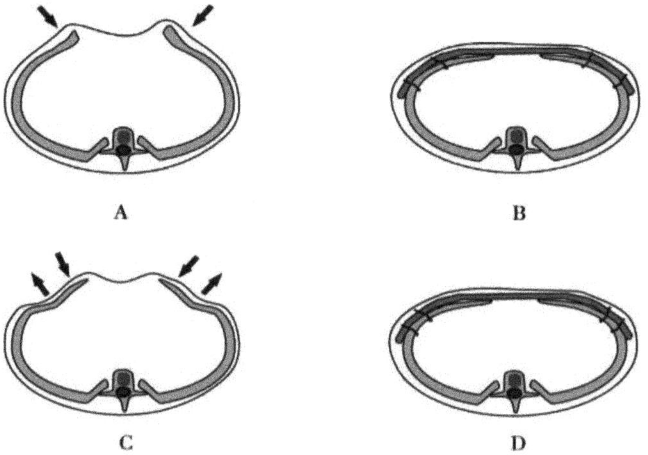

Figure 2-13-4 The Wenlin procedure for rib arch deformities (A. Type I and II rib arch deformities with total or partial anterior convexity of the rib arch; B. The Wenlin procedure requires flattening of all anterior convexity; C. Type III rib arch deformity with convexity of the rib arch combined with localized depressions; D. The Wenlin procedure is performed to flatten the anterior convexity, then to lift the depressions, and ultimately to achieve a template shape).

From the above analysis, it can be seen that Wenlin surgery for rib arch deformity is basically identical to Wenlin surgery for general proptosis thoracic deformity. It is less invasive, easier to perform, and has a satisfactory orthopedics result, making it a more desirable surgical option. However, this operation is not perfect and also has defects. The main drawbacks include: (1) the operation must use a steel plate. The use of steel plates is not uncommon in thoracic deformity surgery. However, the use of a plate at the level of the upper and middle thorax is completely different from the use of a plate at the level of the costal arch. When a plate is used in the upper midsection, the plate is close to the bony structures and does not cause significant discomfort to the patient. At the level of the costal arch, since there is no bony structure in the middle of the costal arch, the plate is equivalent to the presence of the upper part of the

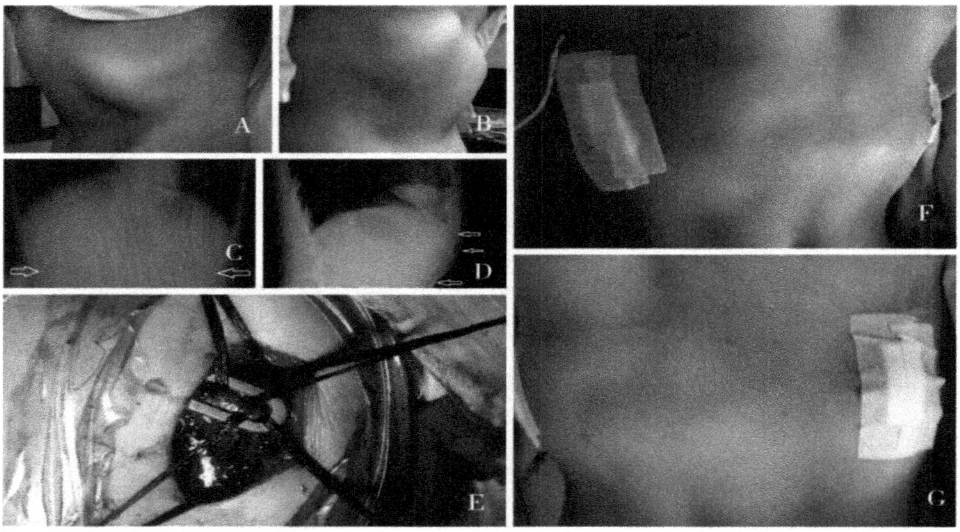

Figure 2-13-5 Type III costal arch deformity treated with Wenlin procedure + Wang procedure (A, B: The deformity covers a wide area of the costal arch, involving both protrusion and depression, with an overall irregular shape; C, D: X-ray images showing the deformity of the costal arch from the lateral view; E: Incision made on the lateral chest wall, with Wenlin and Wang procedures performed; F, G: Postoperative external appearance of the chest, showing that the deformity has essentially disappeared.)

abdominal wall, and the patient will feel significant discomfort. When the rib arch deformity is combined with other thoracic deformities, the management of the rib arch deformity requires an additional plate, which will significantly increase the cost of the surgery, and both the doctor and the patient are reluctant to make such a choice. (2) Complications may occur during plate penetration. As the plate passes through the middle of each rib arch, it may penetrate into the abdominal wall muscles, or it may penetrate deep into the abdominal wall muscles. This is not done under direct visualization, and the plate may enter the abdominal cavity directly during penetration and injure associated structures. This is a serious complication. From the above analysis, it can be seen that the biggest drawback of this procedure is the use of the plate, which would be of great benefit to the patient if it were removed.

(2) Surgery without the use of plates

In order to eliminate the negative effects of the plates, we have devised a special procedure in which a wire is used to directly insert the rib arch towards the center of the rib cage. The correction of proptosis is accomplished by pulling the rib arches together as a means of reducing the height of the rib arch [7]. The rationale for this approach is that, regardless of the type of rib arch deformity, there is anterior convexity, and since there is no bony structure in the middle of the rib arch on both sides, the whole structure is relatively free and has good mobility. When the two rib arches are drawn together toward the median, their height is significantly reduced and the proptosis is eliminated. We have operated on a large number of patients with rib arch deformity using :
this method, and the results have been satisfactory. However, this operation also has certain defects: (1) this operation requires an incision in the center, and it is difficult to complete the operation through the lateral chest wall incision; (2) this operation can only complete the correction of anterior convexity deformity, and it cannot treat the depression; (3) it is not easy to control the strength of pulling together. If the pull is too loose, the orthopedics effect is not good; if the pull is too tight, the rib arch may be broken, resulting in failure of the operation. Compared with the Wenlin procedure, which uses a steel plate, this procedure has obvious advantages because the steel plate is no longer used. However, due to other shortcomings, there is still a need for further improvements.

(3) Scarless surgery

In order to eliminate the drawbacks of the above-mentioned surgery, especially the incision in the center, we designed another surgery, the scarless surgery [7]. This procedure is still designed for the bulging deformity, but it does not require any incision, and the method used is still to make a retraction of the rib arch towards the median. Due to its design, better results can be obtained. However, since it is also only a retraction of the bulge and not a simultaneous treatment of the depression, it can only be used for Type I and Type II deformities, but not for Type III deformities.

(2) Management of rib arch deformity in surgery for other deformities

The anterior projection of the rib arch is a very obvious problem in surgery for some specific deformities, especially funnel chest. Although this problem was not specifically reported in the early years, it is certain that it was treated at that time. This assumption is based on the fact that in those early years the surgery was open and the operation was performed on every detail of the deformity. Once the depression had been eliminated, it would have been impossible to leave the obvious anterior convexity untreated. In fact, it is not difficult to perform this operation in the open state, as long as the local stresses are slightly released and then reasonably fixed.

In 2010, the concept of minimally invasive treatment of rib arch deformity was proposed. The specific method is to cut the skin in the area where the rib arch protrusion is obvious, reveal the structure of the edge of the rib arch, peel off the periosteum of the local osseous structure, excise the protruding portion and the connected structure, and then suture the periosteum for contouring, thus achieving the goal of reshaping the rib arch. Although such an operation is minimally invasive, the specifics of the operation are not different from open surgery, and therefore remain in the realm of open surgery.

In 2016, Park et al. did additional maneuvers in thoracic deformity surgery as a way to do orthopedics for rib arch deformity [11]. A special "Magic string" is inserted into the chest wall through an incision on one side of the chest wall to reach the surface of the raised rib arch, and then passed through the incision on the opposite side of the chest wall. After the suture has been passed through the chest wall, it is secured to a steel plate at both ends, and then the raised rib arch is flattened with the suture by tightening the suture. This is an ingenious approach, but it can only be used as an add-on procedure and not as a stand-alone surgery for costal arch deformity.

Although all of the above methods have been tried in clinical practice, it is clear that they are not ideal. In practice, the methods used in stand-alone arch deformity surgery should be considered, and all three of them can be used in combined arch deformity surgery for all types of deformities. The presence of a deformity surgical incision will greatly facilitate the performance of all three procedures (Figures 2-13-6 and 2-13-7).

As previously mentioned, in the correction of costal arch deformities, the Wenlin procedure requires the additional use of a steel plate, which increases the burden on both the surgeon and the patient. Considering the various postoperative discomforts, this approach is clearly not the ideal option. In contrast, the other two surgical methods appear to be more reasonable. However, in cases of Type III costal arch deformity, the Wenlin procedure remains the preferred choice.

8. Complications

As with any deformity correction surgery, procedures for costal arch deformities are not exempt from complications. The primary complications are generally similar to those seen in other thoracic deformity surgeries. However, due to the involvement of the upper anterior abdominal wall at the midline of the costal arch, additional procedure-specific complications may occur. Special care must be taken during the placement of the steel plate to minimize the risk of these complications as much as possible.

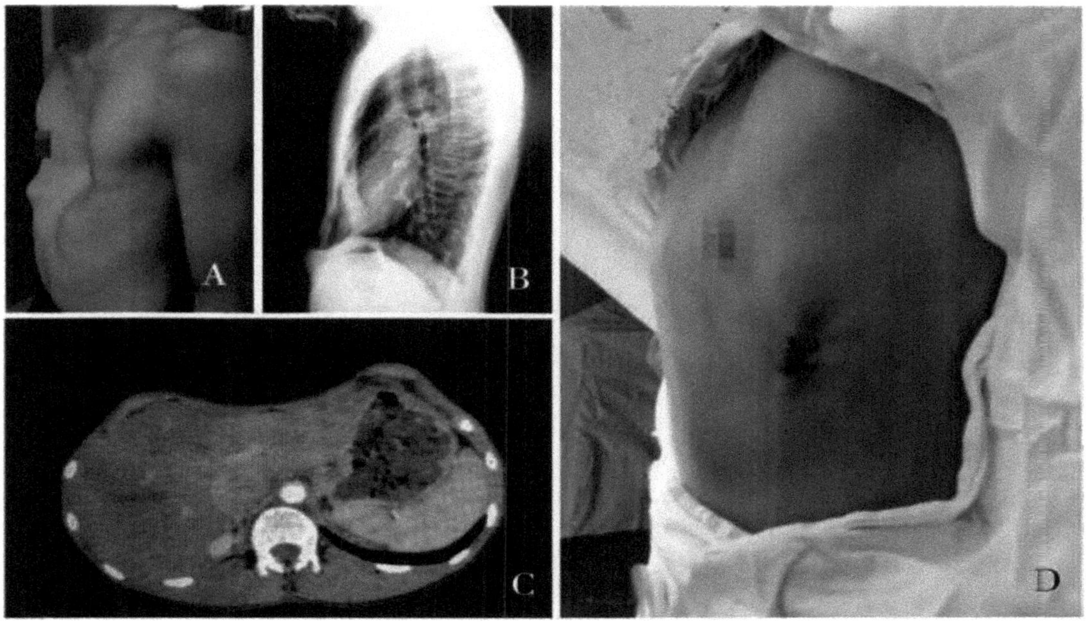

Figure 2-13-6 Funnel chest combined with rib deformity (correction of the funnel chest was accomplished with the Wung procedure, followed by the Wenlin procedure for correction of the rib arch deformity. A. Preoperative appearance of the chest wall, with a markedly depressed deformity and anteriorly projecting rib arches; B, C. Imaging suggests anterior chest wall depression combined with anteriorly projecting rib arches; D. Postoperative appearance of the chest, with a complete disappearance of the deformity).

9. Prognosis

Coastal arch deformities exhibit a variety of morphologies, but they are generally not severe. Moreover, due to the high mobility of the bony structures in this region, correction is typically relatively straightforward. As long as the appropriate surgical method is selected and properly executed, a satisfactory outcome can usually be achieved. However, these procedures demand high precision in technical details; if such details are not well managed, surgical outcomes may be compromised, potentially leading to failure

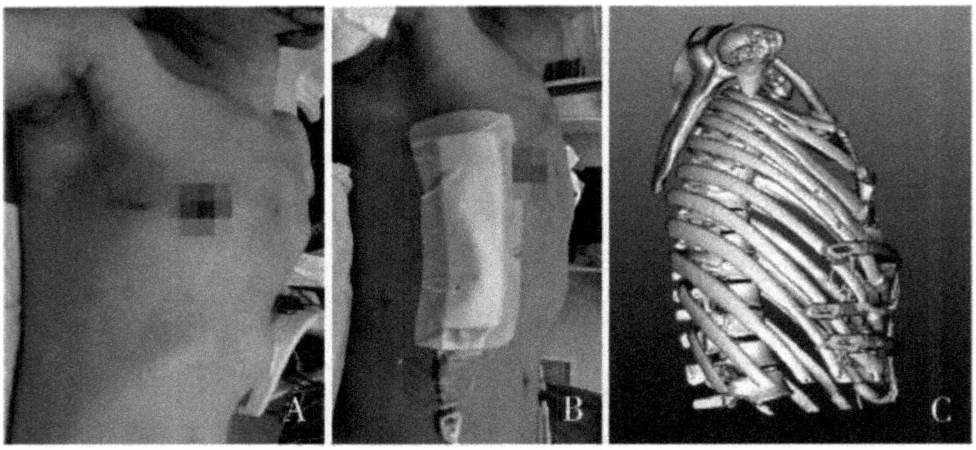

Figure 2-13-7 Surgery for secondary costal arch deformity (This is a patient who had a failed chicken breast surgery. The first surgery was performed with a single plate, which did not eliminate the proptosis. In the second operation, the plate from the first operation was removed and the Wenlin operation was performed with a new plate. During the operation, one plate was used to compress the anterior convexity deformity, and a depression appeared underneath, and a second plate was used to perform the Wung operation. After completion of the operation, the rib arch was found to be anteriorly convex, manifesting a type II costal arch deformity, and the Wenlin operation was performed with a third plate, with satisfactory results. A. Chest wall appearance after the first operation, with the anterior chest wall anteriorly convex at the upper part, slightly concave below, and the rib arches slightly anteriorly convex, with an obsolete surgical scar. B. Thoracic appearance after the second operation, with the deformity basically disappeared. C. Postoperative three-dimensional reconstruction image showing the three steel plates' locations. The top one is Wenlin's surgical plate to correct the anteriorly convex deformity; the middle one is Wung's surgical plate to correct the secondary depressed deformity; and the bottom one is also Wenlin's surgical plate to correct the rib arch deformity).

REFERENCES

[1] Wang, W. L. 2016a. "Surgical Issues of Costal Arch Eversion." *Expert in Thoracic Deformity Surgery*, September 12.

[2] Wang, W. L. 2017a. "Surgical Issues of Costal Arch Deformity." *Expert in Thoracic Deformity Surgery*, August 24.

[3] Wang, W. L. 2018a. "Minimally Invasive Operation for Costal Arch Deformity." *Surgical Case Reports* 1 (2): 1–3.

[4] Wang, W. L. 2016b. "Why Do Young Children with Pectus Excavatum Have Costal Arch Protrusion?" *Expert in Thoracic Deformity Surgery*, September 13.

[5] Wang, W. L. 2021a. "The Wang Procedure for Costal Arch Depression Deformity." *Expert in Thoracic Deformity Surgery*, October 12.

[6] Wang, W. L. 2018b. "Management of Costal Arch Protrusion after Pectus Excavatum Surgery." *Expert in Thoracic Deformity Surgery*, June 14.

[7] Wang, W. L. 2021b. "Surgical Issues of Costal Arch Deformity." *Today's Headlines*, November 6.

[8] Wang, W. L. 2018c. "Minimally Invasive Surgery for Pectus Excavatum Combined with Costal Arch Deformity." *Expert in Thoracic Deformity Surgery*, January 31.

[9] Wang, W. L. 2018d. "Severe Pectus Excavatum with Costal Arch Deformity: Tubeless Minimally Invasive Surgery." *Expert in Thoracic Deformity Surgery*, February 7.

[10] Wang, W. L. 2017b. "Another Success over the Weekend: Successful Correction of Severe Complex Costal Arch Deformity." *Thoracic Deformity Surgery Expert*, June 9.

[11] Park, H. J., and K. S. Kim. 2016. "The Sandwich Technique for Repair of Pectus Carinatum and Excavatum/Carinatum Complex." *Annals of Cardiothoracic Surgery* 5 (5): 434–439.

Chapter 14

POLAND SYNDROME

Poland syndrome is an ancient disease that was first discovered in 1841 by a British medical student named Alfred Poland during a cadaver dissection. In 1962, Clarkson encountered a similar case in clinical practice and named the deformity Poland syndrome [1-3]. Some have found that this condition was actually mentioned even before Poland discovery [3] but unfortunately it was Poland who received the naming credit, not others. Poland syndrome is a complex and variable disease, characterized mainly by abnormalities in the bony structures and soft tissues of the chest wall, accompanied by deformities of the ipsilateral upper limb (Figure 2-14-1) [4,5]. In earlier times, there was limited awareness of Poland syndrome, and thus very few patients sought medical help. With continuous improvements in diagnostic and treatment techniques, more and more patients have been identified and treated, so its incidence rate has been gradually changing. Reports in the literature vary widely, with incidence rates ranging from 1/ 20,000 to 1/7,000. It is more common in males, with a male-to-female ratio of about 2:1 to 3:1 [1-3] Lesions are mostly unilateral, more commonly affecting the right side—accounting for 60% - 70% of cases. The left side is less commonly affected, and bilateral cases are rare [1].In the past, this condition was mainly treated by hand surgeons, plastic surgeons, or cosmetic surgeons, while thoracic surgeons were hardly involved in its treatment. In recent years, we have gradually begun performing surgeries specifically for Poland syndrome patients and have continuously refined these procedures, ultimately establishing this condition as one of the diseases treated by chest wall surgery [6-11]. One of the main lesions of Poland syndrome is the chest wall deformity, whether it involves bony structures or soft tissue abnormalities—making it suitable for treatment by thoracic (chest wall) surgeons. The advantages of this specialty are clearly superior to those of other specialties. For this reason, as the concept of treating Poland syndrome with chest wall surgery continues to spread, more and more patients have begun to receive surgical treatment from thoracic surgeons.

1. Pathogenesis

The pathogenesis of Poland syndrome is relatively complex. Although many researchers have conducted extensive studies, no definitive explanation has been established to date. Based on previous viewpoints, there are four main hypotheses [1,2]: . Some authors explain the disease from an embryological perspective, suggesting that the deformity is mainly caused by injury during the

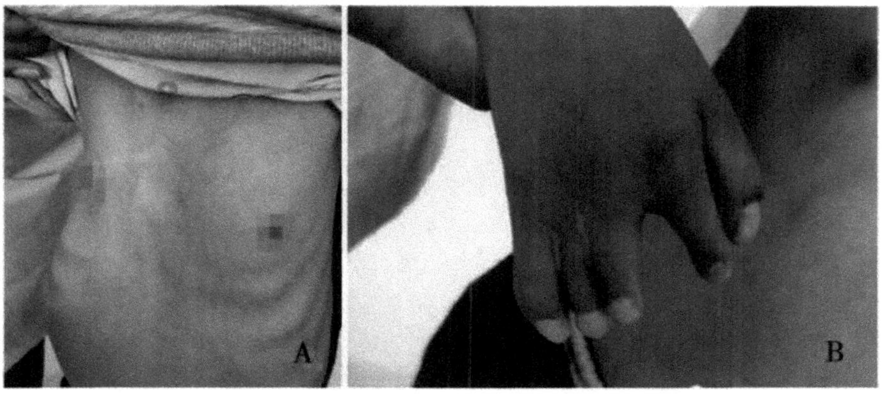

Figure 2-14-1 Poland syndrome (A. Hypoplasia of the soft tissue and bony structures of the right chest wall; B. Syndactyly of the right hand)

splitting of the embryonic chest bud in the sixth week of embryonic development.2 Others believe it results from abnormal differentiation of the mesoderm between 16 and 28 days after fertilization.3. Another hypothesis attributes Poland syndrome to insufficient blood supply. The main theory is that a branch of the subclavian artery near the internal thoracic artery becomes obstructed for unknown reasons, leading to abnormal blood flow in the affected area and causing the deformity. Since this artery supplies blood to both the upper anterior chest wall and the ipsilateral upper limb, any disruption affects the development of all tissues in these regions, resulting in varying degrees of malformation.4. Some researchers suggest a genetic cause, as clinical evidence shows that Poland syndrome can recur in the same family, and gene mutations have been found in patients' chromosomes, providing direct evidence for hereditary factors. In addition to these four major hypotheses, other possible causes have been suggested clinically, including smoking, autosomal dominant inheritance, single-gene defects, viral infections, trauma, and exposure to abortifacient drugs acting on the uterus. All of these factors are considered potential contributors to the occurrence of Poland syndrome. Most people accept the explanation related to vascular insufficiency. This theory can account for all the pathological changes and clinical manifestations observed in Poland syndrome.

2. Pathological Changes

In typical Poland syndrome, the lesions involve both the chest wall structures and the ipsilateral upper limb, but in clinical practice, cases often show deformities in only some of these structures — both sites may not necessarily be affected at the same time. The chest wall deformity may involve both bony structures and soft tissues [1-3]. Bony structural deformities mainly present as absence, thinning, malformation, or fusion of the ribs and costal cartilages. Absence usually appears first as a lack of costal cartilage, primarily affecting the 1-5th costal cartilages. In severe cases, the ribs themselves may also be involved, but rib absence mostly involves only the anterior part of the ribs; complete absence of an entire rib is rare. When a rib is partially missing, a local defect may form, which can lead to chest wall collapse and lung herniation. In some patients, the ribs and costal cartilages are noticeably thin and show clear signs of underdevelopment. Bony structures may also exhibit abnormal shapes or local fusion. Overall, the chest wall may show localized depression. This depression is generally mild, though a few patients may have a more pronounced sunken chest. Soft tissue deformities mainly involve abnormalities of the pectoralis major and minor muscles and the breast, which may appear underdeveloped or absent. In female patients, early signs may not be obvious, but after puberty, clear asymmetry of one breast may appear. This can include underdevelopment of the nipple and breast, and in severe cases, complete absence. Accessory breasts may also be present, while the unaffected side develops normally [1]. Male patients may show absence of subcutaneous fat. Both bony and soft tissue deformities often coexist, but some patients present only with soft tissue deformities without any bony abnormalities. In rare cases, the lesions may extend to other muscles such as the serratus anterior, latissimus dorsi, or trapezius, which may also show underdevelopment or absence. Patients may also have loss of hair on the affected side of the chest and in the axilla, and some may have axillary deformities. Upper limb deformities usually affect the distal parts and can manifest as various forms of syndactyly (webbed fingers) or brachydactyly (short fingers).

The upper limb deformities often include syndactyly, absence of fingers, absence of phalanges, or malformations such as fusion of the flexor digitorum superficialis and profundo's muscles, carpal bone fusion, and fusion between the ulna and trapezium bones [12]. Additionally, some patients may present with spinal developmental abnormalities, typically manifesting as scoliosis.

In addition to lesions of the chest wall and upper limb, Poland syndrome may be accompanied by certain special comorbidities, such as Moebius syndrome and Klippel-Feil syndrome. The pathogenesis of these conditions is complex but may be related to local vascular abnormalities [1]. Furthermore, Poland syndrome has been associated with various tumors. Reported tumors include leukemia, non-Hodgkin lymphoma, cervical cancer, lung cancer, and breast cancer. Among these, breast cancer has the highest incidence and is often found in the hypoplastic breast tissue, suggesting an intrinsic link between tumor development and Poland syndrome [13]. Additionally, Poland syndrome is related to hypoplasia of some internal organs, such as the heart and kidneys, and may present with certain congenital malformations.

3. Clinical Manifestations

The primary lesions in Poland syndrome patients are located in the chest wall and the ipsilateral upper limb, presenting with a variety of symptoms [12,14]. When there is a significant chest wall depression, the concavity can compress the thoracic organs, leading to respiratory symptoms. The main complaints include chest tightness, palpitations, and shortness of breath, which may worsen with physical activity. Due to multiple deformities affecting different parts of the body, patients often experience emotional distress related to their abnormal appearance. This is especially pronounced in post-pubertal female patients, who may suffer from severe asymmetry of the chest wall and abnormal appearance, leading to profound feelings of low self-esteem and potentially triggering various psychological issues. Additionally, due to the presence of other associated deformities and comorbidities, patients may exhibit other related symptoms.

In Poland syndrome, lesions are typically unilateral on the chest wall. Due to the marked asymmetry between the left and right thoraxes, uneven forces may be exerted on either side of the spine, potentially leading to scoliosis. This condition is similar to what is observed in other types of asymmetric thoracic deformities. In summary, because Poland syndrome is inherently complex and often accompanied by various comorbidities, its clinical manifestations can present in multiple specific forms. When assessing patients with this condition, it is essential to take a detailed medical history to avoid missing any associated abnormalities.

4. Investigations

The physical signs of Poland syndrome are usually obvious, and physical examination can reveal lesions of the chest wall and upper limb. However, due to the complexity of associated abnormalities in Poland syndrome, physical examination alone is often insufficient to obtain complete information. Therefore, a comprehensive systemic evaluation is usually necessary. This evaluation includes imaging studies and necessary laboratory tests, with a focus on assessing lesions of the chest wall, upper limb, and any suspected internal organs. Chest CT scan is the fundamental diagnostic tool, and when possible, three-dimensional reconstruction of the chest should be performed (see Figure 2-14-2).

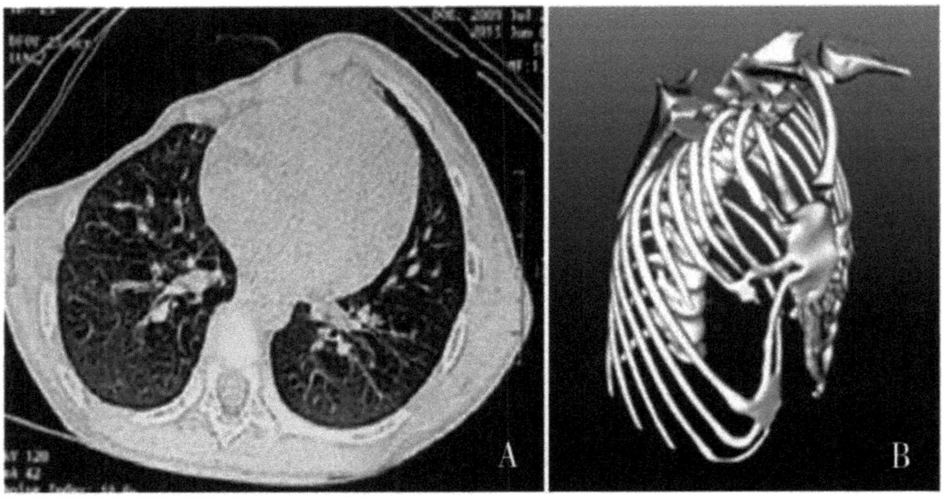

Figure 2-14-2 imaging studies of Poland syndrome: (A. CT cross-sectional image showing hypoplasia of soft tissue and bony structures on one side; B. Three reconstruction images demonstrating absence of bony structures in the chest wall on one side.

5. Diagnosis and Differential Diagnosis

Poland syndrome presents with distinct and relatively fixed anatomical abnormalities, making the diagnosis relatively straightforward. The key diagnostic feature is unilateral underdevelopment of both soft tissue and bony structures of the chest wall, often accompanied by ipsilateral upper limb abnormalities. These chest wall and upper limb deformities may occur simultaneously, or one may appear in isolation. In addition to these primary manifestations, patients may also have associated anomalies in other parts of the body

Poland syndrome should be differentiated from asymmetric high-position pectus excavatum, thoracic dysplasia syndrome, and lateral chest wall depression deformities. In asymmetric high-position pectus excavatum, the chest wall depression may occur in a location similar to that seen in Poland syndrome; however, there is no absence of bony structures or other obvious localized abnormalities, nor is there any associated soft tissue hypoplasia or absence. The only deformity is the depression of the chest wall. The two conditions can be readily distinguished by assessing the internal structure of the chest wall. Thoracic dysplasia syndrome may present with rib defects or fusions, but the abnormalities are primarily located paravertebrally, and patients do not exhibit soft tissue underdevelopment or upper limb anomalies, clearly differentiating it from Poland syndrome. Lateral chest wall depression deformities can occur in the upper chest wall but are fundamentally similar in nature to asymmetric pectus excavatum. These cases lack internal structural abnormalities of the chest wall and are thus relatively easy to distinguish. Deformities of the upper limb and hand also require differential diagnosis; however, since these involve other specialties, they will not be discussed in detail here.

6. Surgical Treatment

The treatment of Poland syndrome has traditionally been managed by specialists from various disciplines. Surgeries involving the fingers and upper limb are typically performed by hand surgeons or plastic surgeons, while thoracic surgeons are primarily responsible for procedures involving the chest wall. Therefore, in the following discussion, we will focus exclusively on surgical treatment of the chest wall, and other aspects will not be addressed here.

(1) Surgical Indications

Patients with Poland syndrome may present with significant symptoms, and surgical intervention should be considered when symptoms are severe. In the absence of major comorbidities, most patients do not exhibit serious clinical symptoms, and the decision to operate is primarily based on the degree of cosmetic deformity. If the patient is dissatisfied with their appearance, surgery should be considered. However, severe functional impairment of other vital organs that renders the patient unable to tolerate surgery constitutes a contraindication, and surgical treatment should not be pursued in such cases.

(2) Timing of Surgery

Surgical treatment of the chest wall in Poland syndrome involves two main components: correction of the bony structures and reconstruction of the soft tissue. Considering the developmental characteristics of the skeletal system, the optimal time for surgery is after puberty. If corrective surgery is performed too early, a second procedure may be required after pubertal growth is complete. Soft tissue reconstruction should also ideally be carried out after puberty—especially in female patients, where achieving symmetry between both sides of the chest wall is critical. The best timing for surgery in such cases is after full breast development. However, in certain special cases, early surgical intervention should be considered: 1. When there is severe chest wall depression causing significant compression and obvious symptoms, necessitating prompt surgery; 2. When the patient is dissatisfied with their appearance and desires early correction; 3. When the chest wall deformity causes uneven mechanical stress on both sides of the spine, potentially leading to scoliosis if surgery is delayed. To prevent such outcomes, early surgical treatment is necessary.

(3) Surgical Methods

Before thoracic surgeons became involved in the treatment of Poland syndrome, the primary management was carried out by plastic or cosmetic surgeons. Different specialties have distinct treatment philosophies and approaches [15,16]. Plastic and cosmetic surgeons mainly focus on the aesthetic appearance and therefore may not address the underlying bony structural abnormalities. Their method typically involves correcting local depressions or abnormal contours using implants or autologous tissue. This approach can achieve a direct and immediate cosmetic improvement. However, because the bony deformities are not corrected, there is a risk of worsening deep structural compression, which may negatively affect respiratory function.

The role of thoracic surgery involves two main aspects: one is the correction of bony structures, and the other is the reconstruction of soft tissues [16]. Correction of bony structures can be divided into two fundamental surgical methods: Remodeling and reconstruction. Remodeling primarily addresses deformities characterized by depressions, while reconstruction targets defects or absent bone.

(1) Correction of Bony Structures

Minimally Invasive Surgery: Poland syndrome's chest wall depression deformity is similar to asymmetric high-position pectus excavatum. However, because the depression usually does not involve the sternum, it is not classified as pectus excavatum but rather falls under the category of lateral chest wall depression deformities.

Considering the varying presentations among patients, we design different surgical approaches based on the individual's specific condition. These approaches may include the Wang procedure [6,8] or the Wenlin procedure, among others surgery[7]. In addition to these two classic surgical methods, we have also designed a special procedure called the Willine procedure [17]. The specific method is as follows: an incision is made on both sides of the chest wall at the level of the deepest depression. First, on the depressed side, the chest wall is dissected to expose the ribs beneath the depression. A tunnel is then created at the planned anchoring point. A tunnel is also created on the opposite side of the chest wall, positioned on the surface of the bony structures but deep to the muscles.A guide device is inserted through the tunnel on the depressed side, passed into the thoracic cavity, looped around the rib at the depression site and brought to the parasternal region, then passed to the surface of the sternum and exited through the tunnel on the opposite side. A steel plate is inserted, flipped into position, and fixed separately on both sides. The incisions are then sutured to complete the procedure (see Figure 2-14-3).

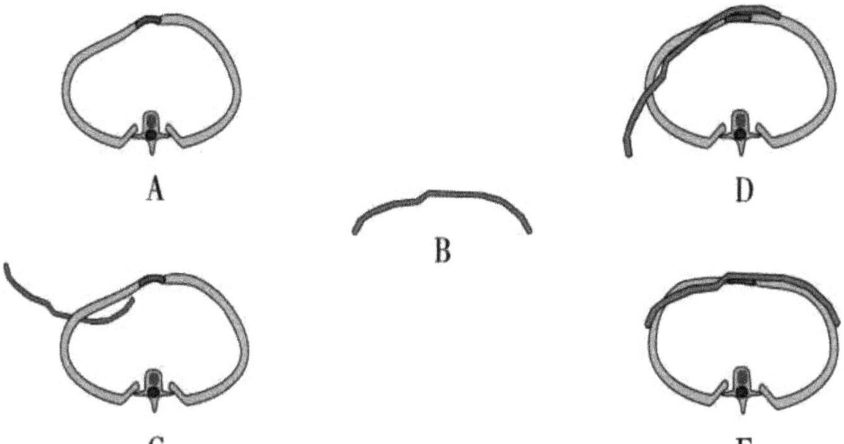

Figure 2-14-3 Schematic diagram of the Willine surgery for Poland syndrome: (A) Cross-sectional view of the thorax, showing a concavity on one side of the chest wall; (B) Specially shaped steel plate; (C) The steel plate enters the thoracic cavity from the edge of the concavity on one side, passes through the bottom of the concavity, and exits the thoracic cavity near the sternal edge of the concavity, reaching the surface of the bony structure of the chest wall; (D) The steel plate proceeds along the surface of the bony structure in front of the sternum toward the opposite chest wall; (E) One end of the steel plate props up the concave side, while the other side presses down on the protruding side, achieving a dual corrective effect

This surgical procedure is fundamentally different from the traditional Nuss procedure. During the operation, because the contralateral chest wall adjacent to the depression is often elevated, there is a downward pressure applied on that side. Therefore, from an overall perspective, this surgery resembles a combination of the Nuss and Wenlin procedures. However, when viewed more broadly in relation to the deformity itself, the operation is more akin to a pure Nuss procedure.

When performing the Nuss procedure for pectus excavatum, the depressed area of the chest wall is the midline sternum, which is a single continuous structure. Therefore, supporting just a part of it can produce good results. However, for lateral chest wall depression deformities, the depressed structures are ribs, and there are no bony connections between different ribs. This means the ribs are independent of each other — lifting one rib does not necessarily lift the others simultaneously, so the overall outcome may not be ideal. This is especially true when the ribs themselves are underdeveloped and relatively thin, which can further affect the surgical result. Given these limitations, when performing this procedure, it is necessary to strictly select appropriate candidates and pay special attention to surgical technique and details.

Overall, this type of surgery is suitable for patients who have only bony structural depressions. If there are defects or underdevelopment of the ribs or costal cartilages, then this technique is not appropriate.

The above surgical method is relatively simple, but during the actual procedure, certain key technical points must be carefully observed; otherwise, it will be difficult to perform the surgery smoothly.

To complete the procedure successfully, these key points must be kept in mind: First, the entry and exit points of the steel plate into and out of the thoracic cavity must be carefully planned to ensure that all the depressed ribs are effectively lifted. Second, the length and curvature of the steel plate must be properly designed; this is critical for success. Third, placement of the steel plate must be done cautiously to avoid injuring important structures such as the internal thoracic artery.

(2) Bony Structure Reconstruction

For patients with localized defects, chest wall reconstruction is required. There are two main types of materials used for reconstruction: autologous materials and artificial materials. Autologous materials have good biocompatibility and do not require removal, but must be harvested from other sites. However, the availability of autologous material is limited, making it insufficient for large defects. Artificial materials, such as Matrix RIB, are commonly used to directly reconstruct ribs and costal cartilages [10,11]. Artificial materials are readily available, do not cause additional harm to the patient, and can meet the needs of large-area defects (Figure 2-14-4). The key point of the reconstructive surgery is the choice of incision. A longitudinal incision can first be made under the axilla to expose the lateral residual part of the defective ribs. Then, a small longitudinal incision is made beside the sternum on the affected side to expose the fixation site. A guide tube is inserted into the reconstruction area, and after introducing the reconstructive material, fixation is performed on both sides. The procedure can thus be easily completed.

The objectives of bony structure reconstruction are twofold: first, to restore the integrity of the bony framework, and second, to reestablish the normal contour of the chest wall. These goals place high demands on the surgical procedure. When using MatrixRIB for reconstruction, it is essential not only to implant and fix the MatrixRIB in the defect area but also to shape it with an appropriate length and curvature to meet the anatomical requirements of the chest wall. Because the intercostal spaces can be relatively wide, when multiple MatrixRIB implants are used for reconstruction, the larger gaps between ribs must be adequately filled.

Additionally, a fibrous membrane is placed over the surface of the reconstruction to serve as padding, thereby enhancing the overall reconstructive outcome

(3) Soft Tissue Reconstruction

Correction of the bony structures is the primary focus of chest wall surgical procedures. After completing this part, combining efforts with plastic surgery for soft tissue reconstruction can achieve optimal aesthetic and functional outcomes. From the perspective of chest wall surgery itself, soft tissue reconstruction is also an integral component of the treatment. Therefore, if technically feasible, this part of the procedure can be performed concurrently by the thoracic surgical team.

Soft tissue reconstruction is divided into two parts [5,15]: chest muscle reconstruction and shaping, and breast reconstruction. Chest muscle restoration can be achieved by two methods: muscle transfer or filler augmentation. The latissimus dorsi muscle is the preferred donor for muscle transfer due to its proximity to the affected area and adequate volume. However, muscle transfer involves significant surgical trauma and long incisions; therefore, if better alternatives exist, they may be preferred. Filler augmentation does not restore the muscle structure itself but aims to achieve an improved aesthetic contour. Traditionally, this procedure was performed by plastic or cosmetic surgeons. With the development of the thoracic surgery specialty, these procedures have become part of routine practice within the field and can be performed independently by thoracic surgeons. Fillers can be autologous fat grafts or synthetic materials. In addition to the technical requirements of muscle reconstruction, an important consideration is breast reconstruction, which is

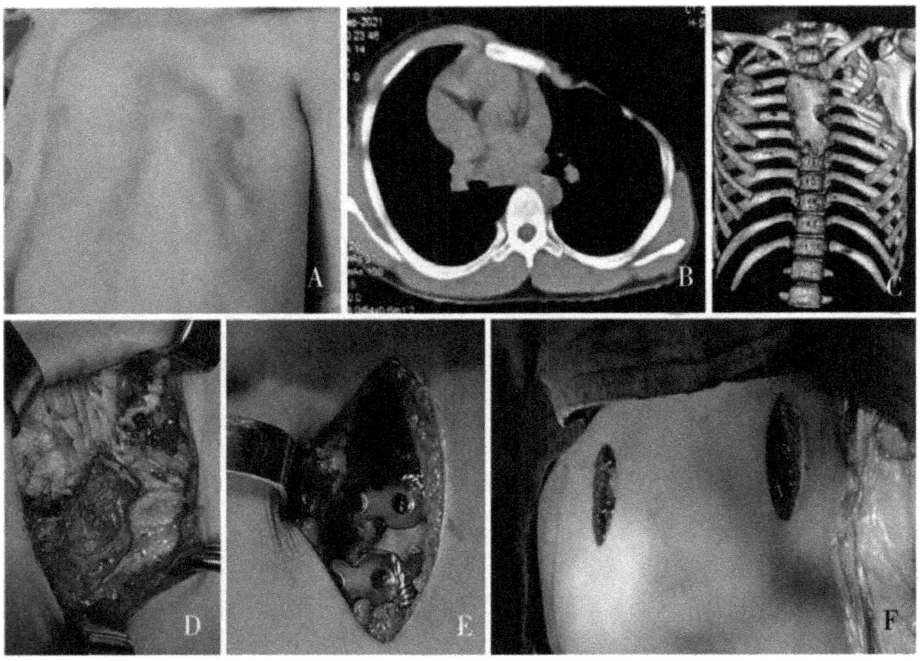

Figure 2-14-4 chest wall reconstruction in a Poland syndrome patient using MatrixRIB (A) preoperative chest wall appearance showing hypoplasia of soft tissue and bony structures on the left side; (B, C) imaging studies demonstrating localized defects of the left ribs and costal cartilages; (D) incision made adjacent to the sternum to expose the chest wall defect; (E) lateral chest wall incision performed for reconstruction of the defect using Matrix RIB; (F) one end of the MatrixRIB implant fixed to the lateral chest wall, the other end secured to the sternum; following fixation, the chest wall contour is effectively restored.

especially critical for female patients. Breast reconstruction can be performed concurrently with muscle reconstruction and may involve direct surgical techniques or implant placement. Such procedures require specialized expertise and are often carried out in collaboration with plastic surgeons or other relevant specialists.

7. Complications

Poland syndrome involves a wide range of deformities and complex surgical procedures. If the surgery is not performed carefully, various complications may arise. In addition to complications transplantation, implant placement, and other procedures. The most frequent complication is surgical failure (see Fig. 2-14-5). To minimize the risk of complications, the following points should be emphasized:1. Establish a multidisciplinary collaborative approach. Procedures that thoracic surgeons are skilled in should be performed independently, but for aspects outside their expertise, close cooperation with other specialties is essential to ensure successful surgery.2. Carefully consider the interrelationships between treatment methods for different affected areas. Surgical planning should be comprehensive and coordinated to avoid negative interactions between procedures and to maximize mutual benefits, thereby improving surgical efficiency.3. Maintain appropriate standards and avoid setting unrealistically high goals. The higher the standards set, the greater the cost and the higher the risk of complications. It is crucial to balance surgical ambition with patient safety

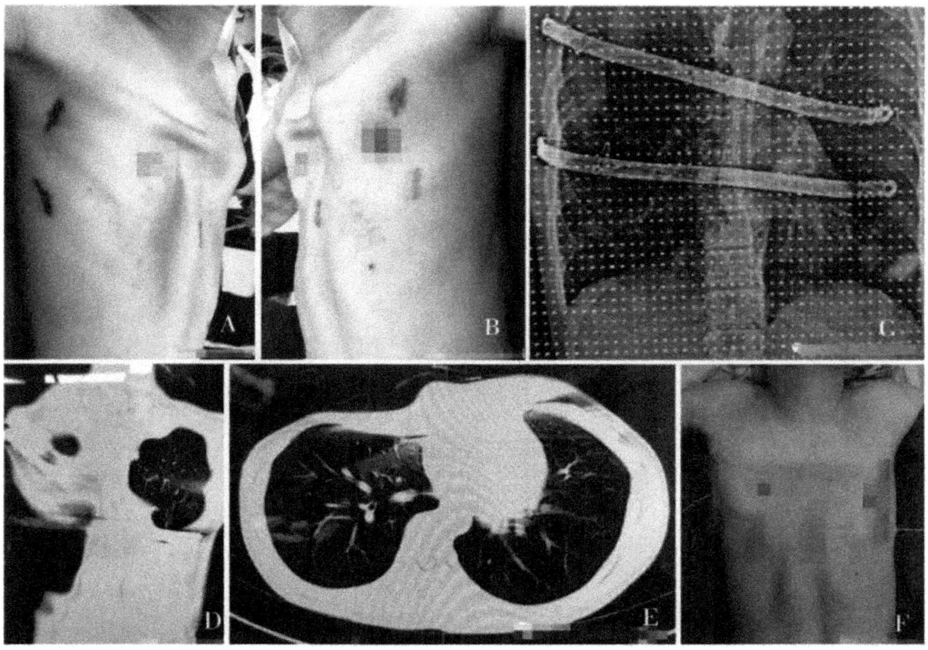

Figure 2-14-5 revision surgery for a patient with failed Poland syndrome surgery (A, B). The patient was initially misdiagnosed and treated as having asymmetric pectus carinatum, resulting in surgical failure. Images show right-sided chest wall depression and left-sided chest wall protrusion, with old scars and outlines of the implanted steel plate visible (C, D, E). Imaging studies demonstrate the position of the steel plate and the chest wall deformity. (F) After removal of the steel plate, a second corrective surgery was performed, resulting in complete resolution of the deformity.

8. Issues Related to Staged Surgery

The chest wall deformities in Poland syndrome involve two fundamentally different types of structures: bony structures and soft tissues, and the surgical approaches for each differ significantly [16]. Ideally, simultaneous surgery addressing both aspects would be the best option for the patient. However, in practice, staged surgery is often necessary. The first stage focuses on correcting the bony structural abnormalities, followed by a delayed procedure to address the soft tissue defects once the bony reconstruction is complete. Although staged surgery requires the patient to undergo multiple operations, it can achieve better overall outcomes, thus justifying its rationale. When performing staged surgery, the key focus is on timing. Since a second surgery is planned, the timing for the bony structural correction can be advanced. Early surgery offers numerous benefits. However, if reconstruction requires the use of synthetic materials, there may be disadvantages that must be carefully weighed during planning. Soft tissue reconstruction should be considered the final procedure, with meticulous surgical planning and execution to avoid the need for additional revision surgeries.

9. Prognosis

Poland syndrome is a complex condition involving multiple disciplines. It is difficult to achieve satisfactory outcomes if treatment is carried out by a single specialty alone. Therefore, the best approach is multidisciplinary collaboration, which is the key to success. However, coordinating care among various specialties can be challenging. For thoracic surgeons, it is essential first to focus on their area of expertise and complete their tasks with the highest quality. At the same time, they should maintain a broad and open mindset to actively cooperate with other specialists. Only by fully leveraging the strengths of different disciplines can the most satisfactory results be achieved.

REFERENCES

[1] Zhang, W., J. T. Li, and W. Tian. 2008. "Poland Syndrome." *Journal of Practical Hand Surgery* 22 (3): 161–163.

[2] Ouyang, Y. J., and C. J. Liu. 2017. "Advances in Diagnosis and Treatment of Poland Syndrome." *Journal of Tissue Engineering and Reconstructive Surgery* 13 (4): 220–223, 237.

[3] Charlier, P., S. Deo, F. M. Galassi, et al. 2019. "Poland Syndrome before Alfred Poland: The Oldest Medical Description (Paris, France, 1803)." *Surgical and Radiologic Anatomy* 41 (10): 1117–1118.

[4] Urschel, H. C. 2009. "Poland Syndrome." *Seminars in Thoracic and Cardiovascular Surgery* 21 (1): 89–94.

[5] Baldelli, I., A. Baccarani, C. Barone, et al. 2020. "Consensus-Based Recommendations for Diagnosis and Medical Management of Poland Syndrome (Sequence)." *Orphanet Journal of Rare*

Diseases 15 (1): 201.
[6] Wang, W. L. 2019a. "Fifth Surgery for a 2.5-Year-Old Child with Poland Syndrome: Wang Procedure." *Chest Wall Deformity Surgery Specialist*, March 22.
[7] Wang, W. L. 2019b. "Minimally Invasive Wenlin Procedure for Poland Syndrome Combined with Anterior Protrusion Deformity." *Chest Wall Deformity Surgery Specialist*, April 3.
[8] Wang, W. L. 2019c. "Wang Procedure for Severe Poland Syndrome." *Chest Wall Deformity Surgery Specialist*, November 20.
[9] Wang, W. L. 2020. "Today's Surgery: Secondary Procedure for Severe Poland Syndrome." *Chest Wall Deformity Surgery Specialist*, March 17.
[10] Wang, W. L. 2021a. "MatrixRIB Remodeling: Secondary Surgery for Wenlin Chest with Poland Syndrome." *Chest Wall Deformity Surgery Specialist*, September 28.
[11] Wang, W. L. 2021b. "Correction of Poland Syndrome Using MatrixRIB." *Chest Wall Deformity Surgery Specialist*, October 23.
[12] Al-Qattan, M. M. 2001. "Classification of Hand Anomalies in Poland's Syndrome." *British Journal of Plastic Surgery* 54 (2): 132–136.
[13] Huang, Y., H. Pang, S. Jin, et al. 2018. "Clinical Characteristics of Poland's Syndrome Associated with Breast Cancer: Two Case Reports and a Literature Review." *Journal of Cancer Research and Therapeutics* 14 (7): 1665–1669.
[14] Vazirnia, A., and P. R. Cohen. 2015. "Poland's Syndrome: A Concise Review of the Clinical Features Highlighting Associated Dermatologic Manifestations." *American Journal of Clinical Dermatology* 16 (4): 295–301.
[15] Chiumariello, S., A. Pica, G. Guarro, et al. 2014. "Poland Syndrome: An Algorithm to Select the Appropriate Chest Wall Surgical Reconstructive Treatment." *Annali Italiani di Chirurgia* 85 (3): 237–243.
[16] Wang, W. L. 2017. "Surgical Strategies for Thoracic Deformity in Poland Syndrome." *Chest Wall Deformity Surgery Specialist*, June 19.
[17] Wang, W. L. 2022. "Willine Procedure for Adult Poland Syndrome." *I Ask Doctor*, May 22.

Chapter 15

THORACIC DYSPLASIA SYNDROME

Thoracic insufficiency syndrome (TIS) was first proposed by Campbell in 1992 [1]. Although Campbell was a spinal surgeon, the condition itself appears more related to thoracic surgery than spine surgery. This has both positive and negative implications. Positively, it highlights the natural connection between the spine and thorax; negatively, the terminology may be inappropriate, potentially affecting disease understanding and management [2,3]. Nonetheless, the concept has helped raise awareness of the disease. While thoracic surgeons largely overlooked this condition, attention from any specialty capable of addressing it has been valuable. Since the introduction of TIS, spinal surgeons worldwide have made significant contributions, but their focus has been on correcting spinal deformities via thoracic procedures rather than addressing thoracic issues directly [4,5]. This specialty bias has limited progress in thoracic management. With the emergence of chest wall surgery, attention to thoracic problems increased, and TIS came into focus. Studies indicate that TIS is better managed by chest wall surgeons [6]. Our extensive work supports this view [7], suggesting TIS is primarily a chest wall disorder rather than a spinal disorder. However, disease classification is influenced by multiple factors, including historical precedence. The substantial research by spine specialists offers valuable insights for chest wall surgeons. Continued collaboration between these disciplines from their respective perspectives will yield improved outcomes.

1. Campbell Classification

From the literal meaning of its name, TIS refers to a defect or abnormality in the overall development of the thoracic cage. By referencing the definition of dysplasia in other anatomical regions, a large number of thoracic deformities can be classified under this condition. Campbell selected several representative deformities and categorized them into three major groups comprising four types (see Figure 2-15-1) [1]: Type I: Rib agenesis associated with scoliosis Type II: Rib synostosis associated with scoliosis Type IIIa: Generalized thoracic cage hypoplasia Type III b: Thoracic cage constriction, also known as Jeune syndrome, or (asphyxiating thoracic dystrophy)

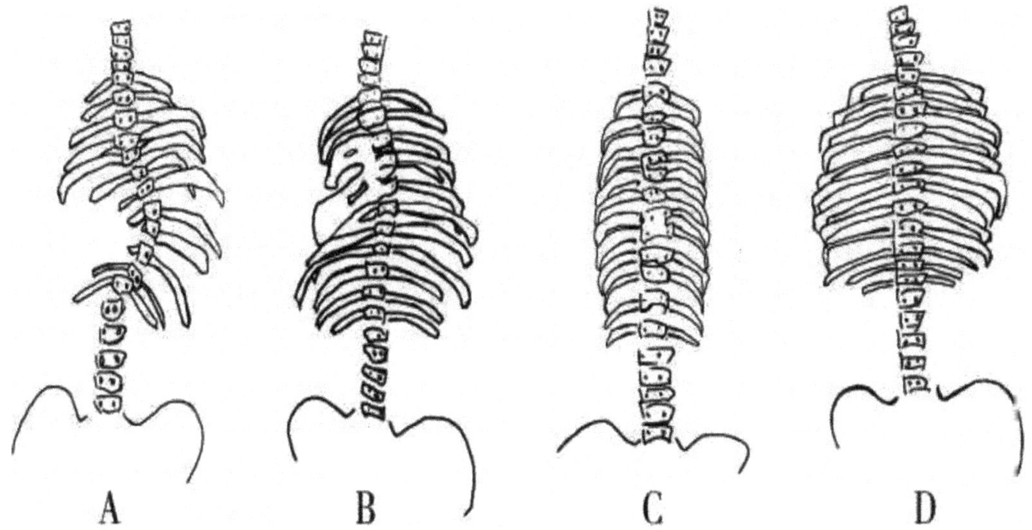

Figure 2-15-1. Campbell classification (A. Type I: rib agenesis with scoliosis; B. Type II: rib fusion with scoliosis; C. Type III A: generalized thoracic cage hypoplasia; D. Type III B: thoracic cage constriction, also known as Jeune syndrome)

The Campbell classification brings together a number of previously unnoticed disorders, gives them a common name, and summarizes their patterns, which is of great importance for the diagnosis and treatment of these disorders. However, there is a big problem with this typology [8]. Firstly, since we are discussing thoracic dysplasia, there should be a wide range of related diseases, such as Poland syndrome, lateral chest wall depression, chest wall defects and even common deformities such as funnel chest and chicken chest, all of them should fall into the category of this disease, but the authors only listed a limited number of diseases, which is suspected of being biased. This approach has the suspicion of generalization. Secondly, there should be a common standard for typing or categorizing, and only when the standard is unified can the classification be reasonable and convincing. type I and type II are categorized according to the shape of the spine and the morphology of the ribs, and there is no problem with the classification. However, the appearance of type III is so incongruous that it is difficult to see the relationship between such a type and types I and II. In the author's treatment, the surgery was designed to deal exclusively with type I and type II diseases. If the criteria for typing are not standardized, the classification system will appear to be unorganized. Thirdly, the authors' purpose of naming and typing is to emphasize thoracic dysplasia or abnormality on the surface, but the focus of treatment is almost entirely on the spine, and the substance of the thorax is not involved throughout, which makes the naming deviate from the original direction. Finally, in the staging process, the authors describe type III, but do not address the treatment of this type. This makes the deformity redundant in this system. When there are completely redundant diseases in a typing system, there is a problem with the typing itself! As can be seen from the analysis as above, Campbell's nomenclature and typology have obvious flaws. However, all the diseases mentioned in the typology are objective, all involve lesions of the thorax, and all warrant discussion from a therapeutic standpoint. For the sake of clarity, this section discusses only type I and type II lesions. Type III involves other diseases of an entirely different nature and will be discussed in a separate section.

2. Pathogenesis

Although the three types of conditions classified under TIS share a common name, the details of the classification reveal that the three types are almost. They are completely independent, and since they are independent, their pathogenesis cannot be the same. In Type I TIS, rib agenesis is a severe defect. Its pathogenesis is still not fully defined, but this absence can directly induce scoliosis. This mechanism is basically clear. Normally, spinal alignment depends on bilateral rib support. When the bilateral support forces are symmetrical, the spinal column remains aligned. If the forces are asymmetrical, scoliosis may occur. In Type I TIS, due to unilateral rib absence, the spinal support on that side is lost, inevitably causing spinal deformity. This is the mechanism for scoliosis in this type. In Type II TIS, rib synostosis is completely different from rib agenesis and has its own specific mechanism. So far, there is also no precise explanation. When multiple ribs are fused on one side, the spinal loading becomes asymmetrical as well, resulting in scoliosis. This mechanism is also relatively clear.

From the perspective of the relationship between the thoracic cage and the spine, the two form an organically integrated whole [10]. The normal shape of the spine depends on the structural support of the thoracic cage, and conversely, the shape of the spine also affects the shape of the thoracic cage. The pathologies of the two are interrelated and can be causally linked. However, for Type I and Type II Thoracic Insufficiency Syndrome (TIS), rib absence and fusion are clearly the primary conditions; spinal scoliosis cannot cause such rib changes. Therefore, in TIS, the relationship between rib pathology and spinal pathology is clear: the primary rib deformities lead to spinal scoliosis. In summary, the pathogenesis of Type I and Type II TIS can be concluded as follows: maintaining the normal shape of the spine requires two factors. The first factor is the physical support of the spine, which comes directly from the ribs and related chest wall structures. When there is an abnormality in the structures on one side of the spine, this support is compromised, affecting spinal

alignment. The second factor is the distribution of mechanical forces on both sides of the spine. This force must be evenly distributed. When there is a structural abnormality in the thoracic cage, the force distribution on both sides of the spine becomes uneven, ultimately affecting the shape of the spine.
In TIS (Thoracic Insufficiency Syndrome), the causal relationship between rib deformities and spinal scoliosis is very clear. However, as an organically integrated whole, once spinal scoliosis occurs, it in turn affects the shape of the thoracic cage. This influence further worsens the chest wall deformity, causing the two conditions to enter a vicious cycle. This is the fundamental reason why the condition of TIS patients progressively deteriorates.

3. Harm

The lesions of TIS involve two main sites, the thorax and the spine, and therefore the harm comes first from these two sites. The first part is the spine. Abnormalities in the shape of the spine can cause harm to the patient in two ways: one is the harm to the physical form and the other is the harm to the physiological function. The physical form of the spine is obvious and has an all-encompassing effect. Physiologic hazards can come from the spine itself and the nervous system, as well as from the effects on surrounding organs and structures. These effects can sometimes be extremely severe and cause great inconvenience to the patient's life. The second area of concern is the thorax, which is a structural abnormality in patients with Type I and Type II TIS. From the outside, the affected side of the thorax may appear to be collapsed and narrowed, and the left and right thorax may be asymmetrical. Structure not only affects the aesthetic appearance of the thorax, but also affects the respiratory system. The impact on the respiratory system is mainly reflected in the restriction of respiratory movements and the impact on the development of lung tissue. The former comes directly from the compression of the thorax and the latter from the narrowing of the thorax.

4. Clinical Manifestations

Although TIS is defined as a group of disorders, the clinical manifestations of the different types of TIS are clearly differentiated. In general, the clinical symptoms are twofold [1,10]. Anomalies in appearance on the one hand, and abnormalities in body function on the other. Appearance anomalies are seen in the spine and thorax. The spine is markedly scoliotic and the thorax is characterized by asymmetry, collapse or narrowing of one side. Functionally, the main abnormality is lung function. Mild abnormalities do not have obvious symptoms. When function is severely impaired, a variety of respiratory symptoms may be manifested.

5. Inspection

Physical examination can broadly characterize the shape of TIS, but imaging is necessary to understand the details of thoracic and spinal lesions. X-ray can clarify the general shape of the spine, but lesions of the ribs are poorly displayed. MRI is helpful in detecting internal thoracic lesions, but is defective in showing overall lesions of the spine and chest wall [11,12]. The commonly used examination is CT examination, which can show the shape of each structure more clearly but lacks the overall effect. The most ideal examination is three-dimensional reconstruction of bony structures, which can clarify the whole picture of the lesions in the spine and thorax, and is important for the diagnosis and treatment of the disease.

6. Diagnosis and Differential Diagnosis

The diagnosis of TIS is relatively easy, and it is basically diagnosed when scoliosis is combined with rib loss or fusion [1]. Thoracic stenosis or narrowing of the thorax, although recognized by Campbell as type III TIS, is not suitable for TIS due to the completely different pathogenesis, clinical manifestations and treatment modalities, and will be discussed as a separate disease.

TIS needs to be differentiated from Poland syndrome, which is characterized by developmental abnormalities of the bony structures and soft tissues of the chest wall on one side, and scoliosis due to the asymmetry of the thorax [13]. There are two main points of differentiation between the two: one is the development of the soft tissue of the chest wall, and the other is the location and nature of the bony structure lesions. In Poland syndrome, the soft tissues of the chest wall are markedly underdeveloped, whereas in TIS, the lesions are limited to the bony structures and do not involve the soft tissues; in Poland syndrome, the bony structures are mainly located in the anterior portion of the costal cartilages and ribs, whereas in TIS, the rib lesions mainly involve the posterior ribs, and are more pronounced closer to the spinal column. Patients with lateral chest wall depression deformity may have depression or collapse of one side of the chest wall, which may be combined with scoliosis of the spine due to the asymmetry of the right and left thorax [14,15]. Cosmetically, it may have similarities with TIS, but the pathologic changes are significantly different. Lateral chest wall depression deformity is usually without rib loss and fusion, which is the most obvious difference from TIS.

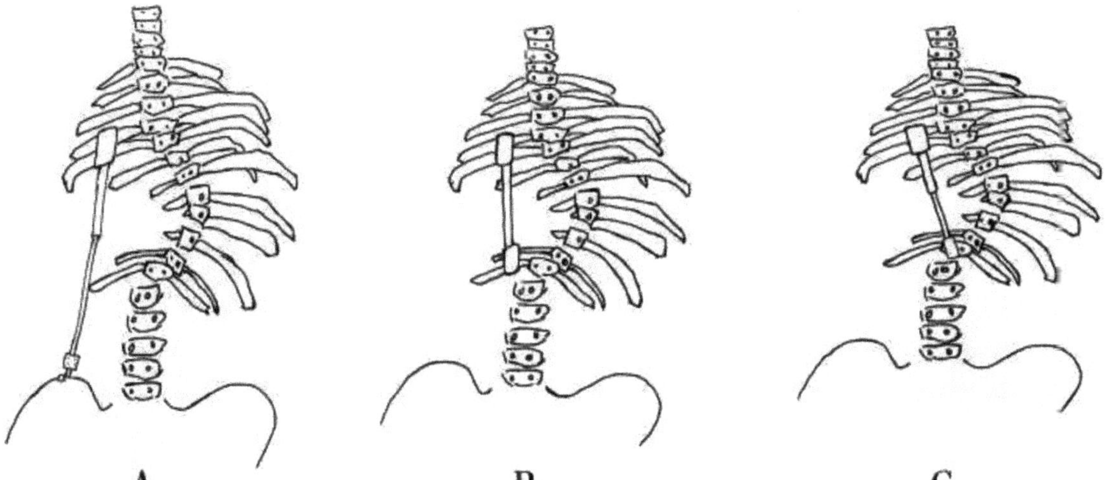

Figure 2-15-2 VEPTR procedure (A. Ribs a dewlap device; B. Ribs a rib device; C. Ribs a lumbar device)

7. Indications for Surgery

TIS lesions are obvious and harmful to patients, therefore, once the diagnosis is clear, all patients should receive treatment. The main contraindications include the following: (1) poor general condition that does not allow surgical treatment; TIS is congenital and has a long history of disease; if it is not effectively treated at an early stage, it may gradually jeopardize the function of many organs and eventually affect the general condition. If the disease is not effectively treated at an early stage, it may gradually jeopardize the function of many organs and eventually affect the general condition. If the vital organs are unable to withstand surgery, surgery is not indicated. (2) The spine itself is severely diseased and there are neurological contraindications. In severe cases of scoliosis, there may be damage to the nerves of the spinal cord, and if surgery could aggravate this damage or cause additional damage to the nerves of the spinal cord, surgery cannot be performed. (3) Lung disease is so severe that it cannot tolerate surgical treatment. Thoracic lesions may be combined with pulmonary lesions. If the lungs are severely diseased, they may not be able to provide the basic conditions for surgery, and surgery cannot be performed.

8. Surgical Treatment

The concept of TIS was developed by spine surgeons and for a long time the surgery was also performed exclusively by spine surgeons. Since 2015, we have been focusing on and implementing treatment for TIS, which is the first time that chest wall surgeons have been involved [16]. Chest wall surgeons implement corrections directly to the primary disease, which is a more rational and definitive procedure, which is significantly better than spinal surgery [6]. However, spine surgery has, after all, done a great deal of basic research and clinical work, and these experiences are worthwhile for chest wall surgeons.

(1) Spinal Surgery

Although TIS has both spinal and thoracic pathologies, if a patient is admitted to spine surgery, there must be only one surgical goal, which is the correction of scoliosis. The correction of scoliosis is usually done directly on the spine. In the case of TIS, however, the spine surgeon designs the surgery to correct the deformity by bracing the ribs. There are good reasons for this approach, and one of those reasons is that the lesions in the rib cage itself are fully taken into account. The spinal surgery was created because the rib cage was structurally abnormal and unsuitable for orthopedics surgery. Such surgery requires a special material, the (vertical expandable prosthetic titanium rib VEPTR) [1,5 17]. This material was developed by Campbell et al. and can be divided into a basal The three materials are fixed at one end to the skeleton, at the other end to the ribs, and at the lumbar vertebrae (Figure 2-15-2). One end of the three materials is fixed to the skeleton, ribs, and lumbar vertebrae, and the other end is fixed to the ribs, which indirectly strengthens the support of the spine through the support of the ribs, and ultimately restores the spine to its normal shape, and provides stabilization and orthopedics effects.

As you can see by how the surgery works, spinal surgery is not directly aimed at correcting scoliosis, but indirectly accomplished by bracing the ribs. This approach certainly has a role to play in the correction of the spine. To illustrate the effect of this approach on the thorax, the spine surgeon

specifically emphasizes that this method expands the thorax, improves the shape of the thorax, and increases the capacity of the thorax. It is undeniable that such an action against the thorax is possible. However, applying external forces directly to the ribs does not improve the shape of the thorax and may result in the deterioration of the local structure. It is clear that spinal surgery is inherently problematic, and it is not an exaggeration to say that the shape of the spine is improved at the expense of the structure and shape of the thorax [18]. While this approach has a clear role to play in terms of the orthopedics aims of spinal surgery, it is by no means an ideal procedure when evaluated holistically. Ideally, the spine should be orthopedically adjusted in conjunction with the thorax.

As mentioned above, since the thoracic lesion is the primary lesion, the focus should be on the correction of the thoracic lesion. When the thoracic problem is completely resolved, not only is the shape of the thorax more satisfactorily restored, but it also serves as a VEPTR-like support. This would be a more rational treatment.

(2) Chest Wall Surgery

The spinal surgery approach to VEPTR is extremely invasive and requires periodic postoperative surgical adjustments to the VEPTR. The patient suffers a great deal of pain throughout the entire treatment process. In addition, there are many complications associated with this procedure. As a result, the spinal surgery approach is not ideal. In contrast, chest wall surgery would be ideal.

(1) Surgical Principles

TIS involves both the thorax and the spine, so it is necessary to operate on both lesions simultaneously, and the general principle of surgery is thoracic reconstruction and spinal correction. The general principle of surgery is thoracic reconstruction with spinal correction. Considering that the basic lesion is thoracic, the final correction should be thoracic reconstruction with spinal correction.

In the implementation of the operation, the surgery is accomplished at two main levels: the first level is the macro level. From the macro level, to see, the thorax of TIS first shows a unilateral depressed deformity. Without considering the local details, it can be treated as a simple concave deformity. The aim of the operation at this point is to make the thorax symmetrical on both sides. This operation does not take into account the details of the deformity or the shape of the spine, but it facilitates the correction of scoliosis because it ultimately results in symmetry of the thorax on both sides. The second level is the microscopic level. In detail, the absence and fusion of the ribs is the most basic lesion, and such a lesion not only leads to an abnormality of the thorax, but also directly affects the shape of the spine. At the microscopic level, it is necessary to correct the details of the rib lesion, so that the thoracic and spinal lesions can be treated at the same time.

(2) Timing of Surgery

TIS has an early onset and some children are diagnosed shortly after birth. Early surgery is generally recommended to minimize the effects of the deformity, especially on the development of lung tissue. However, early surgery has its drawbacks. Problems such as postoperative monitoring and material constraints on the child's development are challenges to early surgery. Therefore, when discussing the timing of surgery, decisions need to be made on a case-by-case basis. In general, if the thoracic lesion is severe enough to interfere with respiratory function, surgery should be performed as soon as possible; if the lesion is not severe enough, surgery can be performed at an earlier age.

(3) Surgical Procedures

(1) Corrective surgery for lateral chest wall depression deformity [19, 20]. This procedure does not address the detailed rib pathology directly, but instead targets the collapse or depression of the lateral chest wall for correction. There are multiple correction methods available. By using special molding materials, the overall shape of the thoracic cage can generally be significantly improved, achieving bilateral symmetry (see Figure 2-15-3).

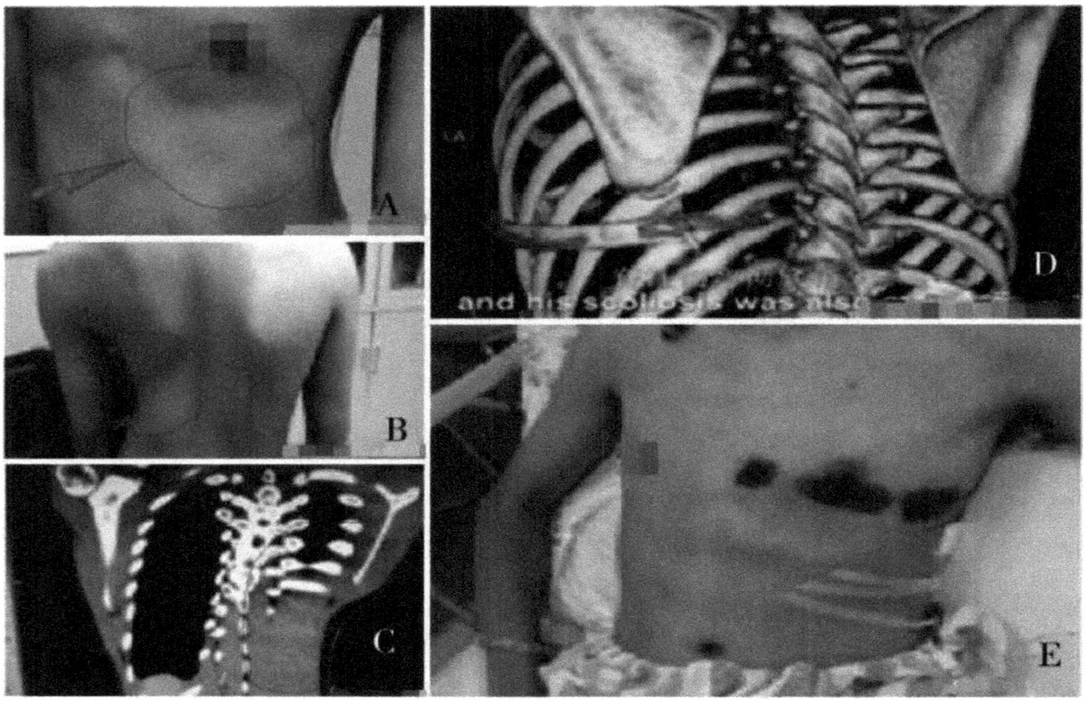

Figure 2-15-3 Corrective surgery for lateral chest wall depression deformity using a specially designed metal plate: (A, B) Hypoplasia of the left chest wall; (C) CT scan shows left chest wall deformity with scoliosis; (D) Local elevation of the chest wall performed using a “C”-shaped metal plate; (E) Postoperative result shows resolution of the deformity and restoration of normal thoracic contour.

(2) Chest Wall Reconstruction Absence or fusion of the ribs indicates severe structural disruption of the thoracic cage. To achieve correction, it is necessary to reconstruct the affected structures.

Absence of ribs is, in essence, a defect of the chest wall; the only difference is that the defect's extent and shape are irregular. For such defects, the fundamental approach is reconstruction. Since the missing structures are ribs, bony structural reconstruction is required. There are various methods for this. Because the reconstructed chest wall must bear the load of supporting the spine, there are special requirements for the reconstruction materials and techniques. The most ideal method is to perform the reconstruction using MatrixRIB [18,21]. This approach not only restores the basic shape of the thoracic cage but also directly provides robust support to the spine, helping it maintain a satisfactory alignment. During the procedure, if reconstruction of a single rib is insufficient to support the spine, MatrixRIB elements can be vertically positioned between ribs and reconstruction segments, acting similarly to VEPTR devices (Figure 2-15-4). Because the reconstruction directly restores the rib structure, its effect is significantly superior to using VEPTR alone.

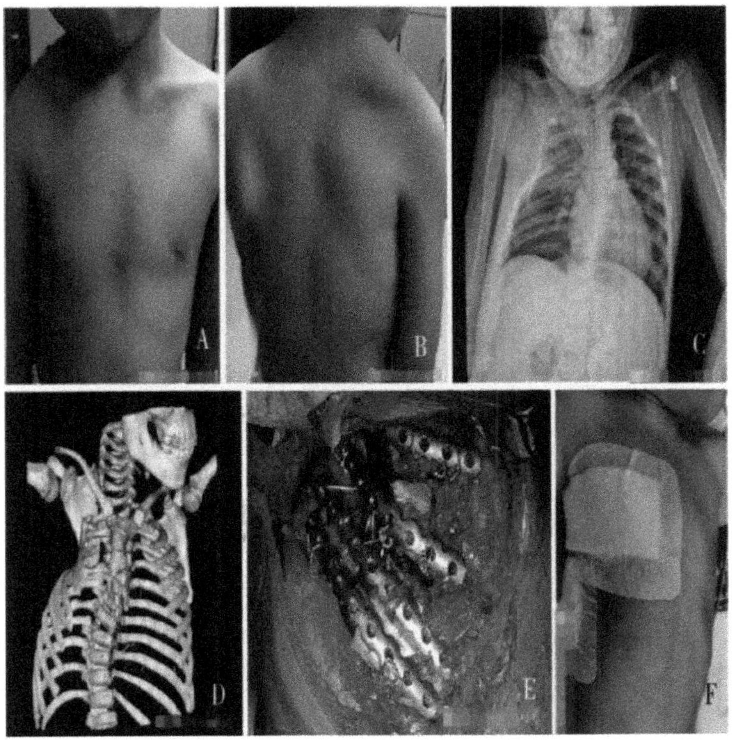

Figure 2-15-4 Correction surgery for thoracic deformity using MatrixRIB (A, B) Preoperative external appearance of the thorax C, D Imaging shows significant costal cartilage pathology on the right side and spinal scoliosis; (E) Local deformity of the chest wall corrected with MatrixRIB, restoring the normal shape of the thoracic cage; (F) Postoperative external chest wall appearance, basically restored to normal.

For Type II TIS patients, due to the presence of rib fusion, there will be a large amount of abnormally shaped bone in the rib region. Such abnormal bone structures likewise affect the shape of the thoracic cage and, of course, also impact the alignment of the spine. Addressing and managing these abnormal bony structures is therefore essential. This is challenging. The general principle is that these deformed bony structures must not be allowed to compromise the shape and size of the thoracic cage. If they do have an impact, correction should be performed through reshaping or even complete reconstruction. Such reconstruction is highly complex, and the key to surgical success is having the appropriate materials. MatrixRIB can be used not only for rib defect reconstruction but also for the reconstruction of fused ribs. During surgery, a personalized design can be implemented to achieve a satisfactory reconstruction result. Considering the need for spinal support, vertical placement of MatrixRIB material may also be employed if necessary.

It must be emphasized that in cases of rib fusion, there is no actual loss of bony structure; instead, the ribs exist in an abnormal shape. In such situations, using MatrixRIB for support provides more anchoring points due to the presence of these irregular structures, which can lead to a more satisfactory outcome. Although the abundance of abnormal bone may make reconstruction results less ideal than with simple defects, a well-planned design can still achieve good results.

(4) Staged Surgery

Children with TIS often develop the condition at a young age, and some patients require surgical intervention during early childhood. However, due to the continuous development of bony structures, it is difficult to complete the surgical correction in a single procedure — in most cases, repeat surgeries are needed. Repeat operations are technically challenging and demand a high level of surgical expertise. Nevertheless, as long as the fundamental principles are well understood and applied, achieving good outcomes is not difficult.

(5) Trauma Issues

If a surgical procedure is designed to correct unilateral chest wall collapse or depression, a minimally invasive approach can be used. However, if the procedure targets rib absence or rib fusion, it will inevitably involve greater surgical trauma. This is especially true for repeat surgeries, where significant trauma is often unavoidable

(6) Collaboration With Spine Surgery

TIS involves pathological changes in both the thoracic cage and the spine. From a professional standpoint, the optimal management should ideally be carried out through collaboration between specialists in both fields. This approach allows each specialty to contribute its strengths, ensuring the best possible outcomes. Currently, thoracic wall surgeons make maximum efforts to address deformities within their domain, while spine surgeons often approach spinal deformities indirectly by manipulating the ribs rather than addressing the spine itself. This situation suggests that there is still significant potential for further development within spine surgery. If more direct and effective methods targeting spinal deformities can be established, the treatment of TIS will undoubtedly reach a new level

9. Prognosis

This is a very unique condition. Its particularity lies not only in the deformity of the thoracic cage but also in the associated spinal deformity. Among all thoracic deformities, those involving spinal malformations are generally more complex and troublesome. When the thoracic deformity itself is not simply an abnormality of shape but rather a significant structural anomaly of its components, the treatment becomes even more challenging. From the management of TIS, it is clear that this is a highly complex disease. Precisely because of this complexity, it is difficult to achieve fully satisfactory results [1,4,17]. To date, both spinal surgery and thoracic wall surgery have limitations that are difficult to completely overcome and require continued efforts to improve treatment strategies. A reality that must be acknowledged is that structural deformities are an exceptionally challenging category of conditions. Some deformities can achieve good outcomes through technological and surgical advancements, but some cannot reach completely satisfactory results no matter the technique used. This is not purely a technical limitation but rather an objective reality. Faced with this, physicians can only strive through their expertise and innovation to approach ideal results as closely as possible — but true perfection is rarely attainable.

REFERENCES

[1] Campbell, R. M. 2013. "VEPTR: Past Experience and the Future of VEPTR Principles." *European Spine Journal* 22 (Suppl 2): 106–117.

[2] Wang, W. L. 2021a. "On Thoracic Insufficiency Syndrome." *Thoracic Deformity Surgery Expert*, September 19.

[3] Wang, W. L. 2021b. "Dr. Campbell's Thoracic Insufficiency Syndrome." *Thoracic Deformity*

Surgery Expert, September 19.
[4] Chatterjee, A. D., K. Hassan, and M. P. Grevitt. 2012. "Congenital Kypho-Scoliosis: A Case of Thoracic Insufficiency Syndrome and the Limitations of Treatment." *European Spine Journal* 21 (6): 1043–1049.
[5] Joshi, A. P., M. K. Roth, J. W. Simmons, et al. 2015. "Expansion Thoracicoplasty for Thoracic Insufficiency Syndrome Associated with Jarcho-Levin Syndrome." *JBJS Essential Surgical Techniques* 5 (2): e1–e2.
[6] Wang, W. L. 2018a. "The Disciplinary Attribution Issue of Thoracic Insufficiency Syndrome." *Expert on Thoracic Deformity Surgery*, February 5.
[7] Wang, W. L. 2018b. "Treatment of Thoracic Insufficiency Syndrome: Returning to Rationality." *Expert on Thoracic Deformity Surgery*, February 22.
[8] Wang, W. L. 2018c. "Thoracic Insufficiency Syndrome: Drawbacks of the Campbell Classification." *Expert on Thoracic Deformity Surgery*, February 10.
[9] Wang, W. L. 2018d. "Thoracic Insufficiency Syndrome: How Does Rib Absence Lead to Scoliosis?" *Expert on Thoracic Deformity Surgery*, December 9.
[10] Canavese, F., and A. Dimeglio. 2013. "Normal and Abnormal Spine and Thoracic Cage Development." *World Journal of Orthopedics* 4 (4): 167–174.
[11] Udupa, J. K., Y. Tong, A. Capraro, et al. 2020. "Understanding Respiratory Restrictions as a Function of the Scoliotic Spinal Curve in Thoracic Insufficiency Syndrome: A 4D Dynamic MR Imaging Study." *Journal of Pediatric Orthopedics* 40 (4): 183–189.
[12] Tong, Y., J. K. Udupa, J. M. McDonough, et al. 2019. "Quantitative Dynamic Thoracic MRI: Application to Thoracic Insufficiency Syndrome in Pediatric Patients." *Radiology* 292 (1): 206–213.
[13] Wang, W. L. 2017. "Successful Surgery on a 10-Year-Old Patient with Poland Syndrome." *Expert on Thoracic Deformity Surgery*, July 19.
[14] Wang, W. L. 2025. "The Wang Procedure for Lateral Chest Wall Depression Deformity." *Expert on Thoracic Deformity Surgery*, October 25.
[15] Wang, W. L. 2015. "Terminology for Localized Lateral Chest Wall Depression." *Expert on Thoracic Deformity Surgery*, May 25.
[16] Wang, W. L., C. M. Chen, W. G. Long, et al. 2015. "Unilateral Corrective Techniques for Asymmetric Thoracic Deformities." *Journal of Practical Medicine* 31 (5, Suppl): 434–435.
[17] Studer, D., and C. C. Hasler. 2020. "Long-Term Outcome of Vertical Expandable Prosthetic Titanium Rib (VEPTR) Treatment in Children with Early-Onset Scoliosis." *Annals of Translational Medicine* 8 (2): 25.
[18] Wang, W. L. 2018e. "Drawbacks of VEPTR Surgery for Thoracic Insufficiency Syndrome." *Expert on Thoracic Deformity Surgery*, December 7.
[19] Wang, W. L. 2021c. "Correction of Poland Syndrome Using MatrixRIB." *Expert on Thoracic Deformity Surgery*, October 13.
[20] Wang, W. L. 2021d. "MatrixRIB Shaping: Revision Surgery for Wenlin Chest with Poland Syndrome." *Expert on Thoracic Deformity Surgery*, September 28.
[21] Wang, W. L. 2018f. "Application of MatrixRIB Implants in Complex Chest Wall Surgeries." *Expert on Thoracic Deformity Surgery*, April 17.

Asphyxiating thoracic dystrophy (ATD), also known as Jeune syndrome, was first reported by Jeune in 1955[1,2], and is a severe form of thoracic deformity. This condition is characterized by distinct anatomical features and is recognized as a separate disease entity. In 1992, spine surgeon Campbell introduced a different condition, which he named Thoracic Insufficiency Syndrome (TIS). Campbell proposed a classification system for TIS and included ATD within this framework, designating type III b deformity as equivalent to Jeune syndrome [3,4]. However, for spine surgeons to name a condition that appears to fall under the domain of thoracic surgery is inherently controversial. Moreover, incorporating a well-established clinical diagnosis like ATD already widely recognized and extensively studied—into a new disease classification has naturally led to debate. The most immediate issue is the confusion it causes between ATD and TIS. This confusion is evident not only in their English terminology but also in their Chinese translations. In clinical practice, very few physicians are able to clearly differentiate between these two terms. This reality suggests that TIS is not a scientifically rigorous diagnostic term, and forcibly classifying ATD under the umbrella of TIS is neither scientifically valid nor clinically necessary is an independent disorder that was recognized well before Campbell's introduction of TIS. There is no compelling reason to subsume it within the TIS classification system.

ATD (Asphyxiating Thoracic Dystrophy) is an extremely rare condition, with an estimated incidence of 1/130,000 – 1/100,000 live births [1,5]. It is an autosomal inherited disorder associated with genetic mutations [6,7]. The disease can affect multiple organ systems, with its hallmark being abnormal structure and morphology of the thoracic cage. In addition to thoracic deformities, skeletal abnormalities, renal involvement, and gastrointestinal manifestations may also occur [6]. The most critical complication of ATD is thoracic constriction, which restricts pulmonary development. As a result, affected infants may present with severe respiratory insufficiency shortly after birth. If respiratory compromise cannot be promptly addressed, the condition often proves fatal in the neonatal period, making ATD a highly life-threatening disease. Over the years, physicians around the world have made continuous efforts to explore treatment strategies for ATD. However, due to the severity and complexity of the disease, therapeutic outcomes have remained suboptimal. When studying Asphyxiating Thoracic Dystrophy (ATD), it is important to distinguish between two concepts: primary ATD and secondary ATD.

Secondary ATD refers to thoracic constriction deformities that develop as a consequence of previous thoracic deformity surgery [5]. These patients typically underwent open surgical procedures for chest wall deformities. During such surgeries, the costal cartilages were removed, and postoperative regeneration of the residual thoracic structure was often inadequate. This resulted in progressive thoracic narrowing, leading to chronic compression of intrathoracic organs, which in turn impaired various physiological functions. In the past, when open surgical techniques were more commonly employed, secondary ATD was relatively frequent. However, with the widespread adoption of minimally invasive techniques, cases of secondary ATD have become increasingly rare. This section will focus primarily on primary ATD.

1.Classification

Thoracic deformity is the primary pathological feature of ATD and the root cause of multiple functional impairments, most notably characterized by thoracic narrowing. We classify Asphyxiating Thoracic Dystrophy (ATD) into two types: Type I, corresponding to Type IIIa in the Thoracic Insufficiency Syndrome (TIS) classification system [3,4], is characterized by generalized thoracic constriction deformity. Patients exhibit underdevelopment of the entire thoracic cage, with both the transverse (lateral) diameter and anteroposterior diameter significantly smaller than normal. The upper lateral chest wall appears intact, while a distinct depression is observed in the lower lateral chest wall, located at the junction between the costal cartilage and ribs (Figure 2-16-1A). Type II, corresponding to Type III b in the TIS classification [3,4] is a specialized form of thoracic constriction. It is mainly characterized by a broad depression at the costochondral junction, caused by abnormal growth orientation of the costal cartilages and ribs. This depression involves multiple ribs along the lateral chest wall, and frequently extends to include the costal arch (Figures 2-16-1B and 2-16-2)[5,6].

2.Pathogenesis

The pathogenesis of Asphyxiating Thoracic Dystrophy (ATD) remains unclear. Traditionally, it has been widely believed that arrested or delayed development of the bony thoracic structures leads to thoracic constriction, and this view has long been considered the primary pathogenic mechanism of the disease [7,8]. However, recent in-depth studies on this deformity have revealed significant issues with this explanation. In Type I ATD, where there is generalized thoracic constriction and marked delayed development of the ribs and costal cartilages,

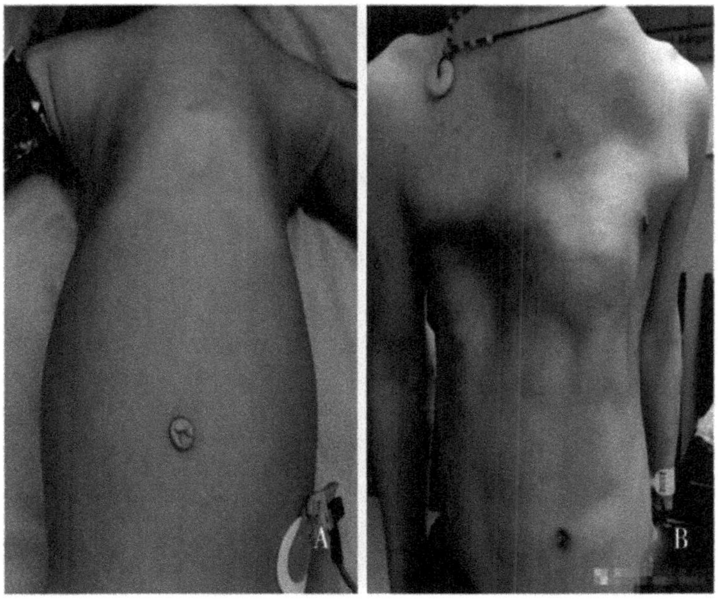

Figure 2-16-1. Classification of ATD (A) type I: generalized thoracic constriction B type II: thoracic constriction with marked lateral chest wall depression

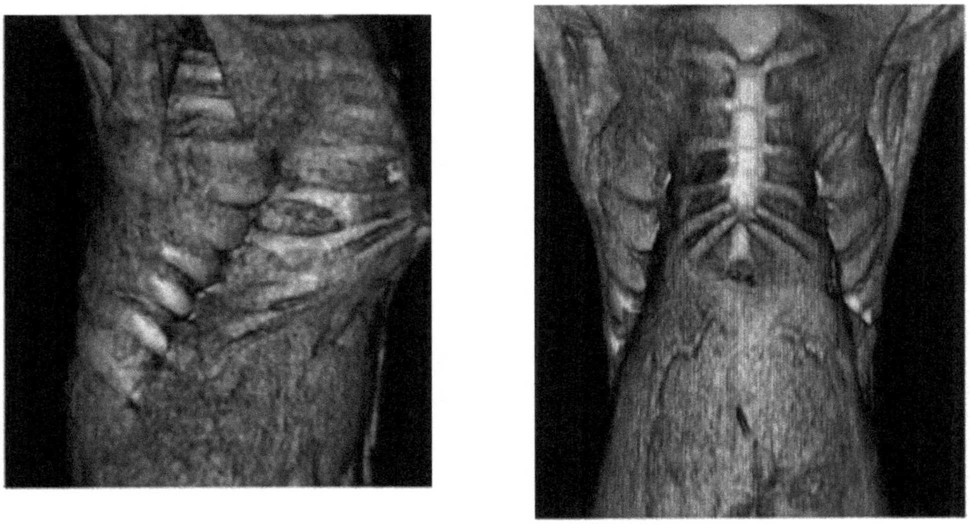

Figure 2-16-2. Three-dimensional reconstruction of the thorax in type ii ATD. lateral chest wall depression, with the deepest point located at the costochondral junction.

This traditional explanation holds some validity. However, in Type II ATD, the growth of ribs and costal cartilages is not arrested; on the contrary, their developmental pace can be comparable to or even exceed that of normal skeletal growth. The fundamental cause of the constricted thorax in these patients lies in the abnormal growth direction of the bones. Under normal circumstances, the ribs and costal cartilages grow outwardly and laterally, allowing synchronized expansion that shapes the thorax properly. In ATD, however, the growth direction of both the ribs and costal cartilages is simultaneously inward toward the thoracic cavity. This aberrant orientation causes the junction between ribs and costal cartilages to form a protrusion projecting into the thoracic cavity. The faster the growth of these structures, the more pronounced the inward protrusion becomes, resulting in severe compression of the lungs (Figure 2-16-3). As patients age, the pressure exerted by the ribs and costal cartilages on the lungs intensifies. This progressive worsening of thoracic constriction with age is the fundamental reason for the increasing severity of symptoms in many patients and constitutes the greatest life-threatening aspect of ATD.

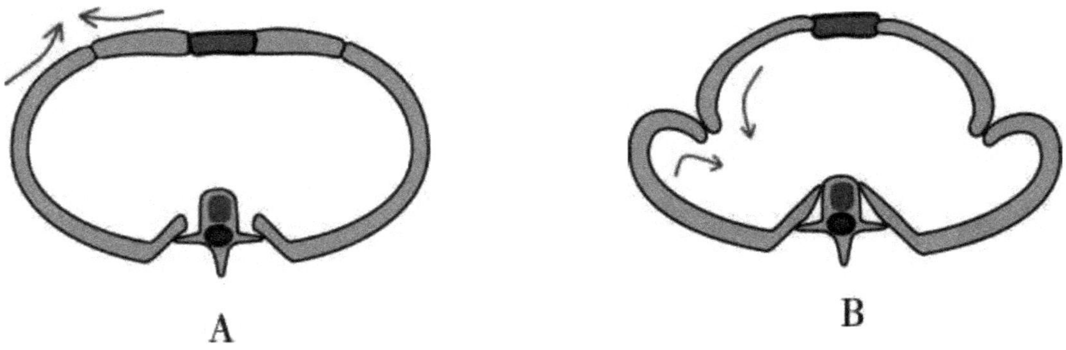

Figure 2-16-3. Schematic illustration of the pathogenesis of ATD. (A) Under normal conditions, the ribs and costal cartilages grow in opposite outward directions, resulting in overall thoracic expansion. (B) In ATD, the growth direction of the ribs and costal cartilages is abnormal, both growing inward toward the thoracic cavity, causing reduced thoracic volume and lung compression. As development progresses, the deformity worsens

3. Complications

ATD can cause two fundamental types of harm [5,7]: one is the impact on the overall shape of the thorax, and the other is the effect on physiological function. Patients with ATD exhibit obvious thoracic deformities, which may even influence the shape of other skeletal structures. The pronounced external deformity can also have psychological effects on the patient. Thoracic constriction and depressions exert direct pressure on the lungs, leading to impaired respiratory function. Many affected infants present with hypoxia immediately after birth. Due to the lungs' inability to expand normally, localized infections often develop, further exacerbating hypoxia. As a result, 60% - 80% of patients die from hypoxia shortly after birth [8]. The remaining patients who survive the high-risk early years often succumb before reaching adolescence. Given the already low incidence of the disease, combined with its extremely high mortality rate, clinical cases seen in practice are exceptionally rare.

4.Clinical Manifestations

The clinical manifestations of ATD vary depending on the severity of the deformity. Most affected children present with severe symptoms, primarily hypoxia, which in serious cases requires mechanical ventilation support [7,8]. Due to continuous lung compression, patients often suffer from significant pulmonary diseases. Early-stage changes may be limited to simple inflammation, but as the patient ages, these can progress to chronic inflammation and even consolidation, leading to irreversible pathological damage and further exacerbation of hypoxia. Chronic hypoxia inevitably impairs physical development. Most patients exhibit short stature compared to their peers, along with disproportionate and shortened limb growth. In addition to respiratory abnormalities, ATD patients may present with multi-organ involvement, which can affect organ function through various mechanisms [6,7]. In terms of physical signs, ATD patients exhibit distinctive thoracic features. Type I patients have a columnar-shaped thorax, which is overall reduced in size with a nearly circular cross-section. Type II patients display a prominent anterior protrusion at the midline of the chest with depressions on both sides, resulting in an overall constricted thorax (Figure 2-16-1).

5.Examinations

Physical examination can provide a preliminary diagnosis of ATD, but detailed structural information requires imaging studies. X-ray imaging typically shows horizontally oriented ribs and thoracic constriction. CT scans reveal a narrowed thorax. In Type I patients, CT cross-sectional images show an irregularly constricted, roughly circular thorax, while in Type II patients, the thorax exhibits a characteristic “convex” shape (Figure 2-16-4). The heart is positioned at the midline, flanked by two lateral depressions, with the deepest point of these depressions located at the costochondral junction. Three-dimensional reconstructions of the bony thoracic structures clearly display the details of the deformity (Figure 2-16-5).

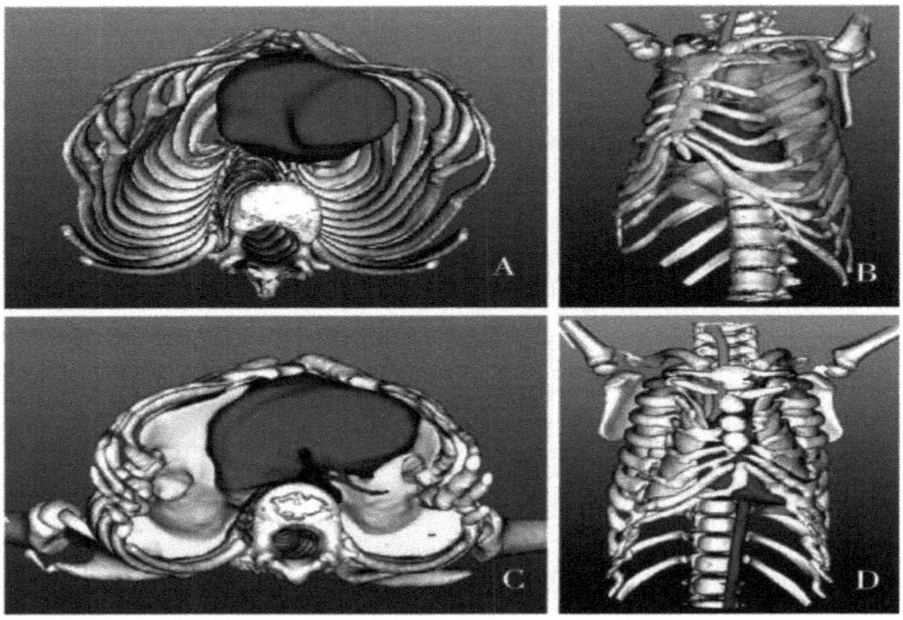

Figure 2-16-4. CT findings in ATD. (A) CT cross-sectional image of type I ATD showing overall thoracic constriction (B) CT cross-sectional image of type II ATD demonstrating the characteristic "convex" shape deformity.

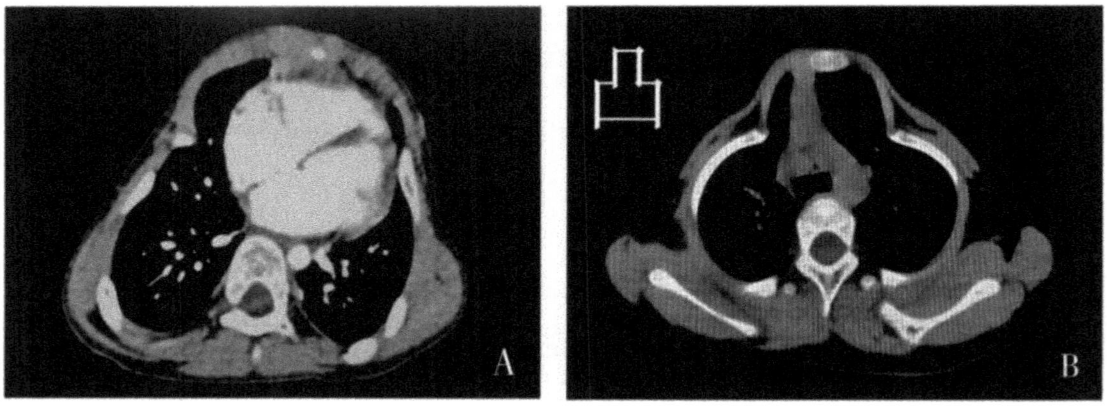

Figure 2-16-5. Three-dimensional reconstruction images of ATD. (A, B) features of type I ATD; (C, D) features of type II ATD.

Diagnosis and Differential Diagnosis:
The diagnosis of ATD is relatively straightforward. Due to the distinct external thoracic features combined with imaging studies, a definitive diagnosis can be

made with relative ease. Differential diagnosis involves two aspects: first, distinguishing ATD conceptually from Thoracic Insufficiency Syndrome (TIS) [3], and second, differentiating ATD from specific thoracic deformities. The distinction from TIS mainly requires clarifying the origin and proper use of terminology to avoid confusion. Differentiation from specific deformities includes distinguishing ATD from pectus excavatum and certain complex mixed deformities. Pectus excavatum is characterized by bilateral depressions of the lower chest wall, with a normal midline segment. This lateral chest wall depression resembles a mild form of Type I ATD, but the primary difference lies in the structure at the base of the depression. In pectus excavatum, the base consists of ribs without significant structural abnormalities, whereas in ATD, the base is at the costochondral junction, forming an angular deformity that protrudes inward toward the thoracic cavity. This represents the most notable distinction between the two conditions [9]. Some complex mixed deformities may present with both protrusions and depressions. When the depression is located on the lateral chest wall, it can resemble ATD. The key point of differentiation again lies in the base of the depression. In complex deformities, the base is generally composed solely
of ribs, whereas in ATD, the base is at the costochondral junction, forming an angular deformity directed inward to the thoracic cavity—a feature generally absent in typical mixed deformities.

6.Surgical Treatment

The concept of ATD encompasses two fundamental elements: first, asphyxiation, and second, thoracic dystrophy. The former defines its high-risk nature, while the latter characterizes the fundamental pathological changes. Since affected children often develop symptoms rapidly after birth and suffer from severe respiratory insufficiency, without appropriate and timely intervention, most will succumb in early life. This is the fundamental cause of the high risk associated with ATD. To eliminate this risk, it is essential to relieve the thoracic compression on the lungs as early as possible, and surgery remains the only effective method to achieve this.

(1).Surgical Principles

The root cause of ATD (Asphyxiating Thoracic Dysplasia) lies in the compression of the lungs, which is due to the narrowing of the thoracic cage. To relieve this compression, the thoracic cage must be expanded. Based on the pathological features of ATD, there are three basic approaches to expand the thoracic cage: 1. Lateral thoracic expansion surgery [10,11]. 2. Median thoracic expansion surgery [12,13], and 3. Depression correction surgery [14].

Lateral thoracic expansion surgery is performed on the lateral chest wall. The basic method is to lengthen the ribs to expand the entire thoracic cage [10,11]. Median thoracic expansion surgery involves splitting the sternum and spreading it open to both sides to achieve chest expansion [12,13]. For Type II patients, there is often a large area of depression on the lateral chest wall, and this depression is the fundamental cause of lung compression and thoracic narrowing. Therefore, eliminating depression can also achieve the goal of expanding the thoracic cage. This is the principle behind depression correction surgery. Like other surgeries for depression-type deformities, there are two main methods for eliminating the depression: the Nuss procedure [14] and the Wang procedure [15]. These two methods correct the deformity through different mechanisms.

In summary, the operating principles of these three basic methods are completely different, and each has its own technical features. In actual clinical practice, the surgical approach must be chosen based on the patient's specific condition only in this way can good treatment outcomes be achieved.

(2) Surgical Methods

(i) Lateral Thoracic Wall Expansion Surgery

Lateral thoracic wall expansion surgery was first proposed by Davis in 1995 [11]. It is performed via a lateral chest wall incision to achieve thoracic expansion. The specific method involves cross-cutting the ribs on the lateral chest wall, then connecting and fixing two adjacent longer rib stumps to increase the thoracic volume. In Type I patients, most ribs and costal cartilages do not exhibit significant directional abnormalities or obvious depressions, making this procedure feasible for them. However, in Type II patients, due to severe depression at the costochondral junction, it is nearly impossible to connect and fix the ribs after cross-cutting. Therefore, this surgical approach is not suitable for treating Type II patients.

(ii) Median Thoracic Expansion Surgery

Median thoracic expansion surgery originated from the procedure developed by Barnes, and it is a widely used surgical approach. In earlier years, many surgeons employed this method [16]. For neonates or young pediatric patients, if no better options are available to save the patient's life, median sternotomy can be considered to expand the entire thoracic cavity and relieve pulmonary compression. This is a relatively effective thoracic expansion technique. However, this method has significant drawbacks. In Type II ATD patients, due to obvious bilateral chest wall depressions, forcibly expanding the thoracic cavity may cause the depressed ribs and costal cartilages to be pushed further inward under external force, leading to increased pulmonary compression. This undoubtedly counteracts the thoracic expansion achieved by sternum spreading. It can be seen that this surgical method is more suitable for the treatment of type I ATD patients and not suitable for type II ATD patients.

(iii) Nuss Operation

The Nuss procedure is a method proposed by Kikuchi, which is based on the principle of the Nuss procedure for the treatment of funnel chest, which is performed on both sides of the chest wall [14] and theoretically, any deformity that has a depression can be supported from the bottom with a material. The ATD has depression, and there is a rationale for treating it in this way. However, it must be clear that the deformity of the ATD is not just a depression, and that the depression is not a funnel chest depression, which is located in the middle of the chest wall. When the structure of the depression itself is very special, the normal Nuss procedure may not be effective, and the special features of ATD are: (1) the depression is a long, narrow groove that extends from the midclavicular line to the lateral side, which is not a pit, but a groove; (2) at the bottom of the depression are longitudinally aligned ribs and associated costal cartilages, which are independent of each other between the ribs, and lack the structure of a sternum to unite them; (3) at the bottom of the depression are longitudinally aligned ribs with attached costal cartilages, which are independent of each other. The chest surface at the bottom of the depression is the connection between the ribs and the costal cartilage, and it is difficult to make the deformity disappear completely if a steel plate is used for indirect contouring without direct contouring of the local area; (4) the depression as a whole is a relative depression, and the surrounding edges are high but not high enough to serve as a pivot point. These characteristics of the ATD lateral chest wall depression indicate that when the Nuss procedure is used to correct it, it is almost impossible to eliminate the depression, let alone eliminate the deformity at its root, and therefore the Nuss procedure is not an ideal procedure.

(iv) Drebov Surgery

The Drebov procedure is a surgical method designed by Drebov. It uses a special wing-shaped material to correct the deformity locally [17]. This method is performed on both sides of the chest wall and directly corrects the deformity locally. It can effectively eliminate depression and expand the chest cavity volume. Compared with the previous three methods, this method has clear advantages, but it also has defects. First, this method only corrects the lateral chest wall depression deformity, and does not treat the median lordosis deformity. The overall shaping effect is not ideal; second, the incision is a transverse incision of the anterior chest wall, which is long, traumatic, and has obvious scars after surgery; third, the material has a large number of holes, and tissue will grow into it after implantation, making it difficult to remove the steel plate

(v) Wenlin Surgery

This method is mainly used to treat type II ATD. The inspiration for using this method for treatment comes from the understanding of the pathogenesis of ATD. As mentioned above, in type II ATD, the development of ribs and costal cartilages has not stopped, but the growth direction has deviated from the normal track. In order to achieve good results, it is necessary to pull the ribs and costal cartilages back to the normal direction, which is a must. In addition, from the overall shape, there are two basic deformities in type II ATD, first the median lordosis deformity, and then the concave deformity of the lateral chest wall. These two deformities not only affect the appearance, but also directly affect the physiological function, so it is necessary to eliminate them. In order to pull the ribs and costal cartilages back to the normal physiological track and then correct the chest deformity as a whole, we refer to the Wenlin operation in the surgery of pigeon chest and barrel chest [18,19] to correct type II ATD. The specific method is to use two steel plates to perform the operation, the steel plates compress the bulge of the anterior chest wall in the middle, and lift the concave on both sides at the same time (Figure 2-16-6). The parts that are lifted are located on both sides of the deepest part of the depression. This operation not only corrects the general deformity, but also makes the depression of the lateral chest wall disappear, and the ribs and costal cartilage return to their normal orbit. This operation is performed on the depression and can also be regarded as a combination of two Wang operations. Its most direct effect is to significantly expand the volume of the chest cavity, and the subsequent effect is to make the chest cavity continue to expand because the ribs and costal cartilage return to their normal orbit

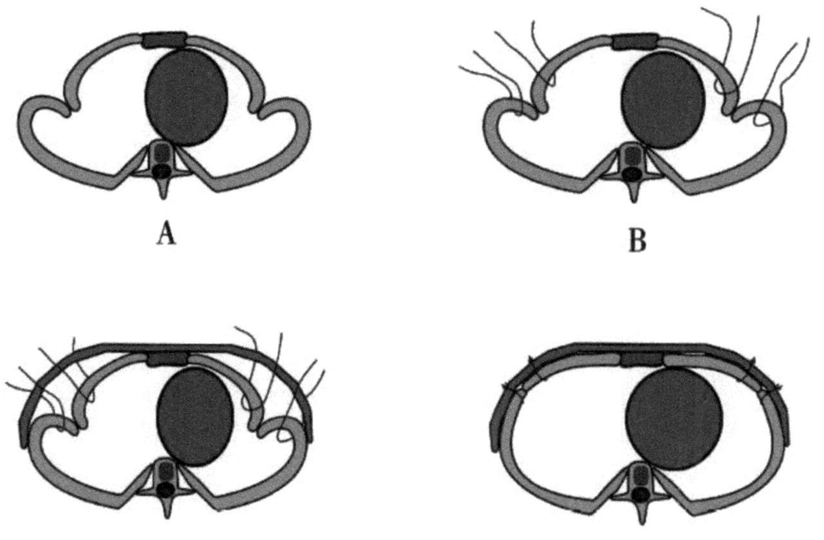

Figure 2-16-6 Schematic of the Wenlin procedure for type II ATD (A. Cross-section of a type II ATD; B. Placement of wires on either side of the depression; C. After placement of the plate, the depressed ribs and costal cartilage are lifted and secured to the plate; D. Postoperative result, the depression is eliminated)

The Wenlin procedure is a two-for-one operation that eliminates both the bulge in the anterior chest wall and the depression in the lateral chest wall. However, since the Wenlin plate can only be placed in the upper part of the chest wall and does not take into account the depression in the lower part of the lateral chest wall, if the Wenlin procedure alone is used to correct the depression, the lower part of the depression will be left behind. In order to correct the depression completely, we used the Wang procedure to correct the lower depression [15,20], in which a short steel plate was placed on the anterior surface of the depression and the depression was lifted and fixed with wires, thus ensuring that all the depressions were corrected and all the ribs and costal cartilages were brought back to the normal track.

The Wenlin procedure is based on a solid theoretical foundation and is scientifically sound. However, it is not easy to lift the depression completely during the execution of the operation. We have found that even in younger children, the ribs are almost completely ossified, so that the bone is almost inelastic and therefore difficult to lift. Although the rib cartilage is flexible, it has a limited range of motion, making it difficult to lift. Because of this, the specifics of the surgery were not easy to perform. In order for the procedure to be successful, a strong pre-contouring has to be performed, which is the key to the success of the procedure [21,22].

(vi) Wang Surgery

Since there is a significant depression in the lateral chest wall in type II patients, we thought that the Wang procedure could also be used for the correction of this deformity. We used MatrixRIB to correct the depression on both sides separately and obtained satisfactory results [23].

7. Prognosis

Due to the extreme rarity of ATD, there are very few surgical reports of this malformation in the literature. To date, the total number of surgeries performed for this malformation abroad is in the single digits, and no surgeries for this malformation have been reported in China, except in our institution. Therefore, the total surgical experience is limited. We have seen a large number of patients with ATD, and up to 6 2023, we have operated on a total of 40 patients with ATD [23]. This is the largest group of surgical cases worldwide. There are three basic approaches to surgery. for type I patients, we used median chest wall enlargement (Figure 2-16-7); for most type II patients, our primary approach was the Wenlin procedure. On top of this, we perform a Wang-like operation for inferiorly confined indentations (Fig. 2-16-8); for a few type II patients, we perform the operation using the Wang procedure alone.

Among all our surgical patients, three patients died, while the other patients had satisfactory postoperative recovery [22]. The deaths were mainly related to postoperative cardiac insufficiency. Upon analysis, the cause was likely excessive pressure on the midline of the anterior chest wall from the steel bar. In later cases, we adjusted the curvature of the steel bar to avoid excessive compression as much as possible, and no further deaths occurred.

The main factor affecting the prognosis after ATD surgery is postoperative monitoring. Since most patients have respiratory dysfunction and other organ function abnormalities, inadequate monitoring after surgery can affect treatment outcomes. In addition, because the patients' lungs are often under long-term compression with some even having localized irreversible lung lesions even though the thoracic cavity volume increases after surgery, recovery of lung function remains a major challenge. To maintain respiratory function, most patients need ventilator support. for patients who cannot be

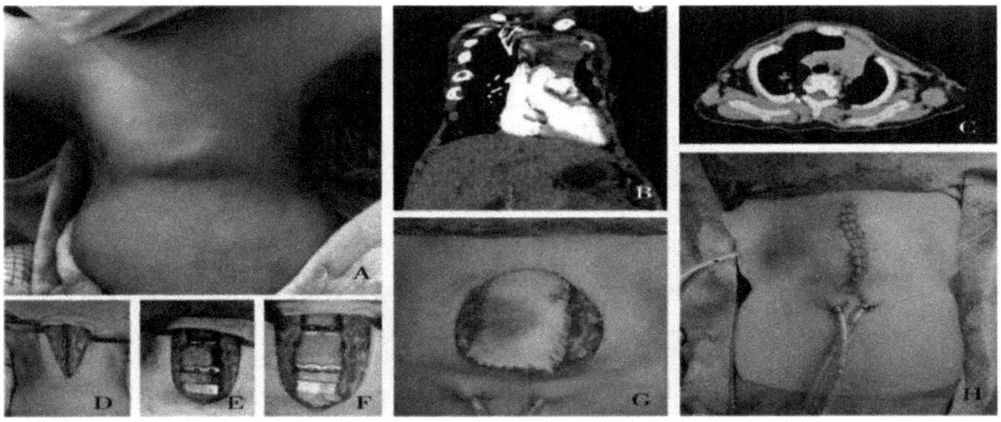

Figure 2-16-7 Median chest wall enlargement in a patient with type I ATD (A. preoperative chest wall appearance; B, C. preoperative imaging suggesting typical thoracic narrowing deformity; D. median incision with splitting of the sternum; E. sternum propped up and securely fastened with a steel plate; F. inner face of the plate lined with fibrous membrane; G. outer surface of the plate lined with fibrous membrane; H. postoperative thoracic appearance, with a significantly enlarged thorax)

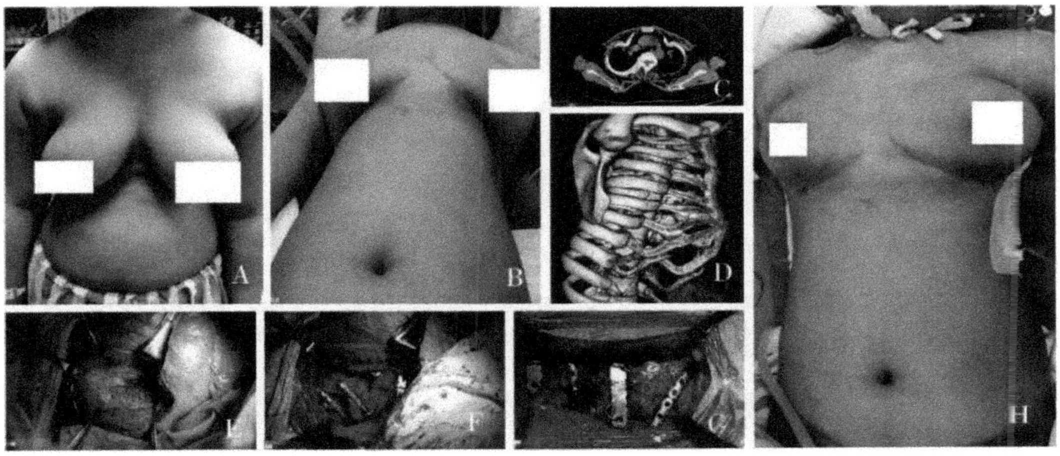

Figure 2-16-8 Wenlin surgery + Wang surgery for patients with type II ATD (A, B. The patient's chest wall appearance before surgery; C, D. Imaging examinations showed typical type II ATD; E. Correction was performed by incision on the lateral chest wall; F, G. Wenlin surgery + Wang surgery was performed with multiple steel plates to correct the concave deformity of the lateral chest wall; H. The appearance of the chest after surgery, the deformity basically disappeared)

Weaned from the ventilator in the short term, we proactively perform tracheotomy, which is more conducive to recovery. The oldest patient we operated on was 36 years old, who is the oldest known surviving patient with this condition worldwide. We performed surgery for this patient and achieved a satisfactory outcome (Figure 2-16-9) [2].

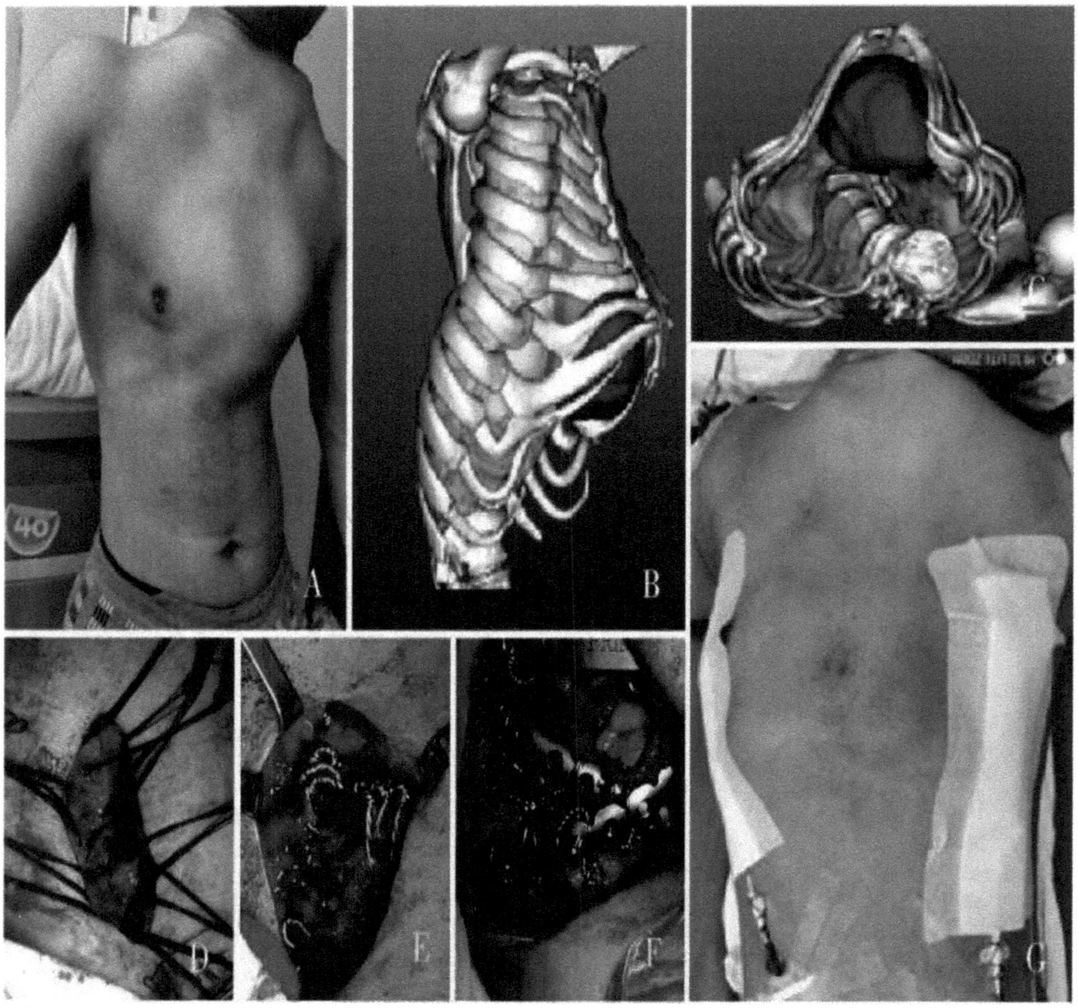

Figure 2 -16 -9 Wenlin + Wang surgeries in a 36-year-old patient with ATD (A. Thoracic appearance, median anterior convexity and bilateral depressions; B, C. 3D reconstruction showing typical type II ATD; D. Incision in the lateral chest wall and placement of wire guide wires; E. Wenlin surgery with two plates lifting the upper chest wall depressions; F. Corrective surgery for the lower depressions with MatrixRIB; G. Postoperative appearance, deformity basically disappeared). G. Postoperative thoracic appearance, deformity almost disappeared).

In summary, ATD is a very complex and specific thoracic deformity that is extremely life threatening due to the extreme severity of the deformity. Surgery is currently the only effective treatment for this deformity. However, due to the limited number of surgical cases, there is a lack of experience in treating this disease worldwide. Although we have performed the largest number of surgeries in the world and have devised some special techniques, these techniques need to be further improved.

REFERENCES

[1] Oberklaid, F., D. M. Danks, V. Mayne, et al. 1977. "Asphyxiating Thoracic Dysplasia: Clinical, Radiological, and Pathological Information on 10 Patients." *Archives of Disease in Childhood* 52: 758–765.

[2] Wang, W. 2022. "Surgical Treatment of a 36-Year-Old Patient with Asphyxiating Thoracic Dysplasia." *Interactive Cardiovascular and Thoracic Surgery* 34 (1): 153–155.

[3] Campbell, R. M. 2013. "VEPTR: Past Experience and the Future of VEPTR Principles." *European Spine Journal* 22 (Suppl 2): 106–117.

[4] Wang, W. L. 2021a. "Dr. Campbell's Thoracic Dysplasia Syndrome." *Thoracic Deformity Surgery Specialist*, September 20.

[5] Phillips, J. D., and J. A. Van Aalst. 2008. "Jeune's Syndrome (Asphyxiating Thoracic Dystrophy): Congenital and Acquired." *Seminars in Pediatric Surgery* 17 (3): 167–172.

[6] Morgan, N. V., C. Bacchelli, P. Gissen, et al. 2003. "A Locus for Asphyxiating Thoracic Dystrophy (ATD) Maps to Chromosome 15q13." *Journal of Medical Genetics* 40 (6): 431–435.

[7] Poyner, S. E., and W. T. Bradshaw. 2013. "Jeune Syndrome: Considerations for Management of Asphyxiating Thoracic Dystrophy." *Neonatal Network* 32 (5): 342–352.

[8] de Vries, J., J. L. Yntema, C. E. van Die, et al. 2010. "Jeune Syndrome: Description of 13 Cases and a Proposal for Follow-Up Protocol." *European Journal of Pediatrics* 169 (1): 77–88.

[9] Wang, W. L. 2018a. "Pathogenesis of Saddle Chest." *Thoracic Deformity Surgery Specialist*, March 15.

[10] Davis, J. T., R. L. Ruberg, D. M. Leppink, et al. 1995. "Lateral Thoracic Expansion for Jeune's Asphyxiating Thoracic Dystrophy: A New Approach." *Annals of Thoracic Surgery* 60 (3): 694–696.

[11] Davis, J. T., J. B. Heistein, R. G. Castile, et al. 2001. "Lateral Thoracic Expansion for Jeune's Syndrome: Midterm Results." *Annals of Thoracic Surgery* 72 (3): 872–878.

[12] Conroy, E., N. Eustace, and D. McCormack. 2010. "Sternoplasty and Rib Distraction in Neonatal Jeune Syndrome." *Journal of Pediatric Orthopedics* 30 (6): 527–530.

[13] Aronson, D. C., J. C. van Nierop, A. Taminiau, et al. 1999. "Homologous Bone Graft for Expansion Thoracoplasty in Jeune's Asphyxiating Thoracic Dystrophy." *Journal of Pediatric Surgery* 34 (3): 500–503.

[14] Kikuchi, N., H. Kashiwa, T. Ogino, et al. 2010. "The Nuss Technique for Jeune Asphyxiating Thoracic Dystrophy Repair in Siblings." *Annals of Plastic Surgery* 65 (2): 214–218.

[15] Wang, W. L., C. M. Chen, W. G. Long, et al. 2018. "Wang Procedure: Novel Minimally Invasive Procedure for Pectus Excavatum Children with Low Age." *Case Reports and Images in Surgery* 1 (1): 1–2.

[16] Barnes, N. D., D. Hull, A. D. Milner, et al. 1971. "Chest Reconstruction in Thoracic Dystrophy." *Archives of Disease in Childhood* 46 (250): 833–837.

[17] Drebov, R. S., A. Katsarov, E. Gagov, et al. 2017. "Is Asphyxiating Thoracic Dystrophy

(Jeune's Syndrome) Deadly and Should We Insist on Treating It? Reconstructive Surgery 'On Demand.'" *Surgery Journal (New York)* 3 (1): E17–E22.
[18] Wang, W. L., W. G. Long, C. M. Chen, et al. 2015. "Ultra-Minimally Invasive Surgery for Pectus Carinatum." *Journal of Practical Medicine* 31 (5): 863–864.
[19] Wang, W. 2018. "Minimally Invasive Surgical Technique for Barrel Chest." *Surgical Case Reports* 1 (2): 1–2.
[20] Wang, W. L. 2019. "MatrixRIB in Surgery for Asphyxiating Thoracic Dysplasia (Jeune Syndrome)." *Thoracic Deformity Surgery Specialist*, April 28.
[21] Wang, W. L. 2021b. "Latest Global Record: 27th Successful Surgery for Asphyxiating Thoracic Dysplasia (Jeune Syndrome)." *Thoracic Surgery Specialist*, September 13.
[22] Wang, W. L., W. G. Long, C. M. Chen, et al. 2021. "Surgical Treatment of Asphyxiating Thoracic Dysplasia." *Chinese Journal of Thoracic and Cardiovascular Surgery* 28 (8): 984–989.
[23] Wang, W. L. 2023. "Successful Surgery of the 40th Asphyxiating Thoracic Dysplasia (Jeune Syndrome)." *Thoracic Surgery Specialist*, June 8.

Verses Kindler Publication

Verses Kindler Publication

Reach us through our website - https://www.verseskindlerpublication.com/
for more information visit our
Instagram or Facebook page.

www.ingramcontent.com/pod-product-compliance
Lightning Source LLC
LaVergne TN
LVHW070524061126
851857LV00024B/2137
* 9 7 8 9 3 4 9 5 3 2 6 8 7 *